SPORTS INJURIES
BASIC PRINCIPLES OF
PREVENTION AND CARE

SPORTS INJURIES

BASIC PRINCIPLES OF PREVENTION AND CARE

VOLUME IV OF THE ENCYCLOPAEDIA OF SPORTS MEDICINE

AN IOC MEDICAL COMMISSION PUBLICATION

IN COLLABORATION WITH THE

INTERNATIONAL FEDERATION OF SPORTS MEDICINE

EDITED BY

P. A. F. H. RENSTRÖM

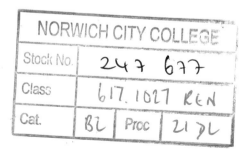
OXFORD
BLACKWELL SCIENTIFIC PUBLICATIONS
LONDON EDINBURGH BOSTON
MELBOURNE PARIS BERLIN VIENNA

© 1993 International Olympic Committee

Published by
Blackwell Publishing
350 Main Street, Malden
MA 02148 5020, USA
9600 Garsington Road, Oxford OX4 2DQ, UK
550 Swanston Street, Carlton,
Victoria 3053, Australia

Other Editorial Offices:
Librairie Arnette SA
2, rue Casimir-Delavigne
75006 Paris
France

Blackwell Wissenschafts-Verlag GmbH
Dusseldorfer Str. 38
D-10707 Berlin
Germany

Blackwell MZV
Feldgasse 13
A-1238 Wien
Austria

First published 1993
Reprinted 2005

Set by Setrite Typesetters, Hong Kong
Printed and bound in India at
Gopsons Papers Ltd., Noida

Part title illustrations by Grahame Baker

DISTRIBUTORS

Marston Book Services Ltd.
PO Box 87
Oxford ox2 0DT
(*Orders:* Tel: 0865 791155
          Fax: 0865 791927
          Telex: 837515)

USA
  Blackwell Scientific Publications, Inc.
  238 Main Street
  Cambridge, MA 02142
  (*Orders:* Tel: 800 759-6102
            617 876-7000)

Canada
  Times Mirror Professional Publishing Ltd
  130 Flaska Drive
  Markham, Ontario L6C 1B8
  (*Orders:* Tel: 800 268-4178
            416 470-6739)

Australia
  Blackwell Scientific Publications Pty Ltd.
  54 University Street
  Carlton, Victoria 3053
  (*Orders:* Tel: 03 347-5552

A catalogue record for this title
is available from the British Library
ISBN 0-632-03331-2

Library of Congress
Cataloging-in-Publication Data

Sports injuries basic principles of
prevention and care/
edited by P.A.F.H. Renstrom.
      p.   cm.
      (The Encyclopaedia of sports medicine; v. 4)
      'An IOC Medical Commission Publication
      in collaboration with the
      International Federation of Sports Medicine'.
      ISBN 0-632-03331-2
      1. Sports-Accidents and injuries.
      I. Renstrom, Per A.F.H. II. Series
      RD97.S733   1993
      617.1.'027-dc20

For further information on
Blackwell Publishing visit our website:
www.blackwellpublishing.com

Contents

V

List of Contributors

H. ALARANTA MD PhD, *Invalid Foundation, Tenholantie 10, SF 00280, Helsinki, Finland*

R.P. BARNES MS ATC, *New York Football Giants, Giants Stadium, East Rutherford, NJ 07073, USA*

T.M. BEST MD, *Department of Orthopaedic Surgery, Duke University Medical Center, Box 3435, Durham, NC 27710, USA*

B.D. BEYNNON PhD, *McClure Musculoskeletal Research Center, Department of Orthopaedics and Rehabilitation, University of Vermont, Burlington, VT 05405, USA*

P.J. BISHOP PhD, *Biomechanics Impact Laboratory, Department of Kinesiology, University of Waterloo, Waterloo, Ontario N2L 3G1, Canada*

P. BRUKNER MBBS DRCOG, *Olympic Park Sports Medicine Centre, Swan Street, Melbourne 3004, Australia*

K.M. CHAN MD, *Department of Orthopaedics and Traumatology, Chinese University of Hong Kong, Prince of Wales Hospital, Shatin, NT, Hong Kong*

T.J. CHANDLER EdD, *Lexington Clinic, Sports Medicine Center, Lexington, KY 40504, USA*

N. CRATON MD, *Pan-Am Sports Medicine, Orthopaedic and Rehabilitation Centre, 75 Poseidon Bay, Winnipeg, Manitoba R3M 3E4, Canada*

M.J. CROSS MD, *North Sydney Orthopaedic and Sports Medicine Centre, 286 Pacific Highway, Crows Nest, NSW 2065, Australia*

W.W. CURL MD, *Department of Orthopaedic Surgery, Bowman Gray School of Medicine, Wake Forest University, Winston-Salem, NC 27157−1070, USA*

V. DAMOISEAUX PhD, *Department of Health Education, Rijksuniversiteit Limburg, 6200 MD Maastricht, The Netherlands*

W.E. GARRETT JR MD PhD, *Department of Orthopaedic Surgery, Duke University Medical Center, Box 3435, Durham, NC 27710, USA*

L.Y. GRIFFIN MD PhD, *2001 Peachtree Road, NW, Suite 705, Atlanta, GA 30309, USA*

S.Y.C. HSU MBBS, *Department of Orthopaedics and Traumatology, Princess Margaret Hospital, Lai King Hill Road, Shatin, NT, Hong Kong*

U. JØRGENSEN MD PhD, *Department of Orthopaedic Surgery, Gentofte Hospital, University of Copenhagen, 2900 Copenhagen, Denmark*

P. KANNUS MD PhD, *Tampere Research Station of Sports Medicine, The Urho Kaleva Kekkonen Institute for Health Promotion Research, SF-33500, Tampere, Finland*

H.A. KEIZER MD PhD, *Department of Movement Sciences, University of Limburg, PO Box 616, 6200 MD Maastricht, The Netherlands*

W.B. KIBLER MD, *Lexington Clinic, Sports Medicine Center, Lexington, KY 40504, USA*

G. KOK PhD, *Department of Health Education, Rijksuniversiteit Limburg, 6200 MD Maastricht, The Netherlands*

H. KUIPERS MD PhD, *Department of Physiology, University of Limburg, PO Box 616, 6200 MD Maastricht, The Netherlands*

W.B. LEADBETTER MD, *Orthopaedic Center, 9711 Medical Center Drive, Rockville, MD 20850, USA*

R. LLOYD-SMITH MD, *Allan McGavin Sports Medicine Centre, University of British Columbia, Vancouver, BC V6T 1Z3, Canada*

G.E. LUTZ MD, *The Hospital for Special Surgery, 535 East 70th Street, New York, NY 10021, USA*

J. MACINTYRE MD, *The Orthopaedic Specialty Hospital and Biomechanics Institute, Salt Lake City, UT 84107, USA*

D.C. MCKENZIE MD PhD, *University of British Columbia, Division of Sports Medicine, John Owen Pavilion, 3055 Westbrook Mall, Vancouver, BC V6T 1W5, Canada*

S.F. McVICAR MD, *Orthopaedic Surgery, Dalhousie University, Nova Scotia B3H 4H7, Canada*

D.F. MARTIN MD, *Department of Orthopaedic Surgery, Bowman Gray School of Medicine, Wake Forest University, Winston-Salem, NC 27157–1070, USA*

W. VAN MECHELEN MD PhD, *Department of Health Science, Vrije University and University of Amsterdam, 1105 AZ Amsterdam, The Netherlands*

J.F. MEYERS MD, *Department of Orthopaedic Surgery, Virginia Commonwealth University, Richmond, VA 23298, USA*

M.T. MOFFROID PhD, *Department of Physical Therapy, University of Vermont, School of Allied Health Sciences, Burlington, VT 05405–0068, USA*

S. MURPHY PhD, *Sport Psychology Department, Division of Sports Science, United States Olympic Committee, Colorado Springs, CO 80909–5760, USA*

B.M. NIGG Dr sc nat, *Human Performance Laboratory, The University of Calgary, Calgary, Alberta T2N 4N1, Canada*

M. O'BRIEN MD, *Department of Anatomy, Trinity College, University of Dublin, Ireland*

L.E. PAULOS MD, *Sports Medicine West, 359 8th Avenue, Suite 206, Salt Lake City, UT 84103, USA*

J.L. PINKOWSKI MD, *Northeastern Ohio Universities College of Medicine, Akron General Medical Center, Akron, OH 44333–2455, USA*

A. PIPE MD, *University of Ottawa Heart Institute and Department of Family Medicine, Ottawa Civic Hospital, Ottawa, Ontario K1Y 4E9, Canada*

M.H. POPE Dr med sc PhD, *McClure Musculoskeletal Research Center, Department of Orthopaedics and Rehabilitation, University of Vermont, Burlington, VT 05405, USA*

P.A.F.H. RENSTRÖM MD PhD, *McClure Musculoskeletal Research Center, Department of Orthopaedics and Rehabilitation, University of Vermont, Burlington, VT 05405, USA*

B. SEGESSER MD, *Praxisklinik Rennbahn, Muttenz CH-4132, Switzerland*

W.D. STANISH MD, *Department of Orthopaedic Surgery, Dalhousie University, Nova Scotia B3H 4H7, Canada*

J.E. TAUNTON MD, *Allan McGavin Sports Medicine Centre, University of British Columbia, Vancouver, BC V6T 1Z3, Canada*

H. TROPP MD PhD, *Department of Orthopaedic Surgery, University Hospital, S581 85 Linköping, Sweden*

T.L. WICKIEWICZ MD, *The Hospital for Special Surgery, 535 East 70th Street, New York, NY 10021, USA*

D. YUKELSON PhD, *Academic Support Center for Student Athletes, The Pennsylvania State University, University Park, PA 16802, USA*

C. ZETTERBERG MD PhD, *Department of Orthopaedics/Occupational Unit, Sahlgren Hospital, S-413 45 Göteborg, Sweden*

Forewords

As President of the International Olympic Committee I welcome the IOC Medical Commission's new publication, Volume IV of the Encyclopaedia of Sports Medicine series, addressing the specific area of injuries in sport, basic principles of prevention and care.

On behalf of the International Olympic Committee I should like to thank all those involved in sports medicine, whose work is highly respected and appreciated by the whole Olympic Family.

JUAN ANTONIO SAMARANCH
Marqués de Samaranch

On behalf of the International Olympic Committee Medical Commission, I thank the contributing authors of this volume of the Encyclopaedia of Sports Medicine for furthering the Olympic spirit by disseminating up-to-date scientific knowledge throughout the world. Our congratulations go to the IOC Medical Commission's Publications Advisory Sub-Committee, and in particular to Professor Per Renström, the editor of Volumes IV and V, which are both devoted to different aspects of injuries in sport. His mastery has been instrumental in making the experts' knowledge accessible to a worldwide audience.

The International Olympic Committee also owes a debt of gratitude to Blackwell Scientific Publications Ltd., which has made a great contribution to the Olympic Movement through its enthusiasm and awareness of the IOC's important task of disseminating knowledge by publishing the Encyclopaedia series.

Baron Pierre de Coubertin showed us through sport how one can surpass oneself within a strict framework. Through our work, this educative message continues to be spread around the world.

PRINCE ALEXANDRE DE MERODE
Chairman, IOC Medical Commission

Note: The International Olympic Committee would like to inform its readership that all revenue obtained from the sale of IOC Medical Commission publications goes towards future Commission publications and the distribution of these free of charge in less developed countries.

Preface

Millions of people around the world participate in sports and physical activities, at different levels, on a regular basis. Sports and physical activities of almost any kind are usually considered beneficial for the individual as well as for society as a whole, as a certain amount of exercise is an important element in health promotion.

The potential risks for injuries in sports seem to increase for all levels of athletes with increasing participation, intensity and demands, as well as longer training periods. Injuries occurring in sports and physical activities are most commonly mild or moderate and seldom serious in nature. In spite of this, injuries cost society billions of dollars in both direct and indirect costs. Furthermore, the athlete and/or the team often experience an injury as a disaster. The incidence of injury levels needs to be reduced and can be achieved by concentrating more on preventative measures.

Through the years there has been some interest in prevention. The sports community itself, by developing protective equipment, helmets, face masks and rule changes, has tried many ways to prevent injuries. In limited areas there has been some success, but more work needs to be done and a comprehensive approach developed.

Prevention will, with time, become increasingly more important. The IOC Medical Commission Publications Advisory Sub-Committee has, therefore, felt the need to collect what is known about the prevention of injuries in sports based on scientific and clinical experience. This material could form a basis for creating preventative strategy programmes and stimulating research in prevention.

It was an honour to have been invited to coordinate this project. The approach has been ambitious and the collected material was extensive. It will, therefore, be published in two volumes. The first volume includes the basic principles behind prevention and care and the second volume will discuss clinical and sport-specific approaches to injury prevention and care.

Measures to prevent sports injuries interact and do not operate by themselves, as discussed in the 35 chapters in this volume. The problems need to be identified and described in terms of incidence and severity of sports injuries. The aetiological risk factors and mechanisms, which play a part in recurrence of sports injuries, also have to be identified. Finally, it is important to introduce measures that are likely to reduce the future risks and/or severity of injuries in sports and physical activities.

Incidence, severity and costs of sports injuries

The overall incidence of injuries in sports is high and seems to be continuously increasing. Some figures need to be mentioned in order to show the magnitude of the problem. The overall sports-injury incidence in The Netherlands was found to be 3.3 injuries per 1000 h spent playing sports (Chapter 1); 1.4 of these injuries were medically treated.

Sports trauma made up 10–15% of all the accidents in West Germany and Finland. Forty years ago, sports injuries formed 1.4% of all injuries seen in emergency rooms, compared to 10% today. Studies from Sweden show that sports injuries make up 17% of all injury visits to emergency clinics at public health-care facilities. The number of treatments of all unintentional childhood (0–19 years) injuries in emergency wards of hospitals in the United States in 1985 caused by sports was 16%, compared to 7.1% traffic-related injuries.

Injuries are traditionally divided into acute and chronic injuries. Acute injuries constitute about 25–40% of all injuries in sports and physical activities. If these injuries are treated accurately and well, which they mostly are, they do not usually give long-lasting problems (Chapter 34). Acute injuries seem to be becoming more serious because of the increasing intensity and demands of most sports.

Chronic or overuse injuries comprise approximately 60–75% of all injuries in sports and physical activities, although the exact incidence is difficult to evaluate. These injuries constitute a diagnostic and therapeutic challenge to everyone active not only in sports medicine but in other branches such as occupational health and family practice as well. Overuse injuries recur in about 20–70% of the cases, especially in sports which include running. It is, therefore, important to use education about pathophysiology, principles of diagnosis and management of overuse injuries in order to stimulate healing and to prevent recurrence of these injuries (Chapter 35). A correct diagnosis is a requirement for successful treatment.

The severity of an injury can be described by the nature and duration of the injury, time spent away from sport and work, permanent damage and costs. Fortunately, serious injuries and permanent damage are relatively rare in sports. The number of sports-injured patients who need operative treatment for an acute or overuse injury varies from 5 to 10%.

The costs for society of treatment and care of sports injuries are huge. It must, however, be remembered that the benefits from sports for society as a whole by far exceed the costs.

Severity in term of costs can include direct costs, such as the cost of medical treatment (e.g. doctor's fee, medicine costs, X-rays) and indirect costs, such as costs incurred in connection with the loss of productivity due to loss of working time. It is, however, very difficult to estimate these economic costs, but some attempts have been made (Chapter 1).

The direct and indirect costs in The Netherlands associated with medically treated sports injuries has been estimated to be US$225 million (1988), and if sick leave is included, US$350 million (Chapter 1). The direct and indirect costs of skiing accidents in Switzerland based on insurance company data from 1978 to 1980, has been calculated to be US$12.9 billion.

The Amateur Softball Association of America has estimated that 40 million people participate in organized softball leagues, which play approximately 23 million games a year. This sport is responsible for the majority of sports injuries seen in emergency room visits. Between 1983 and 1989, the Consumer Products Safety Division documented more than 2.5 million injuries through emergency rooms. This figure does not include non-hospitalization physician visits. Seventy-one percent of all these softball-related injuries sustained in recreational leagues were caused by sliding into a base. Switching from stationary to breakaway bases across the United States could prevent approximately 1.7 million injuries per year, saving more than US$2 billion in medical care, according to analyses performed by the Center for Disease Control in Atlanta.

These huge costs could be reduced if more attention was focused on the prevention of injuries in sports and physical activities. This is an area which is neglected in most societies because it requires a lot of effort and the benefits are not immediately visible. An increased investment in prevention must be part of our long-term medical strategy.

Aetiological risk factors and mechanisms

For effective prevention, it is important to understand the functional anatomy and pathophysiology of injuries of different tissues (Chapters 4–8, 35). For injury prevention it is also necessary to understand the importance of excessive load and how these loads are distributed, sports-injury mechanisms (Chapter 9), and the biomechanical response of body tissues to impact and overuse (Chapter 10).

Physicians commonly treat the symptoms of an injury and not the cause. If the underlying injury-causing mechanism is not analysed and understood, it is not possible to correctly and successfully treat the injury. If the aetiological factors, on the other hand, are well understood it is possible to prevent similar injuries occurring or recurring.

Sports injuries are caused by intrinsic or extrinsic factors, either alone or in combination. It should, however, be stressed that merely to establish the causes of sports injuries is not enough; the mechanisms by which they occur must also be identified. Sports injuries result from a complex interaction of many risk factors of which only a fraction can be identified at the moment; more research is needed.

Common *intrinsic* factors related to overuse injuries include alignment abnormalities, leg-length discrepancy, muscle weakness and imbalance, increased flexibility and joint laxity (Chapter 11), body composition and some predisposing diseases (Chapter 12). There is a higher incidence of overuse injuries among women (Chapter 14). Prevention of injuries in growing individuals is particularly important and interest is focused on secondary and tertiary preventative methods such as protective rules and education (Chapter 13).

The most common *extrinsic* factors related to injuries in sports and physical activities are training errors, environmental malconditions and poor equipment (Chapter 15). Fouls and illegal play are also important factors causing sports injuries. Effective rules and competent officiating are, therefore, crucial in injury prevention (Chapter 16).

It is necessary to understand what factors have to be involved in an injury-prevention strategy for each specific sport (Chapters 2 & 3). In a non-contact sport such as running, previous injury, lack of running experience, running to compete and excessive weekly running distances are significantly associated with injuries (Chapter 15). The dissociation between running injuries and other risk factors such as running frequency, performing warming-up and stretching exercises, body height, malalignment, muscle imbalance, restricted range of motion, level of performance, stability of running pattern, shoes and in-shoe orthoses, and running on one side of the road is judged to be either unclear or backed by contradicting or scarce research findings. Factors not associated with running injuries include age, gender, body mass index, running hills, running hard surfaces, participating in other sports, time of year, and time of day. It is, in other words, important to be aware of what factors are scientifically proven to be efficient.

Preventative measures to reduce the risks of injury and reinjury

Specific preventative activities

These include proper equipment such as well-designed and well-fitting sports shoes (Chapter 32). Face masks have dramatically reduced the rate of facial injuries in college and youth ice-hockey. Helmets have also greatly reduced the number of head injuries seen in many sports such as ice-hockey, American football and Alpine skiing (Chapter 29).

Specific, primary preventative activities also include the use of knee and ankle braces, orthoses (Chapter 30) and ankle and knee taping (Chapter 31). Orthotics are commonly used in injury prevention, compensating for different malalignments (Chapter 33).

Units of Measurement and Terminology*

Units for quantifying human exercise

Mass	kilogram (kg)
Distance	metre (m)
Time	second (s)
Force	newton (N)
Work	joule (J)
Power	watt (W)
Velocity	metres per second $(m \cdot s^{-1})$
Torque	newton-metre (N·m)
Acceleration	metres per second^2 $(m \cdot s^{-2})$
Angle	radian (rad)
Angular velocity	radians per second $(rad \cdot s^{-1})$
Amount of substance	mole (mol)
Volume	litre (l)

Terminology

Muscle action: The state of activity of muscle.
  Concentric action: One in which the ends of the muscle are drawn closer together.
  Isometric action: One in which the ends of the muscle are prevented from drawing closer together, with no change in length.
  Eccentric action: One in which a force external to the muscle overcomes the muscle force and the ends of the muscle are drawn further apart.

* Compiled by the Publications Advisory Sub-Committee, IOC Medical Commission.

Force: That which changes or tends to change the state of rest or motion in matter. A muscle generates force in a muscle action. (SI unit: newton.)

Work: Force expressed through a displacement but with no limitation on time. (SI unit: joule; note: 1 newton × 1 metre = 1 joule.)

Power: The rate of performing work; the product of force and velocity. The rate of transformation of metabolic potential energy to work or heat. (SI unit: watt.)

Energy: The capability of producing force, performing work, or generating heat. (SI unit: joule.)

Exercise: Any and all activity involving generation of force by the activated muscle(s). Exercise can be quantified mechanically as force, torque, work, power, or velocity of progression.

Exercise intensity: A specific level of muscular activity that can be quantified in terms of power (energy expenditure or work performed per unit of time), the opposing force (e.g. by free weight or weight stack) isometric force sustained, or velocity of progression.

Endurance: The time limit of a person's ability to maintain either an isometric force or a power level involving combinations of concentric and/or eccentric muscle actions. (SI unit: second.)

Mass: The quantity of matter of an object which is reflected in its inertia. (SI unit: kilogram.)

Weight: The force exerted by gravity on an object. (SI unit: newton; traditional unit:

kilogram of weight.) (Note: mass = weight/ acceleration due to gravity.)

Free weight: An object of known mass, not attached to a supporting or guiding structure, which is used for physical conditioning and competitive lifting.

Torque: The effectiveness of a force to overcome the rotational inertia of an object. The product of force and the perpendicular distance from the line of action of the force to the axis of rotation. (SI unit: newton-metre.)

Strength: The maximal force or torque a muscle or muscle group can generate at a specified or determined velocity.

PART 1

INTRODUCTION

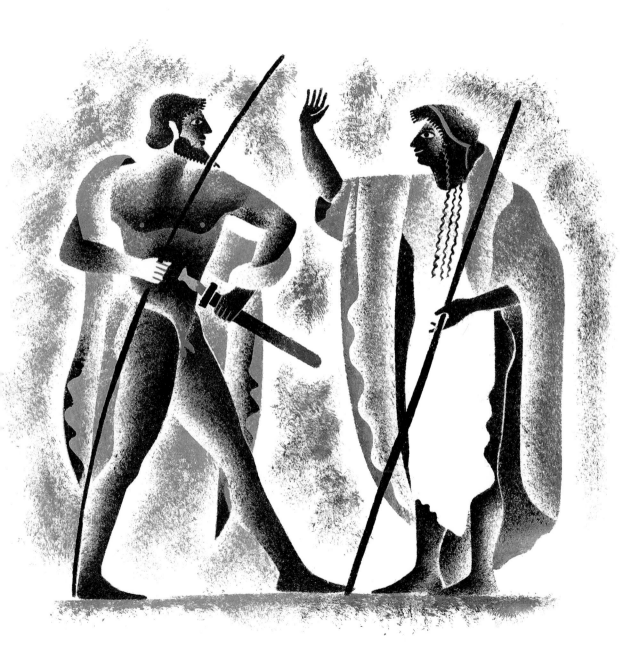

Chapter 1

Incidence and Severity of Sports Injuries

WILLEM VAN MECHELEN

During recent decades both the government and the sports organizations have encouraged sporting activities, as exemplified in The Netherlands for instance by the 'Trim U Fit' (1968), 'Sportreal' (1976), 'Nederland Oké' (1980) and 'Sport, Zelfs ik Doe Het' (1986) campaigns. The Netherlands was not alone in this: witness the 'Sport for All' campaign of the British Sports Council and, again in Britain, the 'Exercise for Health' campaign (Hutson *et al.*, 1983). Underlying these efforts was the supposedly healthy influence of sporting activities on risk factors, in particular those of cardiovascular diseases.

Individual reasons for participating in sport are many and various, but two relatively common ones are health/fitness and pleasure/ relaxation (Manders & Kropman, 1979).

It is becoming increasingly apparent that as well as having a health-giving aspect, sport can present a danger to health in the form of accidents and injuries. An individual who has to give up or cut down his or her sporting activities as a result of a sports injury is unable to pursue some or all of his or her goals. If the injury is serious enough the individual will also have recourse to the medical services to be treated. Lastly, injuries can result in absence from school or work.

Given these unwanted side-effects of sports participation it was recognized within Europe and elsewhere that a preventive approach towards the reduction of sports injuries should have high priority. It was for that reason that, within the 'Health for All by the Year 2000'

policy of the World Health Organization, the Council of Europe launched a European co-ordinated research project 'Sport for All: Sports Injuries and their Prevention' in order to improve the understanding of sports injuries and to develop a scientifically based prevention strategy.

Measures to prevent sports injuries do not stand by themselves. They form part of what might be called a 'sequence of prevention' (Fig. 1.1) (van Mechelen *et al.*, 1987). First the problem needs to be identified and described in terms of incidence and severity of sports injuries. In the second step of the sequence the factors and mechanism which plays a part in the occurrence of sports injuries have to be identified. The third step in the sequence is to introduce a measure likely to reduce the risk and/or severity of sports injuries. This measure should be based on the aetiological factors and the mechanism as identified in the second step. Finally, the effect of the measures must be evaluated by repeating the first step.

In this chapter some aspects of the first step of the sequence of prevention will be discussed.

Sports injury incidence: theoretical considerations

There is little point in discussing possible preventive measures against sports injuries without defining what is meant by sports injury, sports injury incidence and various other terms connected with these phenomena.

3

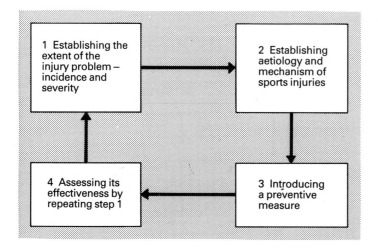

Fig. 1.1 The sequence of prevention. Adapted from van Mechelen *et al.* (1987).

Sports injury

In general 'sports injury' is a collective name for all types of damage received in the course of sporting activities. Various studies of incidence, in which incidence is defined as the number of new sports injuries occurring during a particular period in a particular group of sportspersons, define the term sports injury in different ways (Mueller & Blyth, 1974; LaCava, 1978; Boersma-Slütter *et al.*, 1979; McLatchie, 1979; Hunter & Torgan, 1983; Franke, 1980, Groh, 1962 and Paul, 1982 in Lysens *et al.*, 1984). The different definitions partly explain the differing incidences. The results of these various surveys are therefore not comparable (Kranenborg, 1982).

In some studies, a sports injury is defined as one received during sporting activities for which an insurance claim is submitted (LaCava, 1961 in Brandt Corstius, 1983). In other studies, the definition is confined to injuries treated at a hospital casualty or other medical department (Boersma-Slütter *et al.*, 1979; Edixhoven *et al.*, 1980; Clement & Taunton, 1981; Jaffin, 1981; Jost *et al.*, 1981; Hitchcock & Karmi, 1982; Oh & Schmid, 1983; Kvidera & Frankel, 1983; Schürmeyer *et al.*, 1983; von Steinbrück & Cotta, 1983; Janka & Daxecker, 1984; Maehlum, 1984; Maehlum & Daljord, 1984; Sedlin *et al.*, 1984; von Steinbrück & Rieden, 1984). If sports injur-

ies are recorded through the medical channels, a fairly large percentage of serious, predominantly acute injuries will be observed and less serious and/or overuse injuries will not be recorded. If in research such a limited definition is used, only part of the total sports injury problem is revealed: this 'tip-of-the-iceberg' phenomenon is commonly described in epidemiological research (Last, 1963 in Walter *et al.*, 1985).

To make sports injury surveys comparable and to avoid the tip-of-the-iceberg phenomenon as far as possible, an unambiguous, universally applicable definition of sports injury is the first prerequisite. It should be based on a concept of health other than that customary in standard medicine. In everyday life people are regarded as healthy if they are able to do their daily work. A sportsperson, on the other hand, is not fully recovered unless he or she can take part in his or her sport (training session or match). One of the definitions based on this premise is the one used by the National Athletic Injury Registration System (NAIRS) in the USA. 'The reportable injury is one that limits athletic participation for at least the day after the day of onset' (Powell, 1981). NAIRS classifies injuries, according to the length of incapacitation, into 'minor' (1−7 days), 'moderately serious' (8−21 days) and 'serious' (over 21 days or permanent damage). An example of an even more extensive definition that takes these considerations into account is the one proposed by the Council of Europe, in which a sports injury is defined as any injury as a result of participation in sport with one or more of the following consequences: (i) a reduction in the amount or level of sports activity; (ii) a need for (medical) advise or treatment; and (iii) adverse social or economic effects (van Vulpen, 1989).

But even if one uniform definition is applied in sports injury research, the need remains for uniform agreement on the other terms that make up the sports injury incidence, such as the way in which sports injury incidence is expressed, the ways in which reliable estimates are made of both the number of people engaging in sports and the number of injured sportspersons, etc.

Sports injury incidence

A common indication of disease in the population or a section of the population is incidence. If we substitute 'sports injury' or 'sports accident' for 'disease', incidence can be defined as the number of new sports injuries/accidents during a particular period divided by the total number of sportspeople at the start of the period (= population at risk). Incidence also gives an estimate of risk. If we multiply the figure obtained by 100 we have the percentage rate (Sturmans, 1984). Expressed in this way, sports injury incidence provides a yardstick for the extent of the sports injury problem.

Incidence rate of sports injuries is usually defined as a number of new sports injuries during a particular period (e.g. 1 year) divided by the total number of sportspeople at the start of the period (population at risk). Here again it should be realized that it is important, when interpreting and comparing the various incidence rates, to know what definition of sports injury was used and how comparable the samples were. In this connection, Kranenborg (1980) for instance describes the drawbacks of using data from insurance statistics: 'One of the main limitations is that the sports injury incidences obtained from insurance statistics are always too low, merely representing the tip of the iceberg'. Another drawback of incidence rates lies in the way they are expressed. In some cases, the number of injuries in a particular category of sportspeople per season or per year is taken, or the number of injuries per player per match. In both cases no allowance is made for any differences in exposure (the number of hours during which the person actually runs risk of being injured), despite the fact that this factor certainly influences the risk of injury. Incidence figures that take no account of exposure are therefore, according to Kranenborg (1982), not a good indication of the true extent of the problem, nor can incidence rates for different sports be properly compared. It would be better to calculate the incidence of sports injuries in relation to exposure in days, hours or sports event. This would enable different sports to be compared more fairly in this respect (Kennedy, 1977; Eriksson, 1983; Zemper, 1984; Wallace, 1988). For this purpose injury incidence is expressed as the number of injuries per 1000 h of sports participation by many researchers (e.g. Ekstrand, 1982; Lysholm & Wiklander, 1987; Backx et al., 1990; van Mechelen, 1991). The equation of Chambers (1979) recently adapted by de Loës and Goldie (1988) can be used to calculate injury incidence taking exposure into account:

$$\frac{(n \text{ sports injuries/year}) \times 10^4}{(n \text{ participants}) \times (\text{average h of sports participation}) \times (\text{weeks of season/year})}.$$

De Loës & Goldie (1988) demonstrated very clearly that a league table of 'sports injuries' based on the calculation of incidence without taking exposure into consideration differs from one that does correct incidence for exposure time. The importance of calculating incidence taking exposure time into account was also clearly demonstrated recently by van Galen and Diederiks (1990), who identified major differences in incidence per 1000 h of sports participation according to age, gender and sports.

Lindenfeld *et al.* (1988) proposed that the definition of incidence of sports injuries should be further sharpened by using 'actual exposure time at risk', rather then overall time spent on sports participation. For reasons of practicality until now actual exposure time at risk is not very often used in research.

Research design and research sample

The extent to which sports injury incidence can be assessed does not only depend on the definition of sports injury, nor on the way in which incidence is expressed, but also on the method used to count injuries, on the method to establish the population at risk and on the representativeness of the sample (Kranenborg, 1982). Methods to count injuries can be of a retrospective or prospective nature, using questionnaires or person-to-person interviews. Prospective studies can estimate the absolute risk according to the level of exposure of a sportsperson in relation to risk factors, while retrospective studies can assess the relative risk of injury in various groups, also identifying some risk factors depending on choice of research design (e.g. case-control studies). Depending on the methods used one will be more or less confronted with phenomena such as recall bias with regard to the questions of 'been-injured-or-not', overestimation of the hours of sport participation (Klesges *et al.*, 1990), incomplete response, non-response, validity of injury description in case of an injury, duration and cost of research in terms of money, etc. These aspects will not be further discussed here in depth.

Despite these problems, special attention has to be paid to the method in order to assess the population at risk and to the representativeness of the sample. If the population at risk is not clearly identified, it is not possible to calculate reliable incidence data. With regard to the representativeness of the sample it has to be taken into account that the performance of sports and therefore the incidence of sports injuries, is highly determined by selection. Bol *et al.* (1991) recognized four kinds of selective variables:

1 Self-selection (personal preferences) and/or selection by social environment (parents, friends, school, etc.).
2 Selection by sports environment (trainer, coach, etc.).
3 Selection by sports organizations (organization of competition by age and gender, the setting of participation standards, etc.).
4 Selection by social, medical and biological factors (socioeconomic background, mortality, age, aging, gender, etc.).

To give some examples: (i) within a certain sport competing at a high level enlarges sports injury incidence (Pettrone & Riccardelly, 1987; Jörgensen, 1988; Caine *et al.*, 1989); (ii) in contrast to individual sports, in team sports more injuries are sustained during matches than during training (Ekstrand & Nigg, 1989; Fintelman *et al.*, 1989); (iii) in contact sports, more injuries are sustained in comparison to non-contact sports (Chambers, 1979; de Loës & Goldie, 1988); and (iv) during and shortly after the growth spurt, boys sustain more injuries (Backous *et al.*, 1988; Caine *et al.*, 1989; Stanitski, 1989).

Differences in sports injury incidence between various specific types of sports will be discussed below (see other comparisons).

To sum up, it is very important to realize that the outcome of research on the extent of the sports injury problem is highly dependent on unambiguous definitions of 'sports', 'sports injury' and 'sports injury incidence' and that allowance should also be made for exposure time when calculating incidence. It should be borne in mind that the outcome of such research is also dependent on the applied research design and research methodology, as well as on the representativeness of the sample.

Some results

A case study of sports injury incidence: The Netherlands

In this section some overall sports injury

incidence figures in The Netherlands will be discussed as an example. These figures should be judged in the light of the above-mentioned considerations with regard to the assessment of sports injury incidence.

Dutch incidence rates for sports injuries can be obtained from research by Boersma-Slütter *et al.* (1979) and Kranenborg (1980), who, using different methods, respectively reach annual totals of 560 000 injuries (medically treated) and 1.2 million (medically and non-medically treated), corresponding to yearly rates of 20% and 46.5%. These figures are not directly comparable, since the two surveys differed, in particular with regard to sample, research method and definition of sports injury. Obviously this affects the interpretation of the figures.

Other Dutch data on incidence are those of: (i) Rogmans (1982), who calculated in a survey of accidents in the private sphere that 21% of all accidents took place at sports and recreational locations; (ii) Verbeek *et al.* (1984), who, in a survey of the frequency of and background to sports injuries among schoolchildren, arrived at a rate of 10% a month; and (iii) Inklaar (1985), who, using data from an ongoing survey of morbidity in The Netherlands, calculated an average rate of 2.4% over a period of 4 years.

Recently a representative nationwide study in The Netherlands revealed, on a total population of some 15 million, an allover sports injury incidence of 3.3 (95% confidence limits: 3.1–3.5) injuries per 1000 h spent on sports; 1.4 injuries per 1000 h spent on sports were medically treated (van Galen & Diederiks, 1990). In this study, an absolute number of 2.7 million sports injuries was calculated of which 1.7 million were medically treated. In this study also major sports injury incidence differences per 1000 h spent on sports were discerned with regard to age, gender, specific sport, recreational as opposed to competitive sport, and number of weekly hours spent on sports.

Other comparisons

One way of indicating the relative extent of the sports injury problem is to compare the number of sports injuries with, say, the number of road accidents or accidents at work.

Through the Dutch Home Accidents Surveillance System, for instance, a total of 32 276 accidents were recorded by the casualty departments of the hospitals participating in the scheme during the second 6 months of 1983. Of these, 28.6% related to sport, 14.9% to games, 0.7% to occupational activities and 9.1% to road accidents (Stichting Consument en Veiligheid, 1985). Clearly, sport and games account for the majority.

Davies (1981) noted that more consultations took place at the casualty departments of Glasgow hospitals in 1979 for sports accidents than for road accidents. Williams (1975) estimated, without indicating how, that 5% of injuries treated at casualty departments in Great Britain related to sports accidents. Guyer and Ellers (1990) calculated the number of treatments of all unintentional childhood injuries (ages 0–19 years) in emergency wards of hospitals in 1985 in the USA. Reasons for treatment were: (i) 48.5% not specified; (ii) 23% falls; (iii) 16.3% sports; and (iv) 7.1% traffic-related injuries.

There are also some figures from West Germany. Von Steinbrück and Cotta (1983) estimated the proportion of sports accidents at 10–15% of total accidents and Schürmeyer *et al.* (1983), on the basis of data from other sources, gives the proportion of sports accidents among total in-patient and out-patient cases as 5–10%. In a 1-year prospective study on acute sports injuries in a total population of a municipality with 31 620 inhabitants de Loës (1990) registered all emergency visits to the Public Health Care. 571 sports injuries were registered; they made up 17% of all acute injury visits, whereas acute home injuries, acute work injuries and acute traffic injuries made up 26%, 19% and 7% respectively (31% not defined). In a similar study, Sandelin *et al.* (1987) estimate that in the adult population in Finland about 1.5 million acute medically treated injuries occurred in 1980. Work-related injuries made up 17%, sports injuries 14% and traffic injuries 12%.

The drawback of figures of this kind is that they relate to relatively serious accidents requiring medical attention, ignoring the more chronic injuries and less serious accidents. Nor can reliable incidence rates be calculated from data of this kind, since there are no precise data on the population from which the injured are taken. In many cases the sample is not representative (Walter *et al.*, 1985).

With regard to the representativeness of samples as mentioned earlier it is important to know which sports have higher and which have lower sports injury incidence rates. A report by the Dutch Ministry of Health, Welfare and Cultural Affairs (WVC, 1987) gives a league table based on data concerning in-patient and out-patient treatment. This expresses the risk of sports injuries in terms of the number of injuries per 100 practitioners of each sport. The highest risk is found in soccer (4.2%), the lowest in skating and table tennis (0.1%). Unfortunately, no allowance is made for the fact that the amount of time spent on the various sports can differ, which in itself can affect the risk of receiving an injury. The orthopaedic clinic of the University of Heidelberg treated 8974 injuries to 8204 sportspeople from 1972 to 1981. Von Steinbrück and Cotta (1983) analysed these injuries, calculating a risk factor for each sport from the number of recorded injuries and the total number of organized sportspeople in the region concerned. Here again each sport had a different risk factor, but again no allowance was made for the different lengths of time spent on each sport. Van Galen and Diederiks (1990) made a similar league table taking into account time spent on each sport. In this table, indoor soccer was ranked number 1 with 8.7 injuries per 1000 h, basketball number 10 with 4.4 injuries per 1000 h and swimming number 20 with 1.2 injuries per 1000 h.

Severity of sports injuries

To understand the phenomenon of sports injuries one needs not only a good definition of 'sports injury', 'sports injury incidence' and so on, but one also has to be able to describe the severity of injuries in an efficient and practical manner. There are six important factors here:
1 Nature of sports injury.
2 Duration and nature of treatment.
3 Sporting time lost.
4 Working time lost.
5 Permanent damage.
6 Cost.
The purposes of these descriptions are considered.

Nature of sports injuries

The nature of a sports injury means the type of injury in terms of medical diagnosis. Thorndike (1962 in Hunter & Torgan, 1983) gives the following categories of medical diagnosis: (i) sprain (of joint capsule and ligaments); (ii) strain (of muscle or tendon); (iii) contusion (bruising); (iv) dislocation or subluxation; (v) fracture (of bone); (vi) abrasion (graze); (vii) laceration (open wound); (viii) infection or inflammation; and (ix) concussion.

In order to scale the severity of sports injuries by medical diagnosis in some studies the (abbreviated injury scale) (AIS) is used (de Loës & Goldie, 1988). It is the nature and severity of the injury (Fig. 1.2) that determines whether assistance (medical or otherwise) is sought. It is known, for instance (Kranenborg, 1981), that approximately 50% of injured korfball players seek medical assistance by consulting their GP, taking physiotherapy or attending a hospital casualty department. It is understandable that the other half do not consider medical treatment necessary since the most common injuries in indoor korfball are abrasions and other injuries not requiring medical treatment. In general, the most common injuries are contusions and sprains predominantly located on the lower extremity (Pförringer &

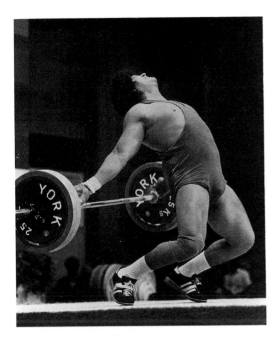

Fig. 1.2 The nature and severity of the injury depends on the type of trauma. Courtesy of the IOC archives.

Keyl, 1978; Hensley & Paup, 1979; Krahl *et al.*, 1980; Shively & Grana, 1981; van Rens, 1982; van Beek & Murphy, 1983; Jüngst *et al.*, 1983; Kristiansen, 1983; von Steinbrück & Cotta, 1983; Maehlum, 1984; Maehlum & Daljord, 1984; von Steinbrück & Rieden, 1984; Sandelin *et al.*, 1987; van Galen & Diederiks, 1990; de Loës, 1990).

This is not true in every sport: fractures are the most common type of injury in horse-riding (Edixhoven *et al.*, 1980; von Steinbrück, 1980), hang-gliding (Penschuck, 1980), parachute jumping (Steinberg, 1988), roller-skating (Jost *et al.*, 1981; Kvidera & Frankel, 1983; Horner & McCabe, 1984) and skiing (Menke *et al.*, 1982).

When assessing literature which takes diagnosis as the yardstick for the severity of injuries, one needs to know where and by whom the injuries are examined. In the case of injuries treated at casualty departments there has already been a kind of preselection: these injuries are of a more serious kind. This could give the impression that sport produces only relatively serious, acute injuries. Overuse injuries (Kowal, 1980; Orava *et al.*, 1985), i.e. injuries that build up gradually, which have become much more common recently with the increasing popularity of recreational sports such as running and fitness training, are not included in casualty department records.

Recording of the nature of sports injuries enables the sports with relatively serious injuries to be identified. The need to prevent serious injuries in a particular sport need not coincide with a high overall incidence of injuries in that sport.

Duration and nature of treatment

Data on the duration and nature of treatment can be used to determine the severity of an injury more precisely, especially if it is a question of which medical bodies are involved in the treatment and what therapies are used. The cost of medical treatment can be estimated (Tolpin *et al.*, 1981), and the effectiveness of different therapies can be compared.

For example in the municipality study of de Loës (1990) during 1 year, 571 acute injuries treated in Public Health Care Clinics were registered. Those 571 injuries led to an average of 1.9 (4% of all, including non-sports injury) visits per injury to the Public Health Care Clinics; fractures required 3.3 visits per injury, while wounds required only 1.1 visits per injury. Of the acute injured sportspersons 8% were hospitalized with an average stay of 3.7 days per patient: 4.8 days per patient for fractures and 2 days per patient for contusions. In this study is was made very clear that the nature of a sports injury and the duration and nature of treatment are strongly related.

In a more global survey amongst 66 804 persons any sports injury noted as such by the interviewed persons was taken down by van Galen and Diederiks (1990): 945 injuries were registered retrospectively over a 4-week recall period. With regard to the first treatment following injury 30% of all injuries were self-treated, 24% were treated by a sports first-aid attendant, 29% were treated by a GP, and 9% by a hospital first-aid ward. Subsequent emergency treatment was given to 119 injuries by a physiotherapist (31%), a first-aid ward (26%), a GP (18%) and a medical specialist (13%). Follow-up treatment was needed for 263 injuries and delivered by a physiotherapist (28%), a GP (26%), a first-aid ward (12%), self-treatment (12%) and a sports first-aid attendant (9%). Average number of subsequent treatments per injury was also calculated: 4.9 for physiotherapy, 3.9 for sport first-aid attendant, 2.6 for medical specialist, 2.3 for first-aid ward and 1.8 for GP.

Sporting time lost

From the individual's point of view it is important to be able to take up sport again as soon as possible after an injury. Sport and exercise play an essential part in people's relaxation nowadays and thus influence their mental well-being. The loss of sporting time is an important factor from the psychosocial point of view (Tsongas, 1981). As pointed out earlier, the term 'health' means something different to a sportsperson than to a non-sportsperson. The length of sporting time lost gives the most precise indication of the consequences of an injury to an individual. Schlatmann *et al.* (1987) classify with regard to sporting time lost the seriousness of injuries in accordance with NAIRS into minor (1–7 days), moderately serious (8–21 days) and serious (over 21 days or permanent damage).

Sporting time lost will be illustrated using the studies of Sandelin *et al.* (1987), de Loës and Goldie (1988) and van Galen and Diederiks (1990) as examples.

In the study of Sandelin *et al.*, 71% of all injuries were classified as minor (absence from sport less than 1 week), 20% as moderate (absence from sport 1–3 weeks) and 9% as severe. In the study of de Loës and Goldie, 20% of all injuries were classified as minor (absence from sport less than 1 week), 50% as moderate

(absence from sport 1–4 weeks) and 30% as severe.

In the van Galen and Diederiks (1990) study, 56% of all medically treated injuries led to a training stop or training reduction, as did 40% of all non-medically treated injuries. In this study there appeared to be a strong relation between sporting time lost and (i) the number of treatments; (ii) injury localization; and (iii) medical diagnosis.

Working time lost

Like the cost of medical treatment, the length of working time lost gives an indication of the financial consequences of sports injuries to society. If official statistics are used, e.g. data from the Industrial Insurance Administration Office and Industrial Insurance Boards, a fairly large number of people, including students, old age pensioners, the disabled, the unemployed, the self-employed, housewives and civil servants, are excluded (Vermeer, 1982). Data of this kind can be used to compare the cost to society of sports injuries with that of other situations involving risks, such as work and traffic (Kranenborg, 1982). The comparison is of particular importance to official bodies wanting to have the consequences of sports injuries covered by a separate insurance scheme.

Sandelin *et al.* (1987) registered in a municipality study medically treated acute sports injuries. Of all registered injuries 29% resulted in sick leave of which 50% did not exceed 1 week.

In her municipality study, de Loës (1990) registered during 1 year on a total of 571 acute medically treated injuries compensated work-related sick leave for 162 (29%) of those injuries, with an average length of sick leave of 21.5 days.

Van Galen and Diederiks (1990) administered on a total of 945 injured sportspersons work time lost as 11% (average duration 8.8 days), study time lost 7% (average duration 5.6 days), and other daily activity time lost 3% (average duration 5.9 days).

It should not be forgotten, however, that sporting activities may reduce the amount of sick leave taken by improving the employees general physical and mental condition of employees. A cost−benefit analysis of the positive and negative effects of sporting activities on loss of working time is needed (Shephard, 1985). According to Sörensen and Sonne-Holm (1980), the adverse socioeconomic effects of sports injuries are negligible in comparison with the positive effects of sporting activities. This last point though should be looked at with some caution. An economic analysis of the effect of sports participation on working time (Van Puffelen et al., 1989) revealed in the age groups 18−34 and 55+ a loss of working time as a result of sports participation rather than a gain. Only in the age group 35−54 could a positive effect on working time be calculated. In this study, however, the overall effect on working time lost was calculated to be negative.

Permanent damage

The vast majority of sports injuries heal without permanent disability. Serious injuries (according to the NAIRS classification) such as fractures, injuries to ligaments and tendons and intra-articulary injuries (Kent, 1982), spinal injuries (Torg et al., 1979) and eye injuries (Vinger, 1981a) can leave permanent damage (residual symptoms). Excessive delay between the occurrence of an injury and the moment at which the sportsperson seeks medical assistance can aggravate the injury (Kent, 1982). If the residual symptoms are slight, they may cause the individual to modify his or her level of sporting activity. In some cases, however, he or she may have to choose another sport or give up sport altogether. Highly serious physical damage can cause permanent disability or death (Koplan, 1979; Dolmans et al., 1985), thus reducing or eliminating the individual's capacity for work. When taking precautions then, priority should be given to measures in sports where such injuries are common, even though the particular sport itself is character-

ized by a low incidence of sports injuries and/or a low absolute number of participants. The government could play a major part here (Tsongas, 1981).

In a study by Sandelin et al. (1987) at follow-up 11% of the patients were found 2 years after injury complaining of some late sequelae from their initial trauma. In the majority of cases the initial trauma having been of a sprain type.

Costs of sports injuries

The calculation of the costs of sports injuries involves essentially the expression of the above-mentioned five categories of seriousness of sports injuries in terms of money.

A general classification of the economic costs of sports injuries is set out by Tolpin et al. (1981). The economic costs are divided into:
1 Direct costs, i.e. the cost of medical treatment (diagnostic expenses such as X-rays, doctor's fee, cost of medicines, admission costs, etc.).
2 Indirect costs, i.e. expenditure incurred in connection with the loss of productivity due to increased morbidity and mortality levels (loss of working time and expertise due to death or handicap).

Another type are the quantifiable and unquantifiable social costs. Quantifiable costs include insurance and legal expenses. Unquantifiable costs are the harmful effects of a sports injury on the psychosocial life of the individual or family, e.g. owing to economic dependence, loss of social status or position, or social isolation. These costs are quantifiable only to the extent that the quality of life is quantifiable (Miles, 1979). In the view of Tolpin et al. (1981) an adequate injury registration system is essential to any assessment of the total cost associated with sports injuries. The system must be reliable and continuous. Any cost analysis must identify the sports which are most 'expensive' for the community (Sörensen & Sonne-Holm, 1980), so that the first interventions can be taken there.

The social consequences can to some extent be expressed in figures, and would seem to be of no small extent. Vermeer (1982), for instance, calculated that compulsorily insured persons alone lost 1073 million working days as a result of sports injuries in 1979. This corresponds to sickness benefit paid out under the compulsory insurance scheme of over 100 million guilders. Vermeer explicitly notes that schoolchildren, students, civil servants, members of the armed forces, old-age pensioners, widows and self-employed people were not included in this calculation.

The direct and indirect cost in The Netherlands associated with medically treated sports injuries have been estimated to run up to some 455 million guilders (den Toom & Schuurman, 1988) ($US1 = approximately 2 Dutch guilders).

In other countries too, large sums are mentioned in connection with the consequences of sports injuries. Von Steinbrück and Cotta (1983) estimated the annual cost of sports injuries in West Germany at over 5000 million marks. Matter et al. (1982) used insurance company data to estimate the direct and indirect cost of skiing accidents in Switzerland from 1978 to 1980 at 9900 000 Swiss francs. Tolpin et al. (1981) calculated that some $US6 million were spent on medical treatment of eye injuries received in the course of sporting activities in the USA in 1980. The total cost of roller-skating accidents in the USA has been estimated at $US100 million per annum (Kvidera & Frankel, 1983). In the USA stationary baseball and softball cause many injuries in base slidings. The average medical cost per base sliding injury was estimated to be $US1223, while it was calculated that the installation of break away bases across the USA would save $US2 billion in medical costs per year (Janda et al., 1990). Guyer and Ellers (1990) estimated the total cost of unintentional hospital in-patient and emergency department treatment of children (0−19 years) in the USA in 1982 as a result of sports injuries to be $US580.8 million on a total of $US7544.9, ranking third after traffic-related injuries $US2785.2 million and injuries as a result of a fall $US809.6. Davison and Ryan (1988) estimate the total cost of treatment by an out-patient

sports injury clinic in the UK to be £89.25 per injury.

One last example: de Loës (1990) calculated an overall mean of direct and indirect cost of $US335 per acute medically treated sports injury, identifying motorcycling, downhill skiing and equine sports as by far the most expensive sports (total cost respectively $US618, 400 and 393).

It should be noted, however, that due to differences in health-care systems and wage compensation systems international comparisons may be hampered. Even at a national level similar injuries may produce different costs in different states as demonstrated by Pritchett (1980) with regard to the high cost of high-school football injuries in the six western states of the USA.

In the earlier mentioned study by Van Puffelen et al. (1989) for The Netherlands an overall positive balance of 155 million Dutch guilders per annum was calculated as a result of sports participation. However, a closer look at the four analysed subcategories of costs presented a diverse picture; there was a 23.3 million guilders positive balance with regard to GP consultation, a 22.1 million guilders negative balance as a result of the consultation of medical specialists, a 286.1 million guilders positive balance for in-patient treatment, and a 130.2 million guilders negative balance due to working time lost.

In a review of the economics of fitness and sport with particular reference to worksite programmes which was not specifically aimed at the description of the costs of sports injuries but at an overall cost−benefit analysis of fitness and sports Shephard (1989) concluded that, particularly with regard to work-site programmes, 'there seems increasing evidence that exercise and fitness programmes are both cost effective and cost beneficial' and that 'many industrial sponsors have concluded that, when exercise is provided in the context of a total package of health promotion, the immediate return is in the range of $US2 to $US5 for every dollar invested'. It should be noted, however, that competitive sports, in which most injuries are sustained, is different from health promotional exercise and fitness programmes.

Conclusion

Incidence and severity provide a yardstick for the first step of prevention of sports injuries. However, in order to get reliable and comparable data uniform definitions and adequate research designs and methodology are needed.

References

Backous, D.D., Friedl, K.E., Smith, N.J., Parr, T.J. & Csarpine Jr, W.D. (1988) Soccer injuries and their relation to physical maturity. *Am. J. Dis. Child* **142**(8), 839–42.

Backx, F.J.G. (1991) *Sports injuries in youth, etiology and prevention*. Thesis, University of Utrecht, The Netherlands.

Backx, F.J.G., Inklaar, H., Koornneef, M. & Mechelen, W. van. (1990) Draft FIMS position statement on the prevention of sports injuries. *Gen. en Sport* special issue May 1990.

Beek, P.A. van & Murphy, P. (1983) Letsel bij volleybal (Injuries in volleyball). *Gen. en Sport* **16**, 59–65.

Boersma-Slütter, W., Broekman, A., Lagra, H.M. & Minderaa, P.H. (1979) Sport, een riskante zaak. *Gen. en Sport* **12**, 41–9.

Bol, E., Schmickli, S.L., Backx, F.J.G. & Mechelen, W. van (1991) *Sportblessures onder de knie* (Sports Injuries of the Knee). Publication No. 38, Netherlands Institute of Sports Health Care, Papendal, The Netherlands.

Brandt Corstius, J.J. (1983) *Het voorkomen van sportblessures — preventie is meer dan vaststellen van incidentie*. Thesis, IFLO, Amsterdam.

Caine, D., Cochrane, B., Caine, C. & Zemper, E. (1989) An epidemiologic investigation of injuries affecting young competitive female gymnasts. *Am. J. Sports Med.* **17**, 811–20.

Chambers, R.B. (1979) Orthopedic injuries in athletes (ages 6–17), comparison of injuries occurring in six sports. *Am. J. Sports Med.* **7**, 195–7.

Clement, D.B. & Taunton, J.E. (1981) A guide to the prevention of running injuries. *Aus. Fam. Phys.* **10**, 156–64.

Davies, J.E. (1981) Sports injuries and society. *Br. J. Sports Med.* **15**, 80–3.

Davison, J. & Ryan, M.P. (1988) A sports medicine clinic in the community. *Br. J. Sports Med.* **22**(2), 75.

Dolmans, I., Pool, J., Erdman-Trip, J.F. & Smith, B.

(1985) Plotse dood bij sport. *Gen. en Sport* **18**(3), 95–9.

Edixhoven, P., Sinha, S.C. & Dandy, J. (1980) Horse injuries. *Injury Br. J. Accid. Surg.* **12**(4), 279–82.

Ekstrand, J. (1982) *Soccer injuries and their prevention*. Linkoping University Medical Dissertations No. 130, Linkoping, Sweden.

Ekstrand, J. & Nigg, B.M. (1989) Surface-related injuries in soccer. *Sports Med.* **8**(1), 56–62.

Eriksson, E.K.G. (1983) *Sports accidents*. Paper presented at Symposium on Accidents in Europe, Sept., England.

Fintelman, L.F.J., Rijks, G.S. & Hildebrandt, V.H. (1989) *Sportblessures bij ervaren competitie-basketballers* (Sports Injuries in Competitive Basketball Players, English summary). TNO Institute for Preventive Health Care, Leiden, The Netherlands.

Galen, W. van & Diederiks, J. (1990) *Sportblessures Breed Uitgemeten* (An Extensive Analysis of Sports Injuries in The Netherlands). De Vrieseborch, Haarlem, The Netherlands.

Guyer, B. & Ellers, B. (1990) Childhood injuries in the United States: Mortality, morbidity and cost. *Am. J. Dis. Child* **144**, 649–52.

Hensley, L.D. & Paup, D.C. (1979) A survey of badminton injuries. *Br. J. Sports Med.* **13**, 156–60.

Hitchcock, E.R. & Karmi, M.Z. (1982) Sports injuries to the central nervous system. *J. Roy. Coll. Surg. Edinb.* **27**(1), 46–9.

Horner, C. & McCabe, M.J. (1984) Ice-skating and roller disco injuries in Dublin. *Br. J. Sportsmed.* **18**(3), 207–11.

Hunter, L.Y. & Torgan, C. (1983) Dismounts in gymnastics: should scoring be reevaluated? *Am. J. Sportsmed.* **11**(4), 208–10.

Hutson, M. (1983) Community health, exercise and injury risk. *Nursing Times* Aug., 22–5.

Inklaar, H. (1985) *De epidemiologie van sportletsels* (Epidemiology of Sports Injuries). Publication No. 16, National Institute of Sports Health Care, Oosterbeek, The Netherlands.

Jacobs, S.J. & Berson, B.L. (1986) Injuries to runners: A study of entrants to a 10 000 meter race. *Am. J. Sportsmed.* **14**(2), 151–5.

Jaffin, B. (1981) An epidemiologic study of ski injuries: Vail, Colorado. *Mount Sinai J. Med.* **48**(4), 353–9.

Janda, D.H., Wojtys, E.M., Hankin, F.M., Benedict, M.E. & Hensinger, R.N. (1990) A three-phase analysis of the prevention of recreational softball injuries. *Am. J. Sports Med.* **18**(6), 632–5.

Janka, Ch. & Daxecker, F. (1984) Augenverletzungen durch Wintersport (Eye injuries during winter sports). *Fortschr. Ophtalmol.* **81**, 71–2.

Jörgensen, U. (1988) The incidence and prevalence of injuries in badminton. In *Proceedings of the Council of Europe, 2nd meeting 1987.* National Institute of Sports Health Care, Oosterbeek, The Netherlands.

Jost, O., Ruland, O. von & Heger, R.A. (1981) Rollschuhfahrersverletzungen (Rollerskating injuries). *Deut. Z. Sportsmed.* **10**, 268−74.

Jüngst, B.K., Keth, R.K., Stopfkuchen, H. & Schranz, D. (1983) Verletzungen im Handballsport, Ergebnisse einer Befragung (Injuries during team handball). *Med. Wschr.* **125**(24), 531−3.

Kennedy, M.C., Vanderfield, G.K. & Kennedy, J.R. (1977) Sport: assessing the risk. *Med. J. Australia* **2**, 253−4.

Kent, F. (1982) Athletes wait too long to report injuries. *Phys. Sports Med.* **10**(4), 127−9.

Klesges, R.C., Eck, L.H., Mellon, M.W., Fulliton, W., Somes, G.W. & Hanson, C.L. (1990) The accuracy of self-reports of physical activity. *Med. Sci. Sports Exerc.* **22**(5), 690−7.

Koplan, J.P., Powell, K.E., Sikes, R.K., Shirley, R.W. & Campbell, G.C. (1982) An epidemiological study of the benefits and risks of running. *JAMA* **248**(32), 3118−21.

Kowal, D.M. (1980) Nature and causes of injuries in women resulting from an endurance training program. *Am. J. Sports Med.* **8**, 265−9.

Krahl, H., Steinbrück, K. von & Cotta, H. (1980) Traumatologie des Sports. In H. Cotta (eds) *Belastungs toleranz des Bewegungsapparates* (Injury Tolerance of the Locomotor Apparatus). Georg Thieme Verlag, Stuttgart.

Kranenborg, N. (1980) Sportbeoefening en blessures (Participation in sports and injuries). *Gen. en Sport* **13**, 89−93.

Kranenborg, N. (1981) Blessures bij micro-korfballers (Injuries during indoor korfball). *Gen. en Sport* **14**, 36−40.

Kranenborg, N. (1982) Sportbeoefening en blessures (Participation in sports and injuries). *Toeg. Soc. Gen.* **60**(9), 224−7.

Kristiansen, B. (1983) Association football injuries in school boys. *Scand. J. Sports Sci.* **5**(1), 1−2.

Kvidera, D. & Frankel, V.H. (1983) Trauma on eight wheels. A study of roller skating injuries in Seattle. *Am. J. Sports Med.* **11**(1), 38−41.

LaCava, G. (1978) Environment, equipment and prevention of sport's injuries. *J. Sports Med. Phys. Fitness* **18**, 11.

Lindenfeld, Th.N., Noyes, E.R. & Marshall, M.T. (1988) Components of injury reporting systems. *Am. J. Sports Med.* **16**(Suppl. 1), 69−81.

Loës, M. de. (1990) Medical treatment of costs of sports-related injuries in a total population. *Int. J. Sports Med.* **11**, 66−72.

Loës, M. de & Goldie, K. (1988) Incidence rate of injuries during sport activity and physical exercise in a rural Swedish municipality: Incidence rates in 17 sports. *Int. J. Sports Med.* **9**, 461−7.

Lysens, R., Lefevre, J. & Ostyn, M. (1984) The predictability of sports injuries. A preliminary report. *Int. J. Sports Med.* **5**(Suppl.), 153−5.

Lysholm, J. & Wiklander, J. (1987) Injuries in runners. *Am. J. Sports Med.* **15**(2), 168−71.

McLatchie, G.R. (1979) Equestrian injuries, a one-year prospective study. *Br. J. Sports Med.* **13**, 29−32.

Maehlum, S. (1984) Football injuries in Oslo: A one-year study. *Br. J. Sports Med.* **18**, 186−90.

Maehlum, S. & Daljord, O.A. (1984) Acute sports injuries in Oslo: A one year study. *Br. J. Sports Med.* **18**, 181−5.

Manders, Th. & Kropman, J. (1979) *Sportdeelname: wat weten wij er van?* (What is known about participation in sports?) Institute voor Toegepaste Sociologie, Nijmegen, The Netherlands.

Matter, P., Spinas, G.A. & Ott, G. (1982) Risiko- und Schweregradentwicklung der aplinen Skiunfaelle und deren soziale Bedeutung (Risks and severity of Alpine skiing injuries and their social impact). *Sozial Praeventivmedizin* **27**, 19−22.

Mechelen, W. van (1991) 25 jaar schade door sport (25 years of sports injuries). *Gen. en Sport* **23**, 196−8.

Mechelen, W. van, Hlobil H. & Kemper, H.C.G. (1987) *How Can Sports Injuries be Prevented?* Publication No. 25E, National Institute of Sports Health Care, Oosterbeek, The Netherlands.

Menke, W. & Muller, E.K. (1982) Sicherheitsskibindung (Safe ski bindings). *Med. Wschr.* **124**(8), 183−4.

Miles, S. (1979) Fit, for anything? *Br. J. Sports Med.* **12**, 173−5.

Mueller, F.O. & Blyth, C.S. (1974) North Carolina high school football injury study: Equipment and prevention. *J. Sports Med.* **2**, 1−10.

Oh, S. & Schmid, U.D. (1983) Kindliche Kopfverletzungen beim Skifahren und ihre optimale Prophylaxe (Children's head injuries in skiing and their optimal treatment). *Z. Kinderchirurgie* **30**, 66−72.

Orava, S., Jaroma, H. & Hulkko, A. (1985) Overuse injuries in cross-country skiing. *Br. J. Sports Med.* **19**(3), 158−60.

Penschuck, C. (1980) Verletzungsursachten beim Drachenfliegen (Causes of hang-gliding injuries). *Chirurg.* **51**, 336−40.

Pettrone, F.A. & Riccardelly, E. (1987) Gymnastic injuries: The Virginia experience 1982−1983. *Am. J. Sports Med.* **15**(1), 59−62.

Pförringer, W. & Keyl, W. (1978) Sportverletzungen beim Squash. Epidemiologie und prevention (Sports injuries in squash. Epidemiology and prevention). *Med. Wschr.* **120**, 1163−6.

Powell, J.W. (1981) National athletic injury/illness reporting system: Eye injuries in college wrestling. *Int. Opht. Clin.* **21**, 47−58.

Pritchett, J.W. (1980) High cost of high school football

injuries. *Am. J. Sports Med.* **8**(3), 197−9.

Puffelen, F. van, Reyman, J.O.N. & Veldhuijzen, J.W. (1989) *Sport en gezondheid, economisch bezien* (Economic aspects of sports and health). Thesis, University of Amsterdam.

Rens, Th.J.G. van (1982) Sport en gezondheid, orthopaedische aspecten (Orthopaedic aspects of sports and health). *Med. Contact* **40**, 1283−8.

Rogmans, W.H.J. & Weerman, A. (1982) *Registratie van ongevalspatienten op de eerste hulpafdeling* (Registration of accident patients treated by first aid departments of general hospitals). Stichting Consument & Veiligheid, Amsterdam.

Sandelin, J., Santavirta, S., Lättilä, R. & Sarna, S. (1987) Sports injuries in a large urban population: Occurrence and epidemiological aspects. *Int. J. Sports Med.* **8**, 61−6.

Schlatmann, H.F.P.M., Hlobil, H., Mechelen, W. van & Kemper, H.C.G. (1987) Naar een Registratiesysteem van Sportblessures in Nederland (Towards a sports injury registration system in The Netherlands). *Gen. en Sport* **20**(5), 179−84.

Schürmeyer, Th., Hiddig, J. & Herter, Th. (1983) Die Bedeutung des Schaedel-Hirn-Traumas im Sport (The significance of skull−brain−trauma in sports). *Deut. Z. Sportmed.* **3**, 86−9.

Sedlin, E.D., Zitner, D.T. & McGinnis, G. (1984) Roller skating accidents and injuries. *J. Trauma* **24**, 136−9.

Shephard, R.J. (1985) The impact of exercise upon medical costs. *Sports Med.* **2**, 133−43.

Shephard, R.J. (1989) Current perspectives on the economics of fitness and sport with particular reference to worksite programmes. *Sports Med.* **7**, 286−309.

Shively, R.A. & Grana, W.A. (1981) High school sports injuries. *Phys. Sportsmed.* **9**, 46−50.

Sörensen, C.H. & Sonne-Holm, S. (1980) Social cost of sports injuries. *Br. J. Sports Med.* **14**, 24−5.

Stanitski, C.L. (1989) Common injuries in pre-adolescent and adolescent children. Recommendations for intervention. *Sports Med.* **7**(1), 32−41.

Steinberg, P.J. (1988) Injuries to Dutch sport parachutists. *Br. J. Sports Med.* **22**(1), 25−30.

Steinbrück, K. von (1980) Wirbelsaulenverletzungen beim Reiten (Vertebral column injuries in riding). Teil I. *Unfallheilkunde* **83**, 366−72.

Steinbrück, K. von & Cotta, H. (1983) Epidemiologie von Sportverletzungen (Epidemiology in sports injuries). *Deut. Z. Sportmed.* **6**, 173−86.

Steinbrück, K. von & Rieden, H. (1984) Verletzungen bei Sportstudenten — Analysen und Konsequenzen (Injuries in sports students — analysis

and consequences). *Deut. Z. Sportmed.* **11**, 335−46.

Stichting Consument & Veiligheid (1985) *Privé ongevallen en registratie systeem*. PORS, Ongevallen 84 (Consumer Safety Institute: Annual report 1984 of the home and leisure time injury registration system). Stichting Consument & Veiligheid, Amsterdam.

Sturmans, F. (1984) *Epidemiologie* (Epidemiology). Dekker & van de Vegt, Nijmegen, The Netherlands.

Tolpin, H.G., Vinger, P.F. & Tolpin, D.W. (1981) Economic considerations. *Int. Ophthal. Clin.* **21**, 179−201.

Toom, P.J. den & Schuurman, M.I.M. (1988) *Een model voor berekening van kosten van ongevallen in de privé-sfeer* (A model for the prediction of the costs resulting from leisure time accidents). Stichting Consument & Veiligheid, Amsterdam.

Torg, J.S., Truex, R., Quendenfeld, T.G., Burstein, A. et al. (1979) The national football head and neck injury registration. Report and conclusions (1978). *JAMA* **241**, 1477−9.

Tsongas, P.E. (1981) The role of government in injury prevention. *Int. Ophthal. Clin.* **21**, 171−7.

Verbeek, A.L.M., Postma, M.A. & Backx, F.J.G. (1984) *De epidemiologie van sportblessures bij de schoolgaande geugd* (The Epidemiology of Sports Injuries in Schoolchildren). National Institute of Sports Health Care, Oosterbeek, The Netherlands.

Vermeer, J.P. (1982) Sport en sociale verzekering (Sports and the social security system). *Toeg. Soc. Gen.* **60**, 222−3.

Vinger, P.F. (1981) Eye and face protection for United States hockey players: A chronology. *Int. Ophthal. Clin.* **21**, 83−6.

Vulpen, A. van (1989) *Sport for All: Sport Injuries and their Prevention*. Council of Europe, National Institute of Sports Health Care, Oosterbeek, The Netherlands.

Wallace, R.B. (1988) Application of epidemiologic principles to sports injury research. *Am. J. Sports Med.* **16**(Suppl. 1), 22−4.

Walter, S.D., Sutton, J.R., McIntosh, J.M. & Connolly, C. (1985) The aetiology of sports injuries. A review of methodologies. *Sports Med.* **2**, 47−58.

Williams, J.P.G. (1975) Sports injuries. The case for specialised clinics in the United Kingdom. *Br. J. Sports Med.* **9**, 22−4.

WVC (1987) *Sports Injuries in The Netherlands*. Ministry of Health, Welfare and Cultural Affairs, Rijswijk, The Netherlands.

Zemper, E.D. (1984) *NCAA injury surveillance system: initial results*. Paper presented at 1984 Olympic Scientific Congress, Los Angeles, USA.

Chapter 2

Types of Injury Prevention

PEKKA KANNUS

Interest in sporting activities has grown in recent years because of the increase in leisure time as well as the belief that general health can be enhanced by improved physical fitness (Devereaux & Lachmann, 1983; Peterson & Renström, 1986). Regular aerobic exercise has been linked quite reliably to a decreased risk of cardiovascular diseases (Paffenbarger et al., 1978); to assistance in reduction of weight (Lewis et al., 1976) and musculoskeletal symptoms (Lane et al., 1987); and possibly also to a decreased morbidity and mortality of aging (Bortz, 1982). As a result, a certain amount of physical activity is considered an important element in health promotion, as has been stated by the American College of Sports Medicine (ACSM, 1978) and the International Federation of Sports Medicine (FIMS, 1989).

With the resultant upsurge in sporting activity there has been an increase in sports injuries, both from acute and overuse trauma (Fasler, 1976; Orava, 1980; Koplan et al., 1985; Sandelin, 1988), and numerous epidemiological studies of sports injuries are available (Robey et al., 1971; Weightman & Browne, 1975; Kvist & Järvinen, 1978; Axelsson et al., 1980; Orava, 1980; Ekstrand, 1982; Devereaux & Lachmann, 1983; Sandelin, 1988). However, due to the fact that the population at risk is extremely difficult to identify, the actual incidences of sports injuries in one society or more specific groups are still almost unknown. In addition, the fact that the population which takes part in physical activity, does so at different levels, and with

considerably different intensity, makes the evaluation even more difficult. Hence, studies analysing sports injuries have not been able to identify athletes at risk or the real risk factors regarding injury, and the aetiological factors have not yet been fully assessed (Ekstrand, 1982). However, in order to develop preventive strategies, epidemiologically valid studies analysing sports injuries have to be performed.

In the 1990s, the number of acute sports injuries treated in hospitals are rather well known. 40 years ago, sports injuries formed 1.4% of all injuries seen at a casualty department (Peräsalo et al., 1955). During the 1970s, this figure varied between 5 and 7% (Vuori et al., 1972; Axelsson et al., 1980), and at the moment about 10% of all traumatic injuries treated in the emergency rooms of hospitals in industrialized countries are sustained in sports (Franke, 1980; Korhonen, 1986; Sandelin, 1988). These numbers, of course, do not represent any real incidence of these injuries, but rather only 'the tip of an iceberg'.

Regarding overuse injuries exact incidence rates are even more difficult to find out. Definitions are more variable, the diagnosis is more difficult to establish, and population at risk is almost always unknown. In addition, these injuries are treated independently in many different places by many different professional and semiprofessional persons. As a matter of fact, the only element, which is certain is that due to the general increase in sporting activities, the absolute number of overuse injuries has increased dramatically during the last decades (Orava, 1980; Peterson & Renström, 1986; Kannus *et al.*, 1987, 1988, 1989). The claim about relative increase (i.e. increase in the incidence) remains without scientific evidence.

Both acute and overuse sports injuries are generally considered to be of relatively mild character (Kvist & Järvinen, 1978; Orava, 1980; Sandelin, 1988). It is estimated that up to 75% of all sports injuries can be classified as mild to moderate requiring only short sick leave and absence from sports (Ekstrand, 1982; Sandelin, 1988). The number of patients requiring further treatment as in-patients because of sports injury appears to be around 10% (Vuori *et al.*, 1972; Axelsson *et al.*, 1980; Watters *et al.*, 1984; Sandelin, 1988). Furthermore, the number of patients needing operative treatment of their acute or overuse injury varies from 5 to 10% (Orava, 1980; Kannus *et al.*, 1987, 1988, 1989).

In spite of the fact that most sports injuries are mild or moderate in nature, the treatment of injured athletes often requires special judgement and experience. The treating physician needs not only special knowledge in sports medicine, but should also be familiar with the sport and its rules and demands. A correct diagnosis, immediate treatment and effective rehabilitation programme are prerequisites for return to the sports arena. Only 100% recovery from injury ensures successful return.

Despite advanced knowledge, modern technology and improved skills in sports medicine, many patients fail to return. Therefore, the prevention of injuries should be a major goal of every physician and other staff working in the field of sports medicine.

Hierarchy of injury prevention

By sports injury prevention we mean all efforts to prevent injuries occurring in connection with physical activity. Efforts may be pitched at individual, group or society level (Fig. 2.1). Injuries may, in turn, be acute or overuse by nature, and connections to sports may be direct or indirect. Furthermore, the level of physical

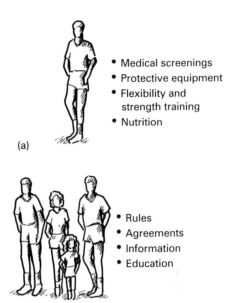

- Medical screenings
- Protective equipment
- Flexibility and strength training
- Nutrition

(a)

- Rules
- Agreements
- Information
- Education

(b)

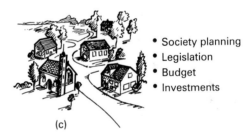

- Society planning
- Legislation
- Budget
- Investments

(c)

Fig. 2.1 Strategies in sport-injury prevention: (a) primary prevention (at individual level); (b) secondary prevention (at group level); and (c) tertiary prevention (at society level). With permission from Renström & Kannus (1992).

activity may vary from mild recreational to strenuous professional.

Primary prevention

The direct or indirect sports injury prevention at individual level can be called 'primary prevention', as is often the case in the prevention strategies in general medicine and health education. Medical preseason examination of a subject, warming-up before the competition, preventive muscle conditioning, avoidance of doping, and usage of protective equipment (helmets, face guards, gum shields, different paddings, safety-release ski-bindings, braces or tape) are typical examples of primary prevention.

In general medicine, an example of primary prevention of lung cancer is an individual decision to stop smoking, or in prevention of atherosclerosis a decision to reduce the consumption of saturated fat rich in cholesterol.

Secondary prevention

Sports injury prevention at group level can be called 'secondary prevention'. The most usual way to carry out secondary prevention is group information and education. Lectures to athletes and coaches about the importance of proper warm-up and cooling down, careful following of the rules (fair play), disadvantages of drugs, alcohol and tobacco, and known risk factors of injuries are typical examples. Any decision within individual sporting events making that particular sport safer can also be seen as secondary prevention. For example, in prevention of cold injuries in cross-country skiing, the demand of cancellation of competition because of very cold weather (under −20°C) is a secondary prevention effort.

Regarding lung cancer and atherosclerosis, a public information campaign against smoking, dangerous foods and unhealthy eating habits on television, radio and other mass media is an excellent way to accomplish secondary prevention.

Tertiary prevention

All efforts undertaken at the society level to prevent sports injuries can be called 'tertiary prevention'. Normally, tertiary prevention is looking far forward, and its consequences will not be seen until years after those strategies were planned and put into effect. Society planning is often seen as a tool in tertiary prevention. Concerning sports injury prevention, an example might be a political decision to build new, safe biking routes to the area and separate them completely from motor vehicle traffic. Also, a legislative decision of one state or country to deny all hits to the head in boxing, or full-contact hits or kicks in karate, can be seen as a tertiary effort of prevention.

In prevention of lung cancer, a typical tertiary action is the decision to increase the price of a packet of cigarettes. In atherosclerosis, a tertiary preventive measure can be a government decision to lower the prices of low-cholesterol products (such as fruits and vegetables) and to improve their public availability throughout the year.

Sports injury prevention can also be seen from different views than those presented here. For example, all these three levels could fit into one individual (Hlobil et al., 1987). In this strategy, prevention of an injury before its occurrence can be called primary prevention. Efforts, which try to prevent reinjuries or existing injuries becoming chronic, can be called secondary prevention, and, finally, prevention of a chronic injury from becoming functionally irreversible can be called tertiary prevention, respectively.

Whatever the view, it is of great importance that the framework of the selected strategy is clear and that everyone involved understands the basic principles of it. If this basis of injury prevention rests on shaky grounds, only disappointing and frustrating results can be expected.

General preventive methods

In practice, the strategies in primary, secondary and tertiary prevention of sports injuries overlap. For example, medical screening before a marathon running competition can be directed to one individual by his or her personal examination, to many people by group examinations, or to whole society by making a legislative decision that every runner should have a medical screening before participation.

General prevention of sports injuries includes all the methods which concern everyone involved in physical activity. Specific preventive methods are directed to specific groups trying to affect the intrinsic and extrinsic predisposing factors of sports injuries. Specific methods are discussed in detail later in this chapter.

Basic physical fitness

Good physical fitness is of the utmost importance in avoiding sports injury. Those whose basic fitness level is below normal are more prone to injury, both from acute trauma and from overuse (Peterson & Renström, 1986). A basic physical fitness level can be achieved by regular exercise and general physical activity throughout the year. General conditioning and training of large muscle groups are of great importance in most sports. Training should progress gradually and this applies above all to those who are no longer young.

Warm-up and cooling down

Warm-up exercises are designed to prepare the body for the ensuing sporting activity (Fig. 2.2). They have two functions: (i) to prevent injury; and (ii) to enhance performance. Regarding injury prevention by warm-up exercise, the most common and important injuries to be prevented are not only muscle strains but also tendon, ligament and other soft tissue injuries. Physical work increases the energy output and the temperature of the muscles, and this in turn leads to improved brain–muscle coordination and cooperation with less likelihood of uncontrolled muscle activities and strain. At the same time, warm-up exercise increases the general alertness providing psychological preparation for the task to come.

  After training or competition, cooling-down exercises are desirable. Cooling down enhances the wash-out of the waste products of muscle metabolism (lactic acid, etc.) shortening the recovery time, respectively. It also offers a unique possibility to stretching exercises, since the

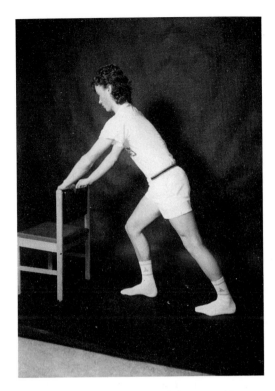

Fig. 2.2 Warm-up exercises, including stretching, are important in avoiding injuries. Courtesy of Dr P.A.F.H. Renström.

muscle temperature is still high and stretching can be performed safely and easily.

Slow progression

The slow progression principle in injury prevention means allowing the musculoskeletal system to gradually adapt to increasing loads. It is well known that at least 50% of all overuse injuries are caused by training errors (James et al., 1978). The majority of these errors are, in turn, due to breaking this slow progression principle.

  Musculoskeletal adaptation to stress is a slow but very potent process. Therefore, to avoid injuries in muscles (e.g. pain, soreness, strain and compartment syndromes), tendons (tendinitis, peritendinitis, tenoperiostitis, tendinosus, and partial or complete ruptures), joints (cartilage softening or avulsion, meniscal ruptures, ligament sprains, synovitis and osteoarthritis), and bones (stress fractures, osteoporotic fractures and apophysitis), special attention is required from athletes and their coaches to understand the importance of slow progression.

Preventive training

Training of the musculoskeletal system is the key to both the prevention of injuries and to a successful recovery after an injury. Repeated, slowly progressive exercises will improve the mechanical and structural properties of the muscles, tendons, joints, ligaments and bones by increasing their mass and tensile strength. Preventive training includes muscle training, mobility and flexibility training, coordination and proprioceptive training, and sports-specific training (Peterson & Renström, 1986).

Medical examinations

Routine physical examinations of recreational or competitive athletes have been widely used as a preventive method. However, they are time consuming and may be costly, and their efficiency in injury or health hazard prevention is questionable (Leach, 1988). If such examinations are to be performed, there must be very good reasons for doing so. In addition, planning and preparation for such examinations should be done long before action.

Generally, the task of the medical examination of athletes is straightforward. It must be determined if there is any physical defect or condition which would jeopardize an athlete playing a particular sport. The question is how effective these examinations can be in injury prevention.

If preseason or preparticipation screenings are performed, they should include a complete orthopaedic evaluation trying to discover possible risk factors such as:

1 Overweight.

2 Previous musculoskeletal diseases like osteoarthritis, osteoporosis and chondromalacia.
3 Malalignments like leg length discrepancy, scoliosis, joint hyperlaxity and foot hyperpronation.
4 Muscle weakness and imbalance.
5 Decreased flexibility.

In most screenings a precise medical history and a physical examination is enough. Further diagnostic tools (radiographs, bone scans, ultrasound and laboratory tests) should be reserved for special cases, or performed only as a further examination of one individual.

Nutrition and diet

In injury prevention, nutrition becomes important in those long-lasting training and competition situations during which the body's carbohydrate (muscle glycogen) stores are emptying. Under normal circumstances, the muscle and liver glycogen stores are sufficient to supply energy for exercises lasting up to 1.5 h, but after that their capability for that task decreases quickly. The performance level, reactions and coordination of the subject impair respectively, and the athlete is then prone to injury.

In injury prevention, other nutritional elements of food (fat, proteins, vitamins and minerals) are of secondary value. Of course, they have a tremendous effect on general well-being, and therefore a well-balanced diet is recommended for every active individual.

Drugs, medication and doping

Basically all athletes taking part in competitions should be healthy and not under medication of any kind. However, if the medication used is really needed, is not under the banned substances list of the International Olympic Committee (IOC), and is prescribed by the athlete's own physician, it obviously enhances the athlete's general well-being and allows him or her to take part in sports and enjoy it. Such drugs like asthma or diabetes medication can only be seen in a positive light, and also as tools of injury prevention in these individuals.

The doping substances are, however, a real problem. The word 'doping' implies all attempts to improve sporting performance in artificial ways, usually with the help of drugs. Every time that the performance is artificially improved, there is an increased risk for acute or overuse injuries as well as many other health hazards, and therefore their use should always be resisted by physicians and other medical staff.

Hygiene

The skin secretes sweat and grease in which dust and dirt may adhere. If the dirt is allowed to accumulate it becomes a breeding ground for bacteria which break down the dirt, and produces unpleasant odours. Rashes, irritation and pimples can occur as a result, which, in turn, may expose the individual to infection or inflammation.

In sports, foot hygiene needs special attention. Inadequate foot care allows dirt to collect between the toes and the cuticles and this becomes a breeding ground for bacteria and fungi. Fungal foot infection is so common among athletes that it has been named 'athlete's foot'. Prevention of athlete's foot is simple: daily washing of the feet with soap and water followed by a socks change, usage of proper shoes, and avoidance of visits to public swimming pools and showers barefoot or during fungal infection.

General preparation for sport

The general preparation includes a rather well-regulated daily life with regular food habits, enough sleep and avoidance of drug abuse. The importance of regular, sound living habits cannot be overemphasized for an individual with athletic aspirations.

The athlete needs not only to be physically well prepared for training and competitions but mentally as well. This includes awareness by the athlete of the requirements of the sport and what it takes to fulfil a race or competition. The requirement for some degree of mental tension varies from sport to sport. Overraised mental tension can cause reactions such as lack of appetite, headaches, and, occasionally, defective coordination which can lead to an increased risk of injury.

Specific preventive methods

Any sports injury can be caused by intrinsic or extrinsic factors, either alone or in combination (Lorentzon, 1988). In acute traumas, extrinsic factors are dominant, while in overuse injuries the reasons are more multifactorial. In overuse injuries an interaction between these two categories is common. In order to achieve effective injury prevention, it is vital to be able to affect these predisposing (risk) factors.

Intrinsic factors

The most usual intrinsic factors related to overuse injuries (Table 2.1) have been suggested to be:
1 Alignment abnormalities.
2 Leg length discrepancy.
3 Muscle weakness and imbalance.
4 Decreased flexibility.
5 Joint laxity.
6 Female gender.
7 Young or old age.
8 Overweight.
9 Some predisposing diseases.
In a recent study of running injuries, Lysholm and Wiklander (1987) found that in 40% of the cases intrinsic predisposing factors were present, but in only 10% were they the only demonstrable factor. However, it should be kept in mind that this area is highly conjectural and many plausible hypotheses at present lack substantiating evidence (Lorentzon, 1988).

Extrinsic factors

By extrinsic predisposing factors we mean all

Table 2.1 Intrinsic factors related to overuse injuries in sports.

Malalignments
  foot hyperpronation/hypopronation
  pes planus/cavus
  forefoot varus/valgus
  hindfoot varus/valgus
  tibia vara
  genu valgum/varum
  patella alta/baja
  femoral neck anteversion
Leg length discrepancy
Muscle weakness/imbalance
Decreased flexibility
Joint laxity
Female gender
Young/old age
Overweight
Predisposing diseases

Table 2.2 Extrinsic factors related to injuries in sports.

Excessive load on the body
  type of movement
  speed of movement
  number of repetitions
  footwear
  surface
Training errors
  over distance
  fast progression
  high intensity
  hill work
  poor technique
  fatigue
Environmental malconditions
  dark
  heat/cold
  humidity
  altitude
  wind
Poor equipment
Ineffective rules

the factors acting externally on the human body (Nigg, 1988). The most common extrinsic factors related to sports injuries (Table 2.2) have been suggested to be:

1 Excessive loads on the body.
2 Training errors.
3 Environmental malconditions.
4 Poor equipment.
5 Ineffective rules.

Extrinsic factors are mainly excessive loads on the body due to training errors. In runners, they are present in 60–80% of the reported injuries (James *et al.*, 1978).

Conclusion

The battle against the increasing number of acute and overuse sports injuries should be concentrated on injury prevention. Preventive work needs a clear strategy, which should include individual, group and society level activities. Accordingly, prevention is best divided into primary, secondary and tertiary preventive efforts, as well as into general and specific preventive methods. General efforts should reach everyone involved in physical activity, while specific methods should be directed at specific groups of people trying to affect the intrinsic

and extrinsic predisposing factors of sports injuries.

Only through well-organized preventive work can encouraging results be expected.

References

American College of Sports Medicine (1978) Position statement on the recommended quantity and quality of exercise for developing and maintaining fitness in healthy adults (Appendix). *Med. Sci. Sports Exerc.* **10**(VII).

Axelsson, R., Renström, P. & Svensson, H.O. (1980) Akuta idrottsskador pa ett centrallasarett (Acute sports injuries in a central hospital). *Läkartidningen* **77**, 3615–17.

Bortz, W.M. (1982) Disuse and aging. *JAMA* **248**, 1203.

Devereaux, M.D. & Lachmann, S.M. (1983) Athletes attending a sports injury clinic — a review. *Br. J. Sports Med.* **17**, 137–42.

Ekstrand, J. (1982) *Soccer injuries and their prevention.* Dissertation, University of Linköping, Sweden.

Fasler, S. (1976) Sportunfalle: statistik 1963–1973 (Sports trauma: statistics 1963–1973). *Sozial Präventivmed.* **21**, 296–301.

Franke, K. (1980) *Traumatologie des Sports* (Traumatology in Sports). Georg Thieme Verlag, Stuttgart.

Hlobil, H., Mechelen, W. van & Kemper, H.C.G. (1987) *How can sports injuries be prevented?* NISGZ Publication No. 25E, Oosterbeek, pp. 1–136.

International Federation of Sports Medicine (1989) Physical exercise — an important factor for health. A position statement. *Int. J. Sports Med.* **10**, 460–1.

James, S.L., Bates, B.T. & Osternig, L.R. (1978) Injuries to runners. *Am. J. Sports Med.* **6**, 40–50.

Kannus, P., Niittymäki, S. & Järvinen, M. (1987) Sports injuries in women: A one-year prospective follow-up study at an outpatient sports clinic. *Br. J. Sports Med.* **21**, 37–9.

Kannus, P., Niittymäki, S. & Järvinen, M. (1988) Athletic overuse injuries in children. A 30-month prospective follow-up study at an outpatient sports clinic. *Clin. Ped.* **27**, 333–7.

Kannus, P., Niittymäki, S., Järvinen, M. & Lehto, M. (1989) Sports injuries in elderly athletes: A three-year prospective, controlled study. *Age Aging* **18**, 263–70.

Koplan, J., Siscovick, D. & Goldbaum, G. (1985) The risk of exercise: A public health view of injuries and hazards. *Public Health Rep.* **100**, 189–97.

Korhonen, K. (1986) *Sports injuries*. Dissertation, University of Kuopio, Finland.

Kvist, M. & Järvinen, M. (1978) Typical injuries at an outpatient sports clinic. *Duodecim* **94**, 1335–45.

Lane, N.E., Bloch, D.A., Wood, P.D. & Fries, J.F. (1987) Aging, long-distance running, and the development of musculoskeletal disability: A controlled study. *Am. J. Med.* **82**, 772–80.

Leach, R. (1988) Medical examination of athletes. In A. Dirix, H.G. Knuttgen & K. Tittel (eds) *The Olympic Book of Sports Medicine*, pp. 572–82. Blackwell Scientific Publications, Oxford.

Lewis, S., Haskell, W.L., Wood, P.H., Monoogian, N., Bailey, J.E. & Pereira, M. (1976) Effects of physical activity on weight reduction in middle-aged women. *Am. J. Clin. Nutrition* **29**, 151–6.

Lorentzon, R. (1988) Causes of injuries: Intrinsic factors. In A. Dirix, H.G. Knuttgen & K. Tittel (eds) *The Olympic Book of Sports Medicine*, pp. 376–90. Blackwell Scientific Publications, Oxford.

Lysholm, J. & Wiklander, J. (1987) Injuries in runners. *Am. J. Sports Med.* **15**, 168–71.

Nigg, B. (1988) Causes of injuries: Extrinsic factors. In A. Dirix, H.G. Knuttgen & K. Tittel (eds) *The Olympic Book of Sports Medicine*, pp. 363–75. Blackwell Scientific Publications, Oxford.

Orava, S. (1980) *Exertion injuries due to sports and physical exercise*. Dissertation, University of Kokkola, Finland.

Paffenbarger, R.S., Wing, A.L. & Hyder, T. (1978) Physical activity as an index of heart attack risk in college alumni. *Am. J. Epidemiol.* **108**, 161–75.

Peräsalo, O., Vapaavuori, M. & Louhimo, I. (1955) Uber die Sportverletzungen. *Ann. Chirurg. Gynaecol. Fenn.* **44**, 256–69.

Peterson, L. & Renström, P. (1986) *Sports Injuries. Their Prevention and Treatment*. Martin Dunitz Ltd, London.

Renström, P. & Kannus, P. (1992) Prevention of sports injuries. In R. Strauss (ed) *Sports Medicine*. WB Saunders, Philadelphia.

Robey, J.M., Blyth, C.S. & Mueller, F.O. (1971) Athletic injuries — application of epidemiologic methods. *JAMA* **217**, 184–9.

Sandelin, J. (1988) *Acute sports injuries. A clinical and epidemiological study*. Dissertation, Helsinki, Yliopistopaino.

Vuori, I., Aho, A.J. & Karakorpi, T. (1972) Injuries sustained in sports and exercise. *Duodecim* **88**, 700–11.

Watters, D., Brooks, S., Elton, R. & Little, K. (1984) Sports injuries in an accident and emergency department. *Arch. Emerg. Med.* **2**, 105–12.

Weightman, D. & Browne, R.C. (1975) Injuries in eleven selected sports. *Br. J. Sports Med.* **9**, 136–41.

Chapter 3

Strategies for Prevention of Musculoskeletal Injuries

MARY T. MOFFROID

Prevention of illness and disability is a renewed focus of modern medicine. The emphasis is appropriate because education about diet, life-style, environment and safety precautions have been shown to greatly reduce direct and indirect costs associated with major killers like heart attack, stroke, cancer and accidents. Until the advent of miracle drugs in the past century, medicine used to focus on consumer education, as in the efforts to abolish unsanitary conditions associated with epidemic infections. But when miracle drugs were discovered and manufactured, the public became passive recipients of health care, exemplifying the 'medical model' described by Brickman in which the individual assumes neither responsibility for contracting illness nor for getting better (Brickman *et al.*, 1982). Research demonstrates that behavioural changes are more likely to occur if the individual does assume responsibility for his or her own treatment regardless of whose fault it was (the compensatory model) or if the individual assumes responsibility for both the treatment and the injury (the moral model). Today, such a change in approach requires education of the health-care practitioner, as well as education of the consumer.

The focus of this chapter is on prevention of musculoskeletal injuries in the athlete, discussed from the viewpoint of related research and slanted towards educating the athlete to assume responsibility for avoiding injuries. An overview of the causes of injury is followed by a discussion of injury prevention in the work-place because of the relatedness of this larger body of literature. General considerations in a programme of injury prevention are then discussed, followed by concerns specific to the musculoskeletal system. Finally, an overall strategy for injury prevention is proposed.

Classification of physical causes of injury

Athletic injuries occur through trauma, overexertion and repetitive motion. These injuries may be classified as extrinsic (trauma) or intrinsic according to Muckle (1978) who states that intrinsic injuries account for about one-third of all sports injuries, but more than half of track and field injuries. Examples of intrinsic and extrinsic injuries pertaining to the four mechanisms of rotator cuff tear would be throwing (intrinsic/overexertion), direct fall (extrinsic/impact), thrust (intrinsic/repetitive motion) and accompanying shoulder dislocation (a combination of factors).

Trauma as an extrinsic event results from a fall, contact with another individual or with an object like a baseball bat. The severity of impact trauma will depend on the momentum, size and direction of the external object, and on one's own body position, stabilization and protective gear.

Overexertion and repetitive motion are intrinsic causes of injury which only pertain to the individual, not to the environment. Examples of overexertion are excessive contractile activity (as when the quadriceps or the soleus becomes painful after a strenuous run), or by excessive stretch (as when the hamstrings become painful after a challenging hurdle). Although contractile and stretch incidents are frequently given as separate examples of overexertion, they both exemplify injury pertaining to eccentric muscle activity. In running, the quadriceps contracts eccentrically to keep the knee from buckling, (a 'contractile' situation), while in the hurdle, the hamstrings muscles contract eccentrically to decelerate the hip flexion and knee extension (a 'stretch' situation). Although eccentric contractions are physiologically efficient, there is frequent microscopic tearing and resultant pain. Injury from eccentric activity relates to the fact that the muscle generates force with increasing sarcomere lengths and disruption of sarcomere alignment (Friden et al., 1986). Overexertion is not a simple problem with muscle strength or length; timing and coordination with the antagonist muscles are also critical factors. In fact, terms like underexertion or misexertion might be as appropriate.

Repetitive motion is the second intrinsic factor related to musculoskeletal injuries. If we were properly aligned so that muscles and ligaments created movement about perfect instant centres of joint rotation, there should not be a problem with repetitive motion. Such is not the case for several reasons. When muscle fatigues (through repetitive activity, vibration, decreased circulation because of cold temperatures or restrictive clothing), the movement pattern is altered and the joint begins to move out of its normal biomechanical alignment, creating abnormal stresses and eventual tissue damage. Poor segmental alignment of body parts produces a similar situation, with potential for injury via repetitive motion. Davies has discussed the effect of the pronated foot which increases medial rotation of the tibia, an increased Q angle of the quadriceps, an increased lateral force on the patella and a resultant patellofemoral pain syndrome (Davies, 1980). Repetitive motion injuries are normally thought to hasten degenerative processes, but Cantu (1981) points out that repetitive motion stresses in youngsters slow growth processes which closes growth plates prematurely.

Prevention of injury: psychosocial factors

Because of the billions of dollars spent in the USA by industry for worker-related injuries, researchers have examined precipitating causes for injury in the workplace. Some of these findings may be very relevant to prevention of injury in sport. For example, a previous injury in the past year is a key warning to potential reinjury, even if the individual has participated in a rehabilitation programme, and is apparently fully recovered. There is no apparent relationship between the severity of the initial injury and the reinjury, but the likelihood of reinjury is sobering because repeat injuries are usually more severe (Horal, 1969).

A worker whose job requirements exceed his or her physical capacity to perform that job is at high risk for injury. 12% of the USA work force have jobs whose lifting requirements exceed the maximal permissable limit (MPL) for lifting as defined by the National Institute of Occupational Safety and Health (NIOSH) (Pope, 1991). Just as job requirements can exceed one's physical capacities to perform them, so some sports can exceed one's capabilities. It is up to the individual to know (or to be counselled) about demands of various sports and whether or not he or she has the physical capability to participate safely.

Other aspects of worksite injury research may also be applicable to injuries in sports, although perhaps not as apparent at first glance. For example, although satisfaction with one's job is a relevant criterion in predicting on-site injury in the workplace (Cats-Baril & Frymoyer, 1991), one might assume that a person would not be engaging in a sport or recreational activity unless motivated. However, with the recent jogging craze and fights with fat, enslaved commitment to an athletic activity may have a lot in common with dissatisfaction in the workplace and hence increased potential for injury.

Environmental considerations are as important on the playing field as in the workplace. Attention to lighting, surface safety, temperature, humidity and pollution are all very relevant to safe performance.

Sometimes in the workplace, a worker may feel the boss or the system has all the responsibility for how things are done, and such abdication of responsibility increases the likelihood of an injury. Although an individual in a sporting activity may not consciously have such an attitude, there is a danger that excess confidence may be placed in the safety of protective gear, in the actions of other team members, or in the timely blowing of the referee's whistle. Knowing and following the rules and codes of sport is an essential component to protecting oneself against injury. Again, to adopt the compensatory or moral model of Brickman, an individual should learn to assume responsibility and have a full understanding of the challenges and of the physical and mental capacity needed to meet the demands.

Another similarity between current practice in the workplace and on the playing field is that someone who is recently injured must rest and reduce physical effort in order to let healing occur. Staying away from a job or a sport is not easy, and is not part of our culture of expectations, but it must be part of management strategy, reinforced by all parties. Running off a minor injury damages surrounding soft tissue, impairs nutrition to the joint and can result in further damage. Mild injuries should not be neglected. Because injury-prone athletes tend to be unduly critical of themselves (Nilsson, 1986), their tendency to prevail and continue playing needs to be countered. Using ice or pain medication to allow continued play presents a real danger because normal cardiovascular and respiratory reflexes are reduced when pain receptors are blocked, creating the potential for further injury (Newham, 1991).

In Western culture, the work ethic conveys that it is good to work, even if we may not feel like working. Grin and bear it, or as Churchill said, much of the world's work is done by people in pain. There is a boundary somewhere between malingering and pressing forward despite the body's warning signs (such as fever, fatigue or distractedness). Such warning signs should preclude participation in sport in order to avoid injury but we have been so schooled in perseverance that these warning signs are often not heeded.

Psychological stress is an added factor contributing to potential injury. Certain personality traits associated with stress contribute to accidents (Yost, 1967). Athletic stress may be biological, physiological, psychological or mixed. Some stress, if recognized, can be managed and ameliorated. Awareness of stressing factors by the athlete, the coach, the trainer and other team mates may help reduce their impact on injury.

Physical growth is a stress to the musculoskeletal system. Since most youngsters are involved in sport, the stresses of a growing system on muscle, ligament, tendon and bone must be taken into account.

Prevention of injury: general factors

Fitness

Overall fitness is prophylactic to injury (Jesse, 1977). Cardiovascular endurance is of primary importance to fitness. The simplest index of cardiovascular fitness is Vo_{2max}, which is an indication of how efficiently the tissues are able to utilize inhaled oxygen. Because of the relationship between Vo_{2max} and distance running (Cooper, 1968), simple tests such as the 12-min run can be used to estimate maximum oxygen uptake. Kulund (1982) states that cardiovascular preseason screening usually identifies serious pathological states. However, a risk factor questionnaire, designed by a physician, should first identify those not be be screened (Schlife, 1982).

Sudden death is a potential hazard of exercise, but short of death, there are still very serious sequelae to overstressing the body. Marathon runners, older kyackers and others have been known to suffer tissue breakdown from overexertion, which in turn prompts auto-immune responses including joint pain and swelling, fever, night sweats and general debilitation lasting for several weeks. Cardiovascular fitness is important, and one should not exceed one's level of fitness.

Arnot summarizes effects which training has on the heart, stating that adults starting training can develop the cardiac system to its full potential in 3 years, whereas younger children take up to 8 years. Heavy training will increase left ventricular wall thickness, whereas endurance training increases end-diastolic volume, left ventricular mass and maybe contractility, but changes in the size of the coronary arteries is debatable. Peripherally, there is reduced resistance to blood flow, which relates to less vasoconstriction of the vessels, and there is also an increase in the capillary networks (Arnot, 1981). Age-based charts, such as those published by the American Heart Association, advising on safe training heart rates, should be followed.

Nutritional status

There are volumes of literature about diet and performance, including discussions of vitamins, supplements, carbohydrates and proteins. Prevention of injury in sports means paying attention to nutritional status and to diet. Anorexia or fasting produces atrophy and weakness of large proximal muscles, which spells trouble for hip joints and shoulder joints if affected individuals engage in vigorous sports.

Lack of vitamins in the normal population is usually not a problem because vitamins are not body builders, and because balanced diets generally include necessary vitamin intakes. However, vitamin C can become depleted in pregnant women, heavy drinkers, high-stress performers and those on high-cholesterol diets

(Kavanagh, 1976). In instances such as these, vitamin C supplements are suggested.

Water intake is essential to body homeostasis. Athletes may lose 1–1.8 kg (2–4 lb) during an event and are advised to take fluids prior to the event. Coffee, tea, colas or cocoa are discouraged because of increased urine production (Kavanagh, 1976).

Obesity is defined as having a fat percentage greater than 20% in males and greater than 30% in females (Wickkiser & Kelly, 1975), and is a condition which is detrimental to the athlete because of the excess weight (Ryan & Allman, 1974). Body fat percentage less than 5% is considered too little for good health. Body fat can be determined by underwater weighing, or by more simple formulae related to skinfold thicknesses at the scapulae, the abdomen, the upper arms and the hips (Jette *et al.*, 1979).

Tissue-specific factors related to injury prevention

Injuries in sports are sport specific (Muckle, 1978), but since all injuries involve the same tissues, tissue vulnerability, assessment and training related to bone, cartilage, ligament, tendon and muscle will follow in this discussion. Skeletal muscle attracts the most attention in rehabilitation, because so much is known about muscle mechanics and changes which can be accomplished with training (Fig. 3.1). In addition, the integrity of the connective tissues (bone, ligament and cartilage) is important to avoiding injury and will also be discussed. Lastly, neurosensory actions and reactions will be addressed because of their important role in safe performance.

Bone

Although we do not normally test bone density or exercise bone tissue consciously, bone is a dynamic tissue which responds to exercise. Geusens and Dequeker (1991) conclude that exercise for at least 14 weeks which loads bone positively influences bone density in both

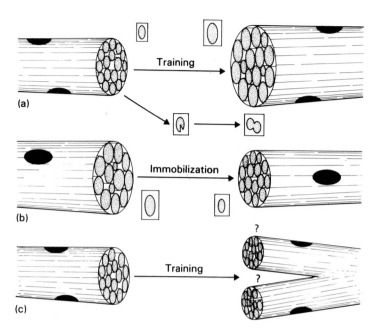

Fig. 3.1 Changes in muscle size that occur in response to strength training and immobilization. (a) With training, cross-sectional fibre area increases in direct proportion to the increases in myofibril size and number. (b) With immobilization, fibre area decreases in proportion to the decrease in myofibril size. (c) Training-induced fibre splitting has been postulated to occur in certain species but it is unlikely that it occurs in adult humans. From MacDougall (1986).

males and females and in both young and old people. Stress fractures are reportedly becoming more common in young adults, reflecting today's increasing demands on juvenile athletes. Such information warrants more study to determine the effects of specific exercises for increasing bone density, preventing stress fractures in athletes, and possibly decreasing the incidence of osteoporosis in later years (Dalsky, 1989).

Cartilage

As an avascular tissue, activity is necessary to maintain the nutritional status and functional integrity of hyaline cartilage which lines all of the articulating surfaces of synovial joints. Although lack of movement reduces overall joint flexibility, and precipitates cartilage fibrosis, activity which is too stressful or too non-physiological will cause excessive wear, softening and ultimate degeneration of cartilage. For example, carrying packs which are too heavy or which are carried for too long will cause ruptures in the hyaline cartilage

lining the end-plates of the vertebral bodies and breakdown of the fibrocartilage in the annulus fibrosis of the intervertebral discs. Preventing these intrinsic injuries is a matter of knowing the demands of the task, training for them, and being adequately fit.

Tendon and ligament

Tendons and ligaments around joints protect against injury, and do not rely on conscious activity or control. When and if muscular activity is insufficient to counteract opposing forces, the ligaments and joint capsule tautness restrain the body segments, like the guy wires which restrain excessive motions of the mast of a sailboat. Such protective action requires these connective tissue structures to be both strong, in order to withstand the magnitude and velocity of opposing forces, and elastic, in order to regain their prestretched state.

Tendons attach muscle to bone. They are passive structures which store energy and contribute up to 50% of the total energy for running (Cavagna & Kaneko, 1977). As with ligaments, tendons can become tight with disuse, over-stretched or ruptured. By the third decade of life, tendons lose their vascular supply and become more vulnerable to rupture with sudden stresses, particularly in middle-aged and older individuals. In younger athletes, sudden stresses are more likely to cause avulsion in which the musculotendinous unit ruptures or in which the tendon separates from bone (Riegger, 1985).

Measures of ligamentous integrity in the human include laxity (length at a specific loading force) and stiffness (change in length with specific change in loading force). Instrumentation for assessing knee joint laxity exists with varying degrees of reliability and varying planes of movement addressed (Hanten & Pace, 1987). Stiffness measures require high levels of force not attained with most instrumentation (or subject consent), so laxity is what is generally measured. Excessively tight ligaments alter normal biomechanics and can precipitate intrinsic injuries related to malalignment (Beynnon, 1991). Increased joint laxity is associated with instability and increased likelihood of injury. Weisman demonstrated increased joint laxity after cyclic loading and inferred that knee injuries in skiing occurred at the end of the day because of the connective tissue fatigue resulting from repetitive stretching after a day of skiing (Weisman et al., 1980).

Much more research is needed in order to determine how best to develop joint structures to protect against injury. One fact is certain, however, and that is that muscle cannot be trained to respond quickly or forcefully enough to avoid many types of injury to ligaments or tendons.

Whether or not the tensile strength of ligaments in humans can be made stronger without surgery is debatable. Animal studies suggest that ligaments respond to dynamic resistive exercise by increasing the amount of collagen and developing increased tensile strength (Tipton et al., 1978). Tensile strength is assessed by the force required to cause rupture, so comparable studies have not been done in vivo,

and it is not known if progressive exercise in humans increases tensile strength of ligaments or capsular tissue. Those who do believe exercise can positively affect the tensile strength of ligaments in humans suggest that a minimum of 12 weeks of training is necessary.

Muscle

Muscle tears may occur microscopically within the muscle cell or macroscopically at the musculotendinous junction. In either case, the precipitating event appears to be during forceful eccentric contractions. Some specific aspects of muscle testing and performance are addressed below.

MUSCLE STRENGTH

Strength is the static or dynamic torque which a muscle can produce at a specific limb position and velocity, and is a function of the muscle's cross-sectional area, number of activated muscle fibres, angle of insertion into the bone and rate of motor unit recruitment. Voluntary effort must be maximal in order to obtain a true maximal measure. Torque of a maximal eccentric contraction is normally 1.5 times greater than that of a concentric effort at a slow speed of testing, but as the testing speed is increased, the difference in torque becomes greater. This is because concentric torque decreases with increasing velocity of motion, whereas eccentric torque stays the same, or increases somewhat (Hortobagyi et al., 1989).

Muscle length is related to muscle strength, and an overstretched muscle may not have adequate torque at the point in the range of motion where it is needed. For example, a lengthened gluteus medius may not be able to generate adequate torque to maintain a level pelvis during running, even though the muscle could attain the target torque level at a more shortened position in the range during muscle testing. The position in which a muscle is tested, and in which it is expected to function, are critical to logical strength assessments during preseason screening.

Muscle strength between opposing muscle groups is thought to be important in preventing injuries in sports events (Burkett, 1970). Although randomized, prospective studies to support this assumption have not been reported, more complete information about muscle strength may eventually demonstrate the optimal muscle balance about various joints for specific sports.

Another expectation about muscle strength of the extremities is that the measures of torque on the right and left sides will be between 10 and 15% of each other. Distal muscles conform to this pattern, with the preferred extremity demonstrating the higher torque levels. More proximally, the torque levels tend to be more similar. There is still no good answer to how much absolute torque is 'normal'. Comparing maximal torque to percentages of body weight is not a good index (Delitto et al., 1989). Calculating specific torque demands for peak velocities specific to expected performance would be more appropriate, but the research is still in its infancy. Because our knowledge about precise training for specific sports is so scant, Zohar (1973) recommends training well beyond the demands of an expected activity.

VELOCITY OF CONTRACTION

Speed is a criterion in many sports. Speed in running, for example, is dependent on inhibiting all but the least necessary eccentric activity of the hip extensors (hamstrings and gluteus maximus) in order to allow rapid acceleration of the advancing limb (Hagood et al., 1990). The balance between that minimal eccentric activity adequate to protect the knee as the tibia advances rapidly, yet insufficient to compromise the desired speed is a delicate balance. Training too quickly or expecting miracles from individuals without such neuromotor capacity invites injury.

A muscle's maximal rate of contraction has an upper physiological limit, dependent on

the length of that muscle's fibres. Exceeding that velocity means the muscle force cannot be generated for protection, leaving passive structures as a last defence. Furthermore, the onset of muscle contraction (reaction time), although responsive to training, also has an upper limit, so one cannot assume that a fit and trained individual is immune to injury. Knowledge of a sport's demands and a body's capabilities allow a compatibility between task demands and task accomplishment to exist which should reduce incidences of injury.

Screening for muscle torque can be done simply with hand dynamometers and manual resistance, or elaborately with isokinetic equipment and electromyography. Many testing procedures and accompanying recording forms are described by Sanders and Eggart (1985).

If deficits in muscle torque production (strength), speed or reaction time are identified, training programmes must be implemented. Pearl and Moran (among many others) have published detailed programmes with good illustrations for a variety of strengthening programmes (Pearl & Moran, 1986; American Academy of Orthopedic Surgeons, 1991).

FLEXIBILITY

A tight muscle with inadequate length poses a problem. In the hurdler, tight hamstrings restrict hip flexion and knee extension, resulting in frequent tears at the musculotendinous junctions during a hurdle event. Less drastic, but also debilitating, is the low back pain which is a predictable sequela to tight hamstrings in males (Biering-Sorensen, 1984).

Flexibility incorporates tendon, ligament and muscle structures. Davies (1985) believes measures of joint range of motion (ROM) should be performed actively by the athlete, not passively by the examiner, because active measures are more functional. Dvorak demonstrated that active ROM testing better characterizes hypomobility, but that passive testing elicits more hypermobility (Dvorak et al., 1988). Therefore, both active and passive ROM testing should be performed. Clarkson and Gilewich (1989) describe details of joint ROM measures with illustrative photographs.

Training programmes to increase flexibility must be specific to the tissue identified as being limited. Muscle responds to slow and progressive stretching, whereas ligaments require deep transverse manipulation and joint capsules require mobilization procedures, as described by Palmer and Epler (1990). Effective stretching programmes for athletes are well described and illustrated by Anderson and Anderson (1980).

MUSCLE ENDURANCE

Repetitive efforts or sustained contractions for any length of time require aerobic mechanisms which utilize the Krebs' cycle. When available oxygen can no longer be supplied to the tissue in adequate quantities, conductivity of muscle fibres slows (Stulen & DeLuca, 1981), and effective muscle tension decreases, despite recruitment of more motor units. Such changes can be assessed by sequential strength testing or quantified by a shift in the centre frequency of a surface electromyogram. Strength decrements after fatiguing eccentric muscle contractions are more noticeable than after fatiguing concentric muscle contractions, and are believed to be due to microscopic muscle tears at the Z-bands which result from the lengthening contractions of the elongated sarcomeres. Muscle endurance can be enhanced with training, but the effects are relatively specific. For example, cross-country skiers may have a high $\dot{V}o_{2max}$ when going with only the legs, but this value drops when arm activity is added, because of the increased peripheral resistance of the lesser trained upper extremities and the body's need to balance blood pressure (Arnot, 1981).

NEUROSENSORY FACTORS

This discussion on muscle would not be complete without addressing the role of the central and peripheral nervous system in governing motor control, and hence in protecting against injury. During voluntary concentric efforts it is known that the small (type I) motor units (supplying mostly slow twitch muscle fibres) are recruited first. However, during eccentric efforts (Nardone & Schieppati, 1988) or during involuntary contractions, as with electrical stimulation (Sinacore et al., 1990), this pattern is reversed and the larger type II motor units supplying fast twitch muscle fibres are recruited first. If the normal physiological pattern is not present, reflexes which occur to counteract falls may not be adequate.

The nervous system is also important to timing of muscle activity, control of force levels, and coordination of synergistic and antagonistic muscles. Some of these activities can be improved with training, but the sports-specific motor performance criteria need to be identified so that an individual trains with specific goals in mind. Even an innocuous act like serving a tennis ball can lead to injury if the server's trunk does not bend laterally during the rotational follow through. Not every potential player cares about the physiological motions of the articular facets of the lumbar vertebrae, nor 'senses' that the lumbar vertebral column needs to bend laterally to the right when the trunk rotates left. Failure to coordinate these movements can be awkward at best and injurious at worst. Some players sense how to move, or have watched enough good players to copy basic moves, but some need to be taught very basic dynamics to prevent injury. The involuntary reflex responses depend on stimuli which may come from skin, joint receptors or muscle receptors. Bracing or taping may alter these cues, but have not been shown to alter normal physiological or functional responses (Karlsson et al., 1992).

Measures of sensation, proprioception and coordination are found on many preseason screening forms and are necessary for a thorough assessment.

Skin

Being the largest organ of the body and one which is vitally important to temperature control and fluid balance, attention to the protection and care of skin is important in injury prevention. Because skin covers proportionately more surface area in younger children, they lose heat more rapidly and are more prone to chilling. Skin is susceptible to carcinoma from ultraviolet exposure and must be protected, particularly where exposure intensity is enhanced by water, ice or snow, ozone depletion and also by increased altitudes. Filtering spectacles or goggles are needed to protect eyes from glare of sun, water and ice.

Posture

Static and dynamic posture reflect the integrated status of the tissues of the musculoskeletal system. Posture is assessed in athletic screening because of a conviction that asymmetries or malalignments portend injury. Bach *et al.* (1985) suggest that muscle tightness represents a likely cause of athletic running injury. Posture should be (among other things) symmetrical, with a 'normal' amount of lordosis (the range of movement has been reported as 20−60°). The toes should be outward 6° and the kneecaps should point straight ahead. Sheehan (1992) contends that failure to attain the ideal posture, particularly with regard to the feet, will lead to injury — either frank overexertion type of injury or more subtle wear and tear injuries due to repetitive motions executed out of alignment. Aside from descriptive reports and testimonials, the research is scant on these assumptions, but runners with pronated feet do report anterior knee pain, and orthotic inserts relieve the symptoms in many cases. Jesse (1977) asserts that excessive toe out is a main cause for foot problems because the posterior tibialis is forced to pull out of alignment when running, so plantar flexor activity is shunted to the peroneal muscles which cannot modify foot pronation in running. Many

theories exist, supported by logic, but not by prospective randomized trials.

Segmental proportions are another consideration in the prevention of injuries in sports. As children grow, the relationships between the lengths of the legs, trunk and arms change. For young children toe-touching is easy but for most adolescents it is impossible, because of the legs being proportionately longer than the arms or trunk. Insistence on toe-touch activities to stretch the hamstrings will only overstretch the upper back, producing a thoracic kyphosis.

Posture and segmental alignment are assessed and recorded on special forms, some of which are described by Kendall *et al.* (1977). Corrective exercises are useful, provided the individual is consistent and provided the problem is not a structural one which cannot be improved with exercise.

Strategies for prevention of injuries

Having considered the classifications for athletic injuries, precipitating psychosocial factors, general factors of fitness and nutrition, and specifics of the musculoskeletal system, we will now turn our attention to an overall strategy for prevention of injuries, of which the component parts are listed below.
1 Identify the demands of the activity.
2 Administer a risk factor questionnaire.
3 Screen the individual related to activity demands.
4 Plan a training programme based on the screening.
5 Warm-up and stretch activities.
6 Training.
7 Cool-down activities.
8 Reassess and modify programme as indicated.

Task identification

The demands of an athletic activity to be identified include the forces, speed and flexibility required. Isometric muscle torque at one joint position does not begin to satisfy demands placed on muscle at various velocities, joint positions or interactions with other muscles. Torque measures of concentric maximal efforts do not relate to eccentric needs encountered when delivering a baseball pitch (shoulder extensors and adductors) or negotiating a mogul on skis (knee and hip extensors).

Because training is specific to performance, identification of tasks within any one sport is critical to proper assessment and planning for safe and rewarding play. Much more needs to be known about the demands of various athletic activities. Research is needed in this endeavour, but what has been accomplished with immunizations can one day be accomplished with preventive training as well.

Identification of the stresses associated with the activity is also relevant to determine if an individual can cope with them, or for developing plans to mediate or accommodate the stress. For example, obtain ear plugs if excessive noise is a stressor. In paediatric sport, avoid competition during examination periods because emotional stress is accompanied by muscle tension, leading to fatigue.

Risk factor questionnaire

A physician-designed risk factor questionnaire should precede the comprehensive screening in order to avoid injury from some of the screening items, such as a heart rate recovery test or a 12-min run.

Screen

A preseason screen test should include measures of cardiovascular fitness, body fat, muscle strength, flexibility, posture and segmental alignment, balance, sensation, coordination and proprioception. A good preactivity assessment, as well as the ongoing pre-event screening, depend on knowing the expected demands of a sport. Such knowledge will indicate more specific tests, such as concentric and eccentric torque measures, open and closed chain performance, reaction time and speed of muscle contraction. Good examples of screening forms are published (Eggart et al., 1985), but each facility should develop its own, specific to its own needs and capabilities.

General factors must also be considered. Previous history is critical. For example, one should appreciate that meniscectomies increase contact forces of the knee joint by 350%, and the articular cartilage degeneration from such an operation will be three times worse if an anterior cruciate ligament deficiency is present (Lynch et al., 1983). Age is an important consideration. Both the younger and the older athlete have unique physical attributes which must be taken into account. Fast growing cells and tissues of youth are most vulnerable to damage or injury. Joint structures and epiphyseal growth cartilages are especially susceptible, and these weaknesses are exacerbated by malnutrition, glandular imbalance, musculoskeletal imbalance or bony deformities (Jesse, 1977).

The screening must occur at least 4–6 weeks prior to competition, because of the time needed for training.

Awareness of personality type is important. Many have written about the injury-prone athlete (Yost, 1967), and contend that aggressiveness, anger, inability to lose, frequent conflict with authority and need for self-punishment are some of the traits contributing to injury. Coaches, trainers and athletes, given the information, will be in a better position to be aware, and thus possibly modify behaviours contributing to potential injury.

Pre-event screening should occur every day. Players with previous injuries, any fever, excessive stress or fatigue should not engage in maximal levels of activity — if any. Individuals, as well as coaches and trainers, must assume the responsibility for requiring optimal fitness prior to participation. Pre-event screening also requires assessment of the environment: temperature conditions, playing surfaces, protective gear and appropriate clothing.

Planning a training programme

Having determined basic requirements of the relevant sport or activity, and having assessed the individual's capabilities and attributes, a training plan can be designed. Attempting to address decreased cardiovascular fitness, tight muscles, weak muscles, low muscular endurance, poor posture, bad nutritional habits and a defensive attitude all at once will not be effective. List the areas which should be addressed, keeping in mind their relevance to the sport to be played. Include aspects of the sport's demands, such as patterned movements and timing. Repetition of an event is essential to lock in proper timing and sequencing of muscle activity. Prioritize the list and define a goal and a time frame. For example, if the individual plans to do hurdles in track and field and has tight hamstrings, stretching the hamstrings would be a priority. Specify that within 2 weeks, the individual should have gained 10° range, as measured by single straight leg raise. Each point of focus in the plan must have a goal and a time frame. The plan is then frequently revised as goals are attained and new objectives are set. Training at the activity itself must be a part of the programme.

Warm-up and stretch

Prior to participation in any sport, and prior to undertaking any designed training plan, warming up is essential. Just as we all know to shower before entering a pool (which we too frequently ignore), we all know to warm up before playing (which we ignore even more frequently). A 20-min warm-up should precede any physically demanding activity.

Once muscles are warmed up, slow stretching should be performed. Stretching must not be used as warm-up. Safran demonstrated in rabbit hindlimbs that warm-ups increased tissue temperature and permitted greater elongation of multijoint muscles (Safran *et al.*, 1988). Warm-ups may be light aerobic work, such as jogging in place, or light resistive exercise with minimal weights or pedalling on a stationary bicycle. The object is to raise internal temperature to reduce the viscosity in muscles. If viscosity is high, muscle resists being lengthened and eccentric efforts require more effort and force, increasing the possibility of an intrinsic injury.

All major muscle groups should be elongated to their normal end ranges. 20-s holds are minimal. Bouncing and ballistic stretching is harmful and ineffective. Specific stretching programmes which focus on those muscles which were identified as tight or short during the screening assessment belongs to the training programme, and not to the warm-up period.

The training programme

Overall fitness is the best prevention from injury. Supreme physical fitness is not inherent in anyone — it must be trained in. Training is not just a dedicated preseason activity. Conscious daily effort towards good nutritional habits and good posture is essential. Slumping stretches ligaments, impairs blood flow and fails to provide good mechanics for action. However, the most well-trained physically fit person is not immune to injury precipitated by stress. Attention to the psychology of sport is essential and developing strategies to cope with the high pressures of athletic performance is essential. Hanley's report that the overall incidence of respiratory infection seemed higher in the most highly trained athletes, compared to the non-athletic population supports Jesse's contention that prolonged emotional tension creates chronic effects which can produce disease.

The training programme must address the goals identified in the plan and establish an order for attainment. Cardiovascular fitness should be the first concern. Firstly, the initial few weeks of training should emphasize aerobic capability. Secondly, focus on muscle strength, particularly in the muscles which have been identified as being weak or overlengthened. Thirdly, include a specific stretching agenda for muscles identified as being tight. The reason for the ordering of the last two is that whereas people normally would stretch out before weight-training, it is better not to have muscles lengthened over both sides of a joint, thereby creating instability of the joint.

Establish a schedule and adhere to it. Training is a year round proposition, so do not embark on an impossible mission. Parsed training is advised, meaning alternating heavy and light training during a week. Overtraining or failure to allow rest periods may lead to depression.

Cardiovascular training should be the first priority. Aerobic tempo training will increase the amount of aerobic work accomplished before anaerobic threshold is reached (Arnot, 1981), but if the training is performed too far below anaerobic threshold, little increase in performance will occur. Distance running, according to Cantu (1981), is not advised in the early phases of cardiovascular training because muscles, which take a long time to develop, are tools for training the heart and such resources should not be overstressed. Training effects are quickly lost by inactivity, such that one can lose up to 50% with a month of inactivity.

Muscle training must take into account how the muscles will be used — open chain, closed chain, concentric, eccentric, endurance, ballistic, precision and any other conditions relevant to the sport or activity (Fig. 3.2). In designing time frames for accomplishment of specific goals for muscle training, recognize that coordination and patterned movements improve readily with practice. Torque increases occur steadily, but the first 6 weeks reflect neural changes in recruitment patterns, not physiological changes in muscle tissue (Moritani & deVries, 1979). Hypertrophy in any given muscle cannot be expected from muscle endurance training, nor from individuals with a preponderance of slow twitch muscle fibres in that given muscle group. Muscle endurance training should be light and repetitive, whereas muscle strength training should be with progressive loading of resistance. If power is required (high torque at high velocities), attention must be given to that demand, but preferably through performance of the activity itself (for example, swimming), not through weightlifting at high velocities.

A stretching programme for targeted muscles may be done according to any number of publications and handouts, provided one pays attention to performing slow, sustained stretches. Hold each position for 20 s and then relax slowly. Ballistic stretching is ineffective and

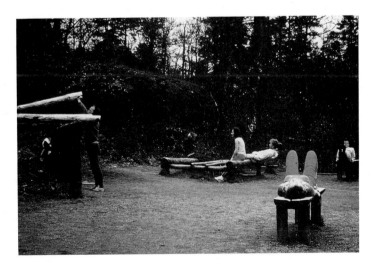

Fig. 3.2 A general warm-up circuit showing that muscle training can be carried out in many ways. Courtesy of Dr P.A.F.H. Renström.

dangerous. Reflex stretching (contracting the muscle group opposite to the tight one) will cause relaxation of the tight muscle group and facilitate stretching, but the position must be attained slowly and held for at least 20 s.

The majority of all running problems, according to Halpern (1984) are created by errors in training. Factors which should be considered include any changes in running surface, shoes, patterns of running, inadequate warm-ups, lower extremity malalignment or weakness, and imbalances of muscle. For example, according to Halpern, running downhill (sometimes used to facilitate running speed) can cause popliteus tendonitis, whereas running on a banked track irritates the pes anserinus (tendons on medial side of knee), and running on a hillside irritates the lateral knee structures, specifically the iliotibial band.

Cool-down

Training and competition efforts should be followed by a gradual cool-down so that the body is not subjected to extreme changes.

Reassess and modify programme

The plan specifies time periods for expected improvements, so that the reassessment schedule is already in place. Measurements taken during the reassessments will guide the modifications to the training programme.

All the good intentions, plans and goals are useless if there is not a unified objective which is endorsed by all parties. The athlete is the responsible party, and it is up to the coach, the trainer and the teacher to provide the resources, information and cohesion to enable the athlete to become an alert and safe consumer. For a thorough discussion of the role and importance of the sports medicine team, the reader is referred to Mueller and Ryan (1991).

In summary the best way to manage a programme for injury prevention is to evaluate, educate and encourage.

References

American Academy Orthopaedic Surgeons (AAOS) (1991) Basic principles of a conditioning program. In AAOS (ed.) *Athletic Training and Sports Medicine*, 2nd edn, pp. 721–50. AAOS Publishers, Park Ridge, IL.

Anderson, B. & Anderson, J. (1980) *Stretching*. Shelter Publications, Bolinas, CA.

Arnot, R.B. (1981) Physical conditioning of the cardiovascular system. In R.C. Cantu (ed.) *Health Maintenance Through Physical Conditioning*, pp. 1–15. PSB Publishing, Littleton, MA.

Bach, D.K., Green, D.S. & Jensen, G.M. (1985) A comparison of muscular tightness in runners and non-runners and the relation of muscular tightness to low back pain in runners. *J. Ortho. Sports Phys. Ther.* **6B**, 315–23.

Beynnon, B.D. (1991) *In vivo biomechanics of the anterior cruciate ligament, reconstruction and application of a mathematical model to the knee joint*. PhD dissertation, University of Vermont.

Biering-Sorensen, F. (1984) Physical measures as risk indicators for low back trouble over a one-year period. *Spine* **9**(2), 106–17.

Brickman, P., Rabinowitz, V.C., Karuza, J. & Coates, D. (1982) Models of helping and coping. *Am. Psych.* **37**(4), 368–84.

Burkett, I.N. (1970) Causative factors in hamstring injuries. *Med. Sci. Sports.* **2**(1), 39–42.

Cantu, R.C. (ed.) (1981) *Health Maintenance Through Physical Conditioning*. PSG Publishing Co., Littleton, MA.

Cats-Baril, W.L. & Frymoyer, J.W. (1991) Identifying patients at risk of becoming disabled due to low back pain: the Vermont Rehabilitation Center Predictive Model. *Spine* **16**(6), 605–7.

Cavagna, C.A. & Kaneko, M. (1977) Mechanical work and efficiency in level walking and running. *J. Physiol.* **268**, 467–81.

Clarkson, H.M. & Gilewich, B.G. (1989) *Musculoskeletal Assessment: Joint Range of Motion and Manual Muscle Strength*. Williams & Wilkins, Baltimore.

Cooper, K.H. (1968) A means of assessing maximal oxygen intake: Correlation between field and treadmill testing. *JAMA* **203**, 201–4.

Dalsky, G.P. (1989) The role of exercise in the prevention of osteoporosis. *Compr. Ther.* **15**, 30–7.

Davies, G.J. (1980) Mechanisms of selected knee injuries. *Phys. Ther.* **60**, 1590–5.

Davies, G.J. (1985) Flexibility screening: techniques for the lower extremities. In B. Sanders & J.S. Eggart (eds) *Guidelines for Pre-season Athletic Participation Evaluation*, 2nd edn, pp. 105–00. American Physical Therapy Association, Alexandria, VT.

Delitto, A., Crandell, C.E. & Rose, S.J. (1989) Peak

torque to body weight ratios in the trunk: a critical analysis. *Phys. Ther.* **69**, 138–43.

Dvorak, J., Froelich, D., Penning, L., Baumgartner, H. & Pahjabi, M.M. (1988) Functional radiographic diagnoses of the cervical spine: flexion extension. *Spine* **13**(7), 748–55.

Eggart, J.S., Leigh, D. & Vergamini, G. (1985) Preseason athletic physical evaluations. In J.A. Gould & G.J. Davies (eds) *Orthopaedic and Sports Physical Therapy*, pp. 605–42. C.V. Mosby, St Louis.

Friden, J., Sfakianos, P.N. & Hargens, A.R. (1986) Muscle soreness and intramuscular fluid pressure: comparison between eccentric and concentric load. *J. Appl. Physiol.* **61**(6), 2175–9.

Geusens, P. & Dequeker, J. (1991) Influence of exercise on bone mineral content and density. In P. Schlapbach & N.J. Gerber (eds) *Physiotherapy: Controlled Trials and Facts*, pp. 61–70. Karger, Basel.

Hagood, S., Solomonow, M., Baratta, R., Zhou, B.H. & D'Ambrosia, R. (1990) The effect of joint velocity on the contribution of the antagonist musculature to knee stiffness and laxity. *Am. J. Sports. Med.* **18**(2), 182–6.

Halpern, A.A. (1984) *The Runner's World Knee Book.* Macmillan, New York.

Hanley, D.F. (1972) Health problems at Olympic games. *JAMA* **221**, 987–90.

Hanten, W.P. & Pace, M.B. (1987) Reliability of measuring anterior laxity of the knee joint using a knee ligament arthrometer. *Phys. Ther.* **67**(3), 357–9.

Horal, J. (1969) The clinical appearance of low back disorders in the city of Gothenburg Sweden. Comparison of incapacitated probands and matched controls. *Acta. Ortho. Scand.* **118**(Suppl.), 1–102.

Hortobagyi, T., Katch, E.I. & LaChance, P.F. (1989) Interrelationships among various measures of upper body strength assessed by different contraction modes. *Eur. J. Appl. Physiol.* **58**, 749–55.

Jesse, J. (1977) *Hidden Causes of Injury, Prevention and Correction for Running Athletes and Joggers.* The Athletic Press, Pasadena, CA.

Jette, M., Gauthier, R. & Mongeon, J. (1979) Simple field procedure for estimating ideal body weight in males. *Res. Q.* **50**, 396–403.

Karlsson, J., Peterson, L., Andreasson, G. *et al.* (1992) The unstable ankle: A combined EMG and biomechanical modeling study. *Int. J. Sport Biomech.* **8**(2), 129–44.

Kavanagh, T. (1976) *Heart Attack? Counter Attack!* Van Nostrand Reinhold, Toronto.

Kendall, H.O., Kendall, E.P. & Boynton, D.A. (1977) *Posture and Pain.* Krieger Publishing, Huntington, NY.

Kulund, D. (1982) *The Injured Athlete.* JB Lippincott, Philadelphia.

Lynch, M.A., Henning, C.E. & Glick, K.R. (1983) Knee joint surface changes: long-term follow-up meniscus tear treatment in stable anterior cruciate ligament reconstruction. *Clin. Orth.* **172**, 148–53.

MacDougall, J.D. (1986) Morphological changes in human skeletal muscle following strength training and immobilization. In N.L. Jones, N. McCartney & A.J. McComas (eds) *Human Muscle Power*, pp. 269–88. Human Kinetics, Champaign, Illinois.

Moritani, T. & deVries, H.A. (1979) Neural factors versus hypertrophy in the time course of muscle strength gain. *Am J. Phys. Med.* **58**(3), 115–30.

Muckle, D.S. (1978) *Injuries in Sport.* John Wright, Littleton, MA.

Mueller, F.O. & Ryan, A.J. (1991) *Prevention of Athletic Injuries. The Role of the Sports Medicine Team.* FA Davis, Philadelphia.

Nardone, A. & Schieppati, M. (1988) Shift of activity from slow to fast muscle during voluntary lengthening contractions of the triceps surae muscles in humans. *J. Physiol.* **395**, 353–81.

Newham, D.J. (1991) Skeletal muscle pain and exercise. *Physiotherapy* **77**(1), 66–70.

Nilsson, S. (1986) Overtraining. In S. Maehlum, S. Nilsson & P. Renström (eds) *An Update on Sports Medicine*, pp. 97–104. Proceedings from the Second Scandinavian Conference in Sports Medicine, Oslo, Norway, 9–15 March, 1986.

Palmer, M.L. & Epler, M. (1990) *Clinical Assessment Procedures in Physical Therapy.* JB Lippincott, Philadelphia.

Pearl, B. & Moran, G.T. (1986) *Getting Stronger: Weight Training for Men and Women.* Shelter Publications, Bolinas, CA.

Pope, M.H. (1991) Spine Seminar II, Burlington, VT, June 3 (Lecture).

Riegger, C.L. (1985) Mechanical properties of bone. In J.A. Gould & G.J. Davies (eds) *Orthopaedic and Sports Physical Therapy*, pp. 3–49. C.V. Mosby, St Louis.

Ryan, A.J. & Allman, F.L. (1974) *Sports Medicine.* Academic Press, New York.

Safran, M.R., Garrett, W.E., Seaber, A.V., Glisson, R.R. & Ribbeck, B.M. (1988) The role of warmup in muscular injury prevention. *Am. J. Sports Med.* **16**(2), 123–7.

Sanders, B. & Eggart, J.S. (1985) *Guidelines for Preseason Athletic Participation Evaluation*, 2nd edn. American Physical Therapy Association, Alexandria, VA.

Schlife, J.E. (1982) Fitness testing in family practice. *Phys. Sports Med.* **10**(10), 142.

Sheehan, G. (1992) Running: Injury pattern and prevention. In D.C. Reid (ed) *Sports Injury Assessment and Rehabilitation*, pp. 1131–58. Churchill Livingstone, New York.

Sinacore, D.R., Delitto, A., King, D.S. & Rose, S.J. (1990) Type II fiber activation with electrical stimulation: a preliminary report. *Phys. Ther.* **70**(7), 416–22.

Stulen, F.B. & DeLuca, C.J. (1981) Frequency parameters of the myoelectric signal as a measure of muscle conduction velocity. *IEEE Trans. Biomed. Eng.* **28**, 515–23.

Tipton, C.M., Martin, R.K. & Matthes, R.D. (1978) Influence of age and sex on the strength of bone–ligament junctions in knee joints of rats. *J. Bone Joint Surg.* **60**, 230–4.

Weisman, G., Pope, M.H. & Johnson, R.J. (1980) The role for cyclic loading in knee ligament injuries. *Am. J. Sports Med.* **8**(1), 24–30.

Wickkiser, J.D. & Kelly, J.M. (1975) The body composition of a college football team. *Med. Sci. Sports* **7**, 199–202.

Yost, C.P. (1967) Total fitness and prevention of accidents. *J. Health, Phys. Educ. Recreation* **38**(3), 32–7.

Zohar, J. (1973) Preventative conditioning for maximum safety and performance. *Scholastic Coach* **42**(9), 65, 113–15.

PART 2

BASIC PRINCIPLES

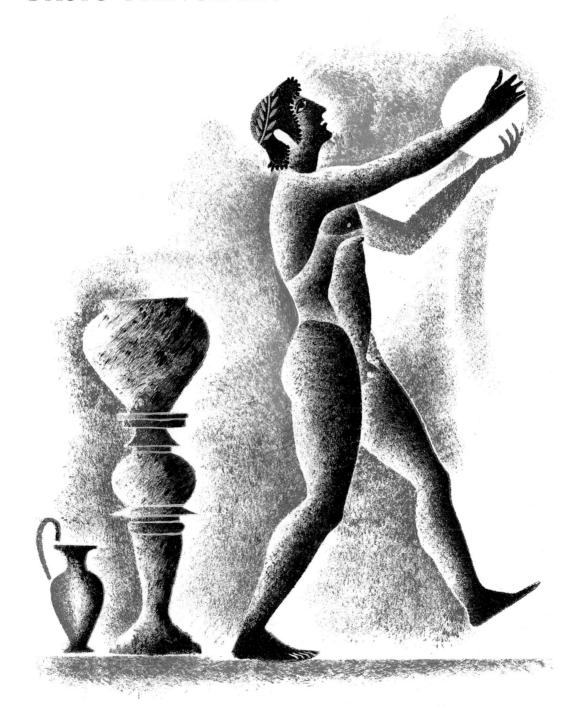

Part 2a

Anatomical, Pathophysiological and Functional Considerations

Chapter 4

Bone Injuries

CARL ZETTERBERG

The skeleton of humans consists of 212 bones with a total mass of 12−14 kg. The element calcium, an important part of the mineral in the bone tissue, comprises 2% of all elements in the body. Together with connective tissue and muscles, the skeleton comprises the supporting and locomotion system of the body. Bone has an excellent capacity for repair and can alter its properties and configuration in response to mechanical demand. There are two types of bone morphology: (i) trabecular (cancellous), and (ii) cortical (compact). The difference is mainly in the degree of porosity. The porosity ranges from 5−30% in cortical bone and from 30 to over 90% in cancellous.

Cortical bone is found in the diaphyses of long bones, skull and mandible, whereas cancellous bone is found in the ends of long bones, metaphyses, vertebrae, inside the bones of the carpus and hindfoot.

Biomechanics of bone

The bone mass, i.e. the amount of mineral in the skeleton, is of importance. A close correlation between measured bone mass of different bones of the body and the strength of the same bones has been shown. The fabric or structure of the bone is also of importance for the mechanical strength and elasticity.

Bone can be considered as a biphasic composite material, with the mineral as one phase and the collagen and ground substance as the other. Composite materials of this type, e.g.

fibreglass, are stronger than either substance alone.

Basic biomechanical concepts

The mechanical load−deformation curve for bone is demonstrated schematically in Fig. 4.1.

The initial straight line is the elastic region,

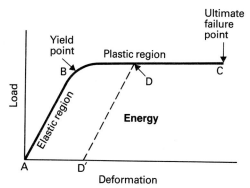

Fig. 4.1 Load−deformation (stress−strain) curve for a structure composed of a somewhat pliable material. If load is applied within the elastic range of the structure (A−B on the curve) and is then released, no permanent deformation occurs. If loading is continued past the yield point (B) and into the structure's plastic range (B−C on the curve) and the load is then released, permanent deformation results. The amount of permanent deformation that occurs if the structure is loaded to point D in the plastic region and then is unloaded is represented by the distance between A and D. If loading continues within the plastic range, an ultimate failure point (C) is reached. Adapted with permission from Nordin & Frankel (1989).

43

where the material returns to its original shape when unloaded. At the yield point, the material starts to fail, and does not regain its original shape when unloaded. This is the plastic region. The area under the curve represents the absorbed energy.

The strength of a structure is determined by:
1 The load that the structure can sustain before failing.
2 The deformation that it can sustain before failing.
3 The energy that it can store before failing.

The more precise mechanical terms for load—deformation is stress—strain. Stress is the load or force per unit area that develops on a plane area within a structure in response to externally applied loads. It is measured in newtons per metre squared ($N \cdot m^{-2}$) or pascals (Pa).

Strain is the deformation, the change in dimension, that develops within a structure in response to externally applied stress. A high strain, without permanent deformation, means a high elasticity and for the different bone types, also a larger capacity for energy storage.

The structure of bone varies between different types of bone, i.e. cancellous and cortical, but also in different planes within the same bone. Thus, the stress—strain curve is different when a bone piece is loaded in different directions, e.g. longitudinal, transverse or shear (anisotrophy) (Fig. 4.2).

Generally bone is strongest in the direction of the most common physiological load.

Bone mechanics

When loaded the bone shows an increased stiffness. This can be accomplished by gravity or muscle pull. Contraction of muscles attached to the bone alters the stress distribution within the bone. Therefore, much higher loads can be sustained by the bone under loaded conditions than unloaded.

This explains why the vertebrae of weightlifters do not fracture as they theoretically would according to *in vitro* tests of vertebral specimens that are not prestressed.

If any load on a skeletal part exceeds the ultimate strength of that bone, a fracture may occur. The load may be a high or low energetic trauma, which rapidly exceeds the strength of the bone, or the load may be a more longstanding, often repetitive overload, inducing a stress fracture (fatigue failure).

The biomechanical behaviour of bone varies with the rate at which the bone is loaded. As the strain rate of bone is increasing, the bone is getting stiffer (absorbs more energy before

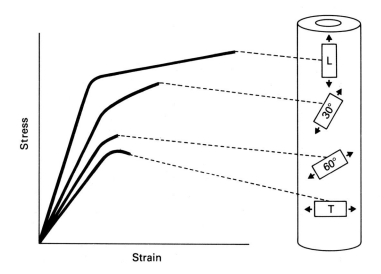

Fig. 4.2 Anisotrophic behaviour of cortical bone specimens from human femoral shaft tested in tension (pulled) in four directions: (i) longitudinal (L); (ii) tilted 30° with respect to the neutral axis of the bone; (iii) tilted 60°; and (iv) transverse (T). Adapted with permission from Nordin & Frankel (1989).

failure). Bone shows an increase of strength severalfold over a few decades of increase in strain rates. This contrasts to soft tissues, e.g. ligaments or tendons, where strain rate sensitivity is less. This explains why the bone, of the ligament–bone unit, fails at low loading rates, leading to avulsion fractures, but ligaments and tendons fail at higher loading rates when the bone is stronger than the soft tissues. The bone of the ligament–bone unit is also weaker in immature bone, which explains why avulsion fractures are relatively more common in younger athletes than in adult athletes.

Bone fatigue

The fatigue effects during cyclic loading of compact bone is more a function of strain range (range of deformation) than that of stress range (range of load).

Stress fractures can be considered as clinical manifestations of bone fatigue, due to increased numbers of load repetitions that are within the normal bone strain range. Thus, only one or a few load cycles induces a tolerable strain, but many repetitions leads to fatigue failure. Load repetitions at a high rate is also more damaging to bone than at a low rate, even if the strain (deformation) at each load cycle is the same.

Fatigue fractures are most often sustained during continuous strenuous exercises, which causes the muscles to fatigue. As a result, the muscles become weaker and fail to neutralize the stress imposed on the bone.

This explains why stress fractures are reported to constitute 15% of running injuries and affect up to 15% of joggers. Animal experiments have shown a fivefold increase in strain values from walking to fast trotting.

In race horses fatigue fractures of the third metacarpal bone are common, up to 70%, during the first year of training. Due to bone remodelling, the strain is decreasing in this bone and so this fracture becomes uncommon in the adult animal.

The bone of younger subjects shows higher strain at a given load than adults with mature bone. They also show fatigue failure after less loading cycles. Thus, immature bone is more sensitive to cyclic loading than mature. Strenuous training during growth may also result in growth arrest and induce bone atrophy and mineral loss, according to animal experiments and clinical studies.

Biomechanics of bone remodelling

The capacity of the skeleton to carry load is achieved and maintained as the result of a continued functional stimulus to the cell population responsible for bone remodelling.

The load sensitive, strain-induced, remodelling of bone has the purpose of decreasing the strain under a certain tolerable level. The strain levels that induce bone remodelling may be considered as an interval. If the upper limit is exceeded, failure of the structure occurs. The bone remodelling brings the strain at a certain load or stress down under this interval. The limits vary in different bones according to their physiological load pattern. The bones of the lower extremity are more highly loaded than those of the upper extremity and may therefore also react with less strain at a given stress level.

Bone remodelling takes time and explains why stress fractures mostly occur during intense periods of training.

Strain memory of bone

One current research question is: how are changes in strain in the bone induced by short periods of loading remembered and a sustained change in bone remodelling induced?

The orientation of the collagen of the bone matrix does not change unless there is physical damage to the tissue.

Very short periods of loading have been shown to affect the rather slow bone remodelling process. Bone has piezoelectric behaviour. Strain induces a steady-state polarization of bone, which can be experimentally observed several days after the test load is removed.

Other experiments have shown that about 50

strain reversals (equalling the number of load cycles), achieves the maximum proteoglycan orientation which has a marked effect on bone remodelling. The change of proteoglycan orientation persists for at least 24 h. This is the so-called 'strain memory' of the bone tissue.

The proteoglycan molecules are highly charged and lie close to the bone cells (osteocytes). The osteocytes have been shown to increase their production of RNA after strain stimulation. Since the osteocytes are located within the bone matrix, they are best placed to sense the strain stimulation. The remodelling is performed by osteoclasts and osteoblasts. The RNA produced by strain stimulation may be a messenger substance to these cells from the osteocyte. Further, osteocytes in cultures have been shown to increase their production of DNA and proliferate when subjected to cyclic mechanical strain.

Another stimulus for bone formation is microdamage to bone. Microdamage has been observed to occur at low strain levels. The bone remodelling of long bones is greatest in the subperiosteal region where the stress is greatest and microdamage most often occurs. Microfractures also occur in the bone trabeculae of cancellous bone.

In summary, there are two known ways for bone remodelling. Either via the electrical events that are started by functionally induced strains, or microdamage, which also induces bone remodelling.

Bone metabolism

Physiology of bone

The skeleton consists of organic and inorganic components. The organic part, 30%, is comprised of collagen, glucoproteins, phosphoproteins, mucopolysaccharides or glycosaminoglycans (GAGs) and lipids.

The inorganic part, 70%, consists mostly of hydroxyapatite crystals ($Ca_{10}(PO_4)_6(OH)_2$) with ceramic physical properties with calcium as the most important component. The recommended daily intake of calcium is about 800 mg day^{-1}. The recommendations differ somewhat between different countries. There is an increased demand during pregnancy and lactation. If the age-dependent loss of bone in the elderly can be decreased by an increased calcium intake, 1000 mg day^{-1} or more is recommended. On the other hand, calcium deficiency leads to mobilization of calcium from the skeleton, since the calcium homeostasis puts the plasma levels in first priority.

Magnesium, sodium, fluoride and other minerals are also parts of the inorganic portion of bone.

The skeleton has the unique capability of rebuilding throughout life. Resorption by the osteoclasts is continuously taking place along with bone formation by osteoblasts (Fig. 4.3). This well-organized remodelling takes place in small units called basic metabolic units (BMUs). In this capability bone is different from other connective tissues in the body.

Osteoblasts have been shown to have a large number of receptors, e.g. oestrogen, progesterone, parathormone (PTH) and other hormonal receptors. There are also other receptors for different growth factors. The osteoclasts have few receptors and are partly regulated by the osteoblasts. Their resorption of bone is stimulated by naked exposed bone surfaces, without lining cells.

Osteocytes are the mature cells within the bones. These show an impressive longevity of 20 years or more. They also participate in the bone remodelling as discussed below.

At any instance about 5% of the bone is in the remodelling phase.

Normal metabolism

During life, the bone mass changes. There is a gain during childhood and adolescence. A peak is reached in adult age. There is some controversy as to whether there is a real peak of bone mass or whether there is merely a plateau from about 20–25 years of age to 35–40 years of age. Anyhow, from this maximum there is a loss of

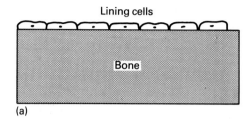

Lining cells

Bone

(a)

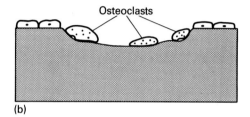

Osteoclasts

(b)

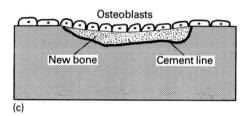

Osteoblasts

New bone   Cement line

(c)

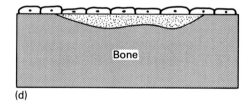

Bone

(d)

Fig. 4.3 Schematic drawing of some stages in the bone turnover. Osteoclasts resorbs bone and osteoblasts deposit new bone. The figure represents a basic metabolic unit. (a) Rest stage; (b) resorbtion; (c) bone formation; and (d) rest stage.

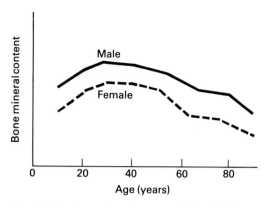

Fig. 4.4 The bone mineral content during life. The somewhat accelerated loss between 45 and 65 years of age is shown.

bone, starting at about 35 years of age, with a rapid phase starting at menopause in women. The annual loss in women is about 1–2%. Men also shows a similar decline of bone mass, but it starts somewhat later, around 45 years of age, and the rate is somewhat less than in women, 0.5–1% annually (Fig. 4.4). The maximum bone mass during life is higher in men than in women. The reasons for this are androgenic hormonal effects, mainly testosterone, greater muscle mass and body mass, which induces an increased load on the skeleton.

At menopause, oestrogen in women begins to decline and the positive effects on the skeleton of this hormone begins to vanish.

Osteoporosis

Osteoporosis and osteoporotic or fragility fractures has become an epidemic in Europe and North America and constitutes a major health problem.

The bone loss that occurs from around 40 years of age can lead to osteoporosis. Osteoporosis can be defined as loss of normal bone to the extent that fractures occur at low energetic trauma. Simultaneously with bone loss, there is a change in the structure of both cortical and cancellous bone.

Cortical bone shows a net loss of bone endosteally, while there is still some gain periosteally. This leads to thinner cortex, but also to an increased diameter. Therefore, the loss of mechanical strength is less than the loss of bone tissue (Fig. 4.5). This is also shown to be the case in preindustrial humans, when physical work load was common during the activities of daily life. In females of modern America, this increase of the outer diameter of long bones has been disputed. Thus, it seems that this

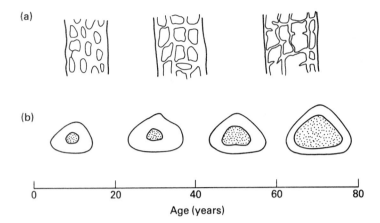

Fig. 4.5 Remodelling of cancellous (trabecular) and cortical (compact) bone during life. (a) In cancellous bone the trabeculae is getting thinner and there is also a loss of trabeculae, especially those not parallel to the main loading axis. (b) Cortical bone shows a widening of the marrow canal, but also an increased outer diameter of the bone, thus preserving the mechanical strength better than cancellous bone.

mechanically advantageous remodelling of cortical bone is load dependent.

Cancellous bone also shows a predominance of loss of transverse bony trabeculae (transverse in relation to the major compressive load direction), while the longitudinal trabeculae along the main mechanical loading direction is better preserved (see Fig. 4.4). The net loss of mechanical strength is greater in cancellous bone. Therefore, fragility or osteoporotic fractures mostly occur in the metaphyseal areas, e.g. distal radius, proximal femur, proximal humerus, ankle and vertebrae. The neck of the femur follows this pattern although it may be considered as a cortical structure (Fig. 4.6).

These fractures occur in the upper age limits, starting around 50 years of age and increases exponentially with age. Typically, the fractures occur with low energy trauma and indoors, e.g. hip and proximal humeral fractures. Some of these fractures are common in more active subjects and occur more often outdoors, i.e. fracture of the distal radius and ankle. Vertebral fractures are the most common, present in about 25% of women and 12% of men, of Caucasian origin, at 70 years of age.

These fractures have shown an increased incidence in recent decades, not explained by the age or gender of the population. One of the important background factors discussed in the literature is lack of physical activity.

People of Scandinavian origin show the highest fragility fracture incidences, while Black people have less osteoporosis and subsequent fractures of this type.

The important preventive question is whether or not a higher peak bone mass leads to a better preserved skeleton in upper age limits and accordingly less fragility fractures.

Physical activity is one important positive factor for bone turnover, and may modify the fundamental biological changes of the bone that is determined by gender, aging, differencies in ethnicity and lifestyle factors.

Bone mineral measurement methods

The bone mineral content can be measured *in vivo*. Ordinary radiography can give an estimate, but the mineral loss has to exceed 30% to be detected. Other methods include photon-absorbtiometry, where mono-energetic energies (photons) from different radioactive isotopes are used. Today, these methods are highly accurate. Continued X-ray energy distribution technique or computerized tomography can also be used.

Physical activity and bone

Muscle action loads the skeleton and bone is rebuilt in proportion to the amount of physical

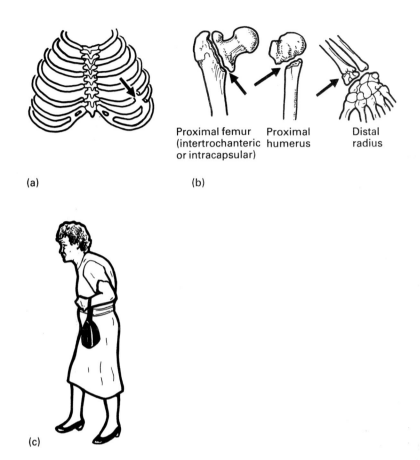

Proximal femur   Proximal   Distal
(intertrochanteric   humerus   radius
or intracapsular)

(a)   (b)

(c)

Fig. 4.6 Common sites for fragility (osteoporosis) fractures: The vertebrae (a) and ends (metaphyses) of long bones (b) are most often affected. (a) Vertebral compression fractures cause continuous (acute) or intermittent (chronic) back pain from the midthoracic to midlumbar (occasionally to lower lumbar) region. Rib fractures are also common. (b) The most common sites of long bone fractures, often caused by minimal trauma. (c). Progressive thoracic kyphosis (dowager's hump) with loss of height and abdominal protrusion. Adapted with permission from CIBA-Geigy, Basle, from Clinical Symposia 39/1 (all rights reserved).

load; Wolff's law. Load on the skeleton can be accomplished either by muscle activity or gravity.

There is a positive correlation between physical activity and the bone mass. However, there are some limitations and many factors influence the bone turnover. The bone mass of an individual is dependent on a large scale of different factors; nutritional factors, diseases, drugs, hormones and anthropometric factors in addition to physical activity. This section summarizes some of the known factors.

Effect of gravity

The body mass is positively correlated to bone mass. This is an expression of the effect of gravity. Weightlessness as experienced by astronauts induces a fast excretion of calcium in the urine and deterioration of bone mineralization. These changes are to some extent reversible and preventable, but not completely. Experiments with vigorous exercises in lying or sitting postures have not prevented bone loss due to the loss of gravity.

Effects of inactivity

Disuse or inactivity has deleterious effects on both muscles and skeleton. Bedrest induces a decrease of the bone mass of about 1% per week. However, not all mineral can be lost, and a steady state is achieved at a loss of about 30–40% of the bone mineral. This loss of mineral from the bone is not necessarily accompanied by a loss of body mass.

The bone atrophy induced by weightlessness or prolonged bedrest is not completely reversible.

Effects of muscle activity

In addition to gravity, muscles load the skeleton. There is evidence for a relationship between muscle activity level and bone strength. The cross-sectional area of the psoas muscle has been shown to correlate positively to the bone mass of the vertebral bodies.

In the elderly, the incidence of fragility fractures of the hip, wrist, proximal humerus and others, have been shown to increase. Studies of such patients using muscle biopsies from the vastus lateralis have shown a disuse atrophy of the muscles, without any signs of disease. Physical activity and coordination have been shown to correlate with calf muscle strength. Further, comparatively lower handgrip strength has been associated with an increased risk of falls and subsequent fractures in the elderly. These examples shows the interrelation between the functional status of the musculature and the quality of the bone of importance for the risk of falls and fractures. This also indicates the preventive effectiveness of physical exercise in the older population.

General skeletal effects of physical activity

A positive correlation between physical activity and the bone mass has been shown in a number of experimental and observational studies. Since the normal bone loss during 1 year only is 0.5–1.5%, and all measurement methods have errors, it is sometimes not possible to prove any effect in prospective studies spanning over a few years due to these methodological errors.

OBSERVATIONAL STUDIES IN ATHLETES

A higher bone density at different measured sites in the body, e.g. proximal, middle and distal femur, distal and middle forearm, humerus, calcaneus, lumbar vertebrae and metatarsus, has been shown in athletes compared to controls.

Long-distance runners have shown up to 20% higher bone mineral content compared with normative controls. Even greater differences has been shown in older active persons; 50–72-year-old long-distance runners had 40% higher bone mineral density compared to inactive controls.

Female college athletes had more mineral in the vertebrae than controls. In postmenopausal physically active women, the difference was even greater.

There seems to be a comparatively greater effect of physical activity on the skeleton over 50 years of age. This may be due to influence on the normally increased bone loss postmenopausally. A dose–response relation has also been shown in some of these studies.

Different parts of the skeleton react to physical activity at different degrees. The effect was greatest in the appendicular trabecular skeleton compared to the axial skeleton in long-distance runners.

The results of several cross-sectional observational studies are consistent and shows the benefit for the bone mass of physical activity at any age.

EXPERIMENTAL STUDIES

There are randomized and non-randomized studies performed prospectively. Due to the difficulties of performing long-term studies over several years, the results of these studies have not shown the same great differencies between the active and inactive study groups as the observational studies. However, a dose—response relation has been shown also in some of these studies. One example is a comparison of the effect of dancing and walking, where dancing preserved the skeleton best in post-menopausal women. However, both activities had a positive effect when compared to inactive controls.

The quantitative results range from 3.5% of increase of bone mineral to a retardation of the normal loss in middle-aged or elderly subjects, but no increase. There is also some evidence of a bone loss initially during training. The reasons for this are unclear, but measurement errors may play a role.

A higher increase of bone mineralization of the order of 5—10% has been observed in the tibia of military recruits after 16 months of training. However, this training dose exceeded the strength of the bone in many cases, as stress fractures were common.

In the elderly, the beneficial effect of physical activity, even at such low doses as walking or training for 1 h twice or more a week, has been shown.

LOCALIZED EFFECTS OF PHYSICAL ACTIVITY

Local increases of the bone mineral content in the loaded areas of the skeleton has been shown in tennis players, the skeleton of the dominant arm being denser than that of the other arm. This localized effect has also been shown in baseball players. It is of some interest that the bone mineral increases in the distal radius of runners. This means that there are also beneficial effects of training in rather unloaded areas of the skeleton.

TRAINING DOSE AND BONE

Generally, measurements of the bone mineral content in the os calcis is more dependent on physical activity than measurements of the axial skeleton, i.e. the vertebrae. The latter seems to

a higher extent dependent on hormonal and other factors.

In adolescents and young adults, the effects of physical activity on the skeleton has to be distinguished from the effects of normal growth. Growth hormone and sexual steroids, both androgens and oestrogens, have a positive influence on the mineralization of the skeleton.

As mentioned earlier, vigorous exercise may induce a loss of bone mineral, stress fractures may occur, or amenorrhoea in females may be of negative importance for the skeleton.

Studies have indicated that bone loss due to calcium deficiency is additive to that of disuse. However, physical activity is also shown to have a protective effect on the skeleton in calcium deficiency.

It seems that a longer daily period of activity gives no extra benefits for the skeleton compared to a shorter. Thus, the dose—response relation between physical activity and bone mineral density seems not to be linear, but rather to reach an optimum level.

The different activities that have been studied include: walking, dancing, aerobic exercise, long-distance and marathon running, strength training, tennis playing, swimming, mixed track and field activities. Lifetime running and tennis playing has been shown to greatly enhance the bone mass in subjects over 50 years of age. In contrast, weightlifters have been shown to lose the gain in bone mineral that they achieved when they were active around 20—25 years of age, when measured around 45 years of age. Therefore, it seems more important for the bone health to continue with any type of physical activity throughout life, than to be very active during a limited phase of life. Thus, a deposit in the bone bank in young adults may not last throughout life.

Hormones, physical exercise and bone

Oestrogens are of great importance for the mineralization of bone in women. Postmenopausal oestrogen substitution has a well-documented bone-retaining effect. Intense training, especially of endurance type may induce amenorrhoea (less than three menstruations per year) or irregularities of menstruation, indicating hormonal aberrations, which may lead to loss of bone mineral. Still, the load of physical activity seems to have some positive effect when non-athlete amenorrhoic females are compared with athletic. However, both groups had lower bone mineral content and serum oestrogen levels than normal females.

The androgenic effect of testosterone and other hormones includes increased muscle mass and also bone mass. The latter may be affected through gravity (increased body mass), increased muscle strength, which increases the load on the skeleton and direct hormonal effects. Anabolic steroids, given as substitution therapy, have been shown to increase the bone mineral in elderly men.

PTH is the hormone that has the greatest effect of all hormones on the serum calcium. PTH has a resorptive effect on the calcium of the skeleton. PTH has an important role in the regulation of a constant serum calcium level.

Lack of vitamin D leads to rickets, which is among other things characterized by bone fragility. The histological picture shows an increased amount of osteid, which fails to be mineralized in a normal fashion. The most active form of the vitamin, 1,25(OH) vitamin D, is formed by sunlight or daylight exposure of the skin.

Growth hormone has a positive effect on the mineralization and normal development of the skeleton in the child and adolescent. Corticosteroids have a well-recognized negative effect on the mineralization of the skeleton.

Bone biopsy, most often transiliacal, is essential in diagnosing metabolic bone diseases.

Factors of negative importance for the skeleton

Inactivity has been mentioned earlier.
1 Smoking. Smoking has been shown to be negative for the mineralization of the skeleton.

In older people, an increased prevalence of vertebral fractures has been shown. Loss of teeth has also been shown to correlate with smoking. The possible mechanisms for these negative effects includes: (i) increased endogenous production of corticosteroids in smokers; (ii) earlier menopause by $3-4$ years are thereby earlier onset of the menopausal oestrogen loss; and (iii) negative influence of the vitamin D turnover, possibly through, among other mechanisms, cadmium deposition in the kidneys.
2 Drugs. Corticosteroids used in the treatment of several diseases have a negative influence on bone mineralization. Diphenylhydantoin, an antiepileptic drug, induces an osteomalacia like deterioration of the mineralization process of bone. Heparin, used over a prolonged period, e.g. during pregnancy, may induce a high degree of bone loss.
3 Diseases. Gastric resection interferes with the normal calcium turnover. Alcoholism is shown to be associated with a decreased bone mass. Many diseases affect the skeleton in different ways, an example of which is diabetes mellitus, which may be complicated by capillary and sensory nerve deficiencies that may lead to stress fractures, especially in the foot. However, physical activity is of benefit for the treatment of the disease itself.

Preventive conclusions

Biomechanical factors

1 The shape of bones are optimized for the normal load pattern. Unphysiological loading directions increases the risk for skeletal injury.
2 When loaded the bone deforms. There is an upper limit at which the bone fails. This is different for different bones of the body.
3 Repetitive load may induce a fatigue failure of bone. The risk is increased with repetitive loading at a high rate.
4 Muscle fatigue decreases the stiffness of bone and increases the risk for fatigue failure.
5 The bones of children and adolescents is less

stiff and shows a higher degree of deformation at a given load than mature bone.

6 The bone in younger people may also be weaker than the attached ligaments or tendons, increasing the risk for avulsion fractures.

Bone physiology

1 Bone remodelling is slow, therefore a training period of high intensity should be preceded by a progressively increased training period to avoid stress fractures.

2 A dose–response relation between physical activity and bone mass has been shown.

3 Excessive training, especially in adolescents, may lead to growth disturbances and also to amenorrhoea in females, with a negative effect on the bone mass.

4 The recommended daily intakes of minerals such as calcium, fluoride and magnesium, vitamins such as vitamin D, should be sufficient for optimal bone turnover. Supplements above this level are not beneficial.

5 Bone is lost during adulthood at a rate of 0.5–1.5% depending on gender and age.

6 One major background factor for osteoporosis and subsequent fragility fractures in the elderly, is lack of physical activity.

7 A short period of physical activity in young adult life does not constitute a deposit to the bone bank that lasts for life. Continuous physical activity throughout life is of greater importance.

8 Even physical activity at low intensity, such as walking, is of benefit for the bone mass.

9 Some diseases and drugs have a negative influence on the skeleton.

10 Smoking and alcoholism leads to a lower bone mass.

Further reading

Black, J. (1988) *Orthopaedic Biomaterials in Research and Practice*. Churchill Livingstone, New York.

Caine, D.J. & Lidner, K.J. (1985) Overuse injuries of growing bones. The young female gymnast at risk. *Phys. Sportsmed.* **13**, 51–65.

Christiansen, C. & Overgaard, K. (eds) (1990) *Osteoporosis 1990*, Vols 1–3. Osteopress ApS, Copenhagen, Denmark.

Cummings, S.R., Kelsey, J.L., Nevitt, M.C. & O'Dowd, K.J. (1985) Epidemiology of osteoporosis and osteoporotic fractures. *Epidemiol. Rev.* **7**, 178–208.

Dirix, A., Knuttgen, H.G. & Tittel, K. (1988) *The Olympic Book of Sports Medicine*, Vol. 1. Blackwell Scientific Publications, Oxford.

Frost, H.M. (1973) *Bone Modelling and Skeletal Modelling Errors*. Charles C. Thomas, Illinois.

Jonson, R. (1988) *Radioanalytical methods for determination of bone mineral and heavy metals in vivo*. PhD Thesis, University of Gothenburg, Sweden.

Micheli, L.J. (1983) Overuse injuries in children's sport: The growth factor. *Orthop. Clin. N. Am.* **14**, 337–59.

Netter, F. (1987) *The CIBA Collection of Medical Illustrations*. Vol. 8, *The Musculoskeletal System*. Part I, *Anatomy, Physiology and Metabolic Disorders*. CIBA-Geigy, New Jersey.

Nordin, M. & Frankel, V.H. (1989) *Basic Biomechanics of the Musculoskeletal System*. Lea & Febiger, London.

Obrandt, K.J., Bengner, U., Johnell, O. & Nilsson, B.E. (1988) Increasing age-adjusted risk of fragility fractures: a sign of increasing osteoporosis in successive generations? *Calc. Tiss. Int.* **44**, 157–67.

Orthopaedic Research Society (1983–1990) *Transactions*, Vols. 8–15. ORS, Illinois.

Riggs, B.L. & Melton, J.L. (1988) *Osteoporosis. Etiology, Diagnosis and Management*. Raven Press, New York.

Wolff, J. (1892) *Das Gesetz der Transformation der Knocken* (The Transformation of Bones). Hirchwald, Berlin.

Zetterberg, C., Nordin, M., Skovron, M-L. & Zuckerman, J. (1990) Skeletal effects of physical activity. *Geritopics* **13**, 17–24.

Chapter 5

Cartilage and Ligament Injuries

KAI-MING CHAN AND STEPHEN Y.C. HSU

Cartilage injury

Cartilage is a firm and translucent tissue of considerable rigidity well adapted for weight-bearing. The bony skeleton is also originally represented by cartilage in the embryo. Like other connective tissues, cartilage consists of cells — chondrocytes and intercellular matrix that contains fibres. The intercellular matrix is chiefly responsible for the properties of cartilage that enables it to restrain a considerable degree of tension, torsion and pressure. At the same time, it shows a certain degree of elasticity. Fully developed cartilage is not supplied by any demonstrable blood vessel, lymphatic or nerve.

Due to the variation of the characteristics of the intercellular matrix, there are three demonstrable types of cartilage:
1 Hyaline cartilage.
2 Fibrocartilage.
3 Elastic cartilage.
The articular cartilage which covers the bony surfaces in all synovial joints represents a slightly modified type of hyaline cartilage in which the fibre in the intercellular matrix is arranged in a regular rather than a random pattern. This is the focus of our attention when we consider sports-related injuries to this important connective tissue in humans.

Structure of articular cartilage

NORMAL ARTICULAR CARTILAGE

This forms a smooth, glistening and slightly elastic covering to the bone end (Bradbury, 1973). It is bluish and translucent in the young, averaging 2–4 mm in thickness. In the elderly, it becomes yellow and more opaque, begins to lose some of the elasticity and is much thinner. Articular cartilage is avascular and has a low metabolic rate.

THE CHONDROCYTES

The articular cartilage cell is a large and ovoid cell usually over 40 μm in diameter surrounded by lacunae of the matrix. The cytoplasm contains glycogen granules, fat droplets and sometimes pigment, and vacuoles are frequently present. There is a large nucleus with one or more nucleoli. Under electronmicroscopy, large amounts of rough surfaced endoplasm recticulum could be identified. The Golgi apparatus is often very large with well-developed vacuoles and there are also numerous particles of glycogen as well as mitochondria. On the border between cartilage and perichondriums, there is usually ordinary undifferentiated fibroblast. The arrangement of cells in the articular cartilage is also characteristic. In the peripheral layer, beneath the perichondrium or near the free joint surface, the cells are flattened in a plane parallel to the surface; deeper down the cells are arranged in groups consisting of two, four or eight along the longitudinal axis.

THE INTERCELLULAR MATRIX

This ground substance appears to be homogeneous when fresh and has a high water content (approximately 70%). It consists of chondromucoprotein, a polymer of mucoprotein together with chondroitin-4-sulphate and chondroitin-6-sulphate. A small amount of the keratin sulphate may also be present.

The intercellular matrix is permeated by a dense network of very fine collagen fibres. Polarization microscopy and electronmicroscopy show that these fibres have a preferential orientation which is coincident with the direction of maximum stress. The central part of the cartilage mass is subject to pressure and hence the chondromucoprotein is particularly concentrated. The collagen fibres are more numerous in the peripheral layer when there is a pulling force.

Since there is no canaliculi in the ground substance, the cartilage cells are nourished by fluid exchange with the intercellular matrix. The nutritive fluid is derived from the blood vessel of the perichondrium. For the articular cartilage, this diffusion of nutrient from the synovial fluid indicates an important functional relationship with joint motion and the integrity of the synovial circulation.

BIOMECHANICS OF NORMAL ARTICULAR CARTILAGE

Articular cartilage exhibits a viscoelastic response when subjected to loads and deformations. It creeps under a constant applied load and stress relaxes under a constant applied deformation. This viscoelastic response of articular cartilage depends on two different physical mechanisms:

1 The intrinsic viscoelastic properties of the macromolecules.

2 The frictional drag arising from the flow of the interstitial fluid.

These two mechanisms together contribute to the overall viscoelastic properties of the articular cartilage under tension, compression and shear. An understanding of these basic structural functional relationships of articular cartilage is important in our further search for the changes in atrophic, osteoarthritic and healing of articular cartilage.

Healing of articular cartilage

HISTORICAL DEVELOPMENT

The subject of articular cartilage healing has been a focus of attention for most basic science investigators for more than 250 years. In 1743, Hunter first noted that '... ulcerated cartilage is a troublesome thing once destroyed it is not repaired' (Hunter, 1743). In 1853, Paget reported that '... no instance in which a lost portion of cartilage has been restored or a wounded portion will be repaired with new and well formed cartilage ...' (Paget, 1853). Throughout the decades, numerous researchers confirm the initial work of Hunter and Paget. However, there are reports that damaged cartilage can heal under certain conditions. But in most instances, the tissue lacks the molecular composition, organization, material properties and the durability of normal articular cartilage (Mankin, 1982). Therefore, specific cartilage healing is unpredictable.

PATHOLOGY OF ARTICULAR CARTILAGE INJURY

Articular cartilage does not undergo independent healing because the matured cartilage cells are incapable of division (Buckwalter, 1983). Any articular cartilage defect is made good by invasion from the perichondrium or the nearest fascia and by deposition of connective tissue. Some of the fibroblasts of this tissue then round up and differentiate into cartilage cells while the intercellular matrix may change into the typical ground substance of the cartilage. Therefore, it is not surprising that in the healing of the articular cartilage, it is quite common to find elastic and white fibre in the matrix. Very often, the healing process stops at this stage and the gap is filled only by dense fibrous tissue (Fig. 5.1).

The loss of matrix proteoglycans is the initial change of a number of conditions notably disruption of the synovial membrane due to trauma, prolonged joint immobilization and other inflammatory processes. Certain kinds of anti-inflammatory agents such as steroids may also predispose to these changes.

When this precipitating process responsible for the loss of matrix is reversible, there is a chance for the chondrocytes to replace the lost

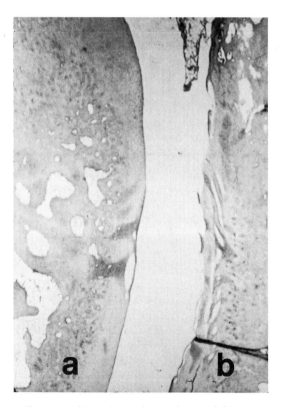

Fig. 5.1 (a) Normal articular cartilage with bluish and translucent character covering the subchondral bone. (b) Degenerated articular cartilage with disrupted edges, pits and fissure formation and disintegration of alignment. Areas of gaps are filled by fibrous tissue. Exposure of subchondral bone may account for the symptom of pain.

matrix components and the cartilage as a whole may regain its normal composition and function. However, if these stimuli continue, the articular cartilage damage may become irreversible. Usually, if the collagen meshwork is intact and the chondrocytes are viable and capable of synthesizing the appropriate proteoglycans, the cartilage can be restored to its normal condition.

TYPE OF INJURY

Closed injury

Closed injury to cartilage occurs frequently in the absence of fractures. It may be a source of significant long-term joint dysfunction. This may be related to the overuse syndrome in sports injury particularly with excessive training programme or injudicious progression of training schedule leading to over-exertion on the joint. It is well-known that impact loading above physiological levels can cause cartilage swelling, increase in collagen fibre size and alteration of the relationship between collagen and proteoglycans. Blunt trauma if extensive and severe enough may produce fracture or fissure of the cartilage matrix, fracture of the subchondral bone, disruption of the collagen network and chondrocyte death.

Open injury

The depth of cartilage injury is important in the consideration of the healing process. There is a zone of calcified cartilage that separates the articular cartilage from the marrow cells and blood vessels that participate in the inflammatory response to injury. When the penetrating injury creates a defect restricted to the substance of the articular cartilage alone, there is a decrease in the healing potential. This is a partial thickness cartilage defect.

Biomechanically, it is also demonstrated by the study of Furukawa *et al*. that the reparative tissue contains an appreciable amount of type I collagen compared with the normal articular cartilage which consists of primary type II collagen (Furukawa *et al.*, 1980). Therefore, it may be concluded that following the articular cartilage injury, the differentiation of fibroblast-like collagen cells into chondrocytes is imperfect and it does not produce a population of chondrocytes whose phenotype is similar to that of chondrocytes in the normal articular cartilage.

That the bone matrix may play a critical role in cartilage healing is also a subject of intense study. There may be a possibility that bone matrix contains growth differentiation factors that may stimulate the formation of hyaline cartilage particularly in the small defects that are within 1 mm in diameter.

Grading of articular cartilage lesion

Over the past few years, several different classification systems for the description of articular cartilage damage have appeared in the literature, each having limitations and deficiencies which may lead to confusion. Noyes and Stabler (1989) proposed a new system which described articular cartilage abnormality in simple terms. This is based on four separate and distinct variables:

1 Description of articular surface.
2 The extent (depth) of involvement.
3 The diameter of the lesion.
4 The location of the lesion.

For comparative study in clinical and basic science research, it is important to have a common language and a universal system of classification. Table 5.1 illustrates the details of the new classification of articular cartilage lesions.

FACTORS AFFECTING ARTICULAR CARTILAGE HEALING

Some athletic injuries cause significant articular cartilage disruption that may lead to pain and disability such as osteochondral fracture and osteochondritis dissecans. Because of the young age of many of these athletes, joint replacement is considered undesirable and various attempts have been made to increase our understanding of full thickness cartilage injury and a search for various methods to improve healing. Broadly speaking, the following two categories of manipulative procedures can be tried to improve articular cartilage healing.

Intrinsic factors

Cellular transplantation. A new population of cells, grown and maintained from cell culture or chondrocytes harvested from another site, can be implanted to the defect and hopefully they may synthesize a new cartilage matrix. There are reports in animal studies that homologous chondrocytes embedded in the resorbable gel while implanted improve the healing process.

Hormonal factor. Various substances that are known to stimulate chondrogenesis have been tried in experimental models to stimulate cartilage repair such as purifiable bovine growth hormone, a 31 kDa bone matrix protein. The potential of these substances is significant but further research is required to identify the most useful factors, the ways of delivering them to the site of injury and to determine the ideal dose−response relationship and quality of the repair tissue.

Artificial scaffold. To potentiate the healing process, filling the defect with collagen or fibrin gel, carbon fibre implant or other synthetic gel substances can be used. It is hoped that mesenchymal cells can invade the scaffold to proliferate and synthesize a new matrix.

Autogenous graft. The use of these grafts provides the approach of introducing a new cell population that participates in the healing of articular cartilage. But there is still doubt as to whether these periosteal or perichondral tissue from skeletally mature individuals have the same facilitating effect as the skeletally immature animals. Also the tissue produced may not have a long-term durability similar to that of normal cartilage.

Table 5.1 New classification of articular cartilage lesions. From Noyes & Stabler (1989).

Surface description	Extent of involvement	Diameter (mm)	Location	Degree of knee flexion
Cartilage surface intact	Definite softening with some resilience remaining	<10 $\leqq15$ $\leqq20$	Patella (A) proximal $\frac{1}{3}$ middle $\frac{1}{3}$ distal $\frac{1}{3}$	Degree of knee flexion where the lesion is in weight-bearing contact (e.g. 20–45°)
	Extensive softening with loss of resilience (deformation)	$\leqq25$ >25	Patella (B) odd facet middle facet lateral facet	
Cartilage surface damaged: cracks, fissures, fibrillation, or fragmentation	$<\frac{1}{2}$ thickness $\geqq\frac{1}{2}$ thickness		Trochlea Medial femoral condyle anterior $\frac{1}{3}$ middle $\frac{1}{3}$ posterior $\frac{1}{3}$	
Bone exposed	Bone surface intact Bone surface cavitation		Trochlea Lateral femoral condyle anterior $\frac{1}{3}$ middle $\frac{1}{3}$ posterior $\frac{1}{3}$ Medial tibial condyle anterior $\frac{1}{3}$ middle $\frac{1}{3}$ posterior $\frac{1}{3}$ Lateral tibial condyle anterior $\frac{1}{3}$ middle $\frac{1}{3}$ posterior $\frac{1}{3}$	

Extrinsic factors

Abrasion arthroplasty. There is ample clinical experience to suggest that arthroscopic shaving or abrasion of fibrillated irregular cartilage may relieve some of the symptoms of degenerative joint diseases. However, the efficacy has not been sufficiently documented in well-controlled long-term clinical studies. On the contrary, there are reports to suggest that shaving may have caused increased fibrillation and cell necrosis in areas adjacent to the original defect.

Spongiolization and drilling. The formation of a fibrin clot and vascular invasion of the repaired tissue after drilling is the basis of this manoeuvre. It is intended that the new cell population entering the defect may produce a more extensive repair response than that found in injury limited to cartilage alone. However, in experimental study, it is found that repair tissue initially has a hyaline appearance but with time it becomes more fibrous and frequently begins to fibrillate and break down. Clinically, drilling occasionally relieves the symptom but the result again is not predictable.

Mechanical stimulation. The classic study by DePalma *et al.* (1966), demonstrated that in small defects (of less than 1 mm) that penetrated the subchondral bone, continuous passive motion might enhance the healing process and produce a tissue that closely resembled hyaline cartilage morphologically and histochemically. However, it is not known whether passive motion had the same efficacy in promoting the healing of larger defects. Moreover, there is no demonstrable beneficial effect of passive motion on the repair of injury limited to articular cartilage alone.

Laser stimulation. It has been found that superficial articular cartilage defect exposed to low-dose laser energy demonstrates a healing process superior to that found in untreated injuries. However, the exact mechanism is un-

clear and the long-term result of laser stimulated healing is uncertain.

Electromagnetic stimulation. Chondrocytes may increase synthesis of cartilage-like proteoglycans when estimated by pulsed electromagnetic fields. But the effect of such manipulation had not been shown to facilitate repair of actual articular cartilage defects.

PROGNOSTIC FACTORS OF ARTICULAR CARTILAGE HEALING

1 The anatomical extent of the injury.
2 The age of the subject.
3 The condition of the joint before injury.
4 Quality, extent and durability of the repaired tissue.
5 The long-term function of the joint.

Normal joint structure

In the normal synovial joint, the bone ends are covered by hyaline articular cartilage and the surface lubricated by synovial fluid produced by the synovial membrane which is supported by the fibrous joint capsule. In the consideration of joint injuries related to sport, it is therefore important to scrutinize the patho-anatomy and pathophysiology of the individual element which may be subject to the traumatic forces.

The synovial membrane is a thin membrane lined by a single layer of spindle cells or one or more layers of ovoid or polygonal cells. These intimal cells are all separated by a basement membrane from the hyaline tissue which may be areolar, densely fibrous or fatty in different parts of the joint. Functionally, two types of intimal cells can be distinguished on electron-microscopy: (i) type A, the more numerous one, is concerned with absorption; while (ii) type B synthesizes mucopolysaccharides such as hyaluronate.

The synovium may be smooth or folded especially at the joint margin to form small villi. It covers virtually the whole of the joint surfaces except the articular cartilage and the menisci. Synovial membrane has a rich network of blood vessels which accounts for its high metabolic activities and is important in the reaction to injuries.

Synovial fluid is a dialysate of blood plasma with the addition of hyaluronic acid which gives the fluid its viscous property. The proportion of hyaluronic acid is believed to diminish with aging. Under normal circumstances, the synovial joint contains less than 1 m of synovial fluid. There is usually 50–400 nucleated cells per mm^3 with a few polymorphs and about 20% of lymphocytes, a few synovial cells and the majority of mononuclear phagocytes derived from the synovial histiocytes. Biochemically, albumin and globulin are present in lower concentrations in the fluid than in plasma with an albumin : globulin ratio of 4 : 1. Glucose level are normally much less than that found in the blood. Synovial fluid is an important element in the nutrition of the articular cartilage. As a response to injury, there is usually a proliferation of synovial fluid (effusion) which distends the joint. It is believed that synovial circulation is an important mechanism in maintaining lubrication of the joint and the nutritional status of the articular cartilage.

The degenerative joint diseases (osteoarthritis) related to sports injuries

PATHOPHYSIOLOGY OF PRIMARY OSTEOARTHRITIS

Articular cartilage

There is a general disruption of this collagen network with decreasing amounts of ground substances in the cartilage matrix often due to an increasing breakdown as a result of the release of lysosomal enzyme from damaged chondrocytes (Cappell & Anderson, 1977). The roughening of the articular cartilage follows due initially to attrition of the superficial layer and later to longitudinal splitting and dis-

integration. Proliferation of small groups of deeper chondrocytes and increased production of ground substances locally at the margin of the degenerated zone may be recognized as an attempt at healing. However, this process is usually ineffectual and may be followed by further loss of cartilage substances with the formation of erosed pits and eventually exposure of the subchondral bone plate. Radiological examination may show the diminution in the joint space which is a helpful diagnostic sign. More recently, the use of magnetic resonance imaging (MRI) may show the early change in the articular cartilage and signals a warning sign to the athlete (Fig. 5.2).

Bone

As the articular cartilage gradually thins, the exposed bone surface will become dense, polished and eburnated, often grooved or scored by irregularity on the opposing joint

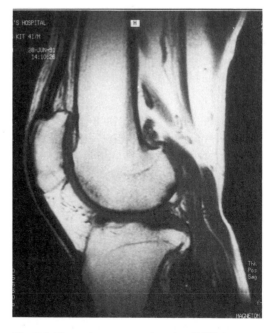

Fig. 5.2 Magnetic resonance imaging (MRI) is an imaging technique which may indicate early changes in soft tissue lesions. MRI can also be helpful in evaluating cartilage changes.

surfaces. Radiologically, it appears as dense sclerotic lines. Fibrocartilaginous metaplasia may occur in any exposed marrow spaces. Marked bone remodelling may change the shape of the joint surface which is particularly obvious in weight-bearing surfaces.

Radiological 'cysts' may be formed in the subchondral bone. These are areas devoid of bone but filled with fatty marrow and degenerated fibrous tissue.

Osteophytes are excrescences from the joint margin formed by proliferation of cartilage, followed by endochondral calcification. It may grow at the margin of the joint, and extend the joint surfaces. This bone outgrowth sometimes breaks off as loose bodies.

Synovium

There is usually a mild inflammatory reaction of the synovium to the irritation of the numerous small fragments of abraded cartilage or bone from the joint surfaces. Usually the synovium capsules are thickened and contracted. Sometimes there is an increased amount of synovial fluid (effusion).

SECONDARY OSTEOARTHRITIS OF THE JOINT

This may be accentuated by a number of sports-related causes that give rise to direct injury to the articular cartilage or fractures with deformity, malalignment and loose bodies. It is therefore of paramount importance to recognize these degenerative changes after sports injuries early in order to minimize the extent of progression that may lead to permanent disability.

Conclusion

The search for all possible means to enhance articular cartilage healing will continue to dominate the scene of basic science research in the coming decades. Until we have a definite solution to this problem, it must be emphasized that prevention is still the mainstay of our strategy to minimize the deleterious effect of acute trauma and overuse injury in sports.

Ligamental injury

Skeletal ligaments had been thought to be composed of only tough fibrous tissues whose sole function was to hold joints in place. In the past decades, a myriad of basic and clinical studies on the anatomical and the pathophysiological aspects of ligamental injuries have appeared that served to put joint ligament under the limelight in the arena of sports injuries. Although there is still a wide gap between the understanding of the basic science of ligamental structure and its clinical implication, scientists and clinicians are continuing to narrow the gap by the many researches and studies that are being undertaken.

Normal anatomy and physiology

GROSS ANATOMY

There are hundreds of ligaments in the human body with a diversity of shapes and sizes. Most of the time, they are strong, white distinct fibrous bands that saddle across joints such as in the cruciate ligaments of the knee. However, sometimes they appear as less distinct sheets of connective tissues such as in the medial collateral ligament of the knee. Since the capsular ligaments subserve functions that are indistinguishable from the more usual type of skeletal ligaments, they may well be included as one of their variants.

The gross appearance of skeletal ligament is quite unremarkable. Often, it appears as an avascular structure with its fibres running parallel between the two points of insertion. The direction of the fibres is remarkably constant among different individuals which illustrates the consistency of the function it serves. Most of the skeletal ligaments are extra-articular though some are intra-articular but extra-synovial such as the cruciate ligaments.

BLOOD SUPPLY

The amount of blood supply to the ligament varies. In the case of medial collateral ligament of the knee, the blood supply comes from at least three sources. It derives its blood supply from the inferior geniculate artery, from the ligament−bone interface and probably from the synovium as well. However, in the case of anterior cruciate ligament of the knee, the main blood supply is thought to come mainly from the synovium.

HISTOLOGY

Histologically, skeletal ligament is composed of parallel collagen fibres between which are spindle-shaped cells called fibrocysts. Vessels are infrequently found along the length of the ligament. Detailed examination of the ligament reveals that the collagen fibres run in the form of waves or 'crimp' (Dale *et al.*, 1972; Diamant *et al.*, 1972). This wave form is thought to allow stretch and elongation of the ligament like a spring. It also allows adjustment of tension and prevents damage to the fibres during physiological load. The site of insertion of the ligament is a specialized zone in its own right. It is composed of a gradual transition from fibrous tissue of the ligament to fibrocartilage, to mineralized fibrocartilage and finally onto bone. This ligament−bone interface is extremely strong and seldom gives way before the ligament does.

BIOCHEMICAL COMPOSITION

A typical skeletal ligament contains approximately 65% by weight of water and 25% by weight of collagen. Most of the collagen is type I. The remainder is composed of elastin, proteoglycans and other biochemical substances. Figure 5.3 shows the biochemical composition of normal ligament. The former gives a limited elasticity to the ligament while the latter holds the water within it (Frank *et al.*, 1983).

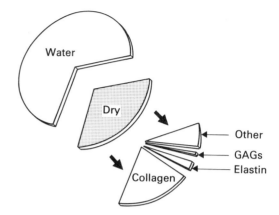

Fig. 5.3 Approximate chemical composition of normal skeletal ligaments by weight. From Frank *et al.* (1983).

BIOCHEMICAL BEHAVIOUR

The skeletal ligament has been extensively tested *in vitro*. It has been found to exhibit some very interesting properties which have direct relevance to the function that it serves (Akeson *et al.*, 1984). The biomechanical behaviour is extremely suitable for it to act as a check-rein for the joint:

1 The stiffness of the skeletal ligament increases with the load that is applied to it up to a certain extent. This allows a certain degree of 'give' in the joint while resisting further displacement when further load is applied.

2 Ligament also exhibits some degree of 'memory' in that it can return to its prestretched length when the load is removed.

3 Ligament possesses the property of stress relaxation in that the tension of the ligament would decrease with time when a constant load is applied.

4 Ligament is strain-rate sensitive. It offers higher resistance when it is loaded faster.

FUNCTIONS OF LIGAMENTS

Although skeletal ligament is a rather inconspicuous structure, its function is severalfold.

1 It is extremely important in aligning the joint and governing the smooth gliding and sliding of joint surfaces. Disruption of any one of the supporting ligaments of the joint will result in malalignment or subluxation of the joint which may lead to premature degeneration (Butler *et al.*, 1980).

2 The ligament is also entrusted with the task of maintaining the physiological pressure on the articular surfaces which is essential in the well-being of the articular cartilage.

3 The skeletal ligament contains proprioceptive nerve endings which provide valuable information to the musculotendinous unit to maintain posture.

4 In some areas such as the foot and the spine, skeletal ligaments help support the skeleton and give the body parts their characteristic shape.

Pathoanatomy and pathophysiology

Ligamental injury is very common in orthopaedic sports medicine practice. It is believed to be the commonest joint injury and accounts for 25–40% of all knee injuries (Dehaven & Lintner, 1986). Although most of these injuries are mild, some will result in significant physical disability and will require surgical intervention eventually. There are some joints that are particularly at risk and these include the knee, ankle, elbow, shoulder, fingers and thumb. Although the aetiology of the so-called 'sprained back' is not entirely clear, it is believed that some of the ligaments in the back are injured most of the time.

CLASSIFICATION OF LIGAMENTAL INJURY

Ligamental injury is clinically divided into three grades: (i) grade 1 includes mild sprain of the ligament without any clinical instability; (ii) grade 2 denotes moderate sprain with mild but not gross clinical instability; and (iii) grade 3 is defined as severe sprain with clinically detectable instability. Most of the ligamental sprains are not severe and less than 15% of the sprains in the knee belongs to grade 3.

MECHANISM OF INJURY

Skeletal ligament may be injured directly or indirectly (DeHaven, 1983). Direct blow to a joint may stretch the ligament beyond its physiological stiffness and result in permanent deformation. More often, because of the long lever arm of the long bones in the limb, bending and twisting force applied distally will also tear the ligament. This commonly occurs during a direct blow to one end of the long bone while the other end is fixed, in deceleration or in sudden change in direction, manoeuvres that frequently occur in most types of sports.

CLINICAL PRESENTATION

Ligamental injury is so common that mild ones are often discharged as joint sprain and never present to the physician. Not uncommonly, the diagnosis is often missed because the athlete can continue to play on the field. However, overt injury is readily recognized by the layperson and professionals alike (Fig. 5.4). The hallmark of acute ligamental injury includes pain, swelling, bruising, giving way and instability of varying degrees. Most of the time, a definite history of trauma can be identified. However, delayed presentation may pose difficulty in the diagnosis. Orthopaedic surgeons are equipped with various clinical stability and function tests to help define subtle instability of the joint. Radiology is only occasionally useful when an avulsion fracture has occurred. Various stress X-rays have been advocated but they are never popular probably due partly to the fact that they require considerable relaxation on the part of the patient which may be too demanding when he or she is in agony. Arthroscopy has broadened the horizon in the identification of intra-articular ligamental injury and some of the problems may even be dealt with through the arthroscope. Figure 5.5 shows the arthroscopic appearance of a normal anterior cruciate ligament. With the advent of high-tech MRI, both clinically occult or obvious ligamental injury should be picked up easily in

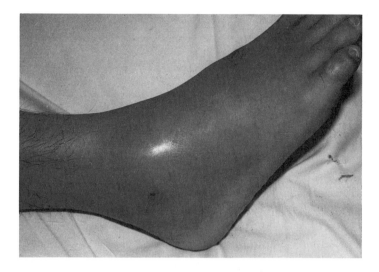

Fig. 5.4 Sprained right ankle.

the future. Figure 5.6 reveals the MRI appearance of the cruciate ligament.

TYPES OF INJURY

Ligamental injury takes on various forms:
1 Uncommonly, the ligament is torn off with

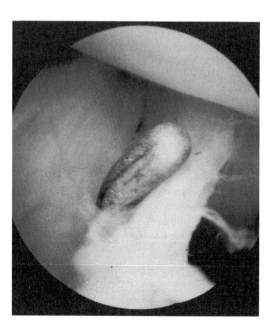

Fig. 5.5 Arthroscopic appearance of anterior cruciate ligament. A hook is pulling on the ligament.

a piece of bone — so-called avulsion fracture. This occurs in the younger population where the ligament itself is relatively stronger than the bone. Figure 5.7 shows a radiograph of avulsion fracture of tibial eminence by the anterior cruciate ligament.

2 Sometimes, the ligament is avulsed from the ligament—bone interface but this is again uncommon because this interface is usually stronger than the ligament and therefore, it seldom gives way first.

3 The midsubstance tear is by far the commonest. The tear may be transverse or oblique, but most frequently, it is a tear at different points along the course of the ligament. This makes direct repair of all the fibres of the ligament virtually impossible.

FUNCTIONAL CONSIDERATIONS

Because skeletal ligament serves a pivotal role in the stability of the joint, it is not surprising that substantial tear of the ligament may have dire consequences. The most direct effect is of course the loss of stability. The functional deficit may be quite variable depending on: (i) the dispensability of the ligament; (ii) the integrity of the other supporting ligaments; (iii) the inherent stability of the joint; (iv) the presence of compensatory adaptive changes in

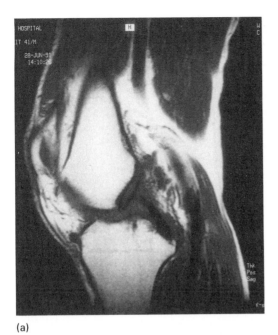

(a)

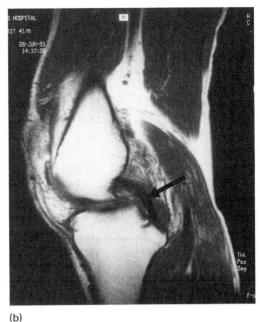

(b)

Fig. 5.6 Magnetic resonance image of (a) the anterior cruciate ligament; (b) the posterior cruciate ligament.

the muscles; and (v) the physical demands of the athlete. The loss of stability of the joint will also lead to changes in the correct axis of movement. This may lead to malalignment of the joint during motion and abnormal contact pressure in certain areas of the joint. Chronic joint instability is found to lead to alteration of the muscular lever arm which may influence the working efficiency of the muscle. Muscular compensation after ligamental injury is a known phenomenon. Whether this would give rise to excessive stress to the joints is being studied. Finally, the loss of proprioception related to ligamental injury also affects the smooth function of the entire musculoligamento-articular system.

LIGAMENTAL HEALING

Healing of the injured ligament is a highly complicated issue (Ross, 1968). Sophisticated and overlapping cellular, biochemical and bio-mechanical events are involved. Ligament healing in an animal model had been studied in detail and could be conceptually divided into four phases:

1 Phase 1: Inflammation. After an acute tear of the ligament, the gap will be readily filled with blood clot. Serous fluid begins to pour into the area and swelling results. White blood cells are attracted to this injured area and fibroblasts whose origin is controversial begin to move in. Capillary buds proliferate and help to make the injured part more vascular.

2 Phase 2: Matrix and cellular proliferation. The fibroblasts now become very active in synthesizing ground matrix and collagen fibrils are laid down. Macrophages and mast cells are abundant. The vascular lumen becomes cannulated and a network of capillaries is established.

3 Phase 3: Remodelling. The number of fibroblasts and inflammatory cells starts to diminish and the activity of these cells also begins to slow down. The density of the collagen increases and the orientation along the length of the ligament improves.

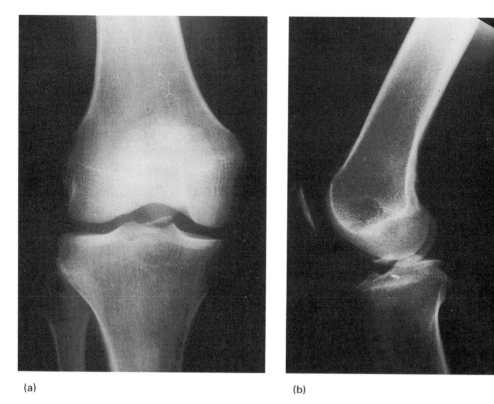

(a)   (b)

Fig. 5.7 Radiographic appearance of fracture of the tibial eminence. (a) Anteroposterior view; (b) lateral view.

4 Phase 4: Maturation. This is a slow process that may take months or even years. The healed ligament becomes stiffer and stronger and starts to possess properties and composition that are more similar to the original ligament. It is in this phase when ligament contracture may take place. This process is ligament-specific and helps restore the healed ligament back to its original physiological length. This phenomenon is thought to be partly due to an increase in the cross-linkage among the collagen fibres and partly due to an active tension applied by cells during the maturation phase.

Functional consideration of ligamental healing

Healing of the ligament does not form pure scar tissue, nor does it produce normal ligamental tissue (Frank, 1983). The resultant ligament is dissimilar to the original ligament in many respects. It has a higher collagen content but a slightly decreased collagen concentration; it contains a higher ratio of type III to type I collagen and the turnover rate of the collagen is also greater. Mechanically, the healed ligament never attains its original strength (50—70% at most) and the deformation is greater even within physiological loading. The cyclic behaviour and stress—relaxation characteristic is also worse than before.

Factors affecting ligamental healing

There are several factors which are conducive to ideal ligamental healing:
1 The torn ends have to be in good opposition. This is seldom the case in clinical practice and often it requires either correct positioning of the joint or surgical repair in order to achieve continuity of the ends.

2 Healing requires blood supply. Avascular ligaments and ligaments that are intra-articular are particularly susceptible to poor healing response.

3 Physiological stress and motion appear to be beneficial and may accelerate the processes of ligamental healing and remodelling. Nevertheless, too early commencement of movement after injury may lead to further haemorrhage and oedema which leads to prolongation of recovery.

4 Protection from excessive stress and motion is definitely desirable in order to avoid eventual laxity. However, prolonged immobilization will lead to decrease in the quantity and quality of the ligament–scar complex. Figure 5.8 shows the histomorphological changes in the anterior cruciate ligament from immobilization. Joint stiffness may be unavoidable (Woo *et al.*, 1982).

Prevention of ligamental injury

Not all ligamental injuries are preventable. However, the incidence may be kept to a minimum if athletes as well as coaches are more aware of the nature of the game, the risk factors involved and the available preventive measures. Probably, too much has been said and done on the pathogenesis and the therapeutics of ligamental injury but prevention has been left out of the limelight. Prevention is much more cost-effective than treatment. Through the close cooperation among athletes, coaches, sports scientists, therapists and doctors, it is hoped that the vulnerability of the athletic population may be diminished.

NATURE OF THE GAME

Different types of sports invite different forms and severity of ligamental injury. Understanding the inherent risk of the game and considering one's suitability for the game would avoid many unnecessary ligamental sprains.

1 High-risk sports. Sports which involve high velocity, high altitude, high energy and high strength are particularly dangerous. Of course, as far as prevention of ligamental injury is concerned, the easy way out is to ban all dangerous sports. Nevertheless, there are people whose thirst to conquer the impossible can never be quenched and therefore, the best policy is to educate the public about the risks and potential hazards of all these sports.

2 Rules of the game. Apart from imparting fairness of competition, another function of the rules of the game is to avoid unnecessary injury. As we become more aware of the aetiology of the various ligamental injuries and their association with certain types of sports, rules have to be modified in order to achieve this goal.

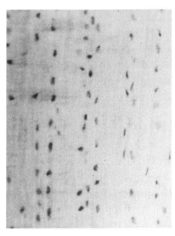 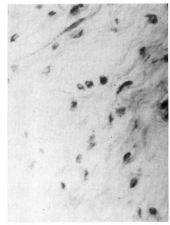

Fig. 5.8 (a) Histological appearance of normal ligament; (b) histological appearance of ligament after immobilization.   (a)   (b)

Having said that, it will require astute observation and tremendous amounts of evidence in order to convince the authorities that certain rules of the game have to change for the well-being of the athletes.

3 Environment. Dangerous terrain and hostile weather are both conducive to injuries. It is the duty of the organizer to decide when and where a competition is safe enough to take place and the athlete should be accountable for his or her own safety. More rules and regulations are necessary in this respect.

4 Equipment and protective devices. The sporting equipment used should not endanger the safety of the participants or the opponents. Those that do should be removed from the market as soon as possible. Protective taping, knee braces, wrist guards and anklets are particularly useful in preventing ligamental sprains and their use should be encouraged.

IDENTIFICATION OF HIGH-RISK FACTORS

There are some factors which make an athlete prone to ligamental injury. Proper identification of these factors may help alter the training technique, put emphasis on strengthening and agility, or even advise the individual to drop that particular sport altogether in order to minimize serious ligamental injury.

1 Proneness to ligamental injury. Athletes who have a history of repeated sprains are particularly prone to further injury. This is partly due to the fact that the injured ligament is usually being stretched beyond its physiological length and joint instability is already established. Another reason is that they have impaired proprioceptive sensation because of damage to mechanoreceptors which would lead to an impairment of the ligamentomuscular reflex. Lastly, it is not uncommon to find that the muscles which assist in stability are usually weak and their function as a dynamic protector of the injured ligament is usually incompetent.

2 Excessive ligamental laxity. Excessive ligamental laxity offers little protection to ligamental sprain. This condition is usually inherent in which case it is usually generalized but it can be acquired locally through repeated stretching and training since a very young age. Although excessive flexibility may be an asset in performance, athletes may become more susceptible to overstretch injury of the ligament.

3 Incompetence of other supportive ligaments. Joint stability is usually contributed by not one but several ligaments. This complementary phenomenon may mean that loss of integrity of one ligament through injury will put the other ligaments in jeopardy. A good example of this is the role of the posterior cruciate ligament in preventing medial and lateral opening up of the knee joint at full extension even when the collateral ligaments are injured.

4 Poor muscle strength. It is well known that good muscle strength is protective in the absence of ligamental integrity. It has been found that patients suffering from anterior cruciate deficiency of the knee are much benefited by strengthening the hamstrings muscles.

5 Intake of alcohol and drugs. Athletes under the influence of alcohol and drugs are found to have a slower reaction time to changes of circumstances. This makes them susceptible to ligamental injury due to poor cerebral control of muscles and impaired proprioceptive input.

PREVENTIVE MEASURES AND DEVICES

Part of the goal of training in sports is to optimize performance during competition but another less well recognized aim is to prevent the occurrence of sports injury. The latter can only be fulfilled by specific conditioning and the use of appropriate protective devices.

1 Proper training and coaching technique. Every sport is inherently dangerous if not properly taught. Although the exact method has to be individualized, the body parts should not be asked to do more than they can. Coaches and athletes should both be responsible for

recognizing the limitations and capability of the human body to perform a certain act or feat.

2 Warming-up and stretching programmes. These programmes have long been recognized as excellent conditioning in the prevention of sports injuries. Apart from preparing the muscles to perform efficiently, these programmes are also essential in tuning the brain in order to achieve controlled movements effectively.

3 Endurance and weight-training. Strong muscle control can take up part of the stress on stretched ligaments. Easy fatigueability is conducive to ligamental injury and this can be avoided by endurance and weight-training.

4 Proprioceptive and agility training. Impairment of proprioception and reflex time always accompanies ligamental injuries. The wobble-board is found to be extremely helpful in regaining the premorbid reflex state and further injuries to the ligaments may be avoided.

5 Protective devices. There are numerous braces and orthotics on the market that claim to be beneficial in the prevention of ligamental injuries. There is not yet an ideal orthotics device that will give complete protection while allowing freedom of movement to the joint. Nevertheless, taping is found to be a good compromise which takes up part of the tension in stretched ligaments while at the same time enhancing the proprioceptive sense of the joint.

References

Akeson, W., Woo, S.L-Y., Amiel, D. & Frank, C. (1984) The biology of ligaments. In F. Funk & L.Y. Hunter (eds) *Rehabilitation of the Injured Knee*, pp. 93–148. CV Mosby, St Louis.

Bradbury, S. (1973) *Hewer's Textbook of Histology*, Vol. 8, pp. 89–97. William Heinemann, London.

Butler, D.L., Noyes, F.R. & Groods, E.S. (1980) Ligamentous restraints to anterior-posterior drawer in the human knee. *J. Bone Joint Surg.* **62A**, 259–70.

Cappell, D.F. & Anderson, J.R. (1977) *Muir's Textbook of Pathology*, Vol. 22, pp. 750–816. Edward Arnold, London.

Dale, W.D., Baer, E., Keller, A. & Kohn, R.R. (1972) On the ultrastructure of mammalian tendon. *Experientia* **28**, 1293.

DeHaven, K.E. (1983) Acute ligament injuries and dislocations. In C.M. Evarts (ed) *Surgery of the Musculoskeletal System*, Vol. 4, pp. 3255–82. Churchill Livingstone, New York.

DeHaven, K.E. & Lintner, D.M. (1986) Athletic injuries: Comparison by age, sport, and gender. *Am. J. Sports Med.* **14**, 218–24.

DePalma, A.F., McKeever, C.D. & Subin, D.K. (1966) Process of repair of articular cartilage demonstrated by histology and autoradiography with tritiated thymidine. *Clin. Orthop.* **48**, 229–42.

Diamant, J., Keller, A., Baer, E., Litt, M. & Arridge, R.G.C. (1972) Collagen; Ultrastructure and its relation to mechanical properties as a function of aging. *Proc. Roy. Soc. Lond.* **180**, 293.

Frank, C., Amiel, D. & Akeson, W. (1983) Medial collateral ligament healing — A morphological and biochemical assessment. *Acta Orthop. Scand.* **54**, 917.

Furukawa, T., Eyre, D.R., Koide, S., *et al.* (1980) Biochemical studies on repair cartilage resurfacing experimental defects in the rabbit knee. *J. Bone Joint Surg.* **62A**, 79–89.

Hunter, W. (1743) On the structure and diseases of articulating cartilage. *Philos. Trans. Roy. Soc. Lond.* **9**, 267.

Mankin, H.J. (1974) The reaction of articular cartilage to injury and osteoarthritis: Part I. *N. Engl. J. Med.* **291**, 1285–92.

Mankin, H.J. (1982) The response of articular cartilage to mechanical injury. *J. Bone Joint Surg.* **64A**, 460–6.

Noyes, F. & Stabler, C. (1989) A system for grading articular cartilage lesion at arthroscopy. *Am. J. Sports Med.* **17**(4), 505–13.

Paget, J. (1853) Healing of injuries in various tissues. *Lect. Surg. Pathol.* T, 262.

Ross, R. (1968) The fibroblast and wound repair. *Biol. Rev.* **43**, 51–96.

Woo, S.L-Y., Gomez, M.A., Woo, Y.K. & Akeson, W.H. (1982) Mechanical properties of tendons and ligaments. II. The relationships of immobilization and exercise on tissue remodeling. *Biorheology* **19**, 397.

Further reading

Aaron, R.K., Ciomber, D.M. & Jolly, G. (1987) Modulation of chondrogenesis and chondrocyte differentiation by pulsed electromagnetic fields. *Trans. Orthop. Res. Soc.* **12**, 272–3.

Aaron, R.K. & Plaas, A.A.K. (1987) Stimulation of proteoglycan synthesis in articular chondrocyte cultures by a pulsed electromagnetic field. *Trans. Orthop. Res. Soc.* **12**, 273.

Delaunay, A. & Bazin, S. (1964) Mucopolysaccharides,

collagen, and nonfibrillar proteins in inflammation. *Int. Rev. Connect. Tiss. Res.* **2**, 301–25.

Hart, J.A.L. (1987) *The use of carbon fibre implants for articular cartilage defects.* Presented at the 47th Annual Meeting of the Australian Orthopaedic Association, Melbourne.

Insall, J. (1974) The Pridie debridement operation for osteoarthritis of the knee. *Clin. Orthop.* **101**, 61–7.

McDaniel Jr, W.J. & Dameron Jr, T.B. (1980) Untreated anterior ruptures of the cruciate ligament: A follow-up study. *J. Bone Joint Surg.* **62A**, 696–705.

Magnuson, P.B. (1941) Joint debridement: surgical treatment of degenerative arthritis. *Surg. Gynecol. Obstet.* **73**, 1–9.

Mankin, H.J. (1974) The reaction of articular cartilage to injury and osteoarthritis: Part II. *N. Engl. J. Med.* **291**, 1335–40.

Markolf, K.L., Mensch, J.S. & Amstutz, H.C. (1976) Stiffness and laxity of the knee — The contributions of the supporting structures. *J. Bone Joint Surg.* **58A**, 583–94.

Noyes, F.R. & McGinniss, G.H. (1985) Controversy about treatment of the knee with anterior cruciate laxity. *Clin. Orthop.* **198**, 61–76.

O'Donoghue, D.H. (1955) An analysis of end results of surgical treatment of major injuries to the ligaments of the knee. *J. Bone Joint Surg.* **37A**, 1–13.

O'Driscoll, S.W., Keeley, F.W. & Salter, R.B. (1986) The chondrogenic potential of free autogenous periosteal grafts for biological resurfacing of major-full-thickness defects in joint surfaces under the influence of continuous passive motion: An experimental study in the rabbit. *J. Bone Joint Surg.* **68A**, 1017–35.

Radin, El. & Burr, D.B. (1984) Hypothesis: Joints can heal. *Semin. Arthritis Rheum.* **13**, 293–302.

Salter, R.B., Minster, R.R., Bell R.S., *et al.* (1982) Continuous passive motion and the repair of full-thickness articular cartilage defects: A one-year follow-up. *Trans. Orthop. Res. Soc.* **7**, 167.

Salter, R.B., Simmonds, D.F., Malcolm, B.W., *et al.* (1980) The biological effect of continuous passive motion on healing of full-thickness defects in articular cartilage: An experimental study in the rabbit. *J. Bone Joint Surg.* **62A**, 1232–51.

Schultz, R.J., Krishnamurthy, S., Thelmo, W., *et al.* (1985) Effects of varying intensities of laser energy on articular cartilage: A preliminary study. *Lasers Surg. Med.* **5**, 577–88.

Speer, D.P., Chvapil, M., Volz, R.G., *et al.* (1979) Enhancement of healing in osteochondral defects by collagen sponge implants. *Clin. Orthop.* **144**, 326–35.

Vailas, A.C., Tipton, C.M., Matthes, R.D., *et al.* (1981) Physical activity and its influence on the repair process of medial collateral ligaments. *Connect. Tiss. Res.* **9**, 25–31.

Chapter 6

Muscle–Tendon Unit Injuries

THOMAS M. BEST AND WILLIAM E. GARRETT Jr

Soft-tissue injuries continue to challenge the investigative efforts of both the clinician and the basic scientist. Injury to the muscle–tendon unit resulting from athletics can occur via a number of mechanisms. An understanding of the basis for these injuries represents an important first step towards prevention. The following discussion outlines our current understanding of the pathophysiology, anatomical and functional considerations regarding athletic injuries to the muscle–tendon unit.

Structure

Skeletal muscle constitutes the single largest tissue mass in the body comprising 40–45% of the total body weight. In general, muscle originates from bone or dense connective tissue, either directly, or from a tendon of origin. The muscle fibres themselves pass distally, usually to a tendon of insertion which will connect with bone. A muscle–tendon unit can cross one, two or more joints. In general, muscles which cross one joint are located close to bone and are frequently more involved in postural or tonic activity, e.g. soleus. Morphologically, they are broad and flat possessing a decreased speed of contraction but increased strength (force output) when compared with the two-joint muscles. The two-joint or phasic muscles lie more superficial within a compartment. Examples include the gastrocnemius which is more superficial than the soleus and the rectus femoris which is the most superficial of the quadriceps group. Compared with one-joint muscles they have a greater speed of shortening and capacity for length change, however they are less effective in producing tension over the full range of motion.

Architecture

The muscle fibre is the basic structural unit of skeletal muscle and the sarcomere is the smallest contractile unit of the fibre. These fibres are grouped into small bundles or fascicles which are usually oriented obliquely to the longitudinal axis. Consequently, fibre arrangement within the muscle is quite variable and a large number of configurations can be seen including: (i) fusiform; (ii) parallel; (iii) unipennate; (iv) bipennate; and (v) multipennate. In general, fusiform muscles permit the greatest range of motion. Pennate muscles are typically more powerful (force of contraction) than parallel-fibred muscles of the same weight because their organization allows a larger number of fibres to work in parallel.

A fibrous connective tissue network within the muscle includes the epimysium (whole muscle), perimysium (each bundle of fibres), and the individual fibres themselves (endomysium). This framework is continuous within the muscle and attaches into the tendon of insertion. The muscle–tendon junction (MTJ) represents an essential element in the mechanical linkage between force generating myofilaments and force transmitting collagen fibres.

71

Structural studies have shown that the muscle cell surface is highly folded at its termination in the tendon which leads to a reduction in the stress (force/unit area) at the MTJ (Tidball, 1984). It is also of interest that the sarcomeres near the MTJ are stiffer than those throughout the rest of the muscle fibre (Huxley & Peachey, 1961). This finding has been offered by some as an explanation for the localization of strain injuries to the MTJ.

Ultrastructure

Figure 6.1 is a typical electronmicrograph of skeletal muscle. The banded arrangement is due to the repetition of dark and light bands. By electronmicroscopy the dark bands are seen as thick filaments with small projections or cross-bridges extending from the filament. The primary constituent protein of the thick filament is myosin. The light band is comprised of thin filaments whose chief protein is actin. The A-band gets its name from the fact that it is anisotropic to polarized light while the I-band is isotropic. The basic functional unit of skeletal muscle is the sarcomere which extends from one Z-band to the next and is further divided into I-bands and A-bands. The Z-band is composed of at least four proteins: alpha actinin, desmin, filamin, and zeugmatin. The I-band contains actin, tropomyosin, and troponin; the A-band consists of myosin and the actin–tropomyosin–troponin complex. With contraction and muscle shortening the light bands get narrower a d the dark bands do not change in length. Finally, there is a region near the centre of the A-band termed the H-zone. In the centre of the H-zone is the M-line.

Regulation of skeletal muscle contraction is accomplished primarily by calcium ions stored in the membrane-bound areas of the cytoplasm known as the sarcoplasmic reticulum. The sarcoplasmic reticulum has two distinct units, the longitudinal tubules and the transverse tubular system. The latter bisects the longitudinal tubules which expand out to form two large lateral sacs in the region of the Z-line. The two lateral sacs and their corresponding transverse tubule are collectively referred to as a triad.

An action potential passes over the sarcolemma and into the transverse tubule system. Excitation spreads longitudinally into the sacs resulting in an increase in calcium permeability and a release of calcium ions into the sarcoplasm. This free calcium binds to the regulatory proteins permitting interaction of the thick and thin filaments. When the Ca^{2+} approaches 10^{-5} mol, tropomyosin binds to its target protein, troponin-C, and allosteric conformational changes in the troponin–tropomyosin complex

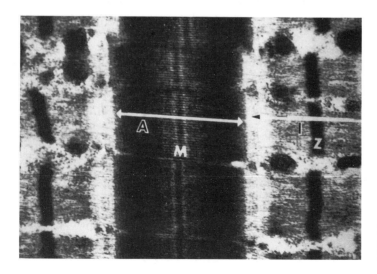

Fig. 6.1 Electron micrograph of skeletal muscle. A, A-band; I, I-band; M, M-line; Z, Z-band.

result with movement of the tropomyosin further back into the grooves. Following completion of the electrical event, relaxation of the muscle occurs by active transport of calcium into the longitudinal tubules of the sarcoplasmic reticulum. This results in calcium dissociation from troponin, allowing the tropomyosin molecule to snap back into the groove, where it prevents any further cross-bridge attachment.

Fibre types

Different striated muscles exhibit significant structural variations at both the histological and ultrastructural levels. There are also differences in innervation, physiology, biochemistry and circulation. Two major classes of fibre types are recognized as being structurally, physiologically and metabolically distinct (Gauthier, 1986). The type I, slow-twitch oxidative fibres (SO), have the slowest contraction time and the lowest content of glycogen and glycolytic enzymes. They are rich in mitochondria and myoglobin and are quite fatigue-resistant. Morphologically, their sarcomeres contain a wide Z-band. The type IIa or fast-twitch oxidative fibres (FOG) have a faster contraction time than the type I fibres. In addition, they have a higher content of mitochondria and myoglobin than type IIb fibres. Physiologically, they are more fatigue-resistant than the type IIb fibres. Also, they have high myosin adenosine triphosphate (ATPase) and glycogen levels, oxidative enzymes, and glycogen content. Morphologically, their Z-bands are slightly narrower than in the type I fibres. The type IIa fibre is termed an intermediate fibre because it possesses both forms of myosin present in the type I and IIb fibres. Most mammalian carnivores, including humans, also possess a type IIc or superfast fibre which is most prominent in the jaw muscles. It possesses a unique myosin that can be distinguished from both the slow and fast types of type I and type II fibres. At birth, up to 10% of muscle fibres can be type IIc; this declines to about 2% after the first year. Therefore, many regard the IIc fibre as an undifferentiated fibre (Gollnick & Saltin, 1989). Interestingly enough, during physical training there may be as many as 10% of these fibres present in some muscles of endurance athletes (Gollnick & Saltin, 1989).

Biochemically, the structural proteins of the sarcomere are also distinct. Myosin, tropomyosin and troponin have distinct isomers in the different fibre types (Lowey & Risby, 1971; Cummins & Perry, 1978). Recent investigations have shown more heterogeneity in these proteins than had been previously expected. Rather than three distinct fibre types, there appears to be a discrete number of basic sets of structural protein isomers for the fast and slow muscles (Gollnick & Saltin, 1989).

Although most muscles in humans have a mean fibre composition of 50% slow-twitch (ST) and 50% fast-twitch (FT), some muscles like the soleus and triceps brachii have a predominance of either ST or FT fibres. The tonic or postural muscles are usually situated closer to the bony skeleton and have a greater proportion of type I fibres, e.g. soleus. In contrast, the phasic or faster contracting muscles lie more on the surface and have a higher proportion of type II fibres (Johnson et al., 1973). These findings have implications regarding human muscular performance. People with higher percentages of type II fibres in the quadriceps are able to generate more knee extensor forces than those with fewer type II fibres (Thorstensson et al., 1976a). Similarly, athletes who demonstrated excellence in sprint events had a relatively higher percentage of type II fibres while élite distance runners had predominantly type I fibres (Komi et al., 1977; Saltin et al., 1977).

Muscle injuries

Skeletal muscle injury can result from both traumatic (e.g. contusion) and atraumatic (e.g. mechanical strain) conditions and can include muscle fibre damage, connective tissue disruption, complete rupture of the muscle, blood vessel damage and occasionally nerve injury.

Muscle cramps

Ordinary muscle cramps are common during and following exercise and are frequent even in healthy young people not involved in athletics. They occur most commonly in the gastro-cnemius complex and their aetiology remains uncertain. It is well known that their onset frequently follows contraction of shortened muscles. The cramp often originates as a fasciculation from a single focus or several distinct foci within the muscle and spreads throughout the muscle in an irregular pattern. Electro-myographic studies reveal fascicular twitching in a single focus followed by very high frequency discharges within the muscle fibres (Denny-Brown, 1953). The electrical activity reveals that the entire motor unit is involved and, therefore, the initiating source is within the motor nerve fibre rather than within individual muscle fibres themselves.

Exercise studies have mainly looked at ultra-endurance athletes. Maughan (1986) followed 90 competitors at the 1982 Aberdeen marathon and found no correlation between hydration status and electrolyte balance and the incidence of muscle cramps. In another study, Kanto-rowska et al. (1990) followed athletes at the 1989 Ironman Championship. Despite more extreme environmental conditions than in Maughan's study, there was no correlation between de-hydration and incidence of muscle cramping.

Excessive sweating or diuresis can cause saline and may produce cramps. Renal failure patients on chronic haemodialysis often have muscle cramps. These conditions may be related by an alteration of sodium concentrations and administration of a saline solution is sometimes helpful. Lowered levels of serum calcium or magnesium have also been implicated (Denny-Brown, 1953). Neither of these ionic disturbances are necessarily present in muscle cramps following exercise.

Clinically, a muscle cramp can usually be interrupted by forceful stretching of the involved muscle or activation of the antagonistic muscle. Following resolution of the knotted and painful contraction, the muscle shows evidence of altered excitability and fasciculations for many minutes following the cramp. The muscle can also be painful for several days after the event. Correction of electrolyte and water disturbances is thought to be helpful. Although adequate water and supplemental sodium may be given empirically, the value of this treatment is not proven.

Delayed-onset muscle soreness

Muscle pain following unaccustomed intense exercise is common and is especially pronounced following initiation or resumption of training after a period of time without training. This should be distinguished from discomfort which occurs during exercise that is often associated with muscle fatigue and is metabolic in origin. Typically, delayed-onset muscle soreness (DOMS) begins a number of hours after exercise and peaks on the second day after activity. The painful areas are noted to be along the tendon or fascial connections within the muscle.

Several pathological mechanisms have been proposed to explain DOMS. Many of the concepts were introduced by Hough who distinguished the pain associated with the immediate fatigue of exercise from the pain in the muscle noted 1–2 days following exercise (1902). The delayed pain did not necessarily follow more fatiguing work and exercise routines producing considerable fatigue did not produce as much delayed-onset muscle pain. However, rhythmic contractions which were marked by high intensity and relatively little fatigue, were much more likely to be associated with delayed soreness. Based on these findings, Hough proposed that DOMS was associated more with the amount of tension developed in the muscle than with fatigue.

Asmussen gave support to the above when negative or eccentric work was shown to produce more DOMS than positive work despite much greater fatigue induced by positive work (1956). It was concluded that the pain was due primarily to mechanical stress rather than fatigue and metabolic waste products. He also felt that the connective tissue within the muscle, rather than the muscle fibres themselves, might be the location of the injury. Abraham (1977) investigated the hypothesis that there might be connective tissue breakdown associated with DOMS by monitoring hydroxyproline levels. It has been shown that excretion of hydroxyproline in the urine is an index of the rate of collagen degradation (Prockop & Sjoerdsma, 1961). Following a weightlifting programme there was a significant increase in urinary hydroxyproline in those subjects experiencing DOMS. Elevated levels of myoglobin excretion were also noted, but the elevated levels occurred in both the subjects who developed pain and in those subjects who did not develop pain. Thus, there was a correlation between muscle soreness and collagen breakdown. In contrast, it has been shown that blood lactic acid concentration measured from the serum is not related to exercise-induced DOMS (Armstrong, 1984). Exercise does create a significant increase in serum muscular enzymes and myoglobin, but these values usually remain within normal limits and are not different in subjects exhibiting soreness and subjects without soreness (Besson et al., 1981). For example, although the release of creatine kinase (CK) from skeletal muscle following eccentric exercise is a commonly observed phenomenon, circulating CK activity is not a quantitative, and, in some cases, a qualitative indication of skeletal muscle damage. An alternative theory of muscle soreness implicates muscle spasm and electrical activity as the cause of the pain rather than connective tissue breakdown (Kraus, 1959; DeVries, 1966).

DeVries proposed that exercise produces ischaemia which subsequently causes pain. Pain initiates reflex tonic muscle contraction prolonging ischaemia and promoting a vicious cycle. Stretching of the muscle diminished the pain and likewise the electromyographic activity. Kraus (1941) advocated the use of surface anaesthesia to interrupt the pain spasm. Abraham (1977) reinvestigated the electromyographic data and was unable to show significant changes in subjects with and without muscle soreness. The weight of the evidence, therefore, seems to be with the advocates of the 'torn tissue' theory of muscle damage as a cause of DOMS. However, it is still possible that electromyographic changes may accompany the tears in the tissue and treatment altering the muscle spasm or electromyographic manifestation might be of benefit in treating DOMS.

Recent studies of DOMS have investigated changes on an ultrastructural level (Fig. 6.2). Electronmicroscopy of muscle in subjects with pain in the vastus lateralis following cycling showed significant changes in the sarcomere and the cross-striated pattern (Friden et al., 1983b). Lesions were localized to the Z-band, suggesting that this area may be the weak link in the chain of contractile units. It was also found that one bout of eccentric exercise produces an adaptation such that the incidence for muscle soreness and myofibrillar lesions is reduced when performing a second bout of the same exercise 2 weeks later (Friden et al., 1983a). Other authors have confirmed similar findings and also noted I-band disorganization and mitochondrial swelling (Armstrong, 1984). T2-weighted magnetic resonance images (MRI) have demonstrated that muscle damage may persist despite a return of muscle function to baseline values (Shellock et al., 1991).

Oxygen-derived free radicals, resulting in increased lipid peroxidation, have recently been suggested as mediators of adaptation to exercise as well as involvement in skeletal muscle damage following eccentric exercise (Jenkins, 1988). Although agents involved in free radical metabolism have been studied to attenuate the development of muscle injury, studies have yielded conflicting results (McBrine et al., 1991; Statt et al., 1991).

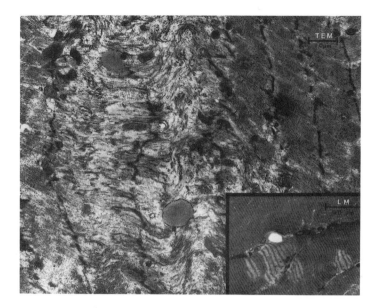

Fig. 6.2 Transmission electron micrograph (TEM) and light microscope (LM) views of injured rat soleus muscle fibres immediately after downhill walking. Note the A-band disruption and Z-band damage. TEM micrograph courtesy of Dr R.W. Ogilvie; LM micrograph courtesy of Dr R.B. Armstrong *et al.*, with permission of publisher.

Muscle contusions

Direct trauma to muscle is a common athletic injury resulting in damage and often partial disruption of muscle fibres with a frequently associated intramuscular haematoma. The quadriceps and gastrocnemius are most prone to these injuries which are typically character-ized by diffuse swelling or a discrete haema-toma, and limitation of motion and strength.

QUADRICEPS CONTUSIONS

Jackson and Feagin (1973) reviewed the quad-riceps injuries occurring in military cadets and found them to be a significant cause of dis-ability. Similar results were reported by Ryan (1969). The possible pathological mechanisms have been described, although there are few scientific data to confirm these hypotheses The treatment regimen generally includes rest and ice with an early return to gentle motion (Jackson & Feagin, 1973). Active and passive motion should be emphasized and care is necessary in therapy to avoid reinjury. A recent study (Aronen *et al.*, 1990) has offered promise for treatment by immobilization in 120° of knee flexion for the first 24 h following the injury. The average time for return to full ath-letic activity was reduced from 18 to 3.5 days.

MYOSITIS OSSIFICANS

An unfortunate complication of muscle con-tusions is myositis ossificans, the calcification or actual ossification of the tissue at the site of injury. The pathogenesis of this heterotopic bone formation is poorly understood. It is radio-logically evident 2–4 weeks following a severe contusion and is often connected to the under-lying bone (Jackson & Feagin, 1973). In one study, heterotopic bone was present in approxi-mately 20% of patients with a quadriceps haematoma (Rothwell, 1982).

The mass may enlarge or be symptomatic for several months before stabilizing. It is im-portant to be aware of the association of the mass and roentgenographic appearance of this condition with a previous contusion because the condition can also mimic osteogenic sar-coma (Fig. 6.3). The histological features may also be similar if a biopsy is performed early in the course of myositis ossificans. The hetero-topic bone may resorb with time. Recovery of normal function is possible even with the pres-ence of myositis ossificans but the recovery

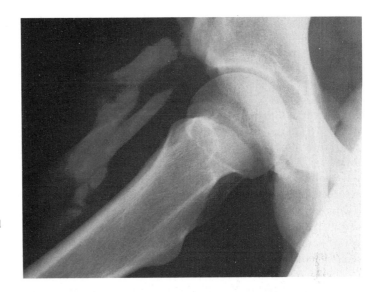

Fig. 6.3 X-ray of myositis ossificans of the rectus femoris. This 22-year-old patient suffered a quadriceps contusion which resulted in the above condition. The resultant heterotopic bone gradually resorbed over time.

period is longer than that following an uncomplicated contusion. No specific treatment is recommended in addition to the treatment for contusions. Specifically, early surgery is to be avoided because it may exacerbate the heterotopic bone formation and prolong disability. Surgery might be considered late in the course of the disease to remove the heterotopic bone if it is causing symptoms (Hughston *et al.*, 1962). In general, surgery should be considered only if the presence of the bone mass is causing symptoms; this does not occur frequently. Surgery should be considered only after the heterotopic bone is mature and no changes are occurring in the orthopaedic and radiological evaluation of the patient.

Compartment syndromes

Much interest has been directed to the diagnosis, management and pathophysiological basis for compartment syndromes. This entity is characterized by increased interstitial pressure within an anatomically confined muscle compartment which interferes with the circulation and function of the muscle and the neurovascular components of the compartment. Most frequently, transient ischaemia is the inciting factor as it causes muscle oedema once circu-

lation is restored. Haemorrhage within the compartment or direct trauma to muscle can also cause pressure elevation or a compartment syndrome. If the entity is recognized then the elevated pressure may be relieved (usually by incising the investing fascia) and the circulation and function of the compartmental muscles and neurovascular components can be restored.

The pathophysiology of compartment syndrome has been investigated by a number of laboratories (Hargens & Akeson, 1981). Increased pressure in the compartment results from increased fluid which can be due to haemorrhage, intracellular or extracellular oedema. Threshold pressures above which significant muscle damage can occur have been proposed to be 30–40 mmHg (Hargens & Akeson, 1981) or to within 10–30 mmHg of diastolic blood pressure (Whitesides *et al.*, 1975).

When the intracompartmental pressure reaches elevated levels, it is felt that capillary perfusion is compromised and the muscle within the compartment is subject to ischaemic injury. The level of pressure necessary to interfere with capillary circulation will not necessarily occlude major arteries running through the compartments. Therefore, the presence of a pulse distal to the compartment will not rule out the presence of a compartment syndrome. Clinical evaluation relies on pain, particularly with active extension of the limb, increased compartment pressure noted with palpation, and altered nervous function as noted by parenthaesias in the sensory distribution of nerves within the compartment. Abnormalities in nerve function with increasing intracompartmental pressure have been demonstrated (Matsen *et al.*, 1977).

Acute compartment syndromes have been associated with a variety of athletic injuries (Kennedy & Roth, 1979). Direct trauma to bone or soft tissue is most frequently noted. Soccer players appear to be at particular risk from direct trauma to the lower extremities. The use of shin guards has been advocated by many as a means of reducing the potential of these injuries. A review by Mubarak (1981) stresses the association of compartment syndromes with fractures. Tibial shaft fractures comprise a large proportion of those fractures leading to compartment syndromes. Direct soft-tissue injury and muscle trauma can also result in elevated pressure and compromise tissue perfusion. The cause of the increased pressure can be oedema, haemorrhage or a combination of the two. In addition to direct trauma, indirect injury due to exertion is well recognized as a cause of compartment syndromes. The indirect injuries can be acute or chronic. They have been well reviewed by Veith (1980) and Mubarak (1981). The acute syndromes are not well understood. Intense muscular activity alone causes a large rise in the interstitial pressure which might prevent normal capillary perfusion. Intermittent pressure levels of greater than 100 mmHg are common during some forms of exercise (McDermott *et al.*, 1982). As a result, muscle perfusion will be possible only intermittently when the pressure falls between muscular contractions. Increasing exercise causes a muscle volume increase which may be as large as 20% associated with increased blood content and intracompartmental fluid accumulation. The increased fluid component will likely raise tissue pressure measurements at rest as well.

Therefore, the combination of intermittent high pressure associated with muscle activity and elevated rest pressure due to compartment fluid expansion can predispose an athlete to an acute compartment syndrome.

Acute exertional or exercise-related compartment syndromes are not common (Mubarak, 1981). They are usually associated with intense muscular activity particularly in individuals unaccustomed to such activity as in military recruits. They are associated with muscle activity and elevated rest pressure due to compartment fluid expansion and can predispose an athlete to an acute compartment syndrome. Treatment should include decompression of the muscle and neurovascular components by fascial release. The *chronic exertional compartment syndromes* are more frequent clinically than the acute form. The presenting complaints are usually those of pain or a deep ache over the anterior or lateral compartments. The discomfort usually occurs after a relatively long exercise period and is usually severe enough to cause the athlete either to cease activity or to reduce the intensity of the exercise. The symptoms are often bilateral (Reneman, 1975; Sudmann, 1979; Rorabeck *et al.*, 1982). Sensory changes may also be present. Occasionally muscle hernias may also be present and the hernias may be near the fascial opening through which the distal branch of the superficial peroneal nerve passes to reach the subcutaneous tissue.

Chronic or recurrent compartment syndrome is a difficult clinical diagnosis. The primary characteristic of the chronic condition is pressure elevation above normal during exercise and a slower return to resting value at the end of exercise (Veith, 1980). Treatment of chronic or recurrent compartment syndrome has been elective fasciotomy of a single compartment if conservative measures and activity alteration are unsuccessful (Veith, 1980; Mubarak, 1981; Rorabeck *et al.*, 1982). Postoperative results in a relatively small number of cases have been gratifying subjectively and pressure measurements have returned close to normal (Rorabeck,

1982). One should be aware that fascial release may adversely affect the strength of a muscle and, therefore, procedures should not be advocated without accurate diagnosis and counselling (Garfin *et al.*, 1981).

Medial tibial syndrome or 'shin splints' refers to exercise-related pain localized to the medial aspect of the distal third of the tibia and had been ascribed to a recurrent deep posterior compartment syndrome (Puranen, 1974; Bryk, 1983). However, objective pressure measurements within the anterior and posterior compartments have not shown any pressure elevation (D'Ambrosia *et al.*, 1977). The entity of 'shin splints' or medial tibial syndrome is most likely due to a stress reaction of the bone or muscle origin from the bone in response to repetitive use. The condition is characterized by pain along the medial aspect of the tibia coursing the junction of muscle and tendon to bone. It is frequently found in athletes running long distances on hard surfaces. It is also more common in athletes with significant hindfoot valgus and midfoot pronation, often called 'flat-footed'.

Muscle strain injuries

The clinical significance of stretch-induced muscle injuries or 'strains' is readily apparent to those treating occupational or sport-related problems and is often cited as the most frequent injury in sports (Ryan, 1969; Krejci & Kock, 1979; Glick, 1980; Peterson & Renström, 1986). Without a firm understanding of the mechanisms and pathophysiology, it has been difficult to find consensus on methods of preventing or treating these often debilitating problems.

Muscle strain injuries are caused by stretching or a combination of muscle activation and stretching. Clinical studies agree that muscle strain injuries occur in response to forcibly stretching a muscle either passively or, more often, when the muscle is activated

(Krejci & Kock, 1979; Zarins & Ciullo, 1983). These injuries most often occur during eccentric activation where the muscle may be more prone to injury for several reasons (Glick, 1980; Peterson & Renström, 1986). If muscle is injured by excessive force development in the muscle—tendon unit, higher forces are possible with eccentric action (Zarins & Ciullo, 1983). It has been shown that active muscle force production can be significantly higher when muscle is being stretched while activated than when muscle is held at the same length or allowed to shorten. In addition, more force is produced by the passive or connective tissue element of muscle as it is being stretched. It is believed that the passive force provides little resistance until enough stretch is applied to the muscle.

Muscles at risk for injury usually include the two-joint muscles, i.e. muscles which cross two or more joints and are therefore subject to stretch at more than one joint (Brewer, 1960). A frequent characteristic of these muscles is their ability to limit the range of motion of a joint because of the intrinsic tightness in the muscle, e.g. hamstring muscles can limit knee extension when the hip is flexed. Similarly, the gastrocnemius can limit ankle dorsiflexion when the knee is extended. Another characteristic of muscles at risk for injury is that they often function in an eccentric manner as they are used in sport. Much of the muscle action involved with running or sprinting is eccentric. For instance, the hamstrings act not so much to flex the knee as to decelerate knee extension during running. Similarly, the quadriceps act as much to prevent knee flexion as to power knee extension in running (Inman *et al.*, 1981).

Epidemiological studies reveal that muscle strain injuries occur most often in sprinting or other activities of high velocity. They are more common in sports and positions requiring bursts of speed or rapid acceleration such as track and field, football, basketball, Rugby or soccer (Peterson & Renström, 1986). Another functional characteristic of the muscles most susceptible to injury is their relatively high percentage of type II fibres (Garrett *et al.*, 1984a).

These muscles are generally more superficial in the extremities and cross two or more joints.

Clinical data are relatively sparse regarding the exact nature of changes in muscle following strain injury. The injury can be partial or complete, the latter characterized by muscle asymmetry at rest when compared to the contralateral contour. With contraction, a muscle will demonstrate a bulge towards the side of the muscle–tendon unit which is still attached to bone.

Muscle strain injuries can be distinguished clinically from DOMS. A strain injury is an acute and usually painful event which is recognized by the patient as an injury. DOMS is a condition characterized by muscle pain often 12–24 h after exercise and usually without a single identifiable injury (Hough, 1902; Armstrong, 1984). The two conditions are alike in that they are more prone to occur with eccentric exercise (Asmussen, 1956; Friden et al., 1983b; Schwane et al., 1983). Incomplete injuries are characterized more by focal pain and swelling. In both injuries, passive stretching and active contraction of the affected region will cause discomfort. DOMS may therefore be a condition that represents an incomplete strain injury at the MTJ.

The location of pathological changes in a muscle following strain injury has only been defined recently. The vulnerable site appears to be near the MTJ or near the tendon–bone junction (Garrett & Tidball, 1987). Injuries involving the muscle belly itself appear to have a strong predilection to occur near the MTJ, but not precisely at the true histological junction. Although surgical exploration of muscle injuries is not routinely performed, there are a number of references regarding the surgical findings. These studies confirm tears near the muscle–tendon junction in:

1 The gastrocnemius medial head (often incorrectly called plantaris rupture) (Durig et al., 1977; Miller, 1977).
2 The rectus femoris muscle (Rask & Lattig, 1972).
3 The triceps brachii muscle (Bach et al., 1987).
4 The adductor longus muscle (Symeonides, 1972).
5 The pectoralis major muscle (Peterson & Stener, 1976).
6 The semimembranosus muscle (Krejci & Koch, 1979).

More recently, high-resolution imaging studies have localized acute hamstring injuries to the region of the muscle–tendon junction (Fig. 6.4). It is often surprising to clinicians to realize the size of the MTJ in humans. The hamstring muscles, for example, have an extended MTJ in the posterior thigh. The proximal tendon and muscle–tendon junctions of the biceps femoris long head and the semimem-

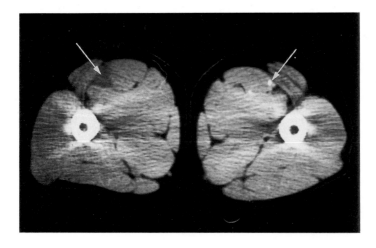

Fig. 6.4 Acute left biceps femoris muscle strain and chronic right hamstring injury. A prone axial CT image of the proximal thighs in this patient demonstrates an area of low density in the region of the long head of the left biceps femoris muscle, typical of an acute muscle strain. Calcifications are noted in the comparable muscle group on the right side likely due to an old injury in this patient. From Garrett et al. (1989).

branosus extend well over half the total length of these muscles.

Bleeding often occurs following muscle strain injuries; however, it usually takes one or more days following the event to detect subcutaneous ecchymosis. Blood collections within the subcutaneous tissue demonstrate that the bleeding is not confined to the muscle proper; rather it escapes through the perimysium and fascia to the subcutaneous space. Computed tomography has shown that there is an inflammatory or oedematous response within the muscle tissue itself (Garrett *et al.*, 1989). In certain instances it appears that bleeding can occur and a haematoma can collect between the muscle tissue and the surrounding fascial compartment (Fornage *et al.*, 1983). In direct muscular contusion bleeding often occurs within the midsubstance (Rothwell, 1982; Rooser, 1988).

Laboratory studies investigating the pathophysiology and mechanisms of muscle strain injury were first performed by McMaster who demonstrated that normal tendon did not rupture in the gastrocnemius muscle—tendon unit of rabbits. Failure occurred at the bone—tendon junction, the myotendinous junction or within the muscle (McMaster, 1933). Initial experiments in our laboratory demonstrated that muscle activation by nerve stimulation alone did not cause complete or incomplete disruption (Almekinders *et al.*, 1984a,b). There was a reduction of force and failure of excitation occurred, but no disruption of the muscle—tendon unit resulted. In order to obtain gross or microscopic muscle injury, stretch of the muscle was required. The forces produced at the time of muscle failure even without muscle activation were several times the maximum isometric force produced by the activated muscles (Garrett *et al.*, 1988b). This demonstrated that passive forces within the muscle might be as important as the active forces involved in muscle strain injury.

The effects of passive stretch in muscle with varied fibre architectural arrangements has been studied (Garrett *et al.*, 1988b). Muscles were stretched from either the proximal or distal tendon at 1, 10 or 100 cm·min^{-1}. Failure consistently occurred near the MTJ, usually distally. A 0.1–1 mm piece of muscle was left attached to the tendon. Subsequent studies have confirmed similar findings at strain rates to 10 cm·s^{-1} (LeCroy *et al.*, 1989). Although the above strain rates may be somewhat slower than those expected in normal locomotion or in sudden limb movements of the rabbit, these findings do indicate the involvement of the MTJ in strain injury.

Classic electrophysiological studies of muscle have demonstrated that the active force production of muscle is proportional to crosssectional area of the muscle fibres while shortening ability is proportional to the length of the muscle fibre. These concepts have been applied to human muscle performance (Wickiewicz *et al.*, 1983). It was felt that the biomechanical factors of muscle in response to stretch might also be related to fibre length. However, the amount of strain based on fibre lengths varied widely from 75 to 225% of the resting fibre length. Previous studies have shown that the ends of the muscle fibres near the MTJ do not undergo as much strain as the more central areas of the fibres (Grana & Schelberg-Karnes, 1983). At this time it is not certain why the ends of the fibres near the MTJ behave differently and are more susceptible to injury. A recent study attempted to localize more accurately the site of injury (Reddy *et al.*, 1991). It was found that 60 min postinjury, ruptured fibres had hypercontracted sarcomeres within 100 μm of the rupture site, both proximal and distal to the injury. Sarcomere length gradually increased away from the rupture site and normalized by about 500 μm. Fibres evaluated 6 h postinjury showed evidence of necrosis prior to transition to normal sarcomere spacing. The presence of severe hypercontraction in the 60-min fibres and eventual necrosis in the 6-h fibres was felt to suggest an ongoing, calcium-induced injury process. Regardless of the time following injury, sarcomere length had normalized by about 500 μm from the site of rupture, suggesting that a protective or reparative barrier effectively restricted the injury response to a small distance from the initial site of rupture. It was concluded that Ca^{2+} influx into the cell was responsible for the injury. This finding is of clinical interest as there is at least one study on patients with unclassified exertional muscle pain syndrome (EMPS) showing that administration of verapamil resulted in an improvement of symptoms in 50% of the patients (Lane *et al.*, 1986).

Experiments have been performed to measure the biomechanical properties of stimulated muscle (Garrett *et al.*, 1988b). The total strain prior to failure did not differ under conditions of tetanic stimulation, submaximal stimulation or passive stretch to failure. The force generated at failure was only about 15% higher in stimulated muscles, however, the energy absorbed was approximately 100% higher in muscles stretched while activated. These data confirm the importance of considering muscles as energy absorbers. This concept helps explain the ability of muscles to reduce injury to themselves as well as the supporting joint structures. There are two components capable of absorbing energy within a muscle. The passive component is not dependent on muscle activation and is a property that is due to the connective tissue elements within the muscle including the muscle fibres themselves and the connective tissue associated with the cell surface as well as between fibres. In addition, there is a further ability to absorb energy based on the contractile mechanism of the muscle. Therefore, conditions which decrease the muscle's contractile ability might diminish the ability of muscle to absorb energy. It has long been felt that conditions which result in muscle fatigue will lead to an increased incidence of muscle injuries (Krejci & Koch, 1979). This theory is supported by two laboratory studies showing that fatigued muscle, defined as an inability to generate contractile force, results in a reduction of load to failure and energy absorption prior to failure properties of the muscle (Chow *et al.*, 1990; Mair *et al.*, 1991).

Previous work has documented the physio-logical and histological recovery of muscle after non-disruptive stretch-induced injury (Nikolaou *et al.*, 1987). Acutely, these injuries are marked by disruption and haemorrhage within the muscle. By 24–48 h after the injury, an inflammatory reaction becomes pronounced and invading inflammatory cells and oedema are present. By the seventh day, the inflammatory reaction is being replaced by fibrous tissue. Although some regenerating muscle fibres are present, normal histology is not restored and scar tissue is persistent. Immediately following the injury, the muscle produced 70% of normal force production. By 24 h only 50% of normal force production was recorded. Recovery then followed and by 7 days was 90% complete (Fig. 6.5). These results were confirmed in a later study evaluating the effect of non-steroidal anti-inflammatory drugs on healing muscle injuries (Obremskey *et al.*, 1988). These studies demonstrate that the recovery of contractile ability is relatively rapid. It may be that the initial loss of function can be attributed to the haemorrhage and oedema at the site of injury.

The tensile strength of muscle following a non-disruptive strain has also been evaluated (Obremskey *et al.*, 1988). Strength of unstimulated muscle recovered to only 77% of normal

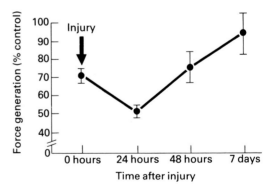

Fig. 6.5 Percent of control force generation over range of frequencies versus time after controlled passive injury: immediately after injury ($n = 30$), 24 hours ($n = 7$), 48 hours ($n = 8$) and 7 days after ($n = 8$). All values +/− s.e.m. From Nikolaou *et al.* (1987).

by 7 days, in contrast to the 90% recovery of active force generating ability. A previous injury may therefore predispose a muscle to further injury. Additional studies are needed to examine these possibilities and to develop sound scientific rationale for our treatment methods.

PREVENTION

Among the factors felt to be important in the behaviour of muscle and the prevention of injury include innate flexibility, warm-up and stretching before exercise. Usually the response of muscle to stretching has been explained on a neurophysiological basis with reference to stretch reflexes (Holt, 1981; Solveborn, 1983). Much less is known about the mechanical behaviour of muscle stretching in a manner that pertains to current athletic and rehabilitation regimens of muscle stretch.

Biological tissues, including skeletal muscle, exhibit complex time- and history-dependent behaviour under applied load. Stress relaxation (a decline in stress over time under a constant deformation) and creep (an increase in deformation over time under a constant load) are important properties of these viscoelastic materials. In addition, the stress−strain history is non-linear. Recent studies have suggested that these properties may have important clinical as well as physiological significance in the prevention of muscle strain injury (Best et al., 1989; Dalton et al., 1990; Taylor et al., 1990).

Stretching is often prescribed as a means of reducing the incidence of muscle injuries during exercise (Beaulieu, 1981; Holt, 1981; Stanish, 1982; Wiktorsson-Moller et al., 1983). Recent laboratory studies have investigated this theory and found that passive stretch of the muscle−tendon unit can alter its failure properties (Best et al., 1989; Dalton et al., 1990; Taylor et al., 1990). Skeletal muscle, like other soft tissues, demonstrates significant stress relaxation. This stress relaxation is greatest during the early part of the applied stretch and approaches an asymptomatic limit with time

(Taylor et al., 1990). The exact mechanism by which these changes occur is unknown, although the adaptation was brought about independent of any reflex influences or other influences mediated by the central nervous system (Taylor et al., 1990). These results suggest that a series of stretches applied over a short period of time would result in greater adaptation than one longer stretch. More work is needed both in the laboratory and clinically to confirm these theories. In another study, a potential mechanism by which passive stretch protects muscle from strain injury has been evaluated (Best et al., 1989). In muscles undergoing a series of stretches, there was an increase in the force required to rupture the muscle as well as an increase in the length at which the muscle failed. Thus, stretching appears to have significant effects on muscle both at physiological lengths where stress relaxation effects predominate, and at highly stretched lengths, where the failure properties of muscle can be altered. These studies offer promise about the potential benefits of stretching and muscle injury prevention. Further studies are needed before specific recommendations can be given.

Acknowledgments

This work was supported in part by a grant from the Medical Research Council of Canada.

References

Abraham, W.M. (1977) Factors in delayed muscle soreness. *Med. Sci. Sports Exerc.* **9**, 11−20.

Almekinders, L.C., Garrett, W.E. & Seaber, A.V. (1984a) Histopathology of muscle tears in stretching injuries. *Trans. Orthop. Res. Soc.* **9**, 306.

Almekinders, L.C., Garrett, W.E. & Seaber, A.V. (1984b) Pathophysiologic response to muscle tears in stretching injuries. *Trans. Orthop. Res. Soc.* **9**, 307.

Armstrong, R.B. (1984) Mechanisms of exercise-induced delayed onset muscular soreness: A brief review. *Med. Sci. Sports Exerc.* **16**(6), 529−38.

Aronen, J.A., Chronister, R., Ove, P. & McDevitt, E.R. (1990) *Thigh contusions: minimizing the length of time before return to full athletic activities with early im-*

mobilization in 120 degrees of knee flexion. Presented at the American Orthopaedic Society for Sports Medicine, Sixteenth Annual Meeting, Sun Valley, Idaho, July 16–19.

Asmussen, E. (1956) Observations on experimental muscular soreness. *Acta Rheum. Scand.* **2**, 109–16.

Bach, B.R., Warren, R.F. & Wickiewicz, T.L. (1987) Triceps rupture: a case report and literature review. *Am. J. Sports Med.* **15**(3), 285–9.

Beaulieu, J.E. (1981) Developing a stretching program. *Phys. Sportsmed.* **9**(11), 59–65.

Besson, C., Rochcongar, P., Beauverger, Y., Dassonvill, J., Aubree, M. & Catheline, M. (1981) Study of the valuations of serum muscular enzymes and myoglobin after maximal exercise test and during the next 24 hours. *Eur. J. Appl. Physiol.* **47**, 47–56.

Best, T.M., Glisson, R.R., Seaber, A.V. & Garrett, W.E. (1989) The response of muscle–tendon units of varying architecture to cyclic passive stretching. *Trans. Orthop. Res. Soc.* **14**, 294.

Brewer, B.J. (1960) *Instructional Lecture, American Academy of Orthopaedic Surgeons*, Vol. 17, pp. 354–8. CV Mosby, St Louis.

Bryk, E. & Grantham, S.A. (1983) Shin splints: A chronic deep posterior ischemic compartmental syndrome of the leg? *Orthop. Rev.* **XII**(4), 29–40.

Chow, G.H., LeCroy, C.M., Seaber, A.V. & Garrett Jr, W.E. (1990) The effect of fatigue on muscle strain injury. *Trans. Orthop. Res. Soc.* **15**, 148.

Cummins, P. & Perry, S.V. (1978) Troponin I from human skeletal and cardiac muscles. *J. Biochem.* **171**, 251–9.

Dalton, J.D., Seaber, A.V. & Garrett Jr, W.E. (1990) The biomechanical effects of passive stretch on muscle–tendon units pulled to failure. *Trans. Orthop. Res. Soc.* **15**(2), 531.

D'Ambrosia, R.D., Zelis, R.F., Chuinard, R.G. & Wilmore, J. (1977) Interstitial pressure measurements in the anterior and posterior compartments in athletes with shin splints. *Am. J. Sports Med.* **5**(3), 127–31.

Denny-Brown, D. (1953) Seminars on neuromuscular physiology. *Am. J. Med.* Sept., 368–90.

DeVries, H.A. (1966) Quantitative electromyographic investigation of the spasm theory of muscle pain. *Am. J. Phys. Med.* **45**(3), 119–34.

Durig, M., Schuppisser, J.P., Gauer, E.F. & Muller, W. (1977) Spontaneous rupture of the gastrocnemius muscle. *Injury* **9**, 143–5.

Edgerton, V.R., Smith, J.L. & Simpson, D.R. (1975) Muscle fibre types populations of human muscles. *Histochem. J.* **19**, 257–66.

Friden, J., Seger, J., Sjostrom, M. & Ekblom, B. (1983a) Adaptive response in human skeletal muscle subjected to prolonged eccentric training. *Int. J. Sports Med.* **4**, 177–83.

Friden, J., Sjostrom, M. & Ekblom, B. (1983b) Myofibrillar damage following intense eccentric exercise in man. *Int. J. Sports Med.* **4**, 170–6.

Fornage, B.D., Tokuche, D.H., Segal, P. & Rifkin, M.D. (1983) Ultrasonography in the evaluation of muscular trauma. *J. Ultrasound Med.* **2**, 549–55.

Garfin, S.R., Tipton, C.M., Mubarak, S.J., Woo, S.L.-Y., Hargens, A.R. & Akeson, W.H. (1981) Role of fascia in maintenance of muscle tension and pressure. *J. Appl. Physiol.* **51**(2), 317–20.

Garrett Jr, W.E., Califf, J.C. & Bassett, F.H. (1984a) Histochemical correlates of hamstring injuries. *Am. J. Sports Med.* **12**(2), 98–103.

Garrett Jr, W.E., Rich, F.R., Nikolaou, P. & Vogler III, J.B. (1989) Computed tomography of hamstring muscle strains. *Med. Sci. Sports Exerc.* **21**(5), 506–14.

Garrett Jr, W.E., Safran, M.R., Seaber, A.V., Glisson, R.R. & Ribbeck, B.M. (1988b) Biomechanical comparison of stimulated and nonstimulated skeletal muscle pulled to failure. *Am. J. Sports Med.* **15**(5), 448–54.

Garrett Jr, W.E. & Tidball, J. (1987) Myotendinous junction: structure, function and failure. In S.L.-Y. Woo & J.A. Buckwalter (eds) *Injury and Repair of the Musculoskeletal Soft Tissues*, pp. 171–201. American Academy of Orthopaedic Surgeons, Park Ridge, Illinois.

Garrick, J.G.K. & Requa, R.K. (1980) Epidemiology of women's gymnastics injuries. *Am. J. Sports Med.* **8**(4), 261–4.

Gauthier, G.F. (1986) Skeletal muscle fiber types. In A.G. Engel & B.Q. Banker (eds) *Myology*, Vol. 1, pp. 255–84. McGraw-Hill, New York.

Glick, J.M. (1980) Muscle strains. Prevention and treatment. *Phys. Sports Med.* **8**(2), 73–7.

Gollnick, P.D. & Saltin, B. (1989) Skeletal muscle physiology. In C.C. Teitz (ed) *Scientific Foundations in Sports Medicine*. B.C. Decker, Inc., Philadelphia.

Grana, W.A. & Schelberg-Karnes, E. (1983) How I manage deep muscle bruises. *Phys. Sports Med.* **11**(16), 123–5.

Hargens, A.R. & Akeson, W.H. (1981) *Pathophysiology of the Compartment Syndrome*. WB Saunders, Philadelphia.

Holt, L.E. (1981) *Scientific Stretching for Sport (3-S)*. Sport Research Ltd, Halifax, Nova Scotia.

Hough, T. (1902) Ergographic studies in muscular soreness. *Am. J. Physiol.* **7**, 76–92.

Hughston, J.C., Whatley, G.S. & Stone, M.M. (1962) Myositis ossificans traumatica (myo-osteosis). *Soc. Med. J.* **55**, 196, 1167–70.

Huxley, A.F. & Peachey, L.D. (1961) The maximum length for contraction in vertebrate striated muscle. *J. Physiol.* **156**, 150–65.

Inman, V.T., Ralston, H.J. & Todd, F. (1981) *Human*

Walking. Williams & Wilkins, Baltimore.

Jackson, D.W. & Feagin, J.A. (1973) Quadriceps contusions in young athletes. *J. Bone Joint Surg.* **55A**, 95–101.

Jenkins, R.R. (1988) Free radical chemistry relationship to exercise. *Sports Med.* **5**, 156–70.

Johnson, M.A., Polgar, J., Weightman, D. & Appleton, D. (1973) Data on the distribution of fibre types in thirty-six human muscles: An autopsy study. *J. Neurol. Sci.* **18**, 111–29.

Kantorowska, P.G., Hiller, W.D.B., Garrett, W.E., Smith, R. & O'Toole, M. (1990) *Cramping studies in 2600 endurance athletes*. Presented at the American College of Sports Medicine 37th Annual Meeting, Salt Lake City, Utah, 24 May.

Kennedy, J.C. & Roth, J.H. (1979) Major tibial compartment syndromes following minor athletic trauma. *Am. J. Sports Med.* **7**(3), 201–3.

Komi, P.V., Rusko, H., Vos, J. *et al.* (1977) Anaerobic performance capacity in athletes. *Acta Physiol. Scand.* **100**, 107–14.

Kraus, H. (1941) The use of surface anesthesia in the treatment of painful motion. *JAMA* **116**, 2582–3.

Kraus, H. (1959) Evaluation and treatment of muscle function in athletic injury. *Am. J. Surg.* **98**, 353–62.

Krejci, V. & Koch, P. (1979) *Muscle and Tendon Injuries in Athletes*. Year Book Medical Publishers, Illinois.

Lane, R.J.M., Turnbull, D.M., Welch, J.L. & Walton, J. (1986) A double-blind, placebo-controlled crossover study of verapamil in exertional muscle pain. *Muscle Nerve* **9**, 635–41.

LeCroy, C.M., Reedy, M.K., Seaber, A.V. & Garrett Jr, W.E. (1989) Limited sarcomere extensibility and strain injury in rabbit skeletal muscle. *Trans. Orthop. Res. Soc.* **14**, 316.

Lowey, S. & Risby, D. (1971) Light chains from fast and slow muscle myosins. *Nature* **234**, 81–5.

McBrine, J.J., Maughan, R.J. & Robertson, J.D. (1991) Lipid peroxidation and anti-oxidant status of red cells following downhill and level running. *Med. Sci. Sports Exerc.* **S147**, 879.

McDermott, A.G.P., Marble, A.E., Yabsley, R.H. & Phillips, D. (1982) Monitoring dynamic anterior compartment pressures during exercise: A new technique using the STIC catheter. *Am. J. Sports Med.* **10**(2), 83–9.

McMaster, P.E. (1933) Tendon and muscle ruptures: Clinical and experimental studies on the causes and location of subcutaneous ruptures. *J. Bone Joint Surg.* **15**, 705–22.

Mair, S.D., Seaber, A.V., Glisson, R.R. & Garrett Jr, W.E. (1991) The role of fatigue in susceptibility to muscle strain injury. *Trans. Orthop. Res. Soc.* **16**, 42.

Matsen, F.A., Mayo, K.A., Krugmire, R.B., Sheridan, G.W. & Kraft, G.H. (1977) A model compartmental syndrome in man with particular reference to the quantification of nerve function. *J. Bone Joint Surg.* **59**, 648–53.

Maughan, R.J. (1986) Exercise-induced muscle cramp: A prospective biochemical study in marathon runners. *J. Sport Sci.* **4**(1), 31–4.

Miller, W.A. (1977) Rupture of the musculotendinous junction of the medial head of the gastrocnemius muscle. *Am. J. Sports Med.* **5**(5), 191–3.

Mubarak, S.J. (1981) Etiologies of compartment syndromes. In S.J. Mubarak & A.R. Hargens (eds) *Compartment Syndromes and Volkmann's Contracture*. WB Saunders, Philadelphia.

Nikolaou, P.K., Macdonald, B.L., Glisson, R.R., Seaber, A.V. & Garrett Jr, W.E. (1987) Biomechanical and histological evaluation of muscle after controlled strain injury. *Am. J. Sports Med.* **15**(1), 9–14.

Obremskey, W.T., Seaber, A.V., Ribbeck, B.M. & Garrett Jr, W.E. (1988) Biomechanical and histological assessment of a controlled muscle strain injury treated with piroxicam. *Trans. Orthop. Res. Soc.* **13**, 338.

Peterson, L. & Renström, P. (1986) Preventive measures. In W.A. Grana (ed) *Sports Injuries: Their Prevention and Treatment*, pp. 86–104. Yearbook Medical Publishers, Illinois.

Peterson, L. & Stener, B. (1976) Old rupture of the adductor longus muscle. *Acta Orthop. Scand.* **47**, 653–7.

Prockop, D.J. & Sjoerdsma, A. (1961) Significance of urinary hydroxyproline in man. *J. Clin. Invest.* **40**, 843–9.

Puranen, J. (1974) The medial tibial syndrome. Exercise ischaemia in the medial fascial compartment of the leg. *J. Bone Joint Surg.* **56B**, 712–15.

Rask, M.R. & Lattig, G.J. (1972) Traumatic fibrosis of the rectus femoris muscle. *JAMA* **221**(3), 368–9.

Reddy, A.S., Reedy, M.K., Best, T.M. *et al.* (1991) Evaluation of strain injuries in rabbit skeletal muscle using a single fiber model. *Surg. Forum* **12**, 44.

Reneman, R.S. (1975) The anterior and the lateral compartment syndrome of the leg due to intensive use of muscles. *Clin. Orthop.* **113**, 69–80.

Rorabeck, C.H., Bourne, R.B. & Fowler, P.J. (1982) The surgical treatment of exertional compartment syndrome in athletes. *J. Bone Joint Surg.* **65A**(9), 1245–7.

Rooser, B. (1988) Quadriceps contusion with compartment syndrome: Evaluation of hematoma in 2 cases. In J.L. Anderson, F.J. George, R.J. Shephard, J.S. Torg & E.R. Eichner (eds) *Year Book of Sports Medicine*, p. 259. Yearbook Medical Publishers, Illinois.

Rothwell, A.G. (1982) Quadriceps hematoma: A prospective clinical study. *Clin. Orthop. Rel. Res.* **171**, 97–103.

Ryan, A.J. (1969) Quadriceps strain, rupture, and charlie horse. *Med. Sci. Sports Exerc.* **1**(2), 106–11.

Saltin, B., Henricksson, J., Nygaard, E. & Anderson, P. (1977) Fiber types and metabolic potentials of skeletal muscles in sedentary man and endurance runners. *Ann. N.Y. Acad. Sci.* **310**, 3–29.

Schwane, J.A., Johnson, S.R., Vandenakker, C.B. & Armstrong, R.B. (1983) Delayed-onset muscular soreness and plasma CPK and LDK activities after downhill running. *Med. Sci. Sports Exerc.* **15**(1), 51–6.

Shellock, F.G., Fukunaga, T., Day, K. *et al.* (1991) Serial MRI and Cybex testing evaluation of exertional muscle injury: Concentric vs. eccentric actions. *Med. Sci. Sports Exerc.* **S110**, 658.

Solveborn, S.-A. (1983) *The Book about Stretching.* Japan Publications, New York.

Stanish, W.D. (1981) Neurophysiology of stretching. In R. D'Ambrosia & D. Drez (eds) *Prevention and Treatment of Running Injuries*, pp. 135–45. Charles B. Slack Inc, New Jersey.

Statt, D.B., Burton, H.W., Cerny, F.J. & Awad, A.B. (1991) The effect of vitamin E on indices of skeletal muscle injury after lengthening contractions. *Med. Sci. Sports Exerc.* **S145**, 869.

Sudmann, E. (1979) The painful chronic anterior lower leg syndrome. *Acta Orthop. Scand.* **50**, 573–81.

Symeonides, P.P. (1972) Isolated traumatic rupture of the adductor longus muscle of the thigh. *Clin. Orthop. Rel. Res.* **88**, 64–6.

Taylor, D.C., Dalton, J.D., Seaber, A.V. & Garrett Jr, W.E. (1990) Viscoelastic properties of muscle–tendon units. The biomechanical effects of stretching. *Am. J. Sports Med.* **18**(3), 300–9.

Thorstensson, A., Grimby, G. & Karlsson, J. (1976a) Force–velocity relations and fiber composition in human knee extensor muscles. *J. Appl. Physiol.* **40**(1), 12–16.

Tidball, J.G. (1984) Myotendinous junction: Morphological changes and mechanical failure associated with muscle cell atrophy. *Exp. Mol. Pathol.* **40**, 1–12.

Veith, R.G. (1980) Recurrent compartmental syndromes due to intensive use of muscles. In F.A. Matsen (ed) *Compartmental Syndromes*. Grune & Stratton, New York.

Whitesides, T.E., Haney, T.C., Morimoto, K. & Harada, H. (1975) Tissue pressure measurements as a determinant for the need of fasciotomy. *Clin. Orthop. Rel. Res.* **113**, 43–51.

Wickiewicz, T.L., Roy, R.R., Powell, P.L. & Edgerton, V.L. (1983) Muscle architecture of the human lower limb. *Clin. Orthop. Rel. Res.* **179**, 275–83.

Wiktorsson-Moller, M., Oberg, B., Ekstrand, J. & Gillquist, J. (1983) Effects of warming up, massage, and stretching on range of motion and muscle strength in the lower extremity. *Am. J. Sports Med.* **11**(4), 249–52.

Zarins, B. & Ciullo, J.V. (1983) Acute muscle and tendon injuries in athletes. *Clin. Sports Med.* **2**(1), 167–82.

Chapter 7

Endocrinological Deregulation and Musculoskeletal Injuries

HANS A. KEIZER AND HARM KUIPERS

Physical exercise has been reported to be a strong stimulus for changing the circulating levels of a wide variety of hormones (Galbo, 1983). Consequently, the homeostasis of the endocrine system may be disturbed for hours or even days after exercise, provided that its duration and intensity was sufficient (Dufaux et al., 1981; Dessypris et al., 1985; Kuoppasalmi & Adlercreutz, 1985; Keizer et al., 1989a).

Although adaptation to training is a not well-understood process yet, there is growing evidence that the endocrine system plays an important role in it. This is exemplified by the growth retardation that has been observed in young tennis players during periods of extreme training (Laron & Klinger, 1989). Growth was progressively retarded but when these boys were badly injured (i.e. did not train for a longer period of time), compensatory acceleration of growth occurred. The growth retardation is most probably caused by an inhibition of the normal episodic secretion pattern of growth hormone during the night. Support for this hypothesis has been found in the disappearance of the normal episodic secretion pattern of another pituitary hormone namely luteinizing hormone (LH) after an exhaustive period of training (Keizer et al., 1989b). Contrastingly, a well-designed training programme seemed to increase the amplitude of the nightly growth hormone peaks, both in hamsters (Borer et al., 1986) and probably in humans. However, in the latter case these increments (accompanied by a higher performance level) only occurred

when training intensity was at or slightly above the level of the so-called anaerobic threshold. It is tempting to speculate, that the endocrine system plays an important role in this adaptation, since several authors (DeMeirleir et al., 1986; Keizer et al., 1987) have shown the close relationship between elevated levels of stress hormones and exercise intensity. Typically, this occurs only at intensities greater than 70% $\dot{V}_{O_{2max}}$, i.e. at or above the lactate threshold. In addition, it has to be mentioned, that the stress hormones, for example catecholamines and cortisol (C), act on catabolism, i.e. they enhance energy liberation to meet the body's increased demands during that type of exercise. In the recovery phase, the body will attempt to restore homeostasis to such an extent, that the same amount of stress is not able to disturb the system anymore.

The endocrine system also plays an important role in energy metabolism after exercise, which is relevant for the rate of the recovery processes. The precise role of the various hormones in mechanisms involved in adaptation, however, has yet to be elucidated. It is not one single hormone that acts either catabolic or anabolic, but the concerted action of the hormone profile that determines the cellular response. At present little is known about whether changes in the function of the endocrine system do contribute to the occurrence of sport injuries. Nevertheless, this chapter will attempt to shed more light hereupon. Since the variety of hormonal responses to exercise and training is tremendous, we will mainly concentrate upon the effects of steroid hormones on muscle and bone tissue.

Steroid hormones and muscle metabolism

Today, there is no doubt that skeletal muscle is a target organ for sex hormones (Krieg, 1976; Seene & Viru, 1982; Carrrington & Bailey, 1985) and C (Mayer et al., 1976; Shoji & Pennington, 1977; Kelly et al., 1986). It has been shown, that both classes of hormones share the same intramuscular receptor (Mayer & Rosen, 1977). In general, sex hormones exert an anabolic action on skeletal muscle, whereas cortisol causes muscle waste and atrophy, especially in the type II muscle (Almon & Dubois, 1990). Thus, in males growth and hypertrophy in skeletal muscle are, among others, induced by testosterone (T) and counteracted by C. Whether there is net growth, or waste and atrophy of muscle depends on the T to C ratio. In females, a concerted anabolic action of both T and oestradiol 17β (E2) is probably involved. Although little is known about the physiological consequences of relatively low plasma sex hormone levels, it has been demonstrated, that when severely depressed as has been found after exhaustive exercise or training (Dufaux et al., 1981; Bonen & Keizer, 1984; Aakvaag & Opstad, 1985; Dessypris et al., 1985; Kuoppasalmi & Adlercreutz, 1985; Loucks & Horvath, 1985; Janssen et al., 1986), the synthesis rate of muscle glycogen may be decreased, whereas increased levels of T and E2 may be paralleled by elevated levels of muscle glycogen (Bergamini, 1975; Carrington & Bailey, 1985). Interestingly, the action of T might be mediated by its conversion to E2 and not by the androgen itself, as recently has been shown in female rats (Van Breda et al., 1990). Furthermore, recent work of Van Breda et al. (1990, 1991) has shown that the concerted action of submaximal endurance training and T administration in female rats potentiated the increased muscle glycogen and the oxidative capacity of soleus muscles

compared to non-T treated animals. Again this action was completely abolished when the conversion to E2 was inhibited. This paracrine action of T, cautions us not to draw premature conclusions from changes in plasma levels of a single hormone.

Increased C levels as we often have observed in élite athletes during very heavy training periods may lower muscle glycogen levels (Bonen et al., 1990), increase protein turnover and cause a net release of amino acids from skeletal muscle (Mayer et al., 1976; Kelly et al., 1986). Although lower glycogen levels do not directly lead to sport injuries, starting strenuous exercise with low glycogen levels will result in early muscle glycogen depletion and premature fatigue. Depletion of muscle glycogen will necessitate a change in the recruitment pattern of the muscle fibres involved in the exercise. This may result in the recruitment of muscle fibres that are usually not involved in a particular type of exercise. Since training effects are highly specific, these fibres may not be well adjusted to a particular exercise and be more vulnerable to damage. Thus, low sex hormone levels may indirectly result in a changed movement pattern, and consequently increase the risk of muscle overuse and overuse injuries.

In conclusion, changed plasma levels of sex hormones are directly related to muscle metabolism, and may indirectly lead to overuse injuries (Fig. 7.1). It is unknown, however, whether changes in plasma hormone concentrations have direct effects on the metabolism of cartilage and connective tissue.

Sex hormones and muscle damage

Muscle damage may occur when unaccustomed exercise is performed. Also in élite athletes muscle damage may occur when they do some type of exercise to which they are not accustomed, especially muscular activities in which an eccentric component or high-peak forces are involved, as these are usually associated with muscle damage. Muscle damage is reflected in delayed-onset muscle soreness (DOMS), stiff-

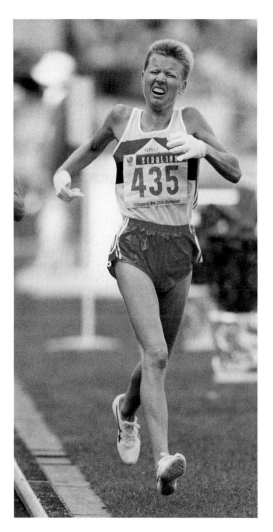

Fig. 7.1 Female runners are more susceptible to overuse injuries. Courtesy of the IOC archives.

ness, decrease in strength, swelling, and a decreased range of motion of the muscle involved. In addition, plasma activity of muscle enzymes increases. Since creatine kinase (CK) is specific for muscle in general the plasma CK activity is used to estimate the amount of muscle damage. However, CK is not only present in skeletal muscle, but isoforms of CK are present in brain, muscle and myocardium. Therefore three isoforms of CK can be distinguished: (i) CK-MM (present in muscle); (ii) CK-MB (present in

myocardium); and (iii) CK-BB (present in brain). For estimating the amount of muscle damage CK-MM is most specific for skeletal muscle (Hortobagyi & Denahan, 1989).

It has been suggested by some investigators that sex hormones play a role in exercise-induced muscle damage. This is based on the finding that after a certain amount of exercise males have higher plasma CK activities than females (Hortobagyi & Denahan, 1989). Based on data obtained in male and female rats, Amelink *et al.* (1988) suggested that females have less exercise-induced muscle damage than males. Later studies by Van der Meulen *et al.* (1991) also demonstrated that female rats have lower plasma CK activities after running than males, although the amount of histological muscle damage was similar in both sexes. This suggests that plasma CK activities do not necessarily reflect muscle damage, but rather changes in membrane permeability. This also explains the finding that males and females who administer anabolic steroids, demonstrate higher plasma CK activity, although signs of muscle damage are absent. Based on these studies it appears that sex hormones do not influence the occurrence of exercise-induced muscle damage, but modify membrane permeability, i.e. androgens enhance CK efflux, while oestrogens inhibit CK efflux (Thomson & Smith, 1980; Amelink *et al.*, 1988; Bär *et al.*, 1988).

Glucocorticoid levels may be increased after exercise depending on its product of duration and intensity, and the level of exhaustion (Dufaux *et al.*, 1981; Dessypris *et al.*, 1985; Kuoppasalmi & Adlercreutz, 1985; Keizer *et al.*, 1989a). Under normal conditions, plasma C levels will normalize within 2–6 h. When, however, the total amount of stress is too high, the adrenohypothalamopituitary axis will be disinhibited, leading to chronically increased C levels (Sapolsky *et al.*, 1986). As in Cushing's syndrome, this probably will result in muscle wasting (Mayer *et al.*, 1976; Kelly *et al.*, 1986) and increased vulnerability to muscle injuries, especially muscle tears. Although exercise has proven to diminish the catabolic effect of hypercortisolism (Falduto *et al.*, 1989; Hickson *et al.*, 1990), there is no doubt, that muscle resistance to lengthening forces is diminished. We found evidence for the existence of such a relation in a female Olympic athlete. She had, in periods of extreme training, exceptionally high basal C levels (Fig. 7.2). When C concentrations peaked to 1500−2000 nmol·l^{-1} (levels which has also been observed in Cushing's syndrome), she injured seriously (muscle tears), whereas when C levels were at nadir, she set personal bests. During the whole observation period (9 months) her T levels remained stable (0.9−1.1 nmol·l^{-1}), whereas her endogenous E2 levels were very low since she used oral contraceptives.

Androgens (no information exists as to oestrogens) may also be able to counteract the negative effects of high C levels on muscle, although the literature does not provide consistent results. For example, Capaccio *et al.* (1987) found that T failed to prevent skeletal muscle atrophy from glucocorticoids in slowly growing, intact female rats. In contrast, Danhaive and Rousseau (1988) showed that RU 486 (a C receptor blocker), T and trenbolone all were effective in attenuating corticosterone-induced retardation of body weight and gain in muscle weight of young, rapidly growing

rats. Furthermore, Seene and Viru (1982) showed that the combination of anabolic steroid administration and exercise was able to prevent glucocorticoid-induced muscle waste in rats. The differences in results of these investigations might be caused by the differences in age (Hickson *et al.*, 1990), endocrine milieu and training status. This needs more research, where the extreme training of élite athletes is mimicked to prove the exact relation between high C levels, normal or elevated sex hormone levels and the occurrence of muscle injuries.

Changes in sex hormones and sport injuries in females

It is well recognized that in female athletes engaging in regular heavy exercise the menstrual cycle may alter and consequently the circulating levels of sex hormones (Baker *et al.*, 1981; Bonen & Keizer, 1984; Loucks & Horvath, 1985; Keizer & Rogol, 1990). In oligomenorrhoeic and amenorrhoeic runners lower plasma oestrogen and chronically elevated C levels over time have been found (Loucks *et al.*, 1989). Together with the training-induced elevations of C, this may render these women more vulnerable for musculoskeletal injuries. Evidence for this hypothesis has been provided by Lloyd *et al.* (1986) who showed an almost three times

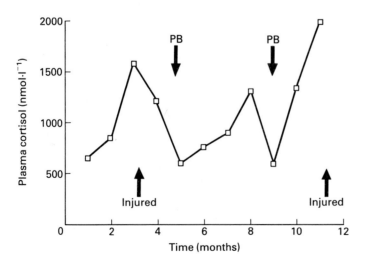

Fig. 7.2 Plasma cortisol levels in an Olympic athlete. The blood samples were taken between 8 and 9 a.m. after an overnight fast during 11 consecutive months. The athlete became injured (muscle tears) after her cortisol peaked at 1558 and 1978 nmol·l^{-1}, respectively. PB, personal best.

higher incidence of musculoskeletal injuries in oligomenorrhoeic/amenorrhoeic runners as compared to their eumenorrhoeic controls. Furthermore, evidence is accumulating that secondary amenorrhoea and oligomenorrhoea is associated with a higher incidence of bone demineralization and stress fractures (Drinkwater *et al.*, 1984; Marcus *et al.*, 1985; Lloyd *et al.*, 1986; Louis *et al.*, 1991).

Although it has been a controversial subject for many years, at present menstrual irregularities are partly considered as an expression of over-training (DeCree, 1990; Keizer & Rogol, 1990). Evidence for this view have been presented by several authors. For example, Bullen *et al.* (1984) showed that moderate endurance exercise for 8 weeks was not able to disturb the menstrual cycle in eumenorrhoeic women. In an extension of that study (Bullen *et al.*, 1985) menstrual cycle alterations were induced in almost all volunteers, when training volume was extremely high (3–4 h·day^{-1}). The authors postulated the hypothesis, that the hypothalamo-pituitary axis might be disturbed. This was supported by Veldhuis *et al.* (1985) who found decreased LH peak frequencies and altered response in gonadotrophin-releasing hormone

in amenorrhoeic athletes. Furthermore, work from Keizer *et al.* (1989b) showed a severely depressed LH pulsatility after exhaustive training (3–4 h·day^{-1} for 3–4 days) in eumenorrhoeic women athletes (Fig. 7.3). Therefore, we conclude, that females engaged in strenuous training who develop menstrual irregularities are prone to develop stress fractures and other overuse injuries. Therefore, these women should be treated with oral contraceptives. In addition, females who develop frequent musculoskeletal injuries should be evaluated on their menstrual status, the training programme and nutrition.

Few data are available about the influence of the phase of the menstrual cycle and the occurrence of sport injuries. Lamont *et al.* (1987) found that basal urinary urea excretion is higher in the midluteal phase compared to the early follicular phase. Landau and Lugibihl (1961) were able to relate this catabolic effect to progesterone. However, very few investigators have studied the relation between the phase of the menstrual cycle and the incidence of injuries. Recently, Möllner-Nielsen and Hammar (1989) demonstrated that female soccer players are more susceptible to traumatic injuries dur-

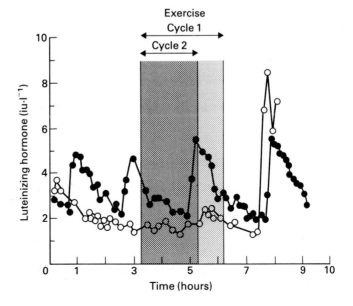

Fig. 7.3 Plasma luteinizing hormone levels in a female hockey player before, during and after exercise. The experiments were performed on day 8 of two consecutive menstrual cycles. In cycle 1, the subject performed light aerobic training (five times per week). In cycle 2, the subject performed intensive and exhaustive training (five times per week) before the experiment. Exercise time was shortened by 52 min, whereas her menstrual cycle lengthened from 31 to 42 days.

ing the premenstrual and menstrual phase. In addition, these investigators observed a lower incidence of traumatic injuries in females who used oral contraceptives. They explain these findings by the fact that the premenstrual and menstrual phase affect coordination and mood state. Oral contraceptives ameliorate most of the premenstrual symptoms.

Exogenous hormones and sport injuries

Drug abuse is widespread in élite sport. Of the various drugs used, hormone substances are frequently used by many athletes. A group of hormones that is used by athletes in many types of sport are anabolic steroids (Wilson, 1988). Numerous studies have demonstrated that these drugs are effective on the one hand (Kuipers et al., 1991), but on the other hand have side-effects (when high doses are used) that increase the risk for developing cardiovascular diseases (Wilson, 1988).

Anabolic steroids can contribute to the development of sport injuries. It has been demonstrated that the use of anabolic steroids can lead to changes in the metabolism of connective tissue (Michina, 1986a), which are associated with dysplasia of collagen fibrils (Michina, 1986b; Laseter & Russell, 1991). A dysplasia of collagen may lead to a decrease in tensile strength and increased risk for rupture (Michina, 1987). In support of this, cases of spontaneous rupture in athletes who used high doses of anabolic steroids have been reported (Hill et al., 1983; Kramhøft & Solgaard, 1986; Bach et al., 1987; Herrick & Herrick, 1987). There is insufficient data on the effect of anabolic steroids on cartilage metabolism. Therefore it remains to be established yet, whether anabolic steroids have a negative influence on joint cartilage and whether there is any relationship between steroid use and joint pathology.

Because of the side-effects, the use of anabolic steroids may also indirectly be associated with the occurrence of sport injuries. Because of the

increased aggressiveness and mood changes during anabolic steroid use (Pope & Katz, 1988), athletes who take these drugs may take more risks and can increase the chances of hurting themselves as well as their opponents.

Corticosteroids and injuries

Another group of hormones used in sports are glucocorticoids. Endurance athletes, such as cyclists use systemic glucocorticoids to enhance performance. Although a positive effect is anticipated, little is known about the influence of glucocorticoids on endurance performance. Hueting (1988) demonstrated in a double-blind study with professional cyclists that the administration of corticosteroids did not improve endurance performance. Nevertheless, this drug is still used by cyclists. Application of corticosteroids has some potentially hazardous side-effects. One of these is that it changes metabolism and enhances protein degradation. Although scientific evidence is lacking, anecdotal evidence suggests that athletes who use glucocorticoids may decline into a severe mental and physical depression after use of these drugs. It is suggested that the risk for infections and injuries is increased after corticosteroid use (Bateman et al., 1989).

Local application of corticosteroids is also used in sport injuries. Corticosteroids suppress the symptoms of inflammation, and for this reason application of this drug is rather popular among athletes. The initial optimism some decades ago has developed into the awareness that corticosteroids do not only suppress the inflammatory process, but also impair the repair potential of the affected tissues (Kennedy & Willis, 1976). Application of corticosteroids in tendons has been shown to be risky. Injection in an injured Achilles tendon does alleviate the symptoms, but increases the risk of developing a rupture of the tendon. For that reason athletes who receive local glucocorticoids should abstain from severe physical exercise for at least 2 weeks (Kennedy & Willis, 1976). Therefore one should have serious reservations about the application of corticosteroids in cases of tendon pathology.

Glucocorticoids may also affect cartilage metabolism. Behrens *et al.* (1976) demonstrated that repair mechanisms of cartilage tissue was impaired after intra-articular glucocorticoid injection. Therefore, joints in which glucocorticoids are injected are more vulnerable for several months after injection and should be spared to avoid premature development of osteoarthritis.

Conclusion

The endocrine system certainly plays an important role in the adaptation to training. In periods of extreme training, often accompanied by mental stress, the endocrine system may be disturbed for a longer period of time. This results in consistently increased levels of stress hormones, even in the recovery phase. In turn, this may lead to muscle wasting, relative muscle atrophy and decrease in bone mass. Secondary to the non-optimal restored muscle glycogen levels, athletes may be more prone to fatigue and consequently musculoskeletal injuries. Special attention should be paid to female athletes, since oligomenorrhoea and secondary amenorrhoea is a proven health hazard.

Future research is needed to uncover the precise role of the endocrine system in the prevalence of musculoskeletal injuries.

References

Aakvaag, A. & Opstad, P.K. (1985) Hormonal responses to prolonged physical strain: Effect of caloric deficiency and sleep deprivation. In K. Fotherby & S.B. Pal (eds) *Exercise Endocrinology*, pp. 25–46. de Gruyter, Berlin.

Almon, R.R. & Dubois, D.C. (1990) Fibre-type discrimination in disuse and glucocorticoid-induced atrophy. *Med. Sci. Sports Exerc.* **22**, 304–11.

Amelink, G.J., Kamp, H.H. & Bär, P.D. (1988) Creatine kinase isoenzyme profiles after exercise in the rat: sex-linked differences in leakage of CK-MM. *Pflügers Arch.* **412**, 417–21.

Bach, B.R., Warren, R.F. & Wickiewicz, T.L. (1987) Triceps rupture: A case report and literature review. *Am. J Sports Med.* **15**, 285–9.

Baker, E.R., Mathur, R.S, Kirk, R.F. & Williamson, H.O. (1981) Female runners and secondary amenorrhea: correlation with age, parity, mileage, and plasma hormonal and sex-hormone binding globulin concentrations. *Fertil. Steril.* **36**, 183–7.

Bär, P.D., Amelink, G.J., Oldenburg, B. & Blankenstein, M.A. (1988) Prevention of exercise-induced muscle membrane damage by oestradiol. *Life Sci.* **42**, 2677–81.

Bateman, A., Singh, A., Kral, T. & Solomon, S. (1989) The immune hypothalamic–pituitary–adrenal axis. *Endocr. Rev.* **10**, 92–112.

Behrens, F., Shephard, N. & Mitchell, N. (1976) Metabolic recovery of articular cartilage after intra-articular injections of glucocorticoid. *Bone Joint Surg.* **58A**, 1157–60.

Bergamini, E. (1975) Different mechanisms in testosterone action on glycogen metabolism in rat perineal and skeletal muscle. *Endocrinology* **96**, 77–84.

Bonen, A. & Keizer, H.A. (1984) Athletic menstrual cycle irregularity: Endocrine response to exercise and training. *Phys. Sports Med.* **12**, 78–94.

Bonen, A., McDermott, J.C. & Tan, M.H. (1990) Glycogenesis and glyconeogenesis in skeletal muscle: Effects of pH and hormones. *Am. J. Physiol.* **258**, E693–700.

Borer, K.T., Nicoski, D.R. & Owens, V. (1986) Alteration of pulsatile growth hormone secretion by growth-inducing exercise: involvement of endogenous opiates and somatostatin. *Endocrinology* **118**, 844–50.

Bullen, B.A., Skrinar, G.S., Beitins, I.Z., Carr, D.B., Reppert, S.M., Dotson, C.O., De Fencl, M. *et al.* (1984) Endurance training effects on plasma hormonal responsiveness and sex hormone excretion. *J. Appl. Physiol.* **56**, 1453–63.

Bullen, B.B., Skrinar, G.S., Beitins, I.Z., Von Mering, G., Turnbull, B.A. & McArthur, J.W. (1985) Induction of menstrual cycle disorders by strenuous exercise in untrained women. *New Engl. J. Med.* **312**, 1349–53.

Capaccio, J.A., Kurowski, T.T., Czerwinski, S.M., Chatterton Jr, R.T. & Hickson, R.C. (1987) Testosterone fails to prevent skeletal muscle atrophy from glucocorticoids. *J. Appl. Physiol.* **63**, 328–34.

Carrington, L.J. & Bailey, C.J. (1985) Effects of natural and synthetic estrogens and progestins on glycogen deposition in female mice. *Hormone Res.* **21**, 199–203.

Danhaive, P.A. & Rousseau, G.G. (1988) Evidence for sex-dependent anabolic response to androgenic steroids mediated by muscle glucocorticoid receptors in rat. *J. Steroid Biochem.* **29**, 575–85.

DeCree, K. (1990) The possible involvement of endogenous opioid peptides and catecholoestrogens in provoking menstrual irregularities in women athletes. *Int. J. Sports Med.* **11**, 329–48.

DeMeirleir, K., Naaktgeboren, N., Steirteghem, A. Van, Gorus, F., Olbrecht, J. & Block, P. (1986) Beta-endorphin and ACTH levels in peripheral blood during and after aerobic and anaerobic exercise. *Eur. J. Appl. Physiol.* **55**, 5–8.

Dessypris, A., Kuoppasalmi, K. & Adlercreutz, H. (1985) Plasma cortisol, testosterone, androstenedione and luteinizing hormone in a non-competitive marathon run. *J. Steroid Biochem.* **7**, 33–7.

Drinkwater, B.L., Nilson, K., Chestnut, C.H., Bremner, W.J., Shainholtz, S. & Southworth, M.B. (1984) Bone mineral content of amenorrheic and eumenorrheic athletes. *New Engl. J. Med.* **311**, 277–81.

Dufaux, B., Assmann, G., Order, U., Holderath, A. & Hollmann, W. (1981) Plasma lipoproteins, hormones, and energy substrates during the first days after prolonged exercise. *Int. J. Sports Med.* **2**, 256–60.

Falduto, M.T., Hickson, R.C. & Young, A.P. (1989) Antagonism by glucocorticoids and exercise on expression of glutamine synthetase in skeletal muscle. *FASEB J.* **3**, 2623–38.

Galbo, H. (1983) *Hormonal and Metabolic Adaptation to Exercise.* Thieme Verlag, Stuttgart.

Herrick, R.T. & Herrick, S. (1987) Ruptured triceps in a powerlifter presenting as cubital tunnel syndrome: A case report. *Am. J. Sports Med.* **15**, 514–16.

Hickson, R.C., Czerwinski, S.M., Falduto, M.T. & Young, A.P. (1990) Glucocorticoid antagonism by exercise and androgen-anabolic steroids. *Med. Sci. Sports Exerc.* **22**, 331–40.

Hill, J.A., Suker, J.R., Sachs, K. & Brigham, C. (1983) The athletic polydrug abuse phenomenon. *Am. J. Sports Med.* **11**, 269–71.

Hortobagyi, T. & Denahan, T. (1989) Variability in creatine kinase: Methodological, exercise, and clinically related factors. *Int. J. Sports Med.* **10**, 69–80.

Hueting, J. (1988) *The Influence of ACTH on Maximal Performance in Professional Cyclists* (in Dutch). De Vrieseborch, Haarlem, The Netherlands.

Janssen, G.M.E., Kuipers, H. & Keizer, H.A. (1986) Plasma CK and AST activity and plasma testosterone after 200 km speed skating. *Med. Sci. Sports Exerc.* **18**(Suppl.), 205.

Keizer, H.A., Janssen, G.M.E., Menheere, P. & Van Kranenburg, G. (1989a) Changes in basal plasma testosterone, cortisol, and dehydroepiandrosterone sulfate in previously untrained males and females preparing for a marathon. *Int. J. Sports Med.* **10** (Suppl. 3), 117–19.

Keizer, H.A., Kuipers, H., De Haan, J., Beckers, E. & Habets, L. (1987) Multiple hormonal responses to physical exercise in eumenorrheic trained and untrained women. *Int. J. Sports Med.* **8**(Suppl. 3), 139–50.

Keizer, H.A., Platen, P., Menheere, P.P.C.A., Biwer, R., Peters, C., Tietz, R. & Wüst, H. (1989b) The hypothalamic/pituitary axis under exercise stress: The effects of aerobic and anaerobic training. In Z. Laron & A.D. Rogol (eds) *Hormones and Sport*, pp. 101–15. Raven Press, New York.

Keizer, H.A. & Rogol, A.D. (1990) Physical exercise and menstrual cycle alterations: what are the mechanisms? *Sports Med.* **10**, 218–35.

Kelly, F.J., McGrath, J.A., Goldspink, D.F. & Cullen, M.J. (1986) A morphological/biochemical study on the actions of corticoids on rat skeletal muscle. *Muscle Nerve* **9**, 1–10.

Kennedy, J.C. & Willis, R.B. (1976) The effects of local steroid injections on tendons: A biomechanical and microscopic correlative study. *Am. J. Sports Med.* **4**, 11–21.

Kramhøft, M. & Solgaard, S. (1986) Spontaneous rupture of the extensor pollicis longus tendon after anabolic steroids. *J. Hand Surg.* **11**, 87–91.

Krieg, M. (1976) Characterization of the androgen receptor in the skeletal muscle of the rat. *Steroids* **28**, 261–5.

Kuipers, H., Wijnen, J.A.G., Hartgens, F. & Willems, S.M.M. (1991) Influence of anabolic steroids on body composition, blood pressure, lipid profile, and liver functions in body builders. *Int. J. Sports Med.* **12**, 413–18.

Kuoppasalmi, K. & Adlercreutz, H. (1985) Interaction between catabolic and anabolic steroid hormones in muscular exercise. In K. Fotherby & S.B. Pal (eds) *Exercise Endocrinology*, pp. 65–156. de Gruyter, Berlin.

Lamont, L.S., Lemon, P.W.R. & Bruot, B.C. (1987) Menstrual cycle and exercise effects on protein catabolism. *Med. Sci. Sports Exerc.* **19**, 106–10.

Landau, R.L. & Lugibihl, K. (1961) The catabolic and natriuretic effects of progesterone in man. *Rec. Prog. Horm. Res.* **17**, 249–92.

Laron, Z. & Klinger, B. (1989) Does intensive sport endanger normal growth and development? In Z. Laron & A.D. Rogol (eds) *Hormones and Sport*, pp. 1–9. Raven Press, New York.

Laseter, J.T. & Russell, J.A. (1991) Anabolic steroid-induced tendon pathology: A review of the literature. *Med. Sci. Sports Exerc.* **23**, 1–3.

Lloyd, T., Triantafyllou, S.J., Baker, E.R., Houts, P.S., Whileside, J.A., Kalenak, A. & Stumpf, P.G. (1986) Women with menstrual irregularities have increased musculoskeletal injuries. *Med. Sci. Sports Exerc.* **18**, 374–9.

Loucks, A.B. & Horvath, S.B. (1985) Athletic amenorrhea: A review. *Med. Sci. Sports Exerc.* **17**, 56–72.

Loucks, A.B., Mortola, J.F., Girton, L. & Yen, S.S.C. (1989) Alterations in the hypothalamic–pituitary–ovarian, and the hypothalamic–pituitary–adrenal axes in athletic women. *J. Clin. Endocrinol. Metab.* **68**, 402–11.

Louis, O., DeMeirleir, K., Kalendar, W., Keizer, H.A., Platen, P., Hollmann, W. & Osteaux, M. (1991) Low vertebral bone density values in young non-élite female runners. *Int. J. Sports Med.* **12**, 214–17.

Marcus, M., Cann, C., Madvis, P., Minkhoff, J., Goddard, M., Bayer, M., Martin, M. *et al.* (1985) Menstrual function and bone mass in élite women runners. *Ann. Int. Med.* **102**, 158–68.

Mayer, M. & Rosen, F. (1977) Interactions of glucocorticoids and androgens with skeletal muscle. *Metabolism* **26**, 937–62.

Mayer, M., Shafir, E., Kaiser, N., Milholland, R.J. & Rosen, F. (1976) Interaction of glucocorticoid hormones with rat skeletal muscle: Catabolic effects and hormone binding. *Metabolism* **25**, 157–67.

Michina, H. (1986a) Organisation of collagen fibrils in tendon: Changes induced by an anabolic steroid. I. Functional and ultrastructural studies. *Virch. Arch. [B]* **52**, 75–86.

Michina, H. (1986) Organisation of collagen fibrils in tendon: Changes induced by an anabolic steroid. II. A morphometric and stereologic analysis. *Virch. Arch. (B)* **52**, 87–9.

Michina, H. (1987) Tendon injuries induced by exercise and anabolic steroids in experimental mice. *Int. J. Orthop.* **11**, 157–62.

Möller-Nielsen, J. & Hammar, M. (1989) Women's soccer injuries in relation to the menstrual cycle and oral contraceptive use. *Med. Sci. Sport Exerc.* **21**, 126–9.

Pope, H.G. & Katz, D.L. (1988) Affective and psychotic symptoms associated with anabolic steroid use. *Am. J. Psychiatr.* **145**, 487–90.

Sapolsky, R.M., Krey, L.C. & McEwen, B.S. (1986) The neuroendocrinology of stress and aging: The glucocorticoid cascade hypothesis. *Endocr. Rev.* **7**, 284–301.

Seene, T. & Viru, A. (1982) The catabolic effect of glucocorticoids in different types of muscle fibres and its dependence upon muscle activity and interaction with anabolic steroids. *J. Steroid Biochem.* **16**, 349–52.

Shoji, S. & Pennington, R.T.J. (1977) The effect of cortisone on protein breakdown and synthesis in rat skeletal muscle. *Mol. Cell. Endocrinol.* **6**, 159–69.

Thomson, W.H.S. & Smith, I. (1980) Effects of oestrogens on erythrocyte enzyme efflux in normal men and women. *Clin. Chimica Acta* **103**, 203–8.

Van Breda, E., Keizer, H.A. & Geurten, P. (1990) Testosterone elicits a glycogen sparing effect in exercising muscle fibres in female rats. *Med. Sci. Sports Exerc.* **22**(Suppl.), S33.

Van Breda, E., Keizer, H.A., Geurten, P., De Jong, Y.F. & Glatz, J.F.C. (1991) Testosterone increases mitochondrial activity in soleus but not in EDL muscle fibres of female rats. *Med. Sci. Sports Exerc.* **23**(Suppl.), S109.

Van der Meulen, J.H., Kuipers, H. & Drukker, J. (1991) Relationship between exercise-induced muscle damage and enzyme release in rats. *J. Appl. Physiol.* **71**, 999–1004.

Veldhuis, J.D., Evans, W.S., Demers, L.M., Thorner, M.O., Wakat, D. & Rogol, A.D. (1985) Altered neuroendocrine regulation of gonadotropin secretion in women distance runners. *J. Clin. Endocrinol. Metab.* **61**, 557–63.

Wilson, J.D. (1988) Androgen abuse in athletes. *Endocr. Rev.* **9**, 181–99.

Chapter 8

Nerve Compression Syndromes

MOIRA O'BRIEN

Anatomical and functional considerations

Nerve compression is a relatively common clinical entity in certain sports such as cycling and back-packing. It also occurs in patients who work in occupations which involve repetitive movements, particularly if they have certain medical conditions, e.g. hypothyroidism, diabetes, malnutrition or pregnancy. Some nerves are more susceptible than others, and may be compressed as a result of anatomical variations, e.g. fibrous bands, accessory muscles, spurs, narrow notches, or anatomical variations of the nerve itself.

Nerve compression syndromes

These occur in areas where nerves are exposed to external forces as they pass through fibro-osseous tunnels, which tend to tether the nerve. Extrinsic causes include oedema, callous formation as a result of a fracture, external compression due to specific movements, or to mechanical compression. The nerve is tender at the site of compression.

The nerve supply of the upper limb

The brachial plexus is derived from the anterior primary rami of the cervical nerves, C5, C6, C7, C8 and T1 (Fig. 8.1). It consists of roots, trunks, divisions and cords. The roots are found be-tween the scalenus anterior and scalenus medius muscles in the neck. The trunks lie in the posterior triangle of the neck. The divisions lie behind the clavicle. The cords are found in the axilla, where they divide into the terminal branches. Branches arise mainly from the roots and the cords. The suprascapular nerve is the only branch from the trunks.

The main nerves from the cords commonly involved in nerve compression syndromes are the axillary, radial, median and ulnar.

Aetiology

Neurovascular syndromes in the upper limb may involve any portion of the brachial plexuses. Compression injuries of the brachial plexus may result from intrinsic or extrinsic causes; the most common symptom complex involves the lowest trunk, with pain and paraesthesia along the medial border of the limb.

Compression at the thoracic outlet affects the nerves and vessels as they pass from the neck to the axilla. Proximally, it is usually due to anatomical anomalies, in the region of the scalene muscles. More distally, it may be due to biomechanical changes.

Due to the mobility of the shoulder, the neurovascular structures may change direction by a full 180°. The coracoid process and the pectoralis minor act as a fulcrum for the change in direction and this is a potential site of compression (Karas, 1990).

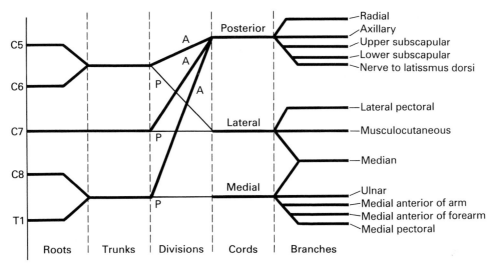

Fig. 8.1 Diagrammatic construction of the brachial plexus. A, anterior; P, posterior.

Congenital and structural anomalies include cervical ribs, scalenus anterior syndrome, fibrous or fibromuscular bands. Cervical ribs are the commonest bony anomalies associated with the thoracic outlet syndrome (Fig. 8.2). Less than 10% of patients with a cervical rib will have symptoms (Brown, 1983; Brown & Charlesworth, 1988). Abnormal development of the scalene muscles or abnormal fibrous bands in the muscles may involve the upper trunk of the brachial plexus (Roos, 1982).

Dynamic compression

Costoclavicular compression is usually dynamic. Elevation of the arm rotates the clavicle at the sternoclavicular and acromioclavicular joints narrowing the costoclavicular space. This will be further narrowed by retraction of the shoulders particularly if carrying a heavy weight as in back-packing. Deep inspiration, which elevates the first rib, narrows the space even further (Lord, 1971). The commonest cause of external injury to the brachial plexus is due to back-packing (Hirasawa & Sakakida, 1983). The straps in the axilla compress the plexuses against the clavicle and the heavy pack pulls the shoulder girdle posteriorly increasing the

traction; it may only involve the axillary or radial nerves, or the whole plexus.

The use of a figure of eight bandage in the early treatment of a fractured clavicle may also compress the brachial plexus.

Specific nerve entrapment in the upper limb

The suprascapular nerve C5, C6 is a branch of the upper trunk of the brachial plexus in the posterior triangle and passes through the suprascapular foramen to enter the supraspinous fossa. Here it gives off muscular branches to the supraspinatus and articular twigs to the shoulder and acromioclavicular joints. It then passes through the spinoglenoid notch to supply the infraspinatus muscle. The suprascapular entrapment may occur at the suprascapular foramen due to a narrow notch, or to a bifid transverse scapular ligament, kinking the nerve, which will affect both the supraspinatus and infraspinatus muscles (Rengachary et al., 1979). In 50% of cases there may be a spinoglenoid ligament, an aponeurotic band, which separates the supraspinatus from the infraspinatus. Entrapment here will only involve the infraspinatus muscle (Rengachary et al., 1979).

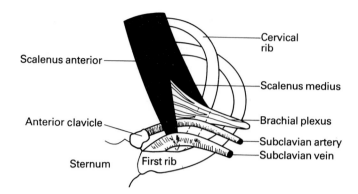

Fig. 8.2 A cervical rib.

Labels: Cervical rib, Scalenus anterior, Scalenus medius, Anterior clavicle, Brachial plexus, Subclavian artery, Subclavian vein, Sternum, First rib

Compression of circumflex nerve

The circumflex or axillary nerve C5, C6 enters the quadrilateral space, which lies below the shoulder joint, and supplies the deltoid and the teres minor muscle. It also supplies the skin over the lower half of the deltoid. It may be damaged in antero-inferior dislocation of the shoulder joint. Osteophytes on the postero-inferior glenoid margin in professional baseball pitchers have resulted in injuries to the nerve. Bennett (1941) and Cahill and Palmer (1983), have reported chronic nerve entrapment and compression of the axillary nerve, and posterior circumflex humeral vessels in the quadrilateral space syndrome.

The radial nerve C6, C7, C8 supplies the long, medial and lateral heads of the triceps, before it enters the radial groove where it gives off the nerve to the anconeus, the lower lateral cutaneous of the arm, and the posterior cutaneous of the forearm. It then pierces the lateral intermuscular septum and supplies the brachialis and the brachioradialis. At the lateral epicondyle, it divides into its superficial and deep (the posterior interosseous) branches. The superficial branch passes down the forearm on the lateral site of the radial artery and pierces the deep fascia between the posterior border of the brachioradialis and the extensor carpi radius longus to become subcutaneous. It supplies the skin over the dorsal aspect of the thumb and the radial three and a half fingers.

The posterior interosseous supplies the supinator and the extensor carpi radialis brevis, and passes between the two heads of the supinator to supply all the other extensor muscles in the posterior compartment of the forearm.

Compression of the radial nerve

The radial nerve can be compressed in the axilla by direct pressure from axillary crutches. In fractures of the middle third of the humerus the radial nerve may be compromised by the fracture itself or by callus formation. Compression at this level does not affect the triceps but does involve the extensor muscles of the forearm. As it passes through the lateral intermuscular septum it may be compromised.

The posterior interosseous nerve passes between the two heads of the supinator. The superficial head may be partly or completely fibrous at its origin from the lateral epicondyle. Compression of the nerve in this region may be due to:
1 A completely fibrous superficial head, this is called the arcade of Frohse (Spinner, 1968).
2 Fibrous bands at the distal border of the supinator (Posner, 1990).
3 Fibrous bands at the sharp tendinous margin along the extensor carpi radialis brevis (Spinner, 1968).
4 A fan (leash) of the radial recurrent vessels (Henry, 1963).

The radial nerve may be compressed due to

traction on the superficial branch of the radial, as it pierces the deep fascia at the wrist (Wartenberg's syndrome) causing pain and paraesthesia over the dorsoradial aspect of the hand and thumb, on flexion and ulnar deviation of the wrist. This problem tends to occur in athletes who repeatedly pronate and supinate and ulnar flex their wrist; wristbands or hand-cuffs may have a similar effect (Reltig, 1990).

Median nerve C5, C6, C7, C8, T1 crosses the elbow joint medial to the brachial artery and the tendon of the biceps, passing under the bicipital aponeurosis. In the cubital fossa it gives off its first branches to the muscles from the common flexor origin and leaves the fossa between the two heads of the pronator teres. In 50% of cases, Johnson *et al.* (1979) found a fibrous band on the dorsal aspect of the superficial head. It passes under the fibrous arch of the flexor digitorum superficialis and just above the wrist, and lies posterolateral to the palmaris longus tendon. The superficial palmar branch passes superficial to the flexor retinaculum and supplies the radial portion of the palm of the hand.

The main nerve passes deep to the flexor retinaculum. Several variations of the median nerve have been described by Lanz (1977) (Fig. 8.3). At the distal border of the retinaculum in 50% of cases the motor branch to the thenar muscles curves back across the tendon of the flexor pollicis longus to supply the thenar muscles, abductor pollicis brevis, opponens pollicis and the superficial head of the flexor pollicis brevis. In 33% of cases it gives off the motor branch under the retinaculum and takes its usual course, but in 20% the motor branch pierces the ligament 2–6 mm proximal to the distal border of the ligament to reach the thenar muscles.

Compression of the median nerve

The median nerve may be compressed in the lower third of the arm by a ligament of Struthers, an abnormally thickened bicipital aponeurosis, but the most frequent site of compression in this region is where the nerve passes between the two heads of pronator teres. It may also be compressed where it passes deep to a fibrous arch, at the proximal margin of the flexor digitorum superficialis. Resisted flexion of the superficialis tendon to the middle finger tends to aggravate the symptoms.

Compression of the anterior interosseous nerve usually occurs deep to the fibrous band of the deep head of the pronator teres or at the tendinous origin of the superficialis (Sharrard, 1968).

Carpal tunnel syndrome

The commonest compression syndrome at the wrist and hand in athletes involves the median nerve as it passes under the flexor retinaculum to supply the thenar muscles and the skin of the radial three and a half fingers. The carpal tunnel syndrome usually presents with pain and paraesthesia of the thumb, index and middle finger. It does not involve the skin of the palm of the hand, and it may progress causing weakness and wasting of the thenar muscles. The pain usually occurs at night or with activity. There is a positive Phalens sign which is achieved by holding both wrists in a fully flexed position for 1–2 min which reproduces the pain. Tinel's sign, i.e. tenderness on pressure over the nerve, is positive. Treatment is to identify the cause, splint the wrists in a dorsiflex position, particularly at night. If this does not relieve the symptoms, an injection of steroid and xylocaine or surgical decompression may be required in a few cases. It is associated with any sport that involves repetitive movements of the wrist.

The ulnar nerve C8, T1 pierces the medial intermuscular septum to enter the posterior compartment of the arm. Thickening of the deep fascia where it pierces the septum may compress the nerve. This is approximately 8 cm above the medial epicondyle. It then passes

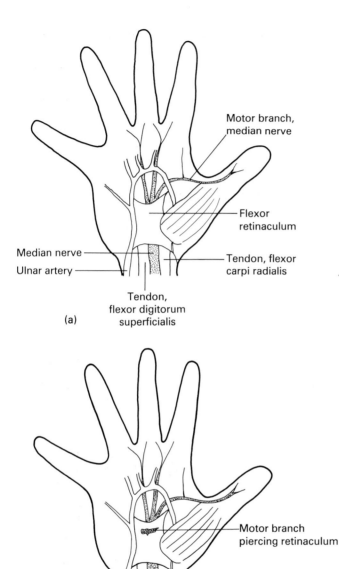

Motor branch,
median nerve

Flexor
retinaculum

Median nerve

Ulnar artery

Tendon, flexor
carpi radialis

Tendon,
flexor digitorum
superficialis

(a)

Motor branch
piercing retinaculum

(b)

Fig. 8.3 Normal (a) and abnormal
(b) variations of the median nerve at
the wrist.

behind the medial epicondyle and enters the
forearm between the two heads of the flexor
carpi ulnaris, which it supplies, to enter the
forearm. The ulnar nerve may be damaged at
the elbow due to traction injuries, as a result of
dynamic valgus forces in athletes, e.g. throwing
a javelin with a rounded elbow or pitching. An
increased valgus stress may be the result of a
previous supracondylar fracture, or injury to

the epiphyseal cartilage. Bony irregularities or
adhesions may tether the nerve causing symptoms. Hypertrophy of the flexor carpi ulnaris
and the medial head of the triceps may also
cause impingement in athletes.

In the forearm, 4.5 cm above the wrist, it gives
off the dorsal cutaneous branch, which supplies
the dorsal aspect of the ulnar one and a half

fingers. The ulnar nerve crosses superficial to the main portion of the flexor retinaculum in Guyon's tunnel, passing medial to the pisiform and lateral to the hamate (Fig. 8.4a). The nerve divides into a superficial cutaneous and a deep motor branch at the distal border of the canal. The superficial branch crosses the hypothenar muscles and is cutaneous to the palmar aspect of the ulnar one and a half fingers. The motor branch goes medial and distal to the hook of the hamate, supplying the hypothenar muscles and most of the small muscles of the hand. Shea and McClain (1969) have described three sites of compression in this area.

Palmar neuropathies are relatively common, particularly in long-distance cyclists (Frontera, 1983) (Fig. 8.4b). Factors that predispose are worn-out gloves, unpadded handlebars and prolonged gripping of dropped handlebars with no change in position (Reltig, 1990). Fractures of the hook of the hamate may involve the motor branch.

Treatment is to identify the cause of the compression. The patient may complain of pain and paraesthesia while throwing the javelin, therefore throwing technique must be analysed and corrected. Compression in Guyon's canal often results in tenderness over the canal and a positive Tinel's sign with radiation into the little finger and ulnar half of the ring finger. There may be weakness of the small muscles of the hand due to involvement of the motor supply. Treatment is rest, ice and splinting, non-steroidal anti-inflammatories, and correcting the position and grip of the handlebars in cyclists. If symptoms do not improve surgical decompression may be required.

The greater occipital nerve C2 pierces the semispinalis capitis and the trapezius to supply the posterior portion of scalp. Compression of the nerve may occur due to increased spasm of the semispinalis capitis and trapezius postwhiplash (Vital *et al.*, 1989).

Specific nerve entrapments in the lower limb

In the lower limb, entrapment syndromes may affect branches of the lumbar and sacral plexus.

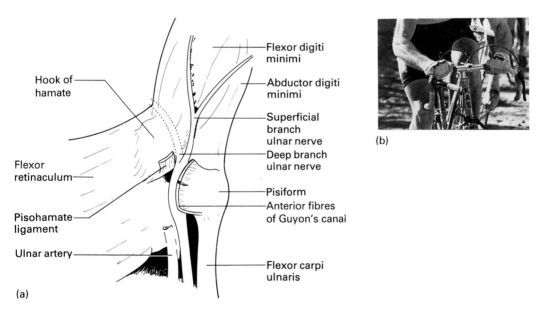

Fig. 8.4 (a) The ulnar nerve crossing the flexor retinaculum in Guyon's canal. (b) The position of the hand when cycling may increase pressure against the ulnar nerve in the palm.

The lateral cutaneous nerve of the thigh L2—L3 enters the thigh, by piercing the inguinal ligament where it lies in a fibrous tunnel. It supplies the anterolateral aspect of the thigh and the anterior portion of the gluteal region (Last, 1978). Entrapment of the nerve in the tunnel or injury to the thigh by the use of asymmetric bars in gymnasts may cause meralgia paraesthetica.

The ilio-inguinal nerve L1 may be trapped in the lower portion of the anterior abdominal wall postsurgery due to adhesions or to poor tone in the muscles (Fig. 8.5).

Tarsal tunnel syndrome

The posterior tibial nerve L4, L5, S1, S2, S3 passes under the flexor retinaculum at the ankle which stretches from the medial malleous of the tibia to the medial margin of the calcaneus (Fig. 8.6). Passing deep to the retinaculum are the flexor tendons and the posterior tibial vessels and nerve. The posterior tibial nerve

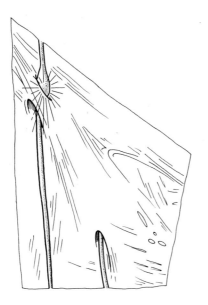

Fig. 8.5 Figure showing the lateral cutaneous nerve of the thigh which is being subjected to pressure from inflammation and swelling. With permission from Peterson & Renström (1985).

gives off the medial calcaneal nerve S1, S2 which pierces the retinaculum to supply the posterior and medial aspect of the heel. It divides into the medial and lateral plantar nerves which run in separate tunnels. The medial plantar nerve L4, L5 divides into digital branches, sensory to the plantar aspect of the medial three and a half toes and motor to the abductor hallucis, the flexor hallucis brevis, the flexor digitorum brevis and the first lumbrical. The lateral plantar S1, S2 is sensory to the lateral one and a half toes and supplies the other intrinsic muscles of the foot.

The posterior tibial nerve may be compressed proximally before it divides, more distally, either the medial or lateral plantar nerves may be involved. The most frequent compression is of the plantar digital branch of the medial plantar nerve to the third cleft, but the digital branch of the fourth cleft may also be affected. People with pronated feet and a depressed transverse arch at the heads of the metatarsals, subject the digital branch to the third cleft to a lot of stress which results in Morton's metarsalgia. In runners and ballet dancers a neuroma may develop. Runners who have a mobile first ray may compress the digital nerve to the second cleft. Compression of the toes in tight shoes will aggravate the pain, which is relieved by removing shoes.

Superficial peroneal nerve L4, L5 is a branch of the common peroneal at the neck of the fibula and it runs in the lateral compartment of the calf. It pierces the deep fascia 10—12 cm above the lateral malleolus. It divides 6 cm above the malleolus into branches which mainly supply the dorsum of the foot. The first cleft is supplied by the deep peroneal nerve. Entrapment occurs where it pierces the deep fascia, particularly if there is herniation of the muscle due to fascial defects (Schon & Baxter, 1990). Chronic ankle strains also stretch the nerve.

The deep peroneal L5 is a branch of the common peroneal at the neck of the fibula which then

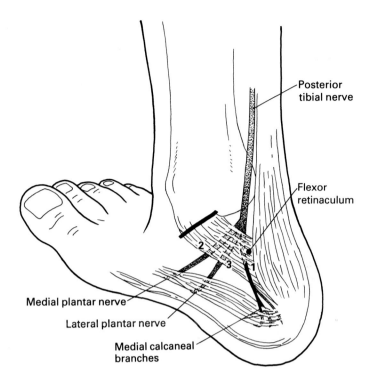

Posterior
tibial nerve

Flexor
retinaculum

Medial plantar nerve

Lateral plantar nerve

Medial calcaneal
branches

Fig. 8.6 Tarsal tunnel syndromes: 1, entrapment of the medial calcaneal; 2, entrapment of the medial plantar; 3, entrapment of the lateral plantar.

runs in the anterior compartment of the calf, and supplies the muscles in the compartment and the skin of the first cleft, passing under the superior and inferior retinacula. The nerve may be compressed due to an anterior compartment syndrome. Entrapment occurs mainly in runners. It also occurs in soccer players, dancers and skiers. It happens most frequently under the inferior extensor retinaculum (Schon & Baxter, 1990). Repetitive ankle-sprains, tight-fitting shoes or trauma may also cause entrapment.

Sural nerve L5, S1, S2 accompanies the short saphenous vein and runs along the lateral border of the foot. It may be entrapped anywhere along its course. It occurs most frequently in runners with a history of ankle sprain.

Treatment principles

Nerve compression may affect a large number of nerves. It is essential in all cases of nerve entrapment to identify the cause. Take a detailed history of the symptoms, particularly what activity or position aggravates the pain. Rule out and treat any medical conditions. X-rays, computerized tomography scan, magnetic resonance imaging, electromyogram and nerve conduction studies may be required in some cases. Relieving the compression may be achieved in some cases by correcting the athlete's technique, ice, splinting or non-steroidal anti-inflammatories, but some may require surgical decompression. An accurate knowledge of the normal anatomy and the common variations is essential to make an accurate diagnosis.

References

Bennett, G.E. (1941) Shoulder and elbow lesions of professional baseball pitchers. *JAMA* **117**, 510–14.
Brown, C. (1983) Compressive, invasive referred pain to shoulder. *Clin. Orthop.* **173**, 55–69.
Brown, S.L.W. & Charlesworth, D. (1988) Results of

excision of cervical rib in patients with thoracic outlet syndrome. *Br. J. Surg.* **75**, 431–3.

Cahill, B.R. & Palmer, R.E. (1983) Quadrilateral space syndrome. *J. Hand Surg.* **8**, 65–9.

Frontera, W.R. (1983) Cyclist palsy. Clinical and electrodiagnostic findings. *Br. J. Sports Med.* **17**, 91–3.

Henry, A.K. (1963) *Extensile Exposure.* Williams & Wilkins, Baltimore.

Hirasawa, Y. & Sakakida, M. (1983) Sports and peripheral nerve injuries. *Am. J. Sports Med.* **11**, 420–6.

Johnson, R.K., Spinner, M. & Shrewsbury, M.M. (1979) Median nerve entrapment syndrome in the proximal part of the forearm. *J. Hand Surg.* **4**, 48–51.

Karas, S.E. (1990) Thoracic outlet syndrome. *Clin. Sports Med.* **9**(2), 297–310.

Lanz, U. (1977) Anatomical variations of the median nerve in the carpal tunnel. *J. Hand Surg.* **2**, 44–53.

Last, R.J. (1978) *Anatomy: Regional and Applied*, 6th edn. Churchill Livingstone, London.

Lord, J.W. & Rosati, L.M. (1971) *Thoracic Outlet Syndrome.* Clinical Symposium, Vol. 23. CIBA Pharmaceuticals Co.

Peterson, L. & Renström, P. (1985) *Injuries in Sport.* Martin Dunitz Ltd, London.

Posner, M.A. (1990) Compressive neuropathy of the median and radial nerves. *Clin. Sports Med.* **9**(2), 343–63.

Reltig, A.C. (1990) Neurovascular injuries in the wrist and hands of athletes. *Clin. Sports Med.* 389–419.

Rengachary, S.S., Neff, J.P., Singer, P.A. *et al.* (1979) Suprascapular entrapment neuropathy. A clinical, anatomical and comparative study. *Neurosurgery* **5**, 441–6.

Roos, D.B. (1982) The place for scalenectomy and first rib resection in the thoracic outlet syndrome. *Surgery* **92**, 1077–85.

Schon, L.C. & Baxter, D.E. (1990) Neuropathies of foot and ankle in athletes. *Clin. Sports Med.* **9**(2), 489–509.

Sharrard, W.J.W. (1968) Anterior interosseous neuritis. *J. Bone Joint Surg.* **50B**, 804–5.

Shea, J.D. & McClain, E.F. (1969) Ulnar nerve compression syndrome at and below the wrist. *J. Bone Joint Surg.* **51A**, 1095–103.

Spinner, M. (1968) The arcade of Frohse and its relationship to posterior interosseous nerve paralysis. *J. Bone Joint Surg.* **50B**, 809–12.

Vital, J.M., Grenier, F., Dautheribes, M., Baspeyne, H., Lavignolle, B. & Senegas, J. (1989) An anatomic and dynamic study of the greater occipital nerve. *Surg. Radiol. Anat.* **II**(3), 205–10.

Part 2b

Basic and Applied Biomechanics

Chapter 9

Excessive Loads and Sports-Injury Mechanisms

BENNO M. NIGG

Load on an athlete's body can be defined as the sum of all the forces and moments acting on it. Load on specific structures of an athlete's body can be defined as the sum of all the forces and moments acting on the specific structure (Nigg & Bobbert, 1990). Load acting on specific structures of the athlete's body during sports activities is one possible stimulus to maintain and/or increase the strength of biological materials such as ligaments, tendons, muscles, bones and articular cartilage. However, if excessive, load may be the reason for microdamage or macrodamage to anatomical structures. Several studies suggest that load is excessive in many sport activities. It has been reported that between 27 and 70% of runners or joggers are injured during the period of 1 year (Clement et al., 1981; Brody, 1982; Jacobs & Berson, 1986; Warren & Jones, 1987; Bahlsen, 1988; Marti et al., 1988) and that between 21 and 52% of tennis players are injured per season (Biener & Caluori, 1977; Nigg & Denoth, 1980). Additionally, injuries related to aerobic activities have been reported for 76% of the instructors and 43% of the participants (Francis et al., 1985; Richie et al., 1985). These numbers suggest that there is a problem and that steps should be taken to reduce the frequency of sport injuries.

Various questions may be of interest in the analysis of sport injuries including the anatomical structure which is damaged (James et al., 1978; Clement et al., 1981), the type of damage to the anatomical structure (Biener & Caluori, 1977), the external forces acting on the athlete's body during movements which may lead to an injury (Cavanagh & Lafortune, 1980; Frederick et al., 1981), the actual internal forces or stresses acting in an anatomical structure before and possibly during an injury (Zernicke et al., 1977; Zernicke, 1981; Renström et al., 1988; Morlock & Nigg, 1991), the factors influencing external and/or internal forces and stresses (Clarke et al., 1983; Snel et al., 1983; Nigg et al., 1987; Stacoff et al., 1988), the material properties of the damaged structures and the critical limits (Yamada, 1970; Noyes & Grood, 1976; Shrive et al., 1988; Stuessi & Faeh, 1988), the factors influencing the material properties and the critical limits (Tipton et al., 1970; Amiel et al., 1982; Woo et al., 1984) and others. However, one of the main goals for research related to sport injuries should be the attempt to reduce the frequency of these injuries.

The purpose of this chapter is to list possible factors influencing the frequency of sport injuries and to discuss possible strategies to reduce forces acting on the athlete's body during sport activities. The following paragraphs concentrate on the discussion of *mechanical* factors responsible for sport injuries.

Possible factors

Whether or not an anatomical structure is injured during a physical activity depends on the material properties of that structure (strength of biomaterial) and the forces acting on that structure (Fig. 9.1, Table 9.1). In order to be able to develop strategies to reduce the occurrence of sport injuries it is important to understand how material properties on one side and acting forces on the other side can be influenced.

Strength of biomaterial

The following paragraphs summarize basic knowledge relevant for the understanding of how material properties of anatomical structures can be influenced. Mechanical properties of materials such as steel or wood are determined following well-defined procedures. Similar protocols are followed when determining the mechanical properties of biomaterials. Mechanical properties of non-living materials remain constant as long as the load applied remains within the elastic limits of these materials. However, mechanical properties of living tissue (biomaterials) change as a function of the applied load. Each load application causes the biomaterial to increase or decrease its mechanical strength. Consequently, the

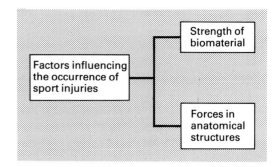

Fig. 9.1 Selected factors responsible for the aetiology of sport injuries.

Table 9.1 Selected experimental results for external vertical impact force (F) peaks in walking and running. The values with an asterisk are calculated using an average body mass of 70 kg. The abbreviation shoe stands for running shoe.

Movement	Footwear	v (m/s)	F_{max} (N)	F_{max}/BW	Author	Year
Walking	Barefoot	1.3	385*	0.55	Cavanagh	1981
	Army boots	1.3	259*	0.37	Cavanagh	1981
	Street shoes	1.3	189*	0.27	Cavanagh	1981
Running (heel)	Shoe	4.5	1540*	2.2	Cavanagh	1980
	Shoe 'hard'	4.0	2000	2.9*	Nigg	1980
	Shoe 'soft'	4.0	1100	1.6*	Nigg	1980
	Shoe	3.4	1365	2.0	Frederick	1982
	Shoe	3.8	1590	2.3	Frederick	1982
	Shoe	4.5	1963	2.9	Frederick	1982
	Shoe	3.0	1345	1.9*	Nigg	1987
	Shoe	4.0	1521	2.2	Nigg	1987
	Shoe	5.0	1799	2.6*	Nigg	1987
	Shoe	6.0	2070	3.0*	Nigg	1987
Running (toe)	Shoe	4.0	300	0.4*	Denoth	1980
Take-off for jump	Spikes	2.0	1000	1.4*	Nigg	1981
	Spikes	4.0	2300	3.3*	Nigg	1981
	Spikes	6.0	3700	5.3*	Nigg	1981
	Spikes	8.0	5700	8.1*	Nigg	1981
	Shoe	2.0	1400	2.0*	Nigg	1981
	Shoe	4.0	2000	2.0*	Nigg	1981
	Shoe	7.0	2900	4.1*	Nigg	1981

BW, body weight.

mechanical properties of biomaterials depend on exercise, immobilization, stretching, nutrition, age and other factors (Fig. 9.2). Selected effects of exercise are summarized for bone, cartilage, ligament, tendon and muscle in the following paragraphs.

BONE

The structural functions of bone include: (i) providing support for the body against gravity; (ii) acting as a lever system to transfer muscular and external forces; and (iii) acting as protection for vital internal organs. Additionally, bone has metabolic functions (e.g. serving as a repository for calcium). More than 100 years ago, Roux (1881) associated changes in the structure of tissue with changes in the pressure applied to the tissue. Wolff (1892) was the first to summarize that physical laws are a major factor influencing bone growth.

Bone health has been studied recently by quantifying bone mineral density and/or bone mass, assuming that these variables are related to bone strength. Significant differences in bone mineral content were found between long-time cross-country runners and sedentary age-

and weight-matched controls (Dalin & Olsson, 1974). However, no differences for bone mineral content were found between sedentary subjects who underwent a 3-month activity programme and their controls. Bone mineral density and total body calcium were compared for post-menopausal women (Aloia *et al.*, 1978) who engaged in 1 h of exercise three times per week over a period of 1 year and a sedentary control group. No differences were found for bone mineral content. However, total body calcium was found to increase significantly during the test period for the subjects involved in the exercise programme and to decrease at the same rate for those who were not involved in the exercise programme.

Several theories are proposed to describe bone remodelling and bone health. The currently available scientific results do not allow a simple description of bone remodelling. However, based on the currently published material one may speculate in a simplistic way that:

1 Light and moderate exercise does not effect bone mineral density while intensive exercise does. Intensive but non-excessive exercise is beneficial for general bone health.
2 Physical activity is beneficial for the transport of nutrients into bone.
3 Limited impact forces are beneficial for the treatment of osteoporotic bone or for the prevention of osteoporosis.
4 Excessive impact forces (peak force and loading rate) are associated with the development of osteoarthritis.
5 Fatigue fractures may be associated with excessive local stress, weak material properties of bone and/or missing vibration stimuli from muscles through tendon onto bone.
Most of these speculations have not been proven and are based on assumptions and/or current beliefs.

CARTILAGE

Hyalin cartilage has two main functions: (i) to provide mobility in the joints (very low friction coefficient); and (ii) to distribute the stress in

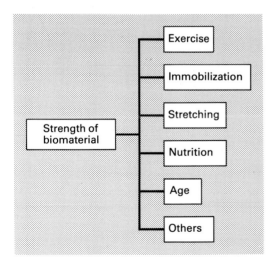

Fig. 9.2 Selected factors influencing the strength of biomaterials.

the joints and thus minimize peak stress to subchondral bone. Exercise may influence the frictional characteristics of cartilage if the applied forces are not within the elastic limits and microdamage or macrodamage result to the cartilage surface. Elastic limits of cartilage for repeated loading with exudation and imbibition of the cartilage's interstitial fluid (Mow & Lai, 1980; Kwan *et al.*, 1984) are much lower than for one single loading cycle (Mow & Rosenwasser, 1987). Repeated joint impact loading is suggested as an additional possible mechanism responsible for the damage of articular cartilage. It is speculated that impact loads (high loads for only a few milliseconds) applied to articular cartilage inhibit the appropriate internal fluid redistribution, resulting in high local forces in the collagen–proteoglycan matrix which may be the reason for possible damage.

This proposed process could explain the dramatic changes (and injuries) in articular cartilage as a consequence of different joint loading found by Radin *et al.* (1984). Furthermore, it has been suggested that an increase in loading rate may be associated with the development of osteoarthritis (Radin *et al.*, 1991). Animal studies (Tammi *et al.*, 1983) suggest that exercise may have positive effects on cartilage when performed properly. Animals were submitted to immobilization, running and increased weight-bearing for 24–27 days. Running increased the proteoglycan content. The ratio of keratin to chondroitin sulphate was found to be maximal at sites of maximum loading. It was concluded that weight-bearing rather than simple joint motion primarily determined cartilage matrix properties. Articular cartilage reacts to loading (exercise) in a short- and long-term way. Articular cartilage increases in thickness by about 10–15% after 10 min of running (Ingelmark & Ekholm, 1948), a result which is suggested to be associated with increased exchange of fluid. Long-term effects are illustrated by the fact that articular cartilage is thicker for trained than untrained animals (Holmdahl & Ingelmark, 1948). An increase in

thickness is commonly accompanied by an increase of elasticity.

Based on the currently available scientific publications one may speculate in a simplistic way that:

1 Cartilage loading is beneficial for the transport of nutrients into cartilage.
2 Cartilage thickness is influenced by cartilage loading and/or exercise.
3 Repeated impact forces are associated with cartilage damage.

The speculation that repeated impact forces are possibly associated with cartilage damage seems plausible. However, there is only limited evidence from animal experiments and no evidence from human studies supporting this speculation.

LIGAMENTS

The main functions of ligaments include: (i) the guidance of movement of two adjacent bones; and (ii) the limitation of the actual range of motion. Additionally, ligaments and capsules are assumed to provide sensory feedback about joint positions (Brand, 1986). Mechanical stress applied to ligaments increases the strength at the junction between ligament and bone and the strength of repaired ligaments (Tipton *et al.*, 1975). Exercise on one side increases the stiffness, ultimate strength and energy to failure of ligaments (Noyes *et al.*, 1984). Stretching, on the other side, increases ligament length. Additionally, exercised ligaments show some increase in ligament mass due to fibre bundle hypertrophy. Injuries to ligaments are associated with excessive movement in joints. Ligament injuries are related to the rate of loading. Ligaments exposed to a slow loading rate show ruptures at the junction between bone and ligaments. If exposed to forces with a high loading rate, midsubstance tear is common.

The current knowledge can be summarized in a simplistic way as follows:
1 Exercise-related loading (as long as it is not

excessive) is beneficial for the strength of ligaments.

2 Mechanical properties of ligaments are influenced by the loading history.

3 Excessive ligament loading is always associated with excessive joint motion.

4 Ligament failure depends on the loading rate of the applied force.

TENDON

The main functions of tendon include: (i) transmitting forces from the muscles to the bones; and (ii) storing energy during human movement, especially during locomotion. Exercise has positive effects on tendon, similar to the ones described for ligaments. The possible negative effects on tendon, however, are not only associated with excessive joint motion as in the case of the ligament ruptures but also with force production in the muscle. Tendon ruptures occur often during maximal muscle contraction. Additionally, the relation of the cross-sectional area of the tendon and the physiological cross-sectional area of the muscle (muscle force) are of importance in the development of possible tendon injuries.

The current knowledge can be summarized in a simplistic way as follows:

1 Exercise-related loading (as long as it is not excessive) is beneficial for the strength of tendon.

2 Mechanical properties of tendon are influenced by the loading history.

3 Excessive tendon loading is associated with excessive joint motion, maximal muscle force and/or the ratio of the cross-sectional areas of tendon and muscle.

MUSCLE

The primary function of muscle is to produce force. Muscles respond to exercise by an increase in the physiological cross-sectional area and by an associated increase in maximal strength. The increase in strength relates to an increase in muscle mass, an improved re-

cruitment pattern and/or a change in fibre orientation. Muscle injuries include cramps, soreness, laceration, contusion and strain/tear. Muscles can be injured by several different mechanisms with specific pathological processes. It has been suggested (Stacoff *et al.*, 1988; Denoth & Stacoff, 1991) that forces in muscles are not only due to muscle contraction but also due to increased angular velocity in the ankle–subtalar joint and related increased loading rates.

The current knowledge can be summarized in a simplistic way as follows:

1 Exercise-related loading of muscles (as long as it is not excessive) is beneficial for the maximal strength of muscles.

2 Muscle injuries may have a complex history and are difficult to isolate with respect to their origin.

3 High muscle loading occurs during eccentric movement.

4 High loading rates are one main reason for excessive loading of muscles.

SUMMARY

Excessive impact and/or active forces, high loading rates, excessive joint movement and malalignment of the skeleton have been suggested as main reasons for the aetiology of sport injuries.

Forces in anatomical structures

Forces in anatomical structures depend on the construction of the athlete's body and on many external factors (Fig. 9.3). The following comments concentrate on the external factors which may be influenced by appropriate strategies since the construction of the athlete's body cannot be changed easily.

The forces acting on specific structures during sport activities depend on the *movement* performed by the athlete. The forces are different for walking and running, take-off in high jump and long jump, boxing and wrestling and for Alpine and cross-country skiing. Most physical

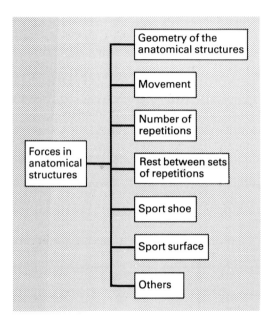

Fig. 9.3 Selected factors influencing the forces acting on an anatomical structure during sport activities.

activities have a number of *repetitions*. Forces in specific anatomical structures act only a few times during a sprint event but many thousand times during a marathon run. The human body consists of living tissue which reacts to loading stimuli in very different ways. The *resting time* between training sessions may influence the biological reaction of bone, tendon, muscle, ligament and cartilage and determine whether or not the reaction is biopositive or bionegative and whether or not a training stimulus improves or weakens the mechanical properties of a structure.

It has been widely documented that the *sport shoe* is one important factor responsible for the development of sport injuries. Sport shoes may alter forces in specific anatomical structures by more than 100% and are considered an important means for the prevention of sport injuries. *Sport surfaces* have been shown to be involved in tripling and quadrupling the frequency of injuries in selected sport activities (Nigg &

Denoth, 1980). Other factors often discussed as possible reasons for sport injuries include weather, temperature, humidity and dirt. They will not be discussed further in this chapter.

SELECTED STRATEGIES

Possible strategies which may be applied to reduce loading of the athlete's body will be discussed for the external factors listed in Fig. 9.3. Some of these strategies apply for élite athletes, others for everyday athletes.

Movement

External and internal forces are significantly influenced by the movement of the athlete. Maximal external active forces in walking are slightly over 1 BW (body weight). Maximal external active forces in running are between 1800 and 2200 N for running speeds from 3 to 6 m·s^{-1}. Maximal impact forces in running increase from about $1200-2300$ N for running speeds from 3 to 6 m·s^{-1} (Nigg *et al.*, 1987). Active forces are sensitive to the type of movement, impact forces to the speed of the movement. Consequently, if forces are excessive one may change the speed (running slower) or change the type of movement (walking instead of running). Such strategies are applicable for everyday athletes. For instance, movement changes from high- to low-impact activities have been introduced in running and aerobics to counter the frequent injuries which have been associated with high-impact loading and running activities have often been replaced with walking activities. The possibility of changing movement in high-performance athletes is rather limited. It may be possible to instruct proper movement techniques in the initial phase of high-performance training. However, in general, movement in hurdling, high jumping, tennis or gymnastics is defined by clear boundary conditions and only small changes are possible.

Number of repetitions and rest between sets of repetitions

Human tissue reaction to load may increase or decrease strength, depending on the number of repetitions of the applied force and the rest between sets of repetitions (exercise periods). The fact that the ultimate strength of bio-materials is significantly smaller for repeated than for single loading suggests that caution is appropriate for long-term cyclic loading. Furthermore, it is suggested that the quality of training is more important than the quantity, assuming that human tissue needs ample rest-ing time to regenerate in order to show a biopositive effect on training. However, clear advice for appropriate numbers of repetitions and rest between sets of repetitions is subject specific and not readily available.

Sport shoe

It has been shown that the type of shoe used for a specific sport activity has an influence on the type and/or frequency of injuries. Torg and Quedenfeld (1971) carried out a retrospective study of knee and ankle injuries of athletes in high school American football leagues. They showed that the frequency and severity of these injuries was higher for athletes using football shoes with seven 19-mm cleats (9.5-mm diameter) than for athletes using shoes with fourteen 9.5-mm cleats (12.5-mm diameter).

Luethi *et al.* (1986) studied the influence of shoes in a prospective study in tennis. They distributed two different shoe models which were available at the time of the experiment to a group of healthy tennis players and monitored the overuse injuries occurring during the fol-lowing 3-month period of tennis activity. They found a significant difference in the relative number of injuries for the two shoe groups (32.6 and 47.1% respectively). Additionally, site and type of injuries were different for the two shoe groups. Both studies indicate that the sport shoe, in fact, does influence site, type and frequency of sport injuries.

Sport shoe construction uses different mid-sole hardnesses (with the help of material and/or constructional solutions) and different geo-metrical forms. Both influence the force devel-opment in a different way:

1 Midsole hardness does not have an effect on the external vertical impact force (Nigg *et al.*, 1987) and the external vertical loading rate (Fig. 9.4). This result is surprising and is not

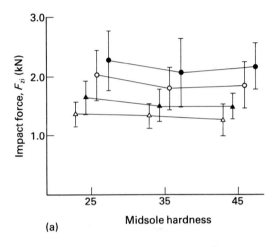

(a)

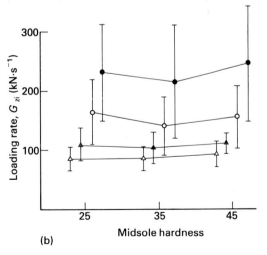

(b)

Fig. 9.4 The influence of midsole hardness on (a) the vertical impact force peaks, F_{zi}, and (b) the vertical loading rate, G_{zi}, for 14 male runners and a running speed of 3 ($\triangle$), 4 ($\blacktriangle$), 5 ($\circ$) and 6 ($\bullet$) m·s^{-1} (mean and SD).

currently completely understood. Ongoing work in our laboratory suggests that internal forces in the major force-carrying structures of the foot during running are not significantly influenced by changes in midsole hardness of the running shoe sole. This suggests that 'cushioning' of the shoe may be more a comfort than a protection function.

2 Geometry and specific construction of the sport shoe has a major effect on movement and, consequently, on external and internal forces. Heel flare, for instance, influences pronation and supination during landing (Nigg & Morlock, 1987). Heel stabilizers and heel counters tend to increase initial pronation and decrease vertical impact forces. Torsional stiffness of the shoe has been demonstrated to influence the elongation of ankle ligaments (Fig. 9.5) and, consequently, load in selected ankle ligaments (Morlock, 1990). In general, one can summarize that increases in levers between shoe and ground tend to increase initial pronation or supination and to decrease impact forces.

Fatigue fractures in the lower extremities are frequent in high-performance athletes. The development of stress fractures in runners has often been linked to a reduction in bone mineral density (Linnell et al., 1984; Martin & Bailey, 1987). It has been demonstrated for six female runners with chronic stress fractures and eight female runners with no history of

stress fractures that runners with stress fractures had significantly greater spinal and femoral neck bone mineral density than runners with no history of stress fractures and that tibial bone mineral density for those two groups did not differ (Grimston et al., 1991). This result suggests that the development of stress fractures is not associated with reduced bone mineral density. However, external forces on the runners' shoes showed differences for the two groups (Fig. 9.6) with the averages for the stress fracture group significantly greater than for the normal group (maximal vertical impact force, 13%; maximal vertical active force, 7%; maximal posterior force, 15%; maximum medial force, 46%; and maximal lateral force, 64%). The extreme differences in the medial forces are the reasons for mediolateral bending moments which may be associated with the aetiology of stress fractures (Fig. 9.6). Since external forces can be influenced with shoe construction it is suggested that stress fractures may preventively be treated with appropriate shoes which reduce the mediolateral force components.

Inappropriate sport shoes may double or triple the pronatory and/or supinatory movement between foot and lower leg compared to barefoot movements (Nigg, 1986). Internal forces may increase accordingly. Furthermore, sport shoes may be used to correct the dynamic alignment of the locomotor system. Canting of

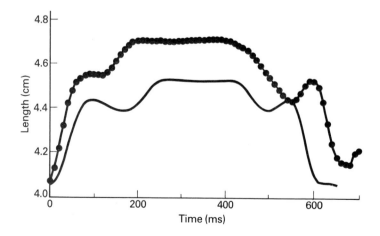

Fig. 9.5 Effect of torsional stiffness of the shoe on ligament length during a sideward jump. ●, Stiff shoe condition; ——, torsion shoe condition. From Morlock (1990).

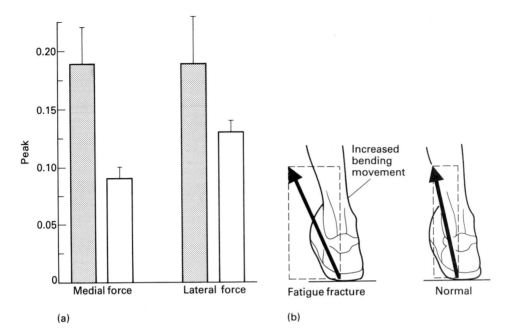

Fig. 9.6 (a) Differences in external forces (mediolateral component) and (b) illustration of these differences for a foot during ground contact. Based on data from Grimston *et al.* (1991).

shoe soles in skiing, orthotics in running or soccer shoes and many other strategies are used to influence the geometric alignment of the skeleton. It is assumed that these manipulations help to prevent sport injuries. However, evidence is often anecdotal in this respect.

SUMMARY

The sport shoe is one of the most important factors in the aetiology and prevention of sport injuries. Excessive levers are assumed to be a primary reason for high internal forces and possible injuries.

Sport surfaces

Sport surfaces have been demonstrated to be associated with the aetiology of sport injuries. Injury frequencies vary significantly for different tennis surfaces (Nigg & Denoth, 1980). In a study with more than 2000 cases (one case = one tennis player during 6 months) the fre-

quency of pain (Table 9.2) was significantly lower for the two surfaces which allowed sliding (clay and synthetic sand) than for the four surfaces which did not allow sliding (synthetic surface, asphalt, felt carpet and synthetic grill). The injury frequencies for surfaces which did not allow sliding were at least 200% higher than the injury frequencies for the two surface types which allowed sliding. Consequently, frictional aspects seem to be of importance for the aetiology of sport injuries.

Long-term retrospective studies on injury frequencies in different sport activities have been published by the National Collegiate Athletic Association (NCAA) (1990–1991). The statistics derive from a retrospective data base which includes millions of practice or game exposures. This data base may be used to compare the influence of natural grass and artificial turf on the frequency of sport injuries. Results from this comparison are summarized in Table 9.3. They suggest that the injury frequency is higher on artificial turf than on

Table 9.2 Frequency of pain and injuries for tennis players on six different surfaces in comparison to the total number of tennis players on a specific surface; f(surface i) is the frequency of pain and injuries on a specific surface i; and f(clay) is the frequency of pain and injuries on clay.

Surface	Frequency of pain and injuries (%)	f(surface i) : f(clay)(%)
Clay	2.2	100
Synthetic sand	3.0	136
Synthetic surface	10.7	486
Asphalt	14.5	659
Felt carpet	14.8	673
Synthetic grill	18.0	818

Table 9.3 Summary of surface-related injuries for American football, soccer and field hockey based on data from the NCAA injury surveillance system reports.

Sport	Gender	Activity	Surface	Percentage of injuries	Years
American football	Male	Practice	Nat. grass	11	1984–1991
			Art. turf	11	
		Game	Nat. grass	7	
			Art. turf	12	
Soccer	Female	Practice	Nat. grass	27	1988–1991
			Art. turf	32	
		Game	Nat. grass	26	
			Art. turf	31	
	Male	Practice	Nat. grass	26	1988–1991
			Art. turf	28	
		Game	Nat. grass	22	
			Art. turf	28	
Field hockey	Female	Practice	Nat. grass	26	1988–1991
			Art. turf	33	
		Game	Nat. grass	21	
			Art. turf	24	

Art., artificial; Nat., natural.

natural grass for American football (71% for games), for male soccer (19% for practice and games), for female soccer (8% for practice and 27% for games) and for female field hockey (27% for practice and 14% for games). The two surfaces do not differ in their injury frequencies for practice activities in American football.

The results of the two discussed studies on injury frequencies suggest that the frictional behaviour of the surface–shoe interface is of great importance for the prevention of sport injuries. Artificial grass, as well as other artificial surfaces, is often softer than natural grass or clay. However, artificial surfaces in the discussed studies do not show a reduced injury frequency. This may lead to the conclusion that cushioning is not the primary protection factor in the discussed sport activities. It is speculated that, for the discussed sports, frictional behaviour is of great importance. Optimal surfaces allow sliding but prevent slipping. Sliding provides an increase in the decelerating distance which corresponds to a reduction in the maximal forces acting on the athletes.

However, there are sports where cushioning is of great importance. Landing in gymnastics activities, for instance, as they are performed nowadays, could not be done without injuries if the landing areas were not cushioned as it is currently. In general, cushioning is of great importance for all movements with a dominant vertical component and friction between surface and shoe is of great importance for all movements with dominant horizontal components. It is suggested for everyday athletes that the translational friction coefficient between surface and shoe be in the order of 0.5−1. However, these friction coefficients may not be the appropriate measure for developing strategies to reduce sport injuries. The critical aspect with respect to friction is that sliding reduces the loading of the athlete's body compared to not sliding. However, external and internal forces will not be influenced by the friction coefficient as long as an athlete does not slide. Furthermore, one must be careful to avoid slipping which, of course, is more likely on a surface which does allow sliding.

SUMMARY

The sport surface is an important factor in the prevention of sport injuries. The sport surface may provide improved cushioning especially during landing from primarily vertical movements and/or frictional properties which allow sliding but prevent slipping.

Conclusion

Sport injuries are of great concern for athletes, coaches and medical specialists. Sport injuries often occur due to excessive mechanical forces acting on a specific structure in the athlete's body. It is proposed that excessive impact and active forces, high loading rates and movement with excessive range of motion are the most important factors to be controlled to prevent sport injuries. Possible strategies to prevent sport injuries include the adjustment of the training quantity and the resting periods between training sessions. Sport shoes and/or sport surfaces can be used to reduce the impact forces and the loading rates of acting forces, to control and restrict motion in joints of the lower extremities, to realign the skeleton and to influence the frictional characteristics between shoe and surface. The problems discussed in this chapter concentrate mainly on lower extremity injuries. Other injuries need different strategies to be applied.

Acknowledgments

This contribution was made possible due to support from NSERC (Canada) and the sport shoe company Adidas.

References

Aloia, J.F., Cohen, S.H., Ostuni, J.A., Cane, R. & Ellis, K. (1978) Prevention of involutional bone loss by exercise. *Ann. Intern. Med.* **89**, 356−8.

Amiel, D., Woo, S.L.-Y., Harwood, F.L. & Akeson, W.H. (1982) The effect of immobilization on collagen turnover in connective tissue: A biochemical−biomechanical correlation. *Acta Orthop. Scand.* **53**, 325−32.

Bahlsen, H.A. (1988) *The etiology of running injuries.* Thesis, University of Calgary.

Biener, K. & Caluori, P. (1977) Tennissportunfaelle (Sports injuries in tennis). *Med. Klinik* **72**, 754−7.

Brand, R.A. (1986) Knee ligaments: a new view. *J. Biomech. Eng.* **108**, 106−10.

Brody, D.M. (1982) Techniques in the evaluation and treatment of the injured runner. *Orthop. Clin. N. Am.* **13**, 541−58.

Cavanagh, P.R. & Lafortune, M.A. (1980) Ground reaction forces in distance running. *J. Biomech.* **13**, 397−406.

Clarke, T.E., Frederick, E.C. & Cooper, L.B. (1983) Effects of shoe cushioning upon ground reaction forces in running. *Int. J. Sports Med.* **4**, 247−51.

Clement, D.B., Taunton, J.E., Smart, G.W. & McNicol, K.L. (1981) A survey of overuse running injuries. *Phys. Sports Med.* **9**, 47−58.

Dalin, N. & Olsson, K.E. (1974) Bone mineral content and physical activity. *Acta Orthop. Scand.* **45**, 170−4.

Denoth, J. & Stacoff, A. (1991) Belastung und Beanspruchung der Muskulatur (Load and stress of muscles). *Sportverl. Sportschad.* **5**, 17–21.

Francis, L.L., Francis, P.R. & Welshons-Smith, K. (1985) Aerobic dance injuries: a survey of instructors. *Phys. Sports Med.* **2**, 105–11.

Frederick, E.C., Hagy, J.L. & Mann, R.A. (1981) Prediction of vertical impact force during running (Abstract). *J. Biomech.* **14**, 498.

Grimston, S.K., Engsberg, J.R., Kloiber, R. & Hanley, D.A. (1991) Bone mass, external loads and stress fracture in female runners. *Int. J. Sports Biomech.* **7**, 293–302.

Holmdahl, D.E. & Ingelmark, B.E. (1948) Der Bau des Gelenkknorpels unter Verschiedenen funktionellen Verhaeltnissen (Construction of articular cartilage for different functional conditions). *Acta Anat.* **6**, 309.

Ingelmark, B.E. & Ekholm, R. (1948) A study on variations in the thickness of articular cartilage in association with rest and periodical load. *Uppsal. Foerhand.* **53**, 61–74.

Jacobs, S.J. & Berson, B.L. (1986) Injuries to runners: a study of entrants to a 10 000 meter race. *Am. J. Sports Med.* **14**, 151–5.

James, S.L., Bates, B.T. & Osternig, L.R. (1978) Injuries to runners. *Am. J. Sports Med.* **6**, 40–50.

Kwan, M.K., Lai, W.M. & Mow, V.C. (1984) Fundamentals of fluid transport through cartilage in compression. *Ann. Biomed. Eng.* **12**, 537–58.

Linnell, S.L., Stager, J.M., Blue, P.W., Oyster, N. & Robertshaw, D. (1984) Bone mineral content and menstrual regularity in female runners. *Med. Sci. Sports* **16**(4), 343–8.

Luethi, S.M., Frederick, E.C., Hawes, M.R. & Nigg, B.M. (1986) Influence of shoe construction on lower extremity kinematics and load during lateral movements in tennis. *Int. J. Sports Biomech.* **2**, 156–65.

Marti, B., Vader, J.P., Minder, C.E. & Abelin, T. (1988) On the epidemiology of running injuries: The 1984 Bern Grand Prix Study. *Am. J. Sports Med.* **16**, 285–94.

Martin, A.D. & Bailey, D.A. (1987) Review: Skeletal integrity in amenorrheic athletes. *Australian J. Sci. Med. Sports* **19**(1), 3–7.

Morlock, M. (1990) *A mathematical model of the ankle and the foot.* Thesis, University of Calgary.

Morlock, M. & Nigg, B.M. (1991) Theoretical considerations and practical results on the influence of the representation of the foot for the estimation of internal forces with models. *Clin. Biomech.* **6**, 3–13.

Mow, V. & Rosenwasser, M. (1988) Articular cartilage: biomechanics. In S.L-Y. Woo & J.A. Buckwalter (eds) *Injury and Repair of the Musculoskeletal Soft Tissues*, pp. 427–63. American Academy of Orthopaedic Surgeons, Illinois.

Mow, V.C. & Lai, W.M. (1980) Recent developments in synovial joint biomechanics. *SIAM Rev* **22**, 275–317.

National Collegiate Athletic Association (1990–1991) *Injury Surveillance System* (football, male; soccer, female and male; field hockey, female). NCAA, USA.

Nigg, B.M. (1986) Experimental techniques used in running shoe research. In B.M. Nigg (ed) *Biomechanics of Running Shoes*, pp. 27–61. Human Kinetics, Illinois.

Nigg, B.M., Bahlsen, H.A., Luethi, S.M. & Stokes, S. (1987) The influence of running velocity and midsole hardness on external impact forces in heel–toe running. *J. Biomech.* **20**, 951–9.

Nigg, B.M. & Bobbert, M. (1990) On the potential of various approaches in load analysis to reduce the frequency of sports injuries. *J. Biomech.* **23**, 1, 3–12.

Nigg, B.M. & Denoth, J. (1980) In B.M. Nigg & J. Denoth (eds) *Sportplatzbelaege* (Playing surfaces). Juris Verlag, Zurich.

Nigg, B.M. & Morlock, M. (1987) The influence of lateral heel flare of running shoes on pronation and impact forces. *Med. Sci. Sports* **19**, 294–302.

Noyes, F.R. & Grood, E.S. (1976) The strength of the anterior cruciate ligament in humans and rhesus monkeys. *J. Bone Joint Surg.* **58**, 1074–82.

Noyes, F.R., Keller, C.S., Grood, E.S. & Butler, D.L. (1984) Advances in the understanding of knee ligament injury, repair and rehabilitation. *Med. Sci. Sports* **16**(5), 427–43.

Radin, E.L., Martin, R.B. & Burr, D.B. (1984) Effects of mechanical loading on the tissues of the rabbit knee. *J. Orthop. Res.* **2**, 221–34.

Radin, E.L., Yank, K.H., Riegger, C., Kish, V.L. & O'Connor, J.J. (1991) Relationship between lower limb dynamics and knee joint pain. *J. Orthop. Res.* **9**, 398–405.

Renström, P., Wertz, M., Incavo, S., Pope, M., Ostgaard, H.C., Arms, S. & Haugh, L. (1988) Strain in the lateral ligaments of the ankle. *Foot Ankle* **9**, 59–63.

Richie, D.H., Kelson, S.F. & Bellucci, P.A. (1985) Aerobic dance injuries: a retrospective study of instructors and participants. *Phys. Sports Med.* **13**, 130–40.

Roux, W. (1881) Der zuechtende Kampf der Teile. In W. Roux (ed) *Theorie der Funktionellen Anpassung* (Theory of Functional Adjustment), p. 137.

Shrive, N.G., Lam, J.C., Damson, E. & Frank, C.B. (1988) A new method of measuring the cross-sectional area of connective tissue structures. *J. Biomech. Eng.* **110**, 104–9.

Snel, J.G., Delleman, N.J., Heerkens, Y.F. & Ingen Schenau, G.J. van (1983) Shock absorbing characteristics of running shoes during actual running. In

D.A. Winter, R.W., Norman, R.P., Wells, K.C., Hayes & A.E., Patla (eds) *Biomechanics IX*, pp. 133–8. Human Kinetics, Illinois.

Stacoff, A., Denoth, J., Kaelin, X. & Stuessi, E. (1988) Running injuries and shoe construction: some possible relationships. *Int. J. Sport Biomech.* **4**, 342–57.

Stuessi, E. & Faeh, D. (1988) Assessment of bone mineral content by *in vivo* measurement of flexural wave velocities. *Med. Biol. Eng. Comput.* **26**, 349–54.

Tammi, M., Saamanen, A.M., Jauhiainen, A., Malminen, O., Kiviranta, I. & Helminen, H.J. (1983) Proteoglycan alterations in rabbit knee articular cartilage following physical exercise and immobilization. *Connect. Tiss. Res.* **11**(1), 45–55.

Tipton, C.M., James, S.L., Mergner, W. & Tscheng, T.K. (1970) Influence of exercise on strength of the medial collateral knee ligaments of dogs. *Am. J. Physiol.* **218**, 894–901.

Tipton, C.M., Matthes, R.D., Maynard, J.A. & Carey, R.A. (1975) The influence of physical activity on ligaments and tendons. *Med. Sci. Sports* **7**, 165–75.

Torg, J.S. & Quedenfeld, T. (1971) Effect of shoe type and cleat length on incidence and severity of knee injuries among high school football players. *Res. Q.* **42**, 203–11.

Warren, B.L. & Jones, C.J. (1987) Predicting plantar fasciitis in runners. *Med. Sci. Sports* **19**, 71–3.

Wolff, J. (1892) *Das Gesetz der Transformatin der Knochen* (The Law of Bone Transformation). August Hirschwald Verlag, Berlin.

Woo, S.L.-Y., Newton, P.O., Gomez, M.A. & Akeson, W.H. (1984) Responses of medial collateral ligament to immobilization and remobilization. *Orthop. Res. Soc.* **9**, 131.

Yamada, H. (1970) *Strength of Biological Materials*. Williams & Wilkins, Baltimore.

Zernicke, R.F. (1981) Biomechanical evaluation of bilateral tibia spiral fractures during skiing—a case study. *Med. Sci. Sports* **13**, 243–5.

Zernicke, R.F., Garshammer, J.J. & Jobe, F.W. (1977) Human patellar tendon rupture: a kinetic analysis. *J. Bone Joint Surg.* **59A**, 179–83.

Chapter 10

Biomechanical Response of Body Tissue to Impact and Overuse

MALCOLM H. POPE AND BRUCE D. BEYNNON

This chapter deals with the response of body tissue to both acute loadings (such as impact) and to chronic or repetitive loadings with special emphasis on the relevance to sports. Some basic biomechanical definitions and issues will be discussed followed by some specifics on the mechanical behaviour of both soft and hard tissues.

Basic biomechanics

If a material is placed under a tensile load, it will elongate. If the elongation is proportional to the load increment (Fig. 10.1), the material is said to behave in an elastic manner. All metals have a largely elastic behaviour whereas all biological materials do not. Figure 10.1a shows the relationship for linear elastic material. In order to normalize for the size of the specimen, the relationship is usually described as stress (load/cross-sectional area) against strain (elongation/original length) as shown in Fig. 10.1b.

Cyclic loading (repetitive loading and unloading) can cause a material to fail at a load lower than that which will usually cause failure. The relationship shown in Fig. 10.2 illustrates the failure versus non-failure regime. Note how failure occurs at progressively lower loads at the higher number of loading repetitions. In some, but not all materials, there is an endurance limit which is a load that can be repetitively applied an infinite number of times without failure. In biological materials, we have two competing processes, the cyclic fatigue process and the healing process. Normally, tissues do not fatigue because of the healing mechanism. However, under athletic training or military marches, the pain signals may be ignored and a fatigue failure (so-called march fracture) of the lower extremity may occur.

Most biological materials are viscoelastic, not

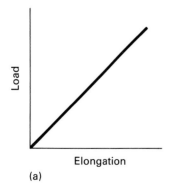

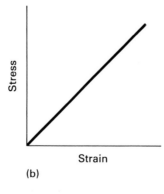

Fig. 10.1 (a) Shows the relationship for linear elastic material. In order to normalize for the size of the specimen, the relationship is usually described as stress (load/cross-sectional area) against strain (elongation/original length) as shown in (b).

120

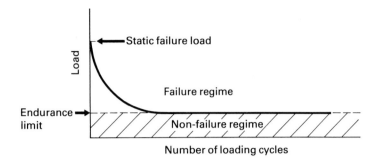

Fig. 10.2 Cyclic loading (repetitive loading and unloading) can cause a material to fail at a load lower than that which will usually cause failure. The relationship shown illustrates the failure versus non-failure regime.

elastic (Fig. 10.3a) and have rheological behaviour represented by the model shown in Fig. 10.3b. The viscoelastic materials have the attributes of strain rate dependency and creep. Strain rate dependency means that the materials have different stiffness and failure loads with different loading rate. Thus, bone may appear brittle at high loading rates but not at lower rates of loading. As we shall see, fracture of bone will have different characteristics at different rates of loading. Creep (Fig. 10.4) means that under continued constant loading, the material will continue to deflect until an equilibrium condition is met. Creep is important in cartilage, meniscus and the intervertebral disc. Krag *et al.* (1990) found that an individual

may lose 17 mm of their total height in the first 2 h after arising due to creep of the intervertebral discs.

Biomechanical background on soft tissues

The biomechanical properties and function of the soft tissues of the human have been extensively studied for many years. Langer (1884), in an interesting early paper, demonstrated the anisotropy of soft tissues by making punctuate marks in the skin of cadavers. Gallie (1924) measured the strength of rabbit connective tissues to see if they could be used for surgical repair in humans. Gritz (1931) measured the strength of fascia lata taken from patients at surgery. In his paper, he made an early study of stress relaxation. Cronkite (1936) measured the tensile strength of tendons and reported considerable variability between cadavers.

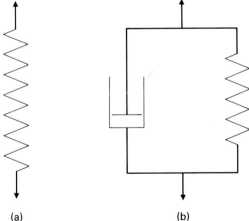

(a)   (b)

Fig. 10.3 Most biological materials are viscoelastic, not elastic (a) and have rheological behaviour represented by the model shown in (b).

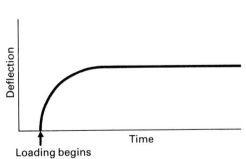

Fig. 10.4 Creep means that under continued constant loading, the material will continue to deflect until an equilibrium condition is met. Creep is important in cartilage, meniscus and the intervertebral disc.

Smith (1954) measured the viscoelastic properties of the anterior cruciate ligaments of rabbits and found that, for loads near failure, the ligaments exhibited a permanent set. Rigby *et al.* (1959) reported on the non-linear stress–strain relation in collagenous tissues and stated that the initial non-linearity coincided with the straightening of the collagen fibres which were previously wavy. Abrahams (1967) was among the first to describe three regions of the stress–strain curve. Up to 1.5% strain, the shape of the curve was due to fibre straightening, between 1.5 and 3% it was due to the reorientation of the fibres, and greater than 3% was due to a linear response of the fully oriented fibres.

Tendons

Tendons are comprised of relatively dense, parallel collagen and elastic fibres interwoven with proteoglycans. Woo (1986) has demonstrated that the proteoglycans, which imbibe water, are responsible for the viscoelastic effects.

Tendons are responsible for the transmission of muscle force to the bones so as to move the joints. It has been suggested by Alexander (1988) that tendons facilitate motion by the storing of elastic energy. In humans, the tensile strength of tendons varies between 45 and 125 MPa with an ultimate strain of 9–30% (Woo, 1986). In common with other soft tissues, tendon exhibits a non-linear stress–strain or load deflection relationship (Fig. 10.5). A curve of this type is indicative of a viscoelastic response. Due to this viscoelastic response, the tendon becomes slightly stiffer with increasing rate of loading and also exhibits some hysteresis. Hysteresis means that the loading curve is different from the unloading curve. The area between the curves represents an energy loss primarily in the form of tendon heating.

According to Kastelic and Baer (1980) tendon diminishes in strength and increases in stiffness with age. This is similar to the changes found with a loss of hydration. This is a finding of importance to the aging athlete who places

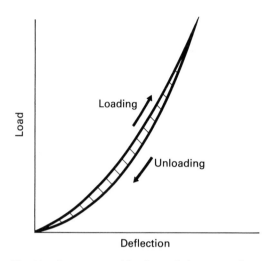

Fig. 10.5 In common with other soft tissues, tendons exhibit a non-linear stress–strain or load deflection relationship. The loading portion of the curve is different from the unloading part (hysteresis). The shaded area between the curves represents an energy loss primarily in the form of tendon heating.

high loads on the tendons. An example might be the high peak forces placed on the Achilles tendon in squash.

Biomechanical testing has been extremely instructive in pointing the direction for the optimal treatment of tendon after injury, repair or after injury to muscle. Akeson (1961) found that immobilization causes a loss of proteoglycans (and thus water content) along with a decrease of strength. Conversely, the same group (Woo *et al.*, 1980) have found that exercise increases collagen fibril size, strength and stiffness. Tendons are widely used in ligament reconstruction. However, Klein and Lewis (1972) found a great deal of collagen turnover. At 3 months, collagen replacement for autografts equalled the loss whereas the allograft had a net loss.

There are three types of tendon injury: (i) avulsion at the insertion site; (ii) in-substance failure; and (iii) laceration. Tendon injuries of the first two varieties can occur in a number of sports due to a violent contraction of the muscle. Laceration injuries are common to the flexor tendons on the hand. Although both conservative and operative treatments can be considered, primary repair ensures the tendon remains at its normal length which can improve function and reduces joint stiffness (Verdan, 1972). These results occur because of the sequence of events after disruption. Scar formation can apparently be minimized if there is good apposition of the ends of the tendon and if that apposition is maintained by the suturing technique. However, scar tissue never regains the strength of the intact soft-tissue structure (Frank et al., 1983).

As in most tissues, tendon repair is a trade-off between loading to stimulate reorganization and strengthening on one hand and immobilization to prevent rerupture. Gelberman et al. (1986) have shown that the tensile strength can be increased by controlled continuous passive motion (CPM) as compared to immobilization. There were also less adhesions on to the flexor tendons in the mobilized groups.

Ligament

Ligaments are primarily composed of collagen (types I and III), hydrated proteoglycans and elastin. Normally, there is 90% type I and 10% type III. Elastin reaches 75% in the ligament nuchae but is usually much less. The collagen fibres in ligaments are not as well organized as they are in tendon and some reorientation is responsible for the non-linear load deflection behaviour. Butler et al. (1983) have demonstrated that significant variations in strain exists along a typical ligament. Likewise, Arms et al. (1983) have found that strains can vary considerably across a ligament as a function of local orientation of fibres.

As in all tissues, age diminishes the strength of ligaments (Noyes & Grood 1976). Woo et al. (1986) found that in rabbits with an open epiphysis, failure was more likely by tibial avulsion whereas, with a closed epiphysis, a midsubstance failure was more common. Similar findings have yet to be confirmed in humans. Other factors are also relevant to the type of failure. Crowninshield and Pope (1976) showed that avulsion failures result primarily at low rates of loading (Fig. 10.6) whereas midsubstance tears occur at high loading rates. Another important consideration in the elderly or inactive population or in those undergoing rehabilitation is that immobilization markedly decreases the strength of the ligament—bone junction (Laros et al., 1971). This effect is particularly important in the collateral ligaments.

Of ligament injuries in athletics, the most common are injuries to the knee ligaments. It is a common sight at athletic events to see participants wearing knee braces. As the interest in fitness continues, there is every indication that the number of these injuries will increase and that the occurrence in older age groups will increase disproportionately. The anterior cruciate ligament (ACL) is the most frequently totally disrupted ligament within the knee. We established that 1.2% of all arriving students at the University of Vermont in 1 year had already

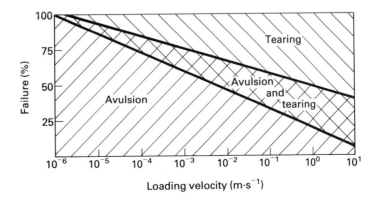

Fig. 10.6 Avulsion failures result primarily at low rates of loading whereas midsubstance tears occur at high loading rates. With permission from Crowninshield & Pope (1976).

sustained a complete disruption of one ACL. The management of the acute ACL injury and the reconstruction of the ACL in the anterior cruciate deficient knee has become synonymous with orthopaedic sports medicine.

For these reasons, there have been many attempts to measure knee ligament function. Edwards *et al.* (1970), Kennedy *et al.* (1977) and Brown *et al.* (1986) utilized mercury filled strain gauges to measure the length of ligaments at various angles of knee flexion. Mutchler *et al.* (1979) used a U-shaped metallic strain gauge to measure strain in the medial collateral ligament (MCL). Other workers have calculated strain by measurement of ligament attachment length under various loads (Wang *et al.*, 1973; Trent *et al.*, 1976; Sidles *et al.*, 1988).

Our approach has been to measure the ACL displacement over a known gauge length and thus compute strain in subjects with normal ACLs (Howe *et al.*, 1990; Beynnon *et al.*, 1992a). This is accomplished, using a Hall effect technique, through a relatively non-invasive arthroscopic procedure with limited risk to the patient. A total of 35 knees from 35 patients were studied. The average age was 25 years, ranging from 18 to 40 years. Strain is defined as the change in ligament length divided by the reference length. The strain reference for these studies were calculated by recording *A/P* load applied to the tibia, ACL displacement and establishing the slack—taut transition length of the ACL.

Figure 10.7 illustrates the averaged strain pattern of the anteromedial bundle (AMB) of the ACL during active range of motion (AROM) (extension of the knee by the subject) and passive range of motion (PROM) (knee extended by the surgeon). During PROM, a decrease in strain occurred from extension to a minimum value reached at 50°. Between the limits of 10 and 110° of flexion the mean ACL strain values remained unstrained. In AROM, the ligament was always load bearing between 48 and 0°, reaching a maximum value at 20° of flexion. In some cases, the AMB was load bearing throughout the AROM activity (Beynnon *et al.*, 1992a).

Knee braces are often prescribed for prevention from and rehabilitation after knee injuries. However, some concern has been voiced as to their efficacy (American Academy of Orthopedic Surgeons, 1988). The authors have evaluated the efficacy of functional knee bracing by measuring ACL strain in subjects with and without knee braces (Beynnon *et al.*, 1992b). Comparisons of ACL strain values between the braced and unbraced knee, were made for both applied anterior shear loading and AROM. A

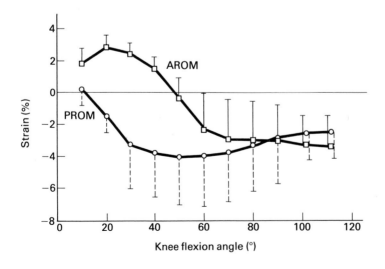

Fig. 10.7 This figure illustrates the averaged strain pattern of the anteromedial bundle of the anterior cruciate during active range of motion (AROM) (extending his or her own knee) and passive range of motion (PROM) (knee extended by surgeon). With permission from Beynnon *et al.* (1992a).

total of seven functional knee braces including three custom and four off-the-shelf designs were evaluated. When compared to the non-braced condition, only two of the seven functional knee braces (Donjoy (Carlsbad, California, USA) and Townsend (Bakersfield, California, USA)) provided a strain shielding effect on the ACL for applied anterior shear loads of 100 N at 30° of knee flexion, a load less than that often predicted to occur in normal activities of daily living. No such effect was observed at 180 N of anterior shear for all the braces tested (a load still less than that predicted to occur during severe activities of daily living). For AROM (ranging between 5 and 110°), application of the knee braces did not alter the ACL strain pattern.

In these studies, we have found significant differences between *in vivo* and *in vitro* experiments, there are many possible explanations but perhaps the most important difference is the function of the muscles and their tendinous attachments. The primary function of the quadriceps mechanism is clearly to extend the knee but, just as importantly, it also controls flexion by antagonizing gravity and the hamstring muscles. Strains were markedly different from the passive curves as compared to those with active extension.

Our *in vivo* testing of the reconstructed ACL (RACL) immediately after fixation indicate that differences between implantation techniques produce different patterns during PROM of the knee joint. The results demonstrate that cyclic PROM does not significantly alter the RACL construct. Where there was an initial increase in RACL length with repeated cycling, the RACL settled into a repeatable pattern by the twentieth cycle. The shape of the RACL percent elongation versus flexion angle curves for the RACL show similarities to the normal ACL data suggesting restoration of normal knee kinematics at the time of ACL reconstruction. Further research is underway to apply arthroscopic strain gauge measurement of the ACL during various activities of daily living. We also plan to use this technique to investigate different continuous passive range of motion machines and compare the strain patterns for the different knee motions and support systems.

The biomechanics of ligament healing is of great interest to the physician. Van der Meulen (1982) has conveniently divided ligament healing into three phases. Phase I, acute inflammation and reaction, is in the first 72 h. Phase II, which is repair and regeneration, is in the time span of 48–72 h up to 6 weeks. Phase III, characterized as remodelling or maturation, lasts from 6 weeks to 1 year. The healing ligament contracts and shows increased tensile strength. Frank *et al.* (1983) report that the strength of the healing ligament only reaches about 50–70% of normal. Clayton *et al.* (1968) and Woo *et al.* (1987a,b) report that immobilization and activity level also affect the outcome. O'Donoghue *et al.* (1971) suggest that primary surgical repair decreases the mass of the scar tissue by changing the healing response to a primary one (analogous to that of bone) and by immobilization of the torn ends and reducing scarring.

Joint immobilization does have a major effect on the insertion site. Tissue–bone junctional strength diminishes with immobilization. Barfred (1971) and Laros *et al.* (1971) found that such failures occurred more frequently in immobilized animals. Woo *et al.* (1987a,b) found increased bone avulsion failure after 9 weeks of knee immobilization. This was explained by subperiosteal resorption of bone, causing disruption of the fibres that attach to bone.

Meniscus

It was Fairbank (1948) who pointed out the degenerative changes (now called Fairbank's changes) that occur after meniscectomy. The changes include osteophyte formation, joint space narrowing and flattening of the femoral articular surface. Jackson (1968) made the link between these changes and the eventual onset of degenerative joint disease.

Several biomechanical studies clearly demonstrated the important clinical role of the meniscus. Krause *et al.* (1976) employed an extensiometer to demonstrate that the meniscus circumferentially displaces as it absorbs the tibiofemoral compressive forces (Fig. 10.8). Furthermore, Kurosawa *et al.* (1980) and Ahmed and Burke (1983) showed that the contact area reduces between 30 and 70% after meniscectomy. For a given load, a contact area reduction of 50% results in an increase of mean contact stress by a factor of two. Ahmed and Burke (1983) concluded that not only is the peak stress increased but also the high pressure areas are located over relatively small regions

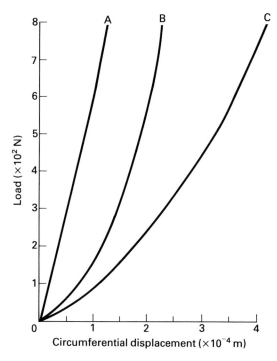

Fig. 10.8 This figure shows how an extensiometer was employed to demonstrate that the meniscus circumferentially displaces as it absorbs tibiofemoral compressive forces. The mean circumferential displacement of the human meniscus tested at: (A) full extension of the knee and 5° of external rotation; (B) 45° of knee flexion and zero external rotation; and (C) full extension of the knee and zero external rotation. With permission from Krause *et al.* (1976).

of the tibial plateau. Bourne *et al.* (1984) found that both partial and complete meniscectomy leads to changes in the strains in the proximal tibia. Some indirect evidence of the importance of this structure comes from the work of Hoch *et al.* (1983) who found that in the meniscectomized rabbit there were changes in mechanical properties of the articular cartilage that were identical to those in human osteoarthritis.

It is also possible, but not proven, that the meniscus has a role in joint lubrication. MacConaill (1932) suggested that since the meniscus provides joint conformity the hydrodynamic lubrication of the knee joint is enhanced. Fluid exudation across the meniscus has not been proven, as it has in articular cartilage, and thus the role of the meniscus in lubrication is unclear.

Injuries to the knee meniscus are quite common in sports that involve running, cutting or some contact. The common aspect of the injuries are that some shear and compression combinations tear the meniscus. Tears often occur through a midplane and this is termed a bucket-handle tear. These tears can often flip over and cause locking of the joint. Non-contact injuries often involve large accelerations associated with a sudden change of direction. External forces (e.g. skiing injury) are often a combination of varus–valgus movements, axial rotation and compression. In such cases, injury to the MCL, ACL and capsule often coexist.

The removal of a damaged meniscus, whole or in part, is still probably the treatment of choice although, some advocate repair or replacement. The ability to repair the meniscus probably resides in the vascularity of the tissue. Under ideal conditions, Arnoczky and Warren (1983) found that small radial tears repair with scar tissue in approximately 10 weeks.

Muscle

Garrett *et al.* (1984) have shown, in many studies, that muscle–tendon units stretched to failure always failed at or near the myotendinous junction. Usually, the tendon avulsed from the muscle with a short length of muscle fibre still attached. Garrett *et al.* (1987) found that muscle activated electrically through the motor nerve led to somewhat higher loads to failure. Stimulated muscle could also maintain a higher force whilst stretching, thus having more ability to absorb energy.

Muscle injury is usually followed by an inflammatory and regenerative phase. In turn, this leads to scarring at the myotendinous junction. According to Williams and Goldspink (1984), immobilization in a lengthened position, which occurs after injury quite frequently, also leads to some reorganization of the so-called passive components of muscle tendon. Jones *et al.* (1985) found that muscle which is immobilized in a shortened position tended to develop less force and had lower strain to failure. It appears that the position of immobilization is one of the most important factors in determining the nature of changes at the myotendinous junction and warrants more study.

Järvinen and Sorvari (1975) found that immediately after muscle injury, an inflammatory reaction and haematoma occurs. Scar formation and some muscle regeneration follows. Järvinen (1976) found more of an inflammatory reaction in mobilized muscle but it disappeared quickly. Biomechanical testing showed that mobilized muscle had a faster recovery of tensile strength. Thus, the evidence seems to favour mobilization as soon as possible.

Nerves

Peripheral nerves are sometimes injured in athletic trauma. These tissues have been completely studied. Although Sunderland and Bradley (1961), in some early work, found that peripheral nerves exhibit a slightly non-linear relationship in tension. Later studies revealed the stress–strain response of rabbit peripheral nerves during tensile testing (Lundborg *et al.*, 1987) (Fig. 10.9). At failure, there is a dramatic drop in strength without obvious loss of struc-

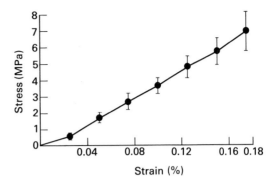

Fig. 10.9 Stress–strain behaviour of rabbit peripheral nerves. Linear stiffness was reached at 3% beyond *in vivo* length. With permission from Lundborg *et al.* (1987).

ture in the nerve trunk. These workers found that the median nerve ruptures at 70–220 N and 70–155 N for the ulnar nerve (Sunderland, 1978). The elastic limit is between 11 and 17% strain whereas, failure is at 15–23% strain. Not all of this strain is 'usable' since some nerves are under some tension *in vivo*. It is noteworthy that if a peripheral nerve is transected, it retracts at between 10 and 20%.

If a nerve is somewhat compressed ischaemia results and there may be some impairment in conduction. At higher pressures, usually in association with acute injuries to extremities, the nerve has some vascular compromise as well as mechanical deformation. This generally affects all parts of the nerve trunk including blood vessels and nerve fibres. A complete conduction block may result.

Rydevik and Lundborg (1977) showed that microvascular damage and the subsequent oedema formation occurs mainly at the edges of the compressed segment. Mathematical modelling by Rydevik *et al.* (1989) has demonstrated that both longitudinal strains and shear stresses are at their maximum at the edges of the compressed nerve. Naturally, a sharp edge produces a greater stress concentration than a rounded edge and thus a sharp edge impinging on a peripheral nerve may have a substantial effect.

Cartilage

The major role of cartilage is to provide a smooth surface, with a low coefficient of friction, so as to enhance joint lubrication. There are numerous theories as to how joint lubrication works but according to Mow and Mack (1987) fluid film lubrication plays some role. McCutchen (1962) suggested that fluid flow out of articular cartilage was the operative mechanism. Mow *et al.* (1984) later provided the mathematical theory to explain such a mechanism. Torzilli *et al.* (1982) explained that cartilage contains 80% water due to the hydrophilic nature of the proteoglycans. Most of this water is freely available to provide the fluid film, at least 25 μm thick, which is adequate for lubrication.

Cartilage is injured in athletic competition in either a chronic overuse syndrome or by acute injury. In the former mechanism, the repetitive loading exceeds the ability of the tissues to respond and the cartilage wears away (osteoarthritis). Acute injuries, on the other hand, can be classified into either those that cause loss of matrix molecules without mechanical damage to cells and matrix and those injuries that do result in mechanical damage. In fact, a continued loss of matrix macromolecules (water binding) will lead to eventual loss of surface cartilage. Conversely, mechanical damage, due to acute or chronic trauma, may release chemical agents that cause matrix degradation. According to Buckwalter (1983) mechanical trauma destroys chondrocytes (that repair injured cartilage) but the overall response to injury seems to depend on the depth of injury. If subchondral bone is involved, the response is more severe. The extent and mechanical quality of the cartilage repair is affected by the amount of surface area affected.

An effective treatment in some cases of osteoarthritis is to change the magnitude or location of joint loading. This can be accomplished, for example, by an osteotomy. Some clinicians also advocate limiting weight-bearing and joint range of motion and suggest that reduction of loads will stimulate cartilage repair. However, DePalma *et al.* (1966) found that early motion and weight-bearing is beneficial. Salter *et al.* (1980) report that continuous passive motion is beneficial in defects of 1 mm diameter that penetrate the subchondral bone. The precise clinical significance of these findings is still unknown.

Intervertebral disc

The intervertebral disc is a complex structure that permits articulation between adjacent vertebrae whilst supporting the loads that pass through the axial skeleton (Pope *et al.*, 1984). The disc is composed of a gel-like nucleus surrounded by collagen sheets. The nucleus is comprised of proteoglycans that are hydrated macromolecules. The collagen sheets in the annulus run at a 30° angle to the adjacent endplate and each sheet crosses at 120°. The nucleus behaves as an osmotic system where the hydrated macromolecules imbibe water and the imposed load tends to force water out.

Disc forces vary from 300 N in the supine position to 700 N in the erect posture (Nachemson, 1976). High disc pressures also occur in twisting and other asymmetric postures largely due to the high levels of antagonistic muscle activity. Adams and Hutton (1982) demonstrated that disc rupture in asymmetric postures such as lateral bend or rotation coupled with usual compression. Axial compression alone will not herniate a disc but will lead to end-plate rupture. Wilder *et al.* (1988) showed that cyclic fatigue will also lead to tracking of the nucleus, particularly if somewhat fibrotic, leading to eventual rupture (Fig. 10.10). These data would suggest that athletes utilizing asymmetric forceful postures such as in tennis, javelin, volleyball or skiing would be at risk for disc herniation. Athletes involved in contact sports would also be at higher risk.

Bone

Compact bone and cancellous bone are the

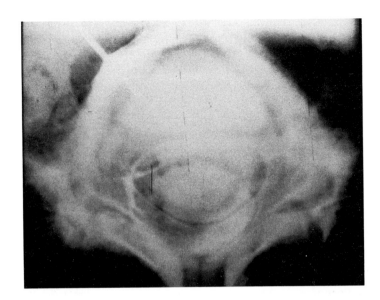

Fig. 10.10 Cyclic fatigue will lead to tracking of the nucleus, particularly if somewhat fibrotic, leading to eventual rupture. With permission from Wilder *et al.* (1988).

basic building blocks of the human frame. Compact bone comprises the midshafts of the long bones whereas cancellous bone makes up the metaphyseal regions and the bulk of the vertebral bodies in the axial skeleton.

Compact bone, when tested mechanically, is found to be anisotropic. This means that bone has different strength and stiffness when tested in different perpendicular directions (Fig. 10.11) (Pope & Outwater, 1972). The anisotropy results from the directionality of bone. Bone behaves like a composite material. The reinforcement, in the case of bone, are the osteons or Haversian systems. Thus, bone is stronger and stiffer in the longitudinal direction as compared to the transverse and is also stronger in compression than tension. For this reason, bone tends to break on the tensile side when bent. Part way across the diaphysis, the fracture front encounters the compressed region and tends to break

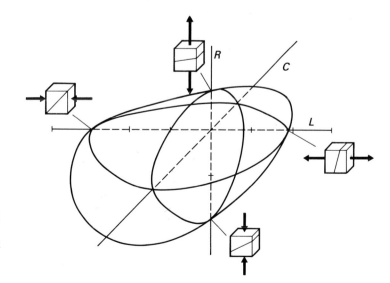

Fig. 10.11 Fracture locus for bone substance from bovine tibia. Specimens were taken from radial (R), circumferential (C) and longitudinal (L) directions. With permission from Pope & Outwater (1974).

in shear, thus giving rise to the transverse oblique fracture. Under torsional loading, a spiral fracture ensues but the angle of the spiral exceeds 45° due to the relative weakness of bone between the osteons directionality.

The properties of bone are also affected by rate of loading as shown in Fig. 10.12 (Crowninshield & Pope, 1974). At higher rates of loading, compact bone becomes slightly stiffer, stronger and suffers less strain to failure. At high rates of loading, the bone exhibits characteristically brittle behaviour. At higher rates of loading, less energy is absorbed prior to failure and the bone has a fracture pattern characteristic of the fracture front moving across the osteons rather than between them (Pope & Outwater, 1972).

Bone is affected by cyclic loading. Clinically, fatigue fractures are known to occur. Reports of such fractures persist in the bones of the lower extremities of athletes and military recruits. Wiltse et al. (1975) were the first to speculate that in patients with spondylolytic defects the fracture of the pars interarticularis may occur secondarily to repetitive loading. Hutton et al. (1977) found in vitro that a cyclic compressive and shear load simulating walking with a 50-kg pack will lend to a fatigue failure of the neural arch. Table 10.1 reports those sports with a higher incidence of spondylolysis. Possible explanations for the higher incidence in this primarily adolescent population include sports that involve repetitive impacts and high repetitive flexion–extension moments.

Cancellous bone has a trabecular pattern based on the loading history on the bone. For example, the trabeculae of the vertebral body appear to be oriented to withstand the vertical compressive forces through the body and the tensile forces of the ligamentous and muscular attachments to the spinous and transverse processes (Fig. 10.13) (Pope et al., 1990). Cancellous bone has an ultimate compressive stress of about 10 MPa compared to 200 MPa for cortical bone and is much less stiff than compact bone (Nordin & Frankel, 1989). The compress-

Table 10.1 Sports associated with higher incidences of spondylolysis.

Sport	Reference
Gymnastics	Jackson et al. (1976), Letts et al. (1986)
Football	Ichikawa et al. (1982)
Weightlifting	Ichikawa et al. (1982)
Judo	Ottolenghi et al. (1985), Ichikawa et al. (1982)
American football	Ferguson (1974)
Sailing	Ottolenghi et al. (1985)
Pole vaulting	Gainor et al. (1983)
Running	Abel (1985)
Ice hockey	Letts et al. (1986)

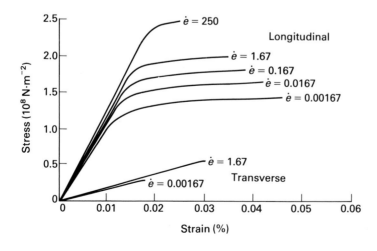

Fig. 10.12 Modulus of elasticity versus strain rate in compact bovine bone.

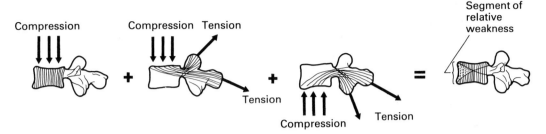

Fig. 10.13 Trabecular directions in the vertebrae. With permission from Pope *et al.* (1984).

ive strength of cancellous bone is markedly affected by the mineral content (Hansson *et al.*, 1985). In the elderly, and particularly the postmenopausal, patient bone mineral content diminishes leading to diminished strength and thus a greater propensity to fractures particularly of the femoral neck or the anterior aspect of the vertebrae. As can be seen in Fig. 10.13, the anterior aspect has a relative paucity of trabecular pattern. Oestrogen therapy (Diddle & Smith, 1984) and exercise (Krolner *et al.*, 1983) is reported to be beneficial in maintaining bone mineral content. Conversely, bedrest will cause a loss of bone mass (Krolner & Toft, 1983).

Bone healing occurs by either primary or secondary healing. Perren (1969) reports that in primary healing, bone heals without an intermediate cartilagenous phase. Blood is first organized into granulation tissue which, by 3 days, shows the first signs of immature (woven) bone. By 2–3 weeks, trabeculae of woven bone have filled the gap. Late remodelling finishes the process. Rigid fixation (e.g. axio-occlusal) is required for primary healing. Secondary bone healing (which occurs if a cast is used) is a process that involves the use of an intermediate cartilagenous phase (callus). Usually, the distinction is made between four zones of callus: bridging, anchoring, uniting and sealing.

Conclusion

This chapter has summarized the mechanical properties of the tissues of the human body as they pertain to impact and overuse in athletic endeavours. An understanding of these basics will enable the sports medicine doctor, the family practitioner, the physical therapist and the athletic trainer to plan strategies to avoid injury and to optimize treatment and rehabilitation. For the graduate student and research colleague, we hope that we have summarized the knowledge adequately so that future research can be planned.

Acknowledgments

We wish to acknowledge the support of the McClure Professorship (MHP), the NIDRR through the Vermont Rehabilitation Engineering Center (USOE H133E80018) and the National Institute of Health (NIH grant Nos PHS R0138630, PHS R0139213 and PHS R0140174).

References

Abel, M.S. (1985) Jogger's fracture and other stress fractures of the lumbar spine. *Skeletal Radiol.* **13**, 221–27.

Abrahams, M. (1967) Mechanical behavior of tendon *in vitro* (a preliminary report). *Med. Biol. Eng.* **5**, 433.

Adams, M.A. & Hutton, W.C. (1982) Prolapsed intervertebral disk: A hyperflexion injury. *Spine* **7**(3), 184–91.

Ahmed, A.M. & Burke, D.L. (1983) *In vitro* measurement of statis pressure distribution in synovial joints — Part I: Tibial surface of the knee. *J. Biomech. Eng.* **105**(3), 216–25.

132   BASIC PRINCIPLES

Akeson, W.H. (1961) An experimental study of joint stiffness. *J. Bone Joint Surg.* **43A**, 1022–34.

Alexander, R.M. (1988) *Elastic Mechanisms in Animal Movement.* Cambridge University Press, Massachusetts.

American Academy of Orthopaedic Surgeons (AAOS) (1988) The use of knee braces. *Am. Acad. Orthop. Surg. Bull.* **36**, 17–18.

Arms, S., Boyle, J., Johnson, R.J. & Pope, M. (1983) Strain measurement in the medial collateral ligament of the human knee: An autopsy study. *J. Biomech.* **15**(7), 491–6.

Arnoczky, S.P. & Warren, R.F. (1983) The microvasculature of the meniscus and its response to injury: An experimental study in the dog. *Am. J. Sports Med.* **11**, 131–41.

Barfred, T. (1971) Experimental rupture of the Achilles tendon: Comparison of experimental ruptures in rats of different ages and living under different conditions. *Acta Orthop. Scand.* **42**(5), 406–28.

Beynnon, B.D., Howe, J.G., Pope, M.H., Johnson, R.J. & Fleming, B.C. (1992a) The measurement of anterior cruciate ligament strain *in vivo*. *Int. Orthop.* **16**, 1–12.

Beynnon, B.D., Pope, M.H., Wertheimer, C.M. *et al.* (1992b) The effect of functional knee braces on anterior cruciate ligament strain *in vivo*. *J. Bone Joint Surg.* **74A**, 1298–312.

Bourne, R.B., Finlay, J.B., Papadopoulos, P. *et al.* (1984) The effect of medial meniscectomy on strain distribution in the proximal part of the tibia. *J. Bone Joint Surg.* **66A**, 1431–7.

Brown, T.D., Sigal, L., Jnus, G.O., Njus, N.M., Singerman, R.J. & Brand, R.A. (1986) Dynamic performance characteristics of the liquid metal strain gage. *J. Biomech.* **19**(2), 165–73.

Buckwalter, J.A. (1983) Articular cartilage. *American Academy of Orthopedic Surgeons Instructional Course Lectures*, Vol. XXXII, pp. 349–70. CV Mosby. St Louis.

Butler, D.L., Grood, E.S., Zernicke, R.R., Hefzy, M.S. & Noyes, F.R. (1983) *Nonuniform surface strains in young human tendons and fascia.* Presented at 29th Orthopaedic Research Society Meeting, Anaheim.

Clayton, M.L., Miles, J.S. & Abdulla, M. (1968) Experimental investigations of ligamentous healing. *Clin. Orthop.* **61**, 146–53.

Cronkite, A.E. (1936) The tensile strength of human tendons. *Anat. Rec.* 173–86.

Crowninshield, R.D. & Pope, M.H. (1974) The response of compact bone in tension at various strain rates. *Ann. Biomed. Eng.* **2**, 217–25.

Crowninshield, R.D. & Pope, M.H. (1976) The strength and failure characteristics of rat medial collateral ligaments. *J. Trauma.* **16**, 99–105.

DePalma, A.F., McKeever, C.D. & Subin, D.K. (1966) Process of repair of articular cartilage demonstrated by histology and autoradiography with tritiated thymidine. *Clin. Orthop.* **48**, 229–42.

Diddle, A.W. & Smith, I.Q. (1984) Postmenopausal osteoporosis: The role of estrogen. *South Med. J.* **77**, 868–74.

Edwards, R.G., Lafferty, J.F. & Lange, K.D. (1970) Ligament strain in the human knee. *J. Basic Eng.* **38**, 131–6.

Fairbank, T.J. (1948) Knee joint changes after meniscectomy. *J. Bone Joint Surg.* **30B**, 664–70.

Ferguson, R.J. (1974) Low back pain in college football linemen. *J. Bone Joint Surg.* **56A**(1), 1300.

Frank, C., Woo, S.L.-Y., Amiel, D. *et al.* (1983) Medial collateral ligament healing: A multidisciplinary assessment in rabbits. *Am. J. Sports Med.* **11**, 379–89.

Gainor, B.J., Hagen, R.J. & Allen, W.C. (1983) Biomechanics of the spine in the polevaulter as related to spondylolysis. *Am. J. Sports Med.* **11**, 53–7.

Gallie, W.E. & leMesurier, A.B. (1924) The transplantation of the fibrous tissues in the repair of anatomical defects. *Br. J. Surg.* **12**, 289–93.

Garrett Jr, W.E., Almekinders, L.C. & Seaber, A.V. (1984) Biomechanics of muscle tears in stretching injuries. *Trans. Orthop. Res. Soc.* **9**, 384.

Garrett Jr, W.E., Safran, M.R., Seaber, A.V. *et al.* (1987) Biomechanical comparison of stimulated and skeletal muscle pulled to failure. *Am. J. Sports Med.* **15**(5), 448–54.

Gelberman, R.H., Botte, M.J., Spiegelman, J.J. *et al.* (1986) The excursion and deformation of repaired flexor tendons treated with protected early motion. *J. Hand Surg.* **11A**, 106–10.

Gritz, C.M. (1931) Tensile strength and elasticity tests on human fascia lata. *J. Bone Joint Surg.* **29**, 334–40.

Hansson, T., Sandstran, B. & Roos, B. (1985) The bone material content of the lumbar spine in patients with chronic low back pain. *Spine* **10**, 158–9.

Hoch, D.H., Grodzinsky, A.J., Koob, T.J. *et al.* (1983) Early changes in material properties of rabbit articular cartilage after meniscectomy. *J. Orthop. Res.* **1**, 4–12.

Howe, J.G., Wertheimer, C.M., Johnson, R.J., Nichols, C.E., Pope, M.H. & Beynnon, B.D. (1990) Arthroscopic strain gage measurement of the normal anterior cruciate ligament. *Arthroscopy* **6**, 198–204.

Hutton, W.C., Stott, J.R.R. & Cryon, B.M. (1977) Is spondylolysis a fatigue fracture? *Spine* **2**, 202–9.

Ichikawa, N., Ohara, Y., Morishita, T. *et al.* (1982) An aetiological study on spondylolysis from a biomechanical aspect. *Br. J. Sports Med.* **16**, 135–41.

Jackson, D.W., Wiltse, L.L. & Cirincione, R.J. (1976) Spondylolysis in the female gymnast. *Clin. Orthop. Rel. Res.* **117**, 68–73.

Jackson, J.P. (1968) Degenerative changes in the knee

after meniscectomy. *Br. Med. J.* **2**, 525–7.

Järvinen, M. (1976) Healing of a crush injury in rat striated muscle. *Acta Pathol. Microbiol. Scand.* **142**, 47–56.

Järvinen, M. & Sorvari, T. (1975) Healing of a crush injury in rat striated muscle: 1. Description and testing of a new method of inducing a standard injury to the calf muscles. *Acta Pathol. Microbiol. Scand.* **83**, 259–65.

Jones, V.T., Garrett Jr, W.E. & Seaber, A.V. (1985) Biomechanical changes in muscle after immobilization at different lengths. *Trans. Orthop. Res. Soc.* **10**, 6.

Kastelic, J. & Baer, E. (1980) *Reformation in tendon collagen: The mechanical properties of biological materials.* Presented at the XXXIV Symposium of the Society for Experimental Biology.

Kennedy, J.C., Haskins, R.J. & Willis, R.B. (1977) Strain gauge analysis of knee ligaments. *Clin. Orthop.* **129**, 225–9.

Klein, L. & Lewis, J.A. (1972) Simultaneous quantification of ^{3}H-collagen loss and ^{1}H-collagen replacement during healing of rat tendon grafts. *J. Bone Joint Surg.* **54A**, 137–46.

Krag, M.H., Cohen, M.C., Haugh, L.D. & Pope, M.H. (1990) Body height change during upright and recumbent posture. *Spine* **15**(3), 202–7.

Krause, W.R., Pope, M.H., Johnson, R.J. *et al.* (1976) Mechanical changes in the knee after meniscectomy *J. Bone Joint Surg.* **58A**, 599–604.

Krolner, B. & Toft, B. (1983) Vertebral bone loss: An unheeded side effect of therapeutic bed rest. *Clin. Sci.* **64**, 537–40.

Krolner, B., Toft, B., Nielsen, S.B. & Tonevold, E. (1983) Physical exercise as prophylaxis against involuntary bone loss: A controlled trial. *Clin. Sci.* **64**, 541–6.

Kurosawa, H., Fukubayashi, T. & Nakajima, H. (1980) Load-bearing mode of the knee joint: Physical behavior of the knee joint with or without menisci. *Clin. Orthop.* **149**, 283–90.

Langer, C. (1884) *Anatomie der ausseren Formen des menschlichen Korpers.* Toeplitz & Deuticke, Wein.

Laros, G.S., Tipton, C.M. & Cooper, R.R. (1971) Influence of physical activity on ligament insertions in the knees of dogs. *J. Bone Joint Surg.* **53A**, 275–86.

Letts, M., Smallman, T., Afanasiev, R. & Grouw, G. (1986) Fracture of the pars interarticularis in adolescent athletes: A clinical–biomechanical analysis. *J. Pediatr. Orthop.* **6**, 40–6.

Lundborg, G., Rydevik, B., Manthorpe, M., Varon, S. & Lewis, J. (1987) Peripheral nerve: The physiology of injury and repair. In S. Woo & J. Buckwalter (eds) *Injury and Repair of the Musculoskeletal Soft Tissues*, pp. 297–352. AAOS, Illinois.

MacConaill, M.A. (1932) The function of intra-

articular fibrocartilages, with special reference to the knee and inferior radio-ulnar joints. *J. Anat.* **66**, 210–27.

McCutchen, C.W. (1962) The frictional properties of animal joints. *Wear* **5**, 1–17.

Meulen, J.C. van der. (1982) Present state of knowledge on processes of healing in collagen structures. *Int. J. Sports. Med.* **3**(Suppl. 1), 4–8.

Mow, V.C., Holmes, M.H. & Lai, W.M. (1984) Fluid transport and mechanical properties of articular cartilage: A review. *J. Biomech.* **17**, 377–94.

Mow, V.C. & Mack, A.F. (1987) Lubrication of diarthrodial joints. In R. Skalak & S. Chien (eds) *Handbook of Bioengineering.* McGraw-Hill, New York.

Mutchler, W., Burri, C. & Claes, L. (1979) *A new possibility of measuring absolute stress and strain of ligaments.* Department of Traumatology, University of Ulm, West Germany.

Nachemson, A. (1976) Lumbar intradiscal pressure. In M. Jayson (ed) *The Lumbar Spine and Low Back Pain*, pp. 257–69. Grune & Stratton, Philadelphia.

Nordin, M. & Frankel, V. (1989) *Basic Biomechanics of the Musculoskeletal System.* Lea & Febiger, Philadelphia.

Noyes, F.R. & Grood, E.S. (1976) The strength of the anterior cruciate ligament in human and rhesus monkeys. *J. Bone Joint Surg.* **58A**, 1074–82.

O'Donoghue, D.H., Frank, G.R., Jeter, G.L. *et al.* (1971) Repair and reconstruction of the anterior cruciate ligament in dogs: Factors influencing long-term results. *J. Bone Joint Surg.* **53A**, 710–18.

Ottolenghi, G., Alessi, G.C., Oggero, P. & Bucelli, R. (1985) Alterazioni del rachide lombosacrale da micropolitraumatismi sportivi. *Minerva Med.* **76**, 2203–12.

Perren, S.M. (1969) The reaction of cortical bone to compression. *Acta Orthop. Scand.* **125**(Suppl.), 19–29.

Pope, M.H., Frymoyer, J.W., Lehmann, M.D. (1984) Structure and function of the lumbar spine. In M.H. Pope, J.W. Frymoyer & G. Anderson (eds) *Occupational Low Back Pain*, pp. 5–38. Prager, New York.

Pope, M.H. & Outwater, J.O. (1972) The fracture characteristics of bone substance. *J. Biomech.* **5**, 457–65.

Pope, M.H. & Outwater, J.O. (1974) Mechanical properties of bone as a function of position and orientation. *J. Biomech.* **7**, 61–6.

Rigby, B.J., Hirai, N., Spikes, J.D. & Eyring, H. (1959) The mechanical properties of rat tail tendon. *J. Gen. Physiol.* **43**, 265–83.

Rydevik, B. & Lundborg, G. (1977) Permeability of intraneural microvessels and perineurium following acute, graded experimental nerve compression. *Scand. J. Plast. Reconstr. Surg.* **11**, 179–87.

Rydevik, B., Lundborg, G. & Skalak, R. (1989) Bio-mechanics of peripheral nerves. In M. Nordin & V.H. Frankel (eds) *Basic Biomechanics of the Musculo-skeletal System*, 2nd edn, pp. 75–87. Lea & Febiger Philadelphia.

Salter, R.B., Simmonds, D.F., Malcolm, B.W. *et al.* (1980) The biological effect of continuous passive motion on healing of full-thickness defects in articular cartilage: An experimental study in the rabbit. *J. Bone Joint Surg.* **62A**, 1232–51.

Sidles, J.A., Larson, R.V., Garbini, J.L., Downey, D.J. & Matsen, F.A. (1988) Ligament length relation-ships in the moving knee. *J. Orthop. Res.* **6**, 593–610.

Smith, J.W. (1954) The elastic properties of the anterior cruciate ligament of the rabbit. *J. Anat.* **88**, 369–81.

Sunderland, S. (1978) *Nerves and Nerve Injuries*, 2nd edn. Churchill Livingstone, Edinburgh.

Sunderland, S. & Bradley, K.C. (1961) Stress–strain phenomena in human peripheral nerve trunks. *Brain*, **84**, 102–19.

Torzilli, P.A., Rose, D.E. & Dethmers, D.A. (1982) Equilibrium water partition in articular cartilage. *Biorheology* **19**, 519–37.

Trent, P.S., Walker, P.S. & Wolf, B. (1976) Ligament length patterns, strength and rotational axes of the knee joint. *Clin. Orthop.* **117**, 263–79.

Verdan, C.E. (1972) Half a century of flexor–tendon surgery: Current status and changing philosophies. *J. Bone Joint Surg.* **54A**, 472–91.

Wang, C.J., Walker, P.S. & Wolf, B. (1973) The effects of flexion and rotation on the length patterns of the ligaments of the knee. *J. Biomech.* **6**, 587–96.

Wilder, D.G., Frymoyer, J.W. & Pope, M.H. (1985) The effect of vibration on the spine of the seated individual. *Automedica* **6**, 5–35.

Wilder, D.G., Pope, M.H. & Frymoyer, J.W. (1988) The biomechanics of lumbar disc herniation and effect of overload and instability. Annual Award of the American Back Society. *J. Spinal Dis.* **1**(1), 16–32.

Williams, P.E. & Goldspink, G. (1984) Connective tissue changes in immobilized muscle. *J. Anat.* **138**, 343–50.

Wiltse, L.L., Widell, E.H. & Jackson, D.W. (1975) Fatigue fracture: The basic lesion in isthmic spondylolisthesis. *J. Bone Joint Surg.* **57A**, 17–22.

Woo, S.L.-Y. (1986) Biomechanics of tendons and ligaments. In G.W. Schmid-Schönbein, S.L.-Y. Woo & B.W. Zweifach (eds) *Frontiers on Biomechanics*, pp. 180–95. Springer-Verlag, New York.

Woo, S.L.-Y., Gomez, M.A., Sites, T.J. *et al.* (1987b) The biomechanical and morphological changes in the medial collateral ligament of the rabbit after immobilization and remobilization. *J. Bone Joint Surg.* **69A**, 1200–11.

Woo, S.L.-Y., Inoue, M., McGurk-Burleson, E. *et al.* (1987a) Treatment of the medial collateral ligament injury: II. Structure and function of canine knees in response to differing treatment regimens. *Am. J. Sports Med.* **15**, 22–9.

Woo, S.L.-Y., Orlando, C.A., Gomez, M.A. *et al.* (1986) Tensile properties of medial collateral liga-ment as a function of age. *J. Orthop. Res.* **4**, 133–41.

Woo, S.L.-Y., Ritter, M.A., Amiel, D. *et al.* (1980) The biomechanical and biochemical properties of swine tendons: Long term effects of exercise on the digital extensors. *Connect Tiss. Res.* **7**, 177–83.

PART 3

RISK FACTORS IN SPORTS INJURIES

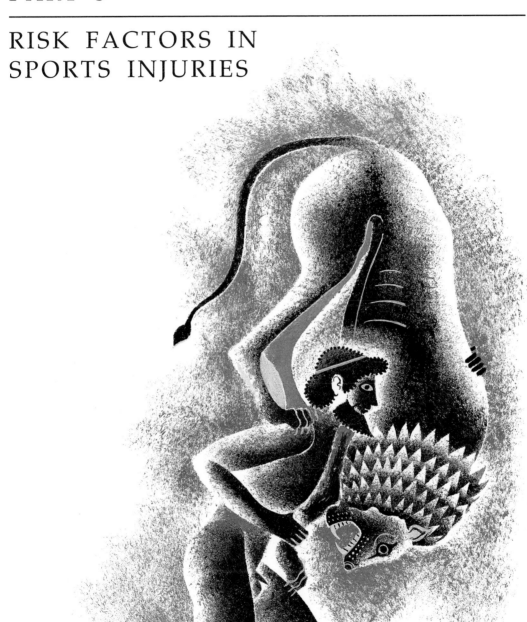

Part 3a

Intrinsic Factors in Injury Prevention

Chapter 11

Overuse Running Injuries

JIM MACINTYRE AND ROB LLOYD-SMITH

An overuse running injury is one of the most common conditions seen by sports-medicine physicians. Knowledge of the factors which influence their genesis and outcome is essential for appropriate treatment, which includes not only relief of the presenting symptoms, but also prevention of further recurrences.

Overuse injuries result from cumulative microtrauma leading to overt tissue injury (Fig. 11.1). They occur when the body is unable to absorb forces generated by repeated cyclical loading of mobile segments or links in the kinetic chain. The site and type of injury are not random occurrences, but are determined by many factors which make a particular site vulnerable to stress.

Running injuries can occur anywhere from the toes to the lumbosacral spine. The vast majority of injuries, however, involve the knee which has reported incidences ranging from 18 to 50% (McKenzie *et al.*, 1985). In a retrospective review of 4173 injuries, the most common individual injuries were patellofemoral pain syndrome, iliotibial band friction syndrome and tibial stress injury with no other injury accounting for greater than 5% of the injuries (Table 11.1) (Macintyre *et al.*, 1991). The study also demonstrated significant differences in injury site when recreational runners were compared with marathon runners and élite middle-distance runners, and this was postulated to be on the basis of differences in the types of musculoskeletal stresses associated with the different activities.

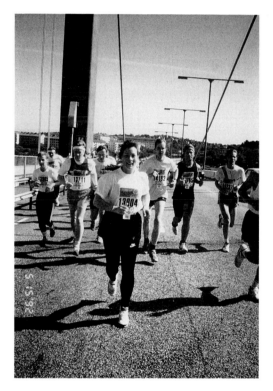

Fig. 11.1 Long-distance running subjects the body to great forces, which can result in injury. Courtesy of Dr P.A.F.H. Renström.

Running injuries are multifactorial in causation with intrinsic and extrinsic factors both important. Extrinsic causes such as inappropriate training methods, poor footwear, and running surface are detailed elsewhere in this

Table 11.1 Most common running injuries.

	Men (%) ($n = 2359$)	Women (%) ($n = 1814$)
Patellofemoral pain	24	30
Iliotibial band friction	7	8
Tibial stress injury	7	11
Plantar fasciitis	5	4
Achilles tendonitis	5	3
Patellar tendonitis	5	3

book, while this chapter focuses on intrinsic factors in overuse injuries.

Intrinsic factors in overuse injuries can be classified as either primary or secondary/acquired dysfunctions, and are listed in Table 11.2. Primary factors are considered those that are inherent to the individual and include such factors as age, gender, fitness level, growth and development, psychological factors, bony alignment, flexibility and strength. These primary factors will be dealt with individually.

There are also secondary or acquired dysfunctions usually resulting from a previous injury. In some cases this will be the result of an acute injury such as a ligamentous or a muscular injury, or following a fracture or surgery. The injury may be at the same site, and merely reflect inadequate rehabilitation from previous injuries. Alternatively, the underlying injury may be at a distant site, and may have occurred at a different time. The failure to compensate adequately for the underlying injury can lead to a mechanical gait dysfunction, resulting in the presenting injury.

This chapter will deal with the basic biomechanics of running and the role of intrinsic biomechanical dysfunction in overuse injuries. It will outline some of the specific clues to dysfunction to be found in the history and physical examination. The primary and acquired factors for overuse running injuries will be discussed individually, and the general principles of treatment and rehabilitation will be outlined. Not all of these concepts have been objectively validated; however, they provide a useful framework for clinical practice. The following information represents an assimilation of epidemiological research, clinical research, and the authors' clinical practice and experience.

Table 11.2 Intrinsic factors in overuse injuries.

Primary	Acquired dysfunctions
Age	Mechanical
Gender	hip/back/sacroiliac joints
Fitness	knee
Growth	ankle
Psychological	subtalar joint
Bony alignment	midfoot/cuboid
leg length	forefoot
pelvis	hallux valgus/rigidis
hip	Muscular
knee	reduced strength
tibia	inflexibility postinjury
foot	imbalance
Muscular development	
anatomical	
flexibility	
strength	
neuromuscular coordination	
Ligamentous	
generalized laxity	

Kinetic chain dysfunction

The kinetic chain is a concept which describes the lower extremity as a series of mobile segments and linkages which allow forward propulsion during gait (Gray, 1989). In a normal individual, the gait cycle consists of a swing and a stance phase. In the stance phase, when the foot is in contact with the surface, the kinetic chain is considered to be closed. When the foot is off the ground, in the swing phase, the kinetic chain is open. Each segment of the chain has a normal movement pattern during both portions of the gait cycle. More detailed summaries of normal biomechanics are presented in other chapters of this book, and in other monographs (Mann, 1982b; Donatelli, 1990b). Anything which interferes with the normal progression and mechanics of force transfer from heel strike to midstance to heel off and toe off, can lead to alterations in gait and compensatory changes in the motion at other sites in the chain (Gray, 1989).

Kinetic chain dysfunction is an important and frequently overlooked factor in the genesis of running injuries. When a runner presents with an injury, it is easy to assume that the injury has occurred in isolation. It is essential, however, to consider that the injury may be secondary to another injury or dysfunction at a site distant from that of the presenting complaint. The underlying injury may have necessitated compensatory changes in joint motion and gait which increased the stress on another segment of the chain, eventually leading to tissue breakdown and overt injury at the vulnerable site. A simplistic analogy can be made to the role of both the culprit and the victim in injury. The presenting injury may merely be the victim which has suffered an injury as a result of an inability to compensate for a primary dysfunction at another site (the culprit).

The complicated nature of kinetic chain dysfunction was illustrated in a study by Kibler *et al.* (1991) who found reduced static and dynamic range of motion, and reduced lower leg strength in individuals with plantar fasciitis. The authors were unsure as to whether these functional deficits were causative or arose as a result of the plantar fasciitis. The presence of these deficits, in addition to the readily apparent clinical entity, demonstrate the need to assess and treat both the presenting pathology and all underlying kinetic chain dysfunctions.

Physicians have traditionally focused on the injury site when dealing with overuse athletic injuries. Yet it is important to recognize that any injury is a manifestation of a dysfunction in the kinetic chain and that the entire chain must be screened to rule out any asymptomatic underlying injury or dysfunction. This is especially important in individuals who have recurrent injuries to the same site or limb. It is not uncommon to have patients present with recurrent injuries to one lower extremity, with episodes of hip, knee, and ankle problems. These may all result from a dysfunction in the kinetic chain that places increased stress on elements of that leg resulting in serial episodes of tissue breakdown and injury. Band-aid treatment of the injuries as they present will not prevent further problems until the underlying problem is treated.

Clinical assessment

History

Like all things in medicine, adequate diagnosis of running injuries requires an appropriate history, physical examination and specific laboratory and imaging studies. The history is essential in documenting the injury. It is important to elicit a complete history of the presenting injury including its site, radiation and other associated symptoms. In order to determine whether the injury has occurred in isolation, or is part of an ongoing dysfunction, it is important to ask about symptoms related to previous injuries or problems with other joints such as the foot, ankle, hip and low back. It is also essential to inquire about previous traumatic injuries, including local injuries to the area as well as recurrent patterns of injury to the same limb which might indicate an underlying kinetic chain dysfunction. A history of falling onto the buttocks or hips, an excessive axial load on a limb, or any hip or pelvic trauma may be an important clue to a sacroiliac (SI) joint injury and dysfunction. It is also useful to ask the patient whether he or she is aware of any abnormality in alignment, motion, flexibility or strength. These are often things that the patient admits to when questioned, but does not volunteer automatically as they often feel that they do not pertain to the injury, especially when they are occurring at a site distant to the problem. Athletic injuries frequently result in complaints of pain and stiffness, and both components must be addressed to allow for a return to normal activity (Maitland, 1991).

Physical examination

Adequate physical examination depends on a complete, systematic examination of the area of the primary presenting problem. It is also essential to do a general scan of the entire kinetic chain. The injured site is often only one link in the complicated locomotory machine and it may be merely reflecting a dysfunction in other areas. It is important to have adequate visibility of the patient. Therefore the patient should always be dressed in shorts and females should wear a halter top so that the low back and general trunk alignment can be examined. Traditionally, physicians have examined these patients lying on a bed, but this is now considered to be an incomplete examination. It is essential to conduct a full functional examination of the individual to test out various linkages in the kinetic chain, especially in runners presenting with recurrent injuries. Running injuries occur with motion and it is thus essential to examine the patient in motion and to determine that the patient has normal functional mobility of all segments of the kinetic chain.

There is a wide range of normal anatomy and alignment. Runners will frequently adapt to any degree to malalignment if they undertake proper training methods and utilize good footwear, thus the mere presence of a malalignment does not automatically lead to injury. It is now apparent, however, that it is much more important to concentrate on the symmetry of the stance and gait, as asymmetries of either a static or dynamic nature will often indicate an underlying dysfunction of the kinetic chain. A prospective study of basketball players showed that asymmetry and side-to-side imbalance were the factors with the greatest predictive value for injuries (Shambaugh *et al.*, 1991). It is the authors' opinion that functional asymmetries are more important than malalignment *per se* in the genesis of overuse running injuries.

The static assessment should first assess the patient from the feet to the shoulders and neck to scan the entire kinetic chain for malalignment, asymmetry or any other clues to dysfunction. A complete scanning examination should detect any potential problems including:

1 Swelling, muscle wasting, inflammation, or other evidence of previous injury.
2 Abnormal resting positions of joints such as varus, valgus, flexion or extension deformities.
3 Asymmetry of the lower limb including knee alignment or abnormal foot positioning such as unilateral out-toeing or in-toeing.
4 Any evidence of rotation through the trunk which can lead to the shoulder girdle and arms being maintained in an asymmetric position.

Many of these asymmetries are subtle, and only careful attention to the individual's side-to-side alignment will detect them, however, with more experience and practice, they become readily apparent.

Following the screening scan, a more thorough examination should be made in a systematic fashion (Table 11.3), with specific techniques detailed in works by Hoppenfeld (1976) and Magee (1987). The individual's foot type and the static positioning should be classified as normally aligned, excessively pronated

Table 11.3 Static examination.

Stance (symmetry)
Pelvic and sacroiliac joint alignment
Muscle wasting
Knee alignment
Patellar alignment
Q-angle
Tibial varum
Foot type
Pronation — static
Subtalar and forefoot varus/valgus
Callous pattern on feet

or supinated. Varus or valgus alignment of the tibia and knees should be noted. Patellar height, orientation, alignment and Q angle are also assessed, with specific note being made of any asymmetry which might indicate other dysfunctions resulting in overall lower limb malalignment. With the patient prone on the examining table, the callous pattern on the soles of the feet is examined, which can give a good indication of where shear stress and weight-bearing is occurring on the foot. The assessment and measurement of subtalar and forefoot alignment and mobility should also be made.

The dynamic assessment is a vital part of the complete functional examination. Abnormalities of body positioning apparent in the static examination may not in fact come into play in the dynamic gait cycle, as individuals will often adapt or compensate for alignment problems when in motion. Feet which are apparently flat and pronated in the static sense may not actually function in a pronated fashion during running, and therefore dynamic assessment is important.

The dynamic assessment can be either indirect or direct. A simple method of indirect assessment is examining the patients' footwear to look for asymmetrical wear and signs of excessive pronation or supination. Patients who pronate excessively will have more marked medial forefoot wear. Patients who supinate excessively and lack pronation may demonstrate a lateral wear pattern of their shoes.

Direct assessment of gait can be done by observing the patient walking up and down the hall, initially normally, then on heels and tiptoes. More detailed assessments can be done with video or cinematographic analysis of the patient running on a treadmill. Other more elaborate assessment can be made through the use of a triplanar electrogoniometer. Some clinicians use an electrodynogram with individual force sensors placed directly on the patients feet, although the accuracy and reliability of these measurements may be questionable. Overall, there is no convenient, accurate office-based gait analysis system available, and for most patients, direct examination remains the most valuable tool.

The dynamic examination should include functional tests for the alignment and movement of the feet, knees and hips and is summarized in Table 11.4. It is important to examine carefully the patient's gait looking for abnormal or restricted movement patterns, limping or other evidence of injury, or asymmetric progression or alignment of the feet and knees. Following a gait assessment, a functional examination of all joint segments is performed, starting with the foot and working proximally.

The first motions to be tested are the cardinal foot movements of plantar flexion, dorsiflexion, pronation and supination. This is first performed with the patient facing the examiner, with the feet at shoulder width apart and aligned in a parallel fashion, and subsequently with the patient facing away from the examiner. These functional tests assess both the degree of

Table 11.4 Dynamic examination.

Gait
Functional foot movements
   plantar flexion
   dorsiflexion
   pronation
   supination
Patellar tracking
Functional sacroiliac joint tests
Leg length (beware of traps!)
Hip range of motion (and symmetry)

motion and the symmetry of motion between the two feet. The patient is first asked to flex the knee and ankles to assess for dorsiflexion of the ankle. Any asymmetry of the degree of pronation should be noted. Next, the patient goes up on tiptoes to assess the degree and range of plantar flexion. The calcaneus normally swings in to a slight degree of inversion during this manoeuvre. To assess functional pronation and supination the individual is asked to rotate the trunk and hips to look first over one shoulder then over the other. This will cause one foot to supinate and the other to pronate, and careful comparison should be made of the symmetry and range of motion. Restricted or exaggerated motion, especially in the presence of asymmetry, can indicate a kinetic chain dysfunction and a problem with joint movement. Testing the joint play and glide of the individual joints can reveal the exact site of the dysfunction, most commonly occurring at the subtalar or tibiofibular joints.

The total range of motion of the foot and ankle is also important to assess. Any restriction of dorsiflexion or plantar flexion can lead to gait abnormalities including early heel off, leading to compensatory stresses on other areas of the lower limb. Flexibility of the gastrocnemius should be assessed separately from that of the soleus. This is done by attempting to passively dorsiflex the foot with knee fully extended. Any restriction will require remedial stretching exercises. Dorsiflexion with the knee flexed tests the mobility of the soleus.

Foot deformities should also be assessed including metatarsus adductus and hallux valgus. Any significant asymmetry should suggest an underlying dysfunction in the kinetic chain, as developmental causes for a unilateral deformity are unlikely.

Patellar tracking is also assessed. This is done by asking the patient to dorsiflex at the ankles and to flex at the knees. In individuals with ideal alignment, the midpoint of the patella tracks approximately over the web space between the first and second toes in this position. If excessive pronation is present, then the mid-

point of the patella often lies medially to the great toe. It is also important to check for the symmetry of this motion, as a marked asymmetry can indicate an underlying kinetic chain dysfunction. Lateral tracking of the patella may be important in the development of patellofemoral pain syndrome.

The function of the SI joint is an important factor in the genesis of running injuries. Any abnormality of SI position or motion can lead to compensatory gait changes and often secondary injury at a distant site. Similarly, problems at other sites can lead to SI joint dysfunction, so that it is frequently difficult to determine which condition started the runner on the path towards injury. In the absence of a clear-cut precipitating injury, the exact causation of a kinetic chain dysfunction can resemble the classical chicken and egg paradox, but it is clear that only the treatment of all dysfunctional sites will allow the runner an injury-free return to activity. More complete discussion of the role of the SI joint in injury can be found in excellent works by Lee (1989), and Schamberger (1991), and examination techniques are also covered by Cibulka (1989), Magee (1987) and Wadsworth (1988). Functional tests of SI joint position and movement are performed to demonstrate hypomobility or hypermobility of the SI joint and pelvic malalignment.

It is also important to examine the individual's leg lengths. This is quite frequently performed, yet often misinterpreted. The adequate examination of leg lengths is a difficult task that is fraught with error, because the land marks that are commonly used for measurement are able to move relative to one another. It is quite difficult to measure from a point on the greater trochanter to the malleoli, yet measurement from the anterior superior iliac spine will introduce any bias created by an SI joint dysfunction into the leg length assessment. Any standing pelvic obliquity may be due to a true anatomic difference in femoral or tibial length, or may be due to an apparent or functional shortening (Fig. 11.2). SI joint dysfunction, unilateral excess pronation, lumbar or hip muscular

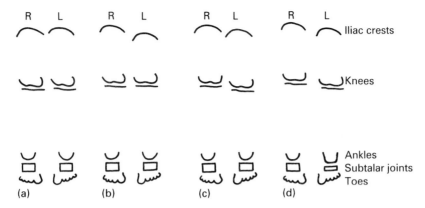

Fig. 11.2 Leg lengths: (a) equal; (b) unequal due to sacroiliac joint dysfunction; (c) unequal due to short left leg; and (d) unequal due to left longitudinal arch collapse.

spasm, contracture or imbalances can all lead to functional shortening (Cibulka, 1989; Donatelli, 1990a).

A simple method of assessing leg length discrepancies is to examine the patient while standing and then while seated on the side of the examination table with hips and knees flexed to 90°. The sitting posture removes any influence of leg lengths on the pelvic girdle, and a persistent abnormality of alignment is an indication of intrinsic SI joint problems. Any standing pelvic obliquity that corrects completely with seating is due to either a true leg length difference, or a functionally short leg resulting from unilateral excessive pronation. Functional shortening due to pronation can be determined by viewing the patient from the front and assessing the longitudinal arch height by palpating the depth that the index finger will slide under the navicular with the volar side up, whereby the finger will slide under the navicular less on the side of the low arch (Cibulka, 1989). If the patient actively corrects the excess pronation, the pelvic obliquity should diminish. The examiner must be aware, however, that unilateral increased pronation may be present as a compensatory mechanism for a true anatomically long leg on that side. It is thus important to perform a complete assessment before reaching any conclusions concerning the exact dysfunction(s).

In order to adequately assess the leg length, it is important to have the pelvis level and the legs relaxed and extended. The patient should lie supine with the knees flexed to 90°. The patient then lifts up their buttocks to extend the hips and then lets their hips flex again as the buttocks are dropped back to the examining table. The examiner then grasps the malleoli and takes the legs out into full extension. It is important to do this passively in order to adequately level the pelvis, as any active motion by the patient can bias the examination results. The easiest assessment is then to examine for the level of the medial malleoli relative to one another. If the examiner is suspicious of a true leg length discrepancy, then it is important to have the patient sit up by flexing at the hips while keeping the knees extended. Assuming this 'long sitting' position will alter the SI joint mechanics such that the results of the leg length discrepancy will often reverse if there is an SI joint dysfunction present. What had previously appeared to be the short leg may now be the apparent long leg (Wadsworth, 1988; Schamberger, 1991).

Any significant degree of true leg length discrepancy will necessitate compensatory changes somewhere else in the kinetic chain, thus the clinical findings often reflect a combination of problems. Occasionally, the clinical picture and physical examination continue to be confusing in sorting through leg length discrepancy, and radiographic measurements of true leg length can be extremely helpful, especially when multiple factors contribute to the discrepancy.

The range of motion of the hips should also be examined. Restriction of hip extension can lead to a short stride length and early heel off and toe off. It is also important to assess the relative range of internal and external hip rotation, and the symmetry from side to side, as an SI joint dysfunction can cause asymmetries of hip range of motion. In these cases the total range of motion from the extremes of external to internal rotation is equal on both sides, but one hip will characteristically show increased internal rotation with restriction of external rotation, while the other hip will show a converse pattern, with decreased internal and increased external rotation.

Even if the examiner is not familiar or adept at the various tests of SI joint function, the detection of marked asymmetry of alignment, a standing and sitting pelvic obliquity, a changing leg length on going from a supine to a long-sitting position, or asymmetric ranges of hip motion are good reasons to suspect an underlying SI joint dysfunction (Table 11.5). These findings, especially in a runner with ongoing injury problems, should necessitate the referral of the patient to someone with greater experience in diagnosing and treating these types of dysfunction.

In summary, it is essential to examine the injured runner for abnormalities of both static and dynamic alignment and function. A high

Table 11.5 Clues to sacroiliac joint dysfunction.

Recurrent ipsilateral injuries
History of hip/pelvic trauma
Asymmetric stance and gait
Pelvic obliquity — maintained with sitting
Apparent change in leg length on moving from
  supine to long-sitting position
Asymmetric hip range of motion
Kinetic tests of sacroiliac function

index of suspicion for kinetic chain dysfunction should be present when assessing individuals with multiple or recurrent injuries. Marked variation from normal alignment, or significant asymmetry may be important clues to diagnosing an intrinsic dysfunction in the kinetic chain which may have predisposed the individual to injury. It is not always essential to be able to determine the exact site and nature of the kinetic chain dysfunction, however, it is most important to determine that a dysfunction is present, and to have the individual assessed by a physician or therapist with experience in these matters especially if the injury patterns persist or recur.

Primary factors

The primary intrinsic factors in running injuries are those which are specific to the individual circumstances of the runner (see Table 11.2). Although research-based information is sparse when considering the primary factors involved in running injuries (Power et al., 1986), one prospective study of 60 competitive runners over a year identified intrinsic factors in 40% of the injuries (Lysholm & Wiklander, 1987).

Age

There is no effect of age on injury rate based on the studies which assess age as a primary factor (Koplan et al., 1982; Marti et al., 1988; Walter et al., 1988). This is a little surprising appreciating the changes that occur in the musculoskeletal system with aging including the decrease in water content, metabolic activity, and collagen turnover of tendons (Hess et al., 1989). Although one might expect an increased injury rate with aging, the fact that this does not occur reinforces the complex interplay of intrinsic and extrinsic factors in the causation of overuse injuries. The role of extrinsic factors is reflected in a study of participants in a 10-km race or run, which showed that a group of older (greater than 30 years) runners had characteristics such as slower pace, fewer recreational activities outside of running, and less tendency to stretch before the race or to run for competition when compared with the younger participants (Walter *et al.*, 1988).

In a retrospective study of overuse injuries, Matheson *et al.* (1989) compared populations with an older mean age, 56.9 years, and a younger mean age, 30.4 years. Metatarsalgia, plantar fasciitis, meniscal injuries and osteoarthritis were more common in the older population. Patellofemoral pain syndrome and tibial stress fractures/periostitis were more common in the younger population. This study suffers from the usual flaws of case series with respect to lack of denominator data.

Gender

Due to the physiological, psychological and social differences between males and females, one might expect gender to influence injury rate (Clement *et al.*, 1981; Grana & Coniglione, 1985). Women, with their wider pelvis, greater genu valgum, less strength, and greater joint flexibility, could be considered more likely to get injured (Kowal, 1980). Although this is felt to be especially true for specific diagnoses such as pelvic stress fracture and patellofemoral pain syndrome, overall women do not seem to be at an increased risk of running injuries when compared to men (Powell *et al.*, 1986; Walter *et al.*, 1988).

Extrinsic factors may play a role in any gender differences, as women tend to run slower and fewer miles per day (Walter *et al.*, 1988). Younger women are more likely to be involved in multiple activities such as swimming, walking, exercise and skiing.

Women with disturbed menstrual function such as secondary amenorrhoea can develop hypo-oestrogenaemia, decreased bone mass and increased risk of stress fracture. This is felt to occur from accumulative stressors suppressing the hypothalamopituitary axis.

Fitness

The individual's fitness level at the time of embarking on a running programme is an intrinsic factor for injury. In a study of female military recruits entering physical training, Kowal (1980) found that those with a lower level of fitness had an increased risk of injury. Additionally, there is an increased risk of injury with increased body weight and body fat. Therefore, the fitness level of the individual must be taken into consideration when planning a running programme.

Growth

Some diagnoses are certainly age and growth dependent. This is evident in the osteochondrotic diseases such as Osgood–Schlatter disease (tibial tubercle), Sinding–Larsen disease (inferior pole of the patella), and Sever's disease (posterior calcaneus), which occur during the rapid growth periods of adolescence.

Rapid periods of growth make the developing athlete more susceptible for overuse injury for two reasons. Firstly, muscle strength lags behind skeletal growth resulting in a relative weakness. This delay can last for months in adolescence until the muscle strength becomes proportional. During this phase of relative weakness, mild biomechanical variations may become more evident resulting in injury. Secondly, with skeletal growth, the muscle–tendon unit is relatively shortened with secondary inflexibility. This may be a factor in the very common patellofemoral pain syndrome and Achilles tendinitis resulting from relative inflexibility of the quadriceps/hamstrings and gastrocnemius/soleus respectively.

Psychological factors

Although sport psychologists have demonstrated the importance of the mind in sports performance, this aspect has been infrequently addressed in sports injury (Kerr & Fowler, 1988). Studies that implicate personality in injury predisposition have been inconclusive (Govern & Koppenhaver, 1965; Brown, 1971; Rotter, 1972; Jackson *et al.*, 1978; Dahlhauser & Thomas, 1979; Valliant, 1980; Passer & Seese, 1983).

However, if one considers psychosocial factors (i.e. interactions between the individual and their social environment), then the studies are more definitive. Bramwell *et al.* (1975) assessed the amount of life change over 1- and 2-year intervals, and athletic injury in college football players. The results showed that injured players had significantly more life changes than the non-injured players using a life stress/change questionnaire to divide the athletes into low, moderate and high risk groups. Their incidence of injury was 30, 50 and 73% respectively. In a similar study modified for high school football players, the risk of injury was five times greater for a player who experienced high object loss (loss of parent of death, separation or divorce) compared to a player who did not experience such a loss (Coddington & Troxell, 1980).

Other studies have also shown a similar relationship between psychosocial factors and risk of injuries in gymnastics, but not in volleyball (Williams *et al.*, 1986; Kerr & Cairns, 1988). Whether this holds true for running remains to be seen, but the concept is interesting and bears investigation.

Bony alignment

The landmark article by James *et al.* (1978) revolutionized the approach of physicians to overuse running injuries. Since that time, great attention has been placed on the importance of lower extremity alignment as an aetiological factor for most, if not all, such injuries (Brody, 1980, 1987; Lutter, 1980; Clement *et al.*, 1981; Taunton *et al.*, 1982; Newell & Bramwell, 1984; Pinshaw *et al.*, 1984; Coniglione, 1985). Careful study to support these clinical impressions is required.

Alignment should be considered not as normal or abnormal, but as variations along the continuum of normal with a parallel continuum of predisposition to injury. One needs only to observe the passing runners in a recreational run, with the wide variation of gaits from very fluid to extremely awkward, to appreciate that there is great biomechanical variability. The runners with an awkward gait may be more prone to injury, but certainly their biomechanics alone do not assure injury.

Biomechanics of running is covered in more detail in Chapter 32. Briefly, the biomechanical propensity to injury occurs during stance phase between heel strike and toe off. Most runners land on the outer aspect of their heel with the foot in supination (plantar flexion, adduction, inversion). Upon landing, the foot passively pronates (dorsiflexion, abduction, eversion) unlocking the subtalar joint, allowing adaptation to the terrain and the dissipation of impact. At midstance, the foot stops pronating and begins supinating to form a more rigid lever for the powerful propulsive toe off. The ideal, perfect foot has neutral subtalar and midtarsal joints at the middle of midstance (Subotnick, 1985). This neutral foot position requires little muscular activity for balance, maximizing that available for shock absorption and propulsion (Subotnick, 1985). The line of force from heel strike to toe off should go from lateral in the rearfoot, medially to the midfoot, and then over between the first and second toes (Fig. 11.3). Biomechanical problems arise from excessive or restricted pronation through midstance. These variations in the lines of force are felt to predispose to injuries when repeated with 600 foot strikes per kilometre.

The rule of three reflects the increased forces of running and proposes that any degree of biomechanical variation has three times the significance in running compared to walking (Subotnick, 1985). If the biomechanical assessment reveals an increase in unweighted rearfoot varus of 5°, then this would function as 5° in walking, but as 15° in running.

The numerous structural variations and their biomechanical effects will be described individually.

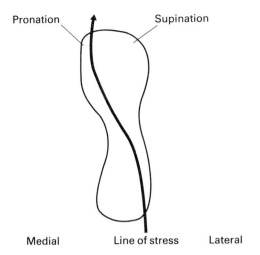

Fig. 11.3 Line of stress from heel strike to toe off. The ideal zone at toe off is between the first and second toe. More medially is excessive pronation and more laterally is excessive supination.

LEG LENGTH

Leg length discrepancy is considered to be an anatomical risk factor in development to lower extremity overuse injury (James *et al.*, 1978; Clement *et al.*, 1981; Subotnick, 1985), which is thought to be mediated through the effects of compensatory excessive pronation or supination. Leg length inequality has also been strongly associated with low back pain (Giles & Taylor, 1981). As previously mentioned, it would be possible to make more definitive conclusions regarding the relationship between leg length and injury, were it not for the confusion and variability between measurers and measurements. It is the authors' experience that the majority of individuals who reportedly have a leg length discrepancy actually have an SI joint dysfunction, either as a primary dysfunction, or as compensation for an anatomical leg length difference. This finding would also account for the high incidence of back pain in this group. Although it is difficult to interpret and generalize from the many studies of leg length discrepancy, any injured runner presenting with a pelvic obliquity should have the underlying dysfunction(s) assessed and corrected as part of the total treatment programme.

HIPS

The bony alignment problems of the hip include coxa vara and femoral neck retroversion and antiversion. Coxa vara is described by the femoral neck—shaft angle being less than the normal 125°. This can occur either congenitally or acquired from slipped capital femoral epiphysis or as a sequelae from a femoral neck or intratrochanteric fracture (Adams, 1976). The effect is an anatomical ipsilateral short leg and impaired efficiency of the hip abductor function due to the approximation of the greater trochanter and the ilium. This may result in a positive Trendelenberg's sign.

Normally the neck of the femur is angled 15° anterior to the long axis of the shaft and the femoral condyle (Hoppenfeld, 1976). Femoral neck anteversion describes greater anterior angulation. In order to accommodate the femoral head in the acetabulum, compensatory changes occur resulting in 'miserable malalignment syndrome'. These changes include excessive internal hip rotation, patellar squint, increased Q-angle, genu valgum, external tibial torsion, pes planus and excessive pronation (Donatelli, 1990a). Femoral neck retroversion, the opposite condition, is rare and is associated with a decreased angulation between the femoral neck and the long axis of the shaft resulting in excessive external hip rotation and limited internal hip rotation (Donatelli, 1990a). There may be compensatory divergent patella, genu varum, and internal tibial torsion that may predispose to excessive supination.

KNEES

Knee alignment is usually evaluated by assessing the degree of standing genu varum or valgum. The closer the knee is to the neutral the better. When coupled with a flexible foot, genu varum can result in a compensatory weighted rear foot valgus and excessive pronation. When coupled with a more rigid foot, genu varum can result in supination. Genu valgum, a component of 'miserable malalignment', can result in excessive pronation.

The most common overuse running injury is patellofemoral pain syndrome, which may be caused by variations in the bony structure of the joint. The local bony factors that have been implicated include patellar dysplasia, patellar malposition and trochlear dysplasia (Fulkerson & Hungerford, 1990). The patellar dysplasias usually involve partial hypoplasia of the medial facet although aplasia, hypoplasia, hyperplasia and fragmentation such as bipartite patella can occur. The patellar malpositions include patella alta and patella baja. Patella alta may occur from increased quadriceps tension, stretching the patellar tendon (Fulkerson & Hungerford, 1990) or rapid femoral growth rate during adolescence causing proximal patellar migration (Micheli et al., 1986). Patella baja is usually iatrogenic from tibial tubercle transfer surgery or stiffness after anterior cruciate ligament reconstruction.

The other important bony variations of the patellofemoral joint involve femoral trochlear dysplasia. These include hypoplasia of the medial condyle, aplasia of the medial trochlea and global dysplasia of the trochlea (Fulkerson & Hungerford, 1990). Concomitant dysplasia of the medial patellar facet usually also exists.

Prominent lateral epicondyles along with genu varum have been implicated as predisposing factors related to iliotibial band friction syndrome.

TIBIA

Structural variations of the tibia include tibial varum plus internal and external tibial torsion. Tibial varum greater than $7°$ is considered excessive and functions biomechanically similar to genu varum. When coupled with a flexible foot, tibial varum can result in a compensatory weighted rear foot valgus and excessive pronation. When coupled with a more rigid foot, tibial varum can result in supination. Tibial valgum may be a sequelae of trauma such as non-union of a tibial fracture and, similar to genu valgum, would contribute to excessive pronation.

Tibial torsion is often a compensation for femoral neck retroversion or anteversion to align the long axis of the foot in a more neutral position. When considered independently, internal tibial torsion should predispose the supination and external tibial torsion to pronation.

FOOT

The foot, as the final linkage to the ground, is considered an important primary factor in the aetiology of running injuries. Although an oversimplification, feet are divided into pes planus (flat) and pes cavus (high arch). The pes planus type foot, found in 20% of the population (Subotnick, 1985), is characteristically flat and flexible resulting in excessive pronation through midstance with a more medial line of force at toe off. Through the gait cycle, pes planus results in excessively weighted rear foot valgus, internal tibial torsion, genu valgum, and internal femoral rotation. This has been implicated in the development of SI joint dysfunction, patellofemoral pain syndrome, iliotibial band friction syndrome, popliteus tendinitis, pes anserine tendinitis/bursitis, tibial stress syndrome, medial tibial periostitis, Achilles tendinitis, posterior tibial tendinitis, plantar fasciitis, tibial and fibular stress fractures, and tarsal stress fractures (Subotnick, 1975a,b, 1979; James et al., 1978; Krisoff & Ferris, 1979; Prost, 1979; Brody, 1980, 1987; Taunton et al., 1982; Andrews, 1983; Viitasalo & Kvist, 1983; Clement et al., 1984; Lutter, 1986; Hunter & Poole, 1987; Matheson et al., 1987; Reilly & Nicholas, 1987; Tiberio, 1987; Torg et al., 1987; Ellis, 1988; Marshall, 1988; Tanner & Marvey, 1988; Cibulka, 1989; Fulkerson & Hungerford, 1990).

Pes cavus type foot, also found in 20% of the population (Subotnick, 1985), is characteristically high-arched, rigid and results in supination with more lateral weight-bearing through midstance and a lateral line of force at toe off. Through the gait cycle, pes cavus results in excessively weighted rear foot varus, reduced internal tibial rotation, increased genu varum and reduced internal femoral rotation. This has been implicated in the development of iliotibial band friction syndrome at the hip and the knee, lateral collateral ligament irritation at the knee, metatarsal stress fracture, peroneal muscle strain/tendinitis and plantar fasciitis (Brody, 1980, 1987; Lutter, 1981, 1986; Taunton & Clement, 1981; Schamberger, 1983; Leach et al., 1986; Kwong et al., 1988; Marshall, 1988; Tanner & Marvey, 1988).

Just as flexibility and collapse of the longitudinal arch can cause problems, so can that of the transverse arch. This can occur with both the pes planus and the pes cavus type feet and result in forefoot pain from sesamoiditis, irritation of the more exposed 2nd or 3rd metatarsal heads or Morton's neuroma.

As mentioned in the introduction, it is important to correlate static foot type and dynamic foot function as assessed by indirect or direct means before making treatment decisions or prescribing orthotics to correct for alignment problems.

In addition to the structural foot types described, structural variations of normal can also predispose to injury. In the rear foot, a prominent posterior calcaneus can result in superficial calcaneal bursitis, insertional Achilles tendinitis and/or retrocalcaneal bursitis. An os trigonum and prominent posterior talar beak can result in posterolateral ankle pain. An os trigonum can also cause tarsal tunnel syndrome by entrapment of the posterior tibial nerve (Murphy & Baxter, 1985).

Bony, cartilaginous or fibrous tarsal coalition between the talus, calcaneus, navicular, cuboid or cuneiforms leads to abnormal subtalar and midtarsal joint motion, which can become symptomatic with the increased impact of running (Donatelli, 1990a).

In the midfoot, an accessory navicular can predispose to medial midfoot pain from an irritation of the pseudoarthrosis with the underlying navicular or bursitis from pressure between the medial side wall of the shoe and a prominent navicular (Micheli, 1987). Stress fracture of the navicular has been associated with short first metatarsus, metatarsus adductus plus limited ankle and subtalar range of motion (Torg et al., 1987).

Along the dorsum of the midfoot, the os intermetatarseum between the proximal 1st and 2nd metatarsus can compress the deep peroneal nerve with subsequent foot pain (Murphy & Baxter, 1985).

In the forefoot, the Morton's foot with the shortened first ray and/or longer 2nd metatarsus can result in pain under the 2nd metatarsal head. This is especially likely if the first ray is hypermobile.

Muscular development

During gait, muscles function to initiate movement, stabilize osseus structures and decelerate movement (Donatelli, 1990b). Muscular abnormalities, specifically those of anatomy, flexibility and strength, are primary factors in the causation of running injuries.

ANATOMY

Variations of normal muscle anatomy can predispose to injury. Piriformis syndrome with sciatic nerve irritation from increased tension in the piriformis is more likely if the nerve courses through the muscle. This exists in approximately 6% of the population (Kopell & Thompson, 1960).

A more frequent clinical scenario involves the role of the quadriceps insertion in the development of patellofemoral pain syndrome. There is variability in the insertion sites of the vastus lateralis obliquus (VLO) and the vastus medialis obliquus (VMO). The more distal the VLO insertion and the more proximal to VMO insertion, the greater the likelihood of excessive patellar lateralization and patellofemoral pain syndrome (Fulkerson & Hungerford, 1990).

Chronic compartment syndromes arise from the inability of the muscle compartment to accommodate for the 20% increase in volume that occurs with exercise (Jones & James, 1987). The existence in some individuals of a 5th compartment in the leg surrounding the posterior tibial muscle and tendon makes them a risk for developing this localized compartment syndrome (Davey et al., 1984). The extension of the tibialis anterior muscle more distally than the usual muscle—tendon junction may predispose to chronic anterior compartment syndrome (Martens & Moeyersoons, 1990).

Posterior ankle pain mimicking Achilles tendinitis has been reported as due to an anomalous soleus muscle, either coursing more distally before attaching on to the Achilles tendon or inserting separately on the posterior calcaneus (Leppilahti et al., 1989).

FLEXIBILITY

Flexibility has been touted as one of the basic aetiological factors in the development of running injuries and overuse injuries in general. Despite all the attention flexibility has received, there is no direct evidence that it is an important factor (James et al., 1978; Shellock & Prentice, 1985). Indeed, one study has shown that runners who stretch more have a greater likelihood of having an injury (Jacobs & Berson, 1986). This may be due to the fact the runner is stretching due to a prior or subclinical problem, but it does question the usual tenets of overuse injury aetiology.

Inflexibility of the gastrocnemius—soleus—Achilles tendon complex can cause problems in both the flexible and the rigid foot. In the flexible foot, restricted ankle dorsiflexion leads to increased movement at the subtalar joint and excessive pronation as the centre of gravity passes anteriorly through the knee from midstance to toe off. The approach to treatment is a stretching programme to address the tight gastrocnemius—soleus mechanism; however, a varus posted orthotic may be required. In the more rigid foot, restricted dorsiflexion can lead

to standing heel varus, with increased strain at the midtarsal joint and the problems characteristic of supination. Treatment will involve stretching and flexibility, and the use of a heel lift to improve functional dorsiflexion.

A number of regional inflexibilities can contribute to injury. Tightness of the iliotibial band can result in irritation at the greater trochanter and/or lateral femoral epicondyle. Since the iliotibial band has a partial insertion on the lateral patellar retinaculum, it can be additive with an inherently tight retinaculum in contributing to excessive patellar lateralization and patellofemoral pain syndrome (Cox, 1985).

The two areas that become inflexible with running are the hamstrings and the calf (D'Ambrosia, 1985). Tightness of the hamstring can result in hamstring strain or pes anserine tendinitis (Cooper & Fair, 1978; Baker, 1984; Reilly & Nicholas, 1987). A tight gastrocnemius—soleus—Achilles tendon complex has also been implicated in the development of Achilles tendinitis and plantar fasciitis due to increased tension within the structures, independent of its role in excess functional pronation (Welsh & Clodman, 1980; Clancy, 1982).

Physiological inflexibility has been described, based on the observation that a fatigued muscle relaxes more slowly and less completely than a non-fatigued muscle (Krause, 1959; Agre, 1985). This suggests the importance of both muscle strength and flexibility for improved performance and reduced injury.

STRENGTH

Similar to inflexibility, muscle strength (or lack thereof) has been described as an important component in the aetiology of running injuries (Clement et al., 1981; Agre, 1985), and there is some evidence to support the association (Kowal, 1980). This relationship is based on the muscle's role in stabilizing the lower extremity and attenuating the forces and impact of running.

Great emphasis has been placed on the relative strength of the different components of the quadriceps muscle in the aetiology of patellofemoral pain syndrome (DeHaven *et al.*, 1979; Gruber, 1979; Insall, 1979). It is proposed that a weak VMO allows excessive patellar lateralization. Therefore, rehabilitation towards a stronger VMO is considered an integral part of successful clinical outcome.

Hip abductor insufficiency is considered a factor in the development of iliotibial band friction syndrome. With running, this weakness allows a dynamic positive Trendelenberg's sign and dropping of the contralateral side of the pelvis. This results in increased tension in the ipsilateral iliotibial band and irritation at either the greater trochanter or the lateral femoral epicondyle.

The role of the hamstring in running is to decelerate the passive knee extension of the swing phase and to allow adequate hip extension in the stance phase (Mann, 1982a, 1982b). Hamstrings strains have been extensively studied with a number of aetiological factors described including an imbalance between the strength of the hamstrings and the quadriceps, and the strength ratio of one hamstrings to the other (Burkett, 1970; Cooper & Fair, 1978; Agre, 1985).

Weakness of the lower leg muscles may predispose to stress fracture due to their important role in both shock absorption and stability.

The posterior tibial muscle is felt to be important in the maintenance of the longitudinal arch height and weakness of this can contribute to excessive pronation and injury (Gray, 1989; Donatelli, 1990a).

NEUROMUSCULAR COORDINATION

Although there is not much written on this in sports injury literature, neuromuscular coordination is considered a factor in hamstrings strain (Glick, 1980; Agre, 1985). The hamstrings' action is to control and oppose quadriceps' action, in the deceleration of knee extension and in knee flexion. A breakdown in the fine balance and motor control between the muscles

can result in injury. A similar model may be applied to the lower leg with the relationship between the gastrocnemius–soleus complex and anterior tibial muscles.

Ligamentous factors

Although known to be at risk for shoulder and patellar dislocation, individuals with a generalized ligamentous laxity may also be at increased risk for certain running injuries. This can be due to subtalar and midtarsal joint laxity resulting in excessive pronation, with the plethora of conditions that can ensue (Donatelli, 1990a). Injury can also be due to local considerations such as increased laxity of the medial retinaculum allowing excessive patellar lateralization to occur, contributing to the development of patellofemoral pain syndrome.

Acquired factors

The primary intrinsic factors have an important and fairly well understood and accepted role in overuse running injuries. The secondary or acquired dysfunctions are equally important, but are much less recognized. These dysfunctions are usually the result of hypomobility or hypermobility of a segment of the kinetic chain following an injury. As mentioned in the introduction, any dysfunction in the kinetic chain can lead to compensatory alterations in stance and gait, which in turn can lead to tissue microtrauma, breakdown and overt injury. It is important to remember that the presenting injury may represent the secondary injury ('victim'), and that the primary dysfunction may have occurred at a distant time or site ('culprit').

The role of acquired dysfunctions in running injuries has only recently been appreciated and remains controversial. There has been much less research into the acquired factors, and although lacking experimental validation, they have proved to be valuable concepts clinically. Increased awareness of their occurrence will result in the recognition of more of these dysfunctions, with resultant improvements in patient care. This section will provide an overview of some specific acquired factors.

Mechanical factors

SACROILIAC JOINT

Dysfunction of the position and motion of the SI joint and lumbosacral complex is a common, frequently overlooked, and almost universally controversial condition.

Conventional medical wisdom frequently maintains that the SI joint is immobile, despite the multitude of studies which have demonstrated that movement does indeed occur. A total description of normal and abnormal function is beyond the scope of this chapter, but a thorough discussion and extensive references describing SI function and dysfunction are available in works by Lee (1989) and Schamberger (1993).

The most common dysfunctions occur with anterior subluxation and rotation of the innominate, leading to an asymmetry in the pelvic ring structure. Some patients will show an upslip pattern where the innominate is subluxed superiorly. Less common are posterior rotations. The presenting dysfunction is usually locking or hypomobility at the involved SI joint. Once the subluxation has been corrected, these patients may demonstrate an underlying hypermobile SI that allows the subluxation and then locking into a position at the extremes of motion.

SI dysfunction can present with pain in either an acute or chronic fashion with the clinical presentation determined by the actual site and type of dysfunction, and the compensatory changes that have occurred in other segments and links of the kinetic chain. There may be a history of some trauma, often a fall onto the buttocks, or an axial load onto one leg, such as can occur with stepping unexpectedly off a curb or into a hole in the ground. It is not uncommon to see SI dysfunction following motor vehicle accidents where the patient has braced their legs against the brake pedal or floor in anticipation of impact.

The pain is often localized to the SI joint itself, but may be found in the buttocks, pubic symphysis, lower abdomen or lateral thigh. Occasionally, there is pain referred to the thigh and lower leg, which can mimic pain of a protruded intervertebral disc, although differing in that there are no associated neurological findings (Coventry & Tapper, 1972). SI joint pain also differs from true sciatica in that the pain is often discontinuous within the leg, and does not radiate in a band-like fashion (Hackett, 1957). Patients with SI dysfunction will often present with a secondary ('victim') injury arising from gait alterations, but will admit to underlying activity-related back pain. Patients will also complain that they feel as if they are out of alignment, and that their gait is abnormal, but many will not admit to this sensation unless specifically questioned.

Dysfunction of the SI joint will lead to compensatory changes at other sites in the axial skeleton, including sacral torsion, rotation of the lumbar vertebrae, and frequently secondary rotations of thoracic and even cervical vertebrae. These can manifest themselves as pain at sites distant from the SI joint, as well as in the characteristic findings of flexible dual scoliosis, and rotations of the upper thorax and shoulder girdle. The pain arising from SI dysfunction can be variously attributed to mechanical stresses on ligamentous structures, facet joints, discs and muscles. Positional and kinetic tests which stress these structures can elicit pain.

Kinetic chain dysfunction will also lead to functional asymmetry of the appendicular skeleton. This can lead to an asymmetrical appearance of the knee alignment, with increased patellar squinting (or divergence) of one side compared to the other. It can also result in compensatory changes and asymmetry of resting foot position, commonly increased pronation one foot relative to the other. Gait and foot function may also be affected, with one study showing improved gait symmetry on a force platform following manipulation of the SI joint (Robinson *et al.*, 1987). In individuals with longstanding SI dysfunction, some of the compensatory changes may be relatively fixed, making it difficult to determine which condition initiated the complex dysfunctional pattern. Anterior rotation of the innominate will also result in increased tension in the ipsilateral hamstrings. Thus, the clinician should always be aware of this potential problem in dealing with a runner with recurrent hamstring injuries, especially when they recur without significant strain, and are associated with low back pain.

Physical examination is directed at the identification of functional asymmetries of the pelvic girdle and SI joint. These tests include static tests of relative positioning of anatomical landmarks on the pelvis, as well as the performance of kinetic tests of SI joint movement as described in the section on the physical examination.

There are several keys to identifying SI joint dysfunctions including:

1 An awareness that they exist, and an understanding of their mechanics.

2 A high index of suspicion when dealing with patients with recurrent injury.

3 A knowledge of the historical clues to their existence.

4 A systematic examination that specifically looks for asymmetry.

5 Familiarity with the indirect clues to their presence.

6 Practice at the specific examination techniques for their detection.

Diagnosing and treating SI dysfunctions can be rewarding for both the patient and clinician, as the patient will often remain in the injury cycle until the kinetic chain function has been returned to normal.

KNEE

Although the knee itself is frequently injured, knee dysfunctions can also lead to other injuries in running sports. Previous trauma or injury

with a knee effusion will lead to reflex inhibition of quadriceps function and possible alteration of gait. Immobilization or incomplete rehabilitation of old injuries can lead to a flexion deformity resulting in increased patellofemoral forces. Similarly, immobilization can lead to tethering and restriction of patellar movement, with resultant injury.

Hypomobility or hypermobility of the proximal tibiofibular joint following injury can result in both local discomfort as well as abnormal pronation and supination of the subtalar joint leading to injury (Maitland, 1991). It is thus important to remember the proximal tibiofibular joint when assessing a patient with lateral knee pain or with abnormal functional foot movements.

FOOT AND ANKLE

The foot and ankle are composed of a complex series of articulations, and dysfunction at any joint can lead to gait changes and injury. Acute trauma can lead to ligamentous injury with corresponding hypermobility and instability. Conversely, immobilization and oedema following injury can lead to fibrosis with adhesion formation and hypomobility, with the loss of normal joint functioning. The degree of abnormal mobility will determine whether the rest of the kinetic chain can compensate for the dysfunction without breakdown. The body may adapt to minor degrees of dysfunction without clinical symptoms, however, severe mobility problems exceed this threshold and lead to overt problems.

When treating foot and ankle injuries, the clinician often focuses on the ankle joint itself, and ignores potential injuries to other joints, even though injuries to the subtalar joint commonly accompany ankle sprains. While there are certainly other causes of persistent ankle pain following inversion injury, it is essential to restore normal joint motion to both the subtalar joint and the ankle joint itself.

Restriction of ankle dorsiflexion can be due to either capsular tightness or tightening of the gastrocnemius–soleus complex following an injury or immobilization. This can lead to compensatory gait changes such as:

1 Increased knee flexion.

2 Hiking and circumduction of the hip to help the foot clear the ground.

3 Early heel off and toe off during stance phase.

4 Increased mobility with pronation at the subtalar and midtarsal joints.

5 Difficulty stabilizing the 1st metatarsal ray.

6 Increased dorsiflexion of the metatarsophalangeal joints with increased tension of the plantar fascia.

These can all lead to tissue overstress and injury (Gray, 1989; Donatelli, 1990a).

Increased mobility or instability of the ankle joint can result from splaying of the anterior or posterior tibiofibular ligaments following a hyperdorsiflexion or external rotation injury (Boytim *et al.*, 1991). Following this type of injury, the talus is less effective as a torque transducer, with resultant abnormal mobility of the rest of the foot. Reduced stability of the talus within the mortice allows it to move readily into either inversion or eversion, and as a result, the subtalar joint will frequently become locked in either pronation or supination depending on subsequent injury and muscle imbalances. This can lead to various patterns of injury corresponding with the distal dysfunction.

Restriction of subtalar motion following ankle sprains can lead to a loss of the normal functional ankle and foot movements. The resting or locked position which the posterior subtalar joint assumes can lead to loss of either pronation or supination on functional testing, and all their attendant problems. Restricted pronation, in the presence of a mobile forefoot, will place increased stress on the midtarsal joints, leading to hypermobility. This can lead to compensatory abduction and eversion of the forefoot and collapse of the medial arch at the talonavicular and navicular cuneiform joints (Donatelli, 1990a). Restricted pronation in the presence of a more rigid forefoot can lead to reduced impact absorption and the inability to

adapt to changes in the terrain, predisposing to recurrent inversion ankle sprains (Donatelli, 1990a). The inability to resupinate at midstance can lead to hypermobility and instability of the forefoot and 1st ray, with increased loading of the 2nd, 3rd and 4th metatarsals (Gray, 1989).

Midtarsal joint injuries can result in a number of dysfunctions with either hypomobility or hypermobility. The clinical picture will depend on the involved joints, the exact mechanical dysfunction and the compensatory changes. Subluxation of the cuboid can occur, usually following an inversion injury. Any such injury which reduces the stability of the calcaneocuboid joint will reduce the efficiency of the peroneus longus and can lead to reduced stability of the 1st metatarsal ray and impaired push off (Donatelli, 1990a).

Hallux limitus is an osteoarthritic condition of the 1st metatarsophalangeal joint leading to subluxation of the proximal phalynx and reduced dorsiflexion, usually resulting from repeated trauma (Magee, 1987; Donatelli, 1990b). The patient will complain of local pain, and will experience an abnormal lateral weight-bearing, possibly leading to overstress injuries.

With foot and ankle injuries, the exact localization of the site of dysfunction is difficult and requires considerable examination skill and experience. The important consideration for the initial clinician is the identification of the presence of a dysfunction, which can be fairly readily ascertained by the discovery of abnormal movements on functional testing. The treating therapist can assess the various glides and tests of joint mobility to determine which joints need treatment. Residual joint dysfunction should always be considered in those individuals with a history of a foot or ankle injury who fail to respond to the usual rehabilitation, especially in the presence of abnormal functional tests of foot movements.

Muscular dysfunctions

Muscle function is essential to absorb impact and stabilize the elements of the kinetic chain.

Overstress and injury can lead to inflammation and pain, which can cause reflex inhibition of muscle function. Once the pain/injury pattern is initiated, the patient enters a vicious cycle of pain—disuse—muscle weakness that tends to perpetuate the problem until both the underlying pathology and the strength deficits have been remedied. Muscle injuries often heal with contracture and resultant inflexibility necessitating compensatory changes in kinetic chain function and gait. Imbalances in strength between agonist and antagonist muscle groups have been identified as a primary cause of injury, and similarly, strength imbalance following injury can lead to further problems. Overall, failure to restore adequately strength, muscle balance and flexibility can lead to further injuries as the kinetic chain dysfunction is perpetuated.

Treatment of acquired dysfunctions

The critical factors in treating overuse injuries are the relief of symptoms and the restoration of normal kinetic chain function. Therefore, the identification of a kinetic chain dysfunction is a crucial part of the treatment. It is all too easy to prescribe rest, ice and anti-inflammatories to treat the overt signs of injury, without discovering the underlying factors which precipitated the injury. This cookbook approach to treatment works very well until the patient attempts to return to activity, at which time the symptoms may recur. Failure to correct the intrinsic or extrinsic factors behind the injury can lead to recurrent injury, patient and physician frustration, and to patients 'doctor shopping' or turning to other health-care providers in search of relief.

It is essential to restore adequate muscular strength, balance, flexibility and coordination. Strength retraining can be performed isometrically or isotonically, using concentric, eccentric or isokinetic exercises. It is the authors' experience that functional, closed kinetic chain exercises are the most useful type of exercise in the rehabilitation of running injuries. Careful attention must also be placed on the restoration of muscle balance and symmetry.

It is also essential to restore normal alignment, mobility and symmetry to the kinetic chain. Dysfunctional joints should be identified, and their normal movements restored. Hypomobile joints should be mobilized or manipulated to allow normal function, and the patient should then be counselled on stretching techniques to maintain normal mobility. Attempts should also be made to stabilize hypermobile joints which are causing recurrent dysfunction. The SI joint can be stabilized through the use of a sacral support brace, and stretching and strengthening exercises. Resistant cases can be treated with prolotherapy, which employs sclerosing injections into the SI ligaments to increase their stability. Proximal or distal tibiofibular joint instability can be stabilized through taping, or the use of an air cast or other functional lower leg brace. Hypermobility of the foot can be controlled through the use of a functional orthotic device.

Prevention

Prevention of running injury is much preferred to diagnosis and treatment. Ideally, an assessment aimed at minimizing injury should occur prior to the onset of a running programme. Other chapters will detail the importance of incorporating training methods, running surfaces and footwear into the safe introduction of a running programme.

Considerations of the individual's age, body composition, menstrual function, fitness level, lower extremity alignment, flexibility, strength and ligamentous laxity can result in a risk of injury profile.

The identification of kinetic chain dysfunction is an integral part of prevention, and involves a directed history and physical examination. The history is aimed at the determination of a pattern of prior overuse injuries, with either recurrent injury at the same site or multiple sites on the ipsilateral lower extremity. A history of prior trauma with potential SI or peripheral joint dysfunction should be elicited. The physical examination is structured to confirm the suspicions found on history taking.

With these factors in mind, it is possible to develop a programme utilizing: (i) adequate warm-up; (ii) appropriate frequency, duration and intensity of training; (iii) proper running surface; (iv) preferred shoes, orthotics and heel lift as required; and (v) specific flexibility and strength exercises, in order to minimize the risk of injury (Kowal, 1980; Agre, 1985; Shellock & Prentice, 1985; Subotnick, 1985; Hess *et al.*, 1989).

Despite the above recommendations, the ability to guarantee injury-free running and accurately predict running injuries is limited. This may reflect the many structural variations of normal that predispose to injury, the presence of important factors that have not yet been determined or the crudeness of the above training programme. More practically applied research in the area is required.

Conclusion

Intrinsic factors play a significant role in the aetiology of overuse running injuries. A knowledge of the primary intrinsic factors can be helpful in determining the cause of an individual injury. Similarly, an awareness of the mechanisms of secondary dysfunction, and a high index of suspicion for their occurrence, can lead to the identification and appropriate treatment of injuries before they become chronic or recurrent.

References

Adams, J.C. (1976) *Outline of Orthopaedics*, 8th edn. Churchill Livingstone, Edinburgh.

Agre, J.C. (1985) Hamstring injuries: Proposed aetiological factors, prevention, and treatment. *Sports Med.* 2(1), 21–33.

Andrews, J.R. (1983) Overuse syndromes of the lower extremity. *Clin. Sports Med.* 2(1), 137–48.

Baker, B.E. (1984) Current concepts in the diagnosis and treatment of musculotendinous injuries. *Med. Sci. Sports Exerc.* 16, 323–7.

Boytim, M.J., Fischer, D.A. & Neumann, L. (1991) Syndesmotic ankle sprains. *Am. J. Sports Med.* 19(3), 294–8.

Bramwell, S., Masuda, M., Wagner, N. & Holmes, T. (1975) Psychological factors in athletic injuries. *J. Hum. Stress* 1, 6–20.

Brody, D.M. (1980) Running injuries. *Clin. Symp.* 32(4), 1–36.

Brody, D.M. (1987) Running injuries. *Clin. Symp.* 39(4), 1–36.

Brown, R. (1971) Personality characteristics related to injuries in football. *Res. Q.* 42, 133–8.

Burkett, L.N. (1970) Causative factors in hamstring strains. *Med. Sci. Sport Exerc.* 2, 39–42.

Cibulka, M.T. (1989) Rehabilitation of the pelvis, hip, and thigh. *Clin. Sports Med.* 8(4), 777–803.

Clancy, W.G. (1982) Tendinitis and plantar fasciitis in runners. In R. D'Ambrosia & D. Drez Jr (eds) *Prevention and Treatment of Running Injuries.* Charles B. Slack, New Jersey.

Clement, D.B., Taunton, J.E. & Smart, G.W. (1984) Achilles tendinitis and perintendinitis: Etiology and treatment. *Am. J. Sports Med.* 12, 179–84.

Clement, D.B., Taunton, J.E., Smart, G.W. & McNicol, K.L. (1981) A survey of overuse running injuries. *Phys. Sportsmed.* 9(5), 47–58.

Coddington, R. & Troxell, T. (1980) The effects of emotional factors on football injury rates — A pilot study. *J. Hum. Stress* 6, 3–5.

Cooper, D.L. & Fair, J. (1978) Trainer's corner: Hamstring strains. *Phys. Sportsmed.* 6(8), 104.

Coventry, M.B. & Tapper, E.M. (1972) Pelvic instability — A consequence of removing iliac bone for grafting. *J. Bone Joint Surg.* 54A(1), 83–101.

Cox, J.S. (1985) Patellofemoral problems in runners. *Clin. Sports Med.* 4(4), 699–715.

Dalhauser, M. & Thomas, M. (1979) Visual disembedding and locus of control as variables associated with high school football injuries. *Perceptual Motor Skills* 49, 254.

D'Ambrosia, R.D. (1985) Orthotic devices in running injuries. *Clin. Sports Med.* 4(4), 611–18.

Davey, J.R., Rorabeck, C.H. & Fowler, P.J. (1984) The tibialis posterior muscle compartment. An unrecognized cause of exertional compartment syndrome. *Am. J. Sports Med.* 12(5), 391–6.

DeHaven, K.E., Dolan, W.A. & Mayer, P.J. (1979) Chondromalacia patellae in athletes — Clinical presentation and conservative management. *Am. J. Sports Med.* 7(1), 5–11.

Donatelli, R.A. (1990a) Abnormal biomechanics. In: R.A. Donatelli (ed) *The Biomechanics of the Foot and Ankle*, pp. 32–65. FA Davis Co., Philadelphia.

Donatelli, R.A. (1990b) Normal anatomy and biomechanics. In R.A. Donatelli (ed) *The Biomechanics of the Foot and Ankle*, pp. 3–31. FA Davis Co.,

Philadelphia.

Ellis, J. (1988) Arch enemy. *Runner's World* **23**, 28.

Fulkerson, J.P. & Hungerford, D.S. (1990) *Disorders of the Patellofemoral Joint*, 2nd edn. Williams & Wilkins, Baltimore.

Giles, L.G.F. & Taylor, J.R. (1981) Low back pain associated with leg length inequality. *Spine* **6**, 510–21.

Glick, J.M. (1980) Muscle strains: Prevention and treatment. *Phys. Sportsmed.* **8**(11), 73–7.

Govern, J. & Koppenhaver, R. (1965) Attempts to predict athletic injuries. *Med. Times* **93**, 421–42.

Grana, W.A. & Coniglione, T.C. (1985) Knee disorders in runners. *Phys. Sportsmed.* **13**(5), 127–33.

Gray, G. (1989) *Chain Reaction: Successful Strategies for Closed Chain Testing and Rehabilitation*. Wynn Marketing, Michigan.

Gruber, M.A. (1979) The conservative treatment of chondromalacia patellae. *Orthop. Clin. N. Am.* **10**, 105.

Hackett, G.S. (1957) *Joint Ligament Relaxation Treated by Fibro-osseous Proliferation. With Special Reference to Low Back Disability — Trigger Point Pain, Referred Pain, and Sciatica–Tendon Relaxation*, 2nd edn. Charles C. Thomas, Illinois.

Hess, G.P., Cappiello, W.L., Poole, R.M. & Hunter, S.C. (1989) Prevention and treatment of overuse tendon injuries. *Sports Med.* **8**(6), 371–84.

Hoppenfeld, S. (1976) *Physical Examination of the Spine and Extremities*. Appleton-Century-Crofts, Connecticut.

Hunter, S.C. & Poole, R.M. (1987) The chronically inflamed tendon. *Clin. Sports Med.* **6**(2), 371–88.

Insall, J. (1979) 'Chondromalacia patellae': Patellar malalignment syndrome. *Orthop. Clin. N. Am.* **10**, 117–27.

Jackson, D., Jarrett, H., Bailey, D., Kausek, J., Swanson, J. & Powell, J.W. (1978) Injury prediction in the young athlete: a preliminary report. *Am. J. Sports Med.* **6**(1), 6–11.

Jacobs, S.J. & Berson, B. (1986) Injuries to runners: A study of entrants to a 10 000 meter race. *Am. J. Sports Med.* **14**(2), 151–5.

James, S.L., Bates, B.T. & Osternig, L.R. (1978) Injuries to runners. *Am. J. Sports Med.* **6**(2), 40–50.

Jones, D.C. & James, S.L. (1987) Overuse injuries of the lower extremity. *Clin. Sports Med.* **6**(2), 273–90.

Kerr, G. & Cairns, L. (1988) The relationship of selected psychological factors to athletic injury occurrence. *J. Sport Exerc. Psychol.* **10**(2), 167–73.

Kerr, G. & Fowler, B. (1988) The relationship between psychological factors and sports injuries. *Sports Med.* **6**, 127–34.

Kibler, W.B., Goldberg, C. & Chandler, J. (1991) Functional biomechanical deficits in running athletes with plantar fasciitis. *Am. J. Sports Med.* **19**(1),

66–71.

Kopell, H.P. & Thompson, W.A. (1960) Peripheral entrapment neuropathies of the lower extremity. *N. Engl. J. Med.* **262**(2), 56–60.

Koplan, J.P., Powell, E., Sikes, R.K., Shirley, R.W. & Campbell, C.C. (1982) An epidemiological study of the benefits and risks of running. *JAMA* **248**(23), 3118–21.

Kowal, D.M. (1980) Nature and causes of injuries in women resulting from an endurance training program. *Am. J. Sports Med.* **8**(4), 265–9.

Krause, H. (1959) Evaluation and treatment of muscle function of the athletic injury. *Am. J. Surg.* **98**, 353–62.

Krisoff, W.B. & Ferris, W.B. (1979) Runners' injuries. *Phys. Sportsmed.* **7**(12), 53, 55–61.

Kwong, P.K., Kay, D., Voner, R.T. & White, M.W. (1988) Plantar fasciitis. *Clin. Sports Med.* **7**, 119–26.

Leach, R.E., Seavey, M.S. & Salter, D.K. (1986) Results of surgery in athletes with plantar fasciitis. *Foot Ankle* **7**, 156–61.

Lee, D. (1989) *The Pelvic Girdle: An Approach to the Examination and Treatment of the Lumbo-pelvic-hip Region*. Churchill Livingstone, New York.

Leppilahti, J., Orava, S., Karpakka, J., Gorra, A., Helal, B., Kvist, M., Peltarri, S. *et al.* (1989) Anomalous soleus muscle as a cause of exertion pain in athletes. *Clin. Sports Med.* **1**, 205–10.

Lutter, L.D. (1980) Injuries to the runner and jogger. *Minn. Med.* **63**(1), 45–51.

Lutter, L.D. (1981) Cavus foot in runners. *Foot Ankle* **1**, 225–8.

Lutter, L.D. (1986) Surgical decisions in athletes' subcalcaneal pain. *Am. J. Sports Med.* **14**, 481–5.

Lysholm, J. & Wiklander, J. (1987) Injuries in runners. *Am. J. Sports Med.* **15**(2); 168–71.

Macintyre, J.G., Taunton, J.E., Clement, D.B., Lloyd-Smith, D.R., McKenzie, D.C. & Morrell, R.W. (1991) Running injuries: A clinical survey of 4173 cases. *Clin. J. Sports Med.* **1**(2), 81–7.

McKenzie, D.C., Clement, D.B. & Taunton, J.E. (1985) Running shoes, orthotics and injuries. *Sports Med.* **2**, 334–47.

Magee, D.J. (1987) *Orthopedic Physical Assessment*. WB Saunders, Philadelphia.

Maitland, G.D. (1991) *Peripheral Manipulation*, 3rd edn. Butterworth–Heinemann, London.

Mann, R.A. (1982a) Biomechanics of running. In R.A. D'Ambrosia and D. Drez Jr (eds) *Prevention and Treatment of Running Injuries*, pp. 1–14. Charles B. Slack, New Jersey.

Mann, R.A. (1982b) Biomechanics of running. In R.P. Mack (ed) *American Academy of Orthopedic Surgeons' Symposium on The Foot and Leg in Running Sports*, pp. 1–29. CV Mosby, St Louis.

Marshall, P. (1988) The rehabilitation of overuse foot

injuries in athletes and dancers. *Clin. Sports Med.* **7**, 175–91.

Martens, M.A. & Moeyersoons, J.P. (1990) Acute and recurrent effort-related compartment syndrome in sports. *Sports Med.* **9**(1), 62–8.

Marti, B., Vader, J.P., Minder, C.E. & Abelin, T. (1988) On the epidemiology of running injuries. *Am. J. Sports Med.* **16**(3), 285–94.

Matheson, G.O., Clement, D.B., McKenzie, D.C., Taunton, J.E., Lloyd-Smith, D.R. & Macintyre, J.G. (1987) Stress fractures in athletes. *Am. J. Sports Med.* **15**(1), 46–58.

Matheson, G.O., Macintyre, J.G., Taunton, J.E., Clement, D.B. & Lloyd-Smith, D.R. (1989) Musculo-skeletal injuries associated with physical activity in older adults. *Med. Sci. Sports Exerc.* **21**(4), 379–85.

Micheli, L.J. (1987) The traction apophysites. *Clin. Sports Med.* **6**(2), 389–404.

Micheli, L.J., Slater, J.A., Woods, E. & Gergino, P.G. (1986) Patella alta and the adolescent growth spurt. *Clin. Orthop.* **213**, 159–62.

Murphy, P.C. & Baxter, D.E. (1985) Nerve entrapment of the foot and ankle in runners. *Clin. Sports Med.* **4**(4), 753–63.

Newell, S.G. & Bramwell, S.T. (1984) Overuse injuries to the knee in runners. *Phys. Sportsmed.* **12**(3), 80–92.

Passer, M. & Seese, M. (1983) Life stress and athletic injuries: Examination of positive versus negative events and three moderator variables. *J. Hum. Stress* **9**, 11–16.

Pinshaw, R., Atlas, V. & Noakes, T.D. (1984) The nature and response to therapy of 196 consecutive injuries seen at a runners' clinic. *S. Afr. Med. J.* **65**, 291–8.

Powell, K.E., Kohl, H.W., Caspersen, C.J. & Blair, S.N. (1986) An epidemiological perspective on the cause of running injuries. *Phys. Sportsmed.* **14**(6), 100–14.

Prost, W.J. (1979) Biomechanics of the foot. *Can. Fam. Phys.* **25**, 827–31.

Reilly, J.P. & Nicholas, J.A. (1987) The chronically inflamed bursa. *Clin. Sports Med.* **6**(2), 345–70.

Robinson, R.O., Herzog, W. & Nigg, B.M. (1987) Use of force platform variables to quantify the effects of chiropractic manipulation on gait symmetry. *J. Manipulative Physiol. Ther.* **10**(4), 172–6.

Rotter, J. (1972) *Applications of a Social Learning Theory of Personality.* Holt, Rhinehart & Winston, New York.

Schambaugh, J.P., Klein, A. & Herbert, J.H. (1991) Structural measures as predictors of injury in basketball players. *Med. Sci. Sports Exerc.* **23**(5), 522–7.

Schamberger, W. (1983) Orthotics for athletes: Attacking the biomechanical roots of injury. *Can. Fam. Phys.* **29**, 1670–80.

Schamberger, W. (1993) *Functional Malalignment — The Hidden Cause of Sports Injuries.* Human Kinetics, Illinois (in press).

Shellock, F.G. & Prentice, W.E. (1985) Warming-up and stretching for improved physical performance and prevention of sports-related injuries. *Sports Med.* **2**, 267–78.

Subotnick, S.I. (1975a) Orthotic control in the overuse syndrome. *Phys. Sportsmed.* **3**(1), 75–9.

Subotnick, S.I. (1975b) *Pediatric Sports Medicine.* Futura, New York.

Subotnick, S.I. (1979) *The Running Foot Doctor.* Anderson World Publications, Mountain View, California.

Subotnick, S.I. (1985) The biomechanics of running: Implications for the prevention of foot injuries. *Sports Med.* **2**, 144–53.

Tanner, S.M. & Harvey, J.S. (1988) How can we manage plantar fasciitis. *Phys. Sportsmed.* **16**, 39–47.

Taunton, J.E. & Clement, D.B. (1981) Iliotibial tract friction syndrome in athletes. *Can. J. Appl. Sports Sci.* **6**, 76–80.

Taunton, J.E., Clement, D.B. & McNicol, K. (1982) Plantar fasciitis in runners. *Can. J. Appl. Sports Sci.* **7**(3), 41–4.

Tiberio, D. (1987) The effect of excessive subtalar joint pronation on patellofemoral mechanics: A theoretical model. *J. Orthop. Sport Phys. Ther.* **9**, 160–5.

Torg, J.S., Pavlov, H. & Torg, E. (1987) Overuse injuries in sport: The foot. *Clin. Sports Med.* **6**(2), 291–320.

Valliant, P. (1980) Injury and personality traits in non-competitive runners. *J. Sports Med. Phys. Fitness* **20**, 341–6.

Viitasalo, J.T. & Kvist, M. (1983) Some biomechanical aspects of the foot and ankle in athletes, with and without shin splints. *Am. J. Sports Med.* **11**(3), 125–30.

Wadsworth, C.T. (1988) *Manual Examination and Treatment of the Spine and Extremities.* Williams & Wilkins, Maryland.

Walter, S.D., Hart, L.E., Sutton, J.R., McIntosh, J.M. & Gauld, M. (1988) Training habits and injury experience in distance runners: Age- and sex-related factors. *Phys. Sportsmed.* **16**(6), 101–13.

Welsh, R.P. & Clodman, J. (1980) Clinical survey of Achilles tendinitis in athletes. *Can. Med. Assoc. J.* **122**, 193–6.

Williams, J., Tonymon, P. & Wadsworth, W. (1986) Relationship of life stress to injury in intercollegiate volleyball. *J. Hum. Stress* **12**, 38–43.

Chapter 12

Body Composition and Predisposing Diseases in Injury Prevention

PEKKA KANNUS

Sports injuries result from a complex interaction of identifiable risk factors at a given point in time (Lysens *et al.*, 1984). Since many factors are involved (extrinsic and intrinsic factors, see Chapter 2), the prevention of sports injuries is a complex problem, and a continuing challenge to preventive medicine.

Any sports injury can be caused by intrinsic or extrinsic factors, either alone or in combination (Lorentzon, 1988). In acute traumas, extrinsic factors play a major role, while in overuse injuries the reasons are more multifactorial, and interaction between these two categories is common. However, in order to achieve an effective injury prevention, it is vital to be able to affect these predisposing risk factors.

Body composition

Weight and height

Many reports suggest that poor physical fitness and lack of practice may lead to an increased incidence of injuries (Nicholas, 1974; Wright, 1979). However, Jackson *et al.* (1978) found in young athletes no relationship between anthropometric data and physical fitness characteristics on the one hand, and sports injuries on the other. Also Lysens *et al.* (1984), in their study in a group of 138 physical education students of the same age, trained in the same conditions, and exposed to quite similar extrinsic factors, found no statistically significant differences

between weight, height, somatotype components and motor fitness characteristics, and acute and overuse sports injuries.

On the other hand, in some studies excessive height and weight have been found to predispose to acute (Blyth & Mueller, 1974) and overuse (Watson, 1981; Kujala *et al.*, 1986; Taimela *et al.*, 1990) injuries. Taimela *et al.* (1990) suggest that the relationship between body size and injuries may be due to the high position of the centre of gravity or to length of the limbs. Greater limb length could produce greater leverage and thus more stress on the limb joints in situations that require rapid change of direction.

Altogether, since the results of the studies have been controversial, we cannot make any definitive conclusions about the relationship between anthropometrics, and acute or overuse sports injuries. Also therefore, preventive measures in this context cannot be seen as very effective.

A completely separate issue is the role of body composition in degenerative musculoskeletal diseases and symptoms. McGoey *et al.* (1990) listed the sites and diagnoses of musculoskeletal symptoms in 105 morbidly obese persons (at least 45 kg overweight). 88% had pain which was severe enough to interfere with the activities of daily living. The areas involved were low back (62%), the hips (11%), the knees (57%), the ankles (34%), and the feet (21%) with the most characteristic diagnoses of mechanical back pain and sciatica (back), patellofemoral chondromalacia or degenerative arthritis, tibiofemoral arthritis and ligamentous laxity (knee), degenerative arthritis and ligamentous laxity (ankle), and metatarsalgia and plantar fasciitis (foot).

Heliövaara (1987) showed quite conclusively that body height and weight are directly correlated with the risk of herniated lumbar intervertebral disc so that the taller and heavier an individual, the higher the risk of disc prolapse. This becomes understandable when it is remembered that the load on lumbar discs is different in different positions of the body (Nachemson, 1966). The load is highest in sitting and lifting (straight knees) positions, and clearly lower when standing or lying. For example, in tall individuals lifting can be extremely strenuous in lumbar segments with forces exceeding many times body weight.

A strong relationship has been found between osteoarthritis (OA) and overweight, especially in knees (Leach et al., 1973; Lawrence, 1975; Hinz & Pohl, 1977; Silberberg, 1979; Hartz et al., 1986; Felson et al., 1988; Davis et al., 1990). However, other weight-bearing joints (hip and foot) have also been shown to be affected more often in obese people than in controls (Bray, 1985; Hartz et al., 1986). Even the OA changes in non-weight-bearing joints (hands) have been more advanced in obese subjects (Acheson & Collant, 1975; Bray, 1985; Davis et al., 1990). The association between OA and obesity has been more clear in women than in men (Hartz et al., 1986; Felson et al., 1988).

In sports injury prevention, overweight may be a problem in full weight-bearing recreational activities, since such activity in an obese individual may not only start the OA process but also significantly accelerate it. Studies trying to find out the effect of weight loss on musculoskeletal pain in the obese have been very scarce. However, a recent prospective study showed that in the morbidly obese, weight reduction (average 44 kg) by vertical banded gastroplasty lead to significant release of musculoskeletal symptoms (McGoey et al., 1990). After losing

weight, 89% of patients had complete relief of pain in one or more joints.

The results of this study are most encouraging for obese patients and their physicians. A low-energy diet and participation in sports events, in which the whole body weight does not stress the lower extremities, are recommended for all overweight people. The final goal is to reduce the weight to 'normal', which according to modern definitions is the body mass index (BMI) under 25 (BMI = $w \cdot h^{-2}$ where w is weight (kg) and h is height (m)) (Pacy et al., 1986).

Bone mass

Decreased bone mass is a well-recognized risk factor for stress fractures of lower extremities in young, active women, and an especially strong risk factor for osteoporotic fractures of hip, spine, proximal humerus, and distal radius in older women (Johnston & Slemenda, 1987; Schoutens et al., 1989; Sinaki, 1989; Bailey & McCulloch, 1990). It has been estimated that in the USA approximately 1.2 million fractures occur each year as a result of this condition, including 530 000 vertebral fractures and 227 000 hip fractures, with annual cost of rehabilitation exceeding \$US6 billion (Johnston & Slemenda, 1987).

The rising fracture rate with age is principally determined by the decrease in bone mass that universally occurs if no intervention is attempted (Fig. 12.1). As the population ages, osteoporosis will become even more important and an expensive problem during the next decades. In addition, even if sports and physical activity have been recommended for prevention of bone loss in young and old, there is an inbuilt risk that increased activities may lead to an increased number of sports accidents and fractures, consequently worsening the problem. In addition, a severe injury may lead to permanent osteoporosis (Fig. 12.2).

Bone density status of the skeleton at any time during life is dependent on bone gained during the growing and early adult years and bone lost with advancing years (Bailey &

Bone density

Low ▮▮▮▮▮▮▮▮▮▮▮▮▮▮▮▮ High

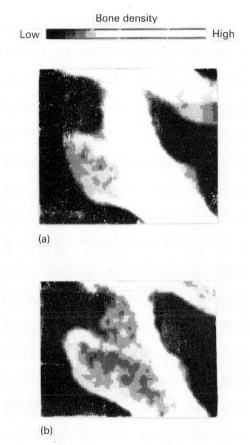

(a)

(b)

Fig. 12.1 (a) A dual energy X-ray absorbtiometric (DEXA) picture from a femoral neck of a 25-year-old female with normal bone density. (b) A DEXA picture from an osteoporotic femoral neck of a 55-year-old female.

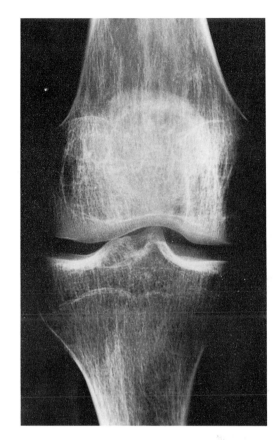

Fig. 12.2 A severe permanent knee osteoporosis 5 years after a complete rupture of the anterior cruciate ligament.

McCulloch, 1990). Total bone mass and bone density increase during adolescence, reaching a maximum in early adulthood. There is, however, significant individual age and sex variation in the development rate, growing pattern and final result of bone mass and density (Christiansen *et al.*, 1975). Peak bone mass and bone density are determined by genetic, mechanical, nutritional and hormonal factors so that women have in general 30% lower peak bone mass than men (Peck, 1984).

After a transient period of stability at peak bone mass, an incessant, age-related loss of

bone begins (Riggs & Melton, 1986; Bailey & McCulloch, 1990). This bone loss is observed in both men and women, but the rate of loss is greater in women. Over their lifetime, women lose about 35% of their cortical bone and 50–60% of their trabecular bone, whereas men lose about 30% less (Mazess, 1982). So, lower peak bone densities with higher losses (especially after menopause) most likely explain the higher fracture rate in females.

After the age of 35, the average rate of cortical bone loss for both sexes is about 0.3–0.5% of peak adult bone density per year. In women, the loss of cortical bone can be as high as 2–3% per year for the first 10 years after menopause (Mazess, 1982). According to Gärdsell *et al.*

(1990), the low initial bone mineral content was the best predictor of fracture in a longitudinal 15-year follow-up of 366 women. The rate of bone loss was not correlated with fracture risk, probably since 'rapid losers' were found only among women with high initial bone mass. Rapid loosing may, however, be a risk factor if it occurs with other risk factors.

While the basic aetiology of age-related bone loss and osteoporosis is unclear, there is a good general agreement that three major factors (which it is possible to affect) are of importance in maintenance of bone integrity:

1 Endocrine status (in women not only oestrogen but also progesterone levels) (Prior, 1990; Prior et al., 1990).
2 Nutritional factors (calcium, vitamin D, proteins).
3 Physical activity.

The relative contribution of each of these factors has not been established, but clearly, physical activity is a dominant player (Bailey & McCulloch, 1990). In the absence of weight-bearing activity, no amount of nutritional or hormonal intervention can maintain bone density (Mazess & Whedon, 1983).

Most of the cross-sectional studies analysing the relationship between physical activity and bone density have reported that people with high levels of physical activity have significantly higher bone density than less active persons (Smith & Gilligan, 1987; Schoutens et al., 1989; Sinaki, 1989; Bailey & McCulloch, 1990). This has also been the case in sport studies involving unilateral activities such as tennis (Dalsky, 1987). Intensive, longstanding exercise can increase bone mineral content as much as 40–50% as described in male junior competitive weightlifters when compared with age- and sex-matched non-athletic controls (Virvidakis et al., 1990). Also in females, weight-training may provide a better stimulus for increasing bone mass than running or swimming (Heinrich et al., 1990).

On the other hand, much lower level activities (e.g. daily walking) have been shown to be effective in reduction of age-related bone loss.

Zylstra et al. (1989) found that both lumbar spine (+0.8% increase per hour of daily walking) and femoral neck (+1.9%) densities were significantly correlated with walking, which was substantial, considering that the age-related rate of bone loss in the same population was 0.7% and 0.5% per year.

Longitudinal studies on the effect of exercise on bone mass and density have been very scarce to date, but those performed seem to confirm the generally positive effects of physical activity that were observed in the cross-sectional literature (Bailey & McCulloch, 1990). In order to be able to give specific recommendations for exercise prescription according to frequency, intensity, duration and type of activity, more prospective, controlled studies are needed.

However, today general recommendations can be confidently given. In order to increase the peak bone mass when young and decelerate the bone loss when older, weight-bearing physical activities of all kinds (including daily walking) are suggested for females as well as males. In this respect, suitable sports are walking, jogging, running, cross-country skiing, calisthenics, aerobics and many ball games. In the elderly, the sport should, however, be safely organized to avoid unnecessary accidents and fractures.

Predisposing diseases

Diseases and disorders of the musculoskeletal system may directly increase the risk for acute or overuse injuries by disturbing the normal structure and function of bone, cartilage, joints, ligament, muscle and tendon. Other diseases may, in turn, predispose to an injury more or less indirectly by affecting balance, coordination, mental concentration, energy supply or vision of the subject.

The most characteristic musculoskeletal diseases which can be seen as risk factors for sports injuries are: (i) OA; (ii) osteoporosis (discussed in detail previously in this chapter); (iii) chondromalacia; (iv) genetic joint hypermobility; (v) rheumatoid diseases; (vi) osteochondroses; (vii) age-related musculotendineal degeneration; and (viii) malalignments, scoliosis, leg length discrepancies, spondylolysis and spondylolisthesis (all of these are discussed elsewhere in this book).

Typical general diseases and conditions which may predispose to sports injuries are: (i) all neurological disorders; (ii) exceptional personality traits; (iii) diabetes and other endocrinological disorders; and (iv) all kinds of eye diseases and disorders (e.g. myopia) which impair visual capacity. This chapter concentrates on the musculoskeletal diseases and disorders as predisposing factors for sports injuries.

Musculoskeletal diseases and disorders

OSTEOARTHRITIS

The definition and criteria for OA have been for many years under discussion and subject to change, and are still not consistent and universally accepted by all (McAlindon & Dieppe, 1989). The definition by the American Rheumatism Association (Altman *et al.*, 1986) is, perhaps, most widely accepted indicating that OA is 'a heterogenous group of conditions that lead to joint symptoms and signs which are associated with defective integrity of cartilage, in addition to the related changes in underlying bone and at the joint margin'. Thus, the definition implies that OA is a group of heterogenous diseases with a similar endpoint: cartilage destruction. Its aetiology is clearly multifactorial, the main factors being: (i) aging; (ii) mechanical stress factors (overload, traumas, biomechanical malalignments), (iii) constitutional factors (female gender, Caucasian race, obesity); (iv) heredity (genetic predisposition); (v) metabolic disturbance; and (vi) inflammation (Peyron 1989).

Clinically, the most characteristic symptoms are pain, stiffness, tenderness, feeling of instability, loss of motion, effusion and crepitus (Cooke & Dwosh, 1986). Radiologically, typical signs are narrowing of the joint space, osteophytes, subchondral sclerosis and subchondral cysts, and, in advanced disease, subluxation, angular deformities, loose bodies and bone remodelling (Kellgren & Lawrence, 1957; Kannus & Järvinen, 1989) (Fig. 12.3). The most frequently affected joints are shown in Fig. 12.4.

Idiopathic (primary) OA is a problem in the elderly (increasingly after the age of 50), while secondary (usually post-traumatic) OA can disturb joint function in the very young. Whatever its cause, OA can be a very irritating and frustrating condition during sports activities, especially those requiring weight-bearing and quick starts, stops, jumpings and cuttings. In the hours subsequent to such activities, the joint usually swells and becomes tender and painful. After a couple of days rest and anti-inflammatory medication, the symptoms subside, but return if activity is tried again. In such a condition, the only way to continue sporting activities is to find a sport in which the whole body weight is not on the lower extremities and the movements are smooth. In this respect, swimming, cycling and rowing are most recommendable.

If OA is due to post-traumatic joint laxity, hard sporting activities may predispose the joint to a new injury (Lysens *et al.*, 1984; Kannus & Järvinen, 1989). In such cases, prophylactic bracing or taping of the affected joint is worth trying.

CHONDROMALACIA

Chondromalacia refers to wear and tear (destruction) of the articular cartilage without signs of OA. Most usually it affects the patellofemoral joint causing a characteristic clinical entity called 'patellofemoral pain syndrome' or 'patellar chondropathy'. Articular cartilage of the patella becomes involved in a process that leads to softening, cracking and wearing away of the surface. This syndrome can occur at any age but is most frequently seen in teenagers and young adults, and its onset is often insidious (Renström, 1988).

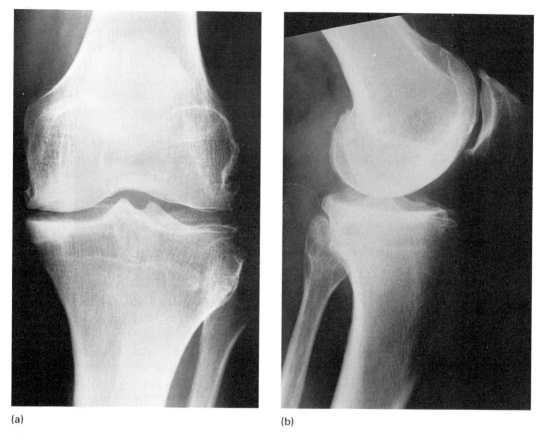

(a)   (b)

Fig. 12.3 Anteroposterior (a) and lateral (b) radiographs taken 15 years after a combined knee ligament rupture, involving the anterior cruciate and medial collateral ligaments and medial meniscus, was conservatively treated. A severe post-traumatic osteoarthritis has developed.

The basic aetiology of chondromalacia is unknown, but overuse or acute patellar contusion can often be found in connection with the onset of symptoms. Many predisposing factors have been found, such as: (i) abnormal distal or proximal placement of the patella; (ii) excessive patellar laxity and subluxation; (iii) lower extremity malalignments (ankle hyperpronation, external tibial torsion, excessive Q-angle, increased femoral anteversion, leg length inequality); and (iv) hypoplastic vastus medialis obliquus of the quadriceps muscle (Fig. 12.5). These factors may predispose the patella to a lateral displacement particularly when vigorous quadriceps contraction occurs (Fig. 12.6).

Clinically, the patient with chondromalacia presents with pain in the front of the knee. It is characteristically aggravated by activities such as running, climbing stairs or kneeling and is relieved by rest (Garrick, 1989). The pain is made worse by prolonged sitting with the knee bent such as when one attends the cinema or theatre (a 'movie sign'). After prolonged sitting, retropatellar pain and stiffness on initiating activity is also typical.

Patellar chondromalacia, when present, typically appears in sporting activities like running and jumping and very often makes continuation impossible. At rest, the symptoms are quickly relieved. These overuse symptoms can be alleviated more permanently by a quad-

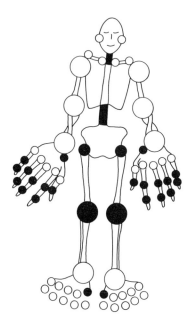

Fig. 12.4 The joints most frequently affected by osteoarthritis.

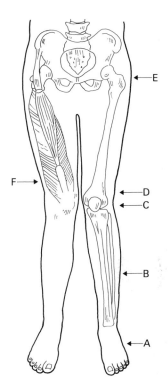

Fig. 12.5 The characteristic factors in knee biomechanics predisposing to chondromalacia patellae; A, foot hyperpronation; B, external tibial torsion; C, patella subluxation; D, excessive Q-angle; E, increased femoral anteversion; F, vastus medialis hypoplasia.

riceps muscle exercise programme, a patellar knee brace and anti-inflammatory medication. If symptoms are extremely severe and persistent, an abnormal patellofemoral tracking mechanism (lateral subluxation) can be treated surgically.

Since patellar chondromalacia is often associated with patellar laxity and subluxation, these patients have an increased risk for a complete luxation of the patella during activity. In prevention of complete luxation, all the above-mentioned conservative measures must be performed. If a complete patellar luxation does occur, surgery is often needed.

GENETIC JOINT HYPERMOBILITY

Genetic joint hypermobility or the 'hypermobility syndrome' is characterized by an excessive range of motion of one or more joints in normal physiological directions of movement, in abnormal directions, or in both (Steiner, 1987; Grahame, 1990). It must be separated from increased flexibility, which is a func-

Fig. 12.6 (a) An abnormal lateral tracking of the patella is a common finding in chondromalacia patellae. (b) Normal patellar tracking.

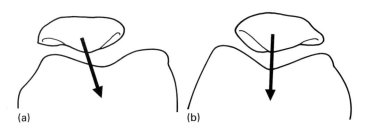

(a) (b)

tion of muscle and tendon tightness, even though there is some overlap between these two categories so that people with joint hypermobility are often quite flexible (Steiner, 1987). A third term in the field is ligamentous laxity which refers to joint distraction and shear and is a function of ligament tightness. A mild laxity is physiological, but a ligamentous injury may lead to an excessive (pathological) joint laxity (usually called instability) causing many residual problems especially in the knee, ankle and shoulder joints.

Hypermobility was first proposed as a cause of joint problems in 1964 by Carter and Wilkinson. Beighton and Horan (1970) created five tests for hypermobility (Fig. 12.7). All of these tests tend to move the joints in their normal planes of motion. In most clinical studies individuals have been classified as hypermobile if they can perform three or more of these manoeuvres (Steiner, 1987).

Depending upon the study criteria used, between 4 and 7% of the population probably can be classified as hypermobile (Steiner, 1987; Grahame, 1990). Hypermobile individuals are clearly more often female than male, and the

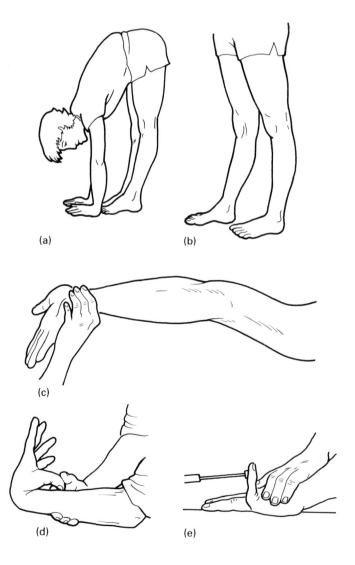

(a)

(b)

(c)

(d)

(e)

Fig. 12.7 Five tests for hypermobility. (a) Forward bending. In a positive case the subject can touch the floor with both palms while keeping the knees straight. (b) Hyperextension of the knee. A positive case is hyperextension more than 10°. (c) Hyperextension of the elbow. A positive case is hyperextension more than 10°. (d) Abduction of the thumb. In a positive case the thumb can touch the forearm. (e) Hyperextension of the 5th metacarpophalangeal joint. A positive case is extension more than 90°.

syndrome is clearly age dependent: almost 50% of toddlers and preschoolers are hypermobile, but this figure drops to about 5% by the age of 6 (Carter & Wilkinson, 1964). Thereafter the proportions remains fairly constant into early adulthood. While it is common knowledge that adults joints become stiffer with age, there are few data to confirm this clinical impression. Hypermobility also has some racial connections. Asians generally show a greater joint range than Negroes, who in turn are more mobile than Caucasians (Grahame, 1990).

Hypermobility is partly inherited as an autosomal dominant trait (Beighton & Horan, 1970; Steiner, 1987). Many extra-articular organs and tissues, which rely for their structural integrity on the tensile strength of normal collagen, may also become disordered in hypermobile subjects. The skin may be thin, soft, hyperextensible and develop striae. Associations with: (i) mitral valve prolapse; (ii) abnominal hernia; (iii) rectal and uterine prolapse; (iv) bone fragility; (v) Marfan's syndrome; (vi) osteogenesis imperfecta; (vii) Ehlers–Danlos syndrome; (viii) Down's syndrome; (ix) hyperlysinaemia; (x) homocystinuria; and (xi) hypermobility has been reported (Grahame, 1990). In the vast majority of individuals with hypermobility, however, the condition is probably just one extreme of the natural variation seen in all human characteristics. Furthermore, the implications of hypermobility may also be highly joint specific.

The role of excessive flexibility training in the development of hypermobility is unclear. It seems possible that through intensive training (especially in childhood and adolescence) ballerinas may permanently increase their spine and hip mobility (Steiner, 1987). On the other hand, in none of these studies has the question of a selection process versus the effects of training been properly answered.

An interesting issue concerns whether genetic hypermobility predisposes an individual to a joint injury (sprain or dislocation). In 1970, Nicholas reported that 72% of the New York Jets football players with hypermobility had major surgery on their knee ligaments over a 5-year period, while only 9% of the players with no positive tests for hypermobility had such surgery over the same period. None of the following studies could, however, confirm his drastic findings (Steiner, 1987). One condition strongly associated with hypermobility is patellar dislocation. Hypermobility is seen in more than half of the individuals with this problem (Runow, 1983). Quadriceps exercises and a patellar knee brace is recommended for these people. A common clinical impression that recurrent anterior shoulder subluxation or dislocation, and recurrent ankle sprains (especially if bilateral) are associated with hypermobility syndrome needs prospective follow-up studies. In the mean time, muscular rehabilitation with coordination and proprioceptive training, bracing and taping can be recommended.

Concerning overuse-type symptoms, there is evidence that joint hypermobility leads to joint pain and swelling during activity even though some researchers have not found correlation between joint problems and hypermobility (Steiner, 1987; Grahame, 1990). Some reports have even indicated that hypermobility may lead to OA (Grahame, 1990). These studies yielded evidence that osteoarthritic patients with hypermobility have more extensive joint disease than those without hypermobility. However, this relationship has not yet been shown to be causal. It may be that hypermobility, while not causing OA, makes the condition worse when the two coexist.

RHEUMATOID DISEASES

Rheumatoid arthritis (RA) is a chronic disease, still largely of unknown origin. It is primarily a joint disease involving inflamed synovial tissue and joint swelling. According to the American Rheumatoid Association (ARA), the main criteria of RA are:

1 Morning stiffness.
2 Tenderness and pain on motion.
3 History or observation of joint swelling.

4 Subcutaneous nodules.

5 Some positive laboratory tests (increased erythrocyte sedimentation rate and C-reactive protein and possibly a positive rheumatoid factor).

6 Some radiographic erosions and histological changes (inflammation) in affected joints (Ekblom, 1985).

RA usually has a gradual onset, with pain, swelling and stiffness of small peripheral joints. The disease begins most commonly between the ages of 25 and 60 years. There is female dominance of 3 : 1 (Lyngberg & Danneskiold-Samsoe, 1988). The progression of the disease is slow, with periods of exacerbation and remission. The inflammatory process involves the joints, leading to a gradual destruction of the joint surface, and finally to OA. It also affects the surrounding joint capsule and ligaments. Furthermore, tendons and skeletal muscles can become affected (inflammation), which is important to remember in exercise prescription of these patients. Since the disease is systemic, symptoms from the cardiovascular (pericarditis, arteritis), pulmonary (pleuritis, fibrosis), nervous (neuropathy, neuritis) and urogenital (nephropathy) systems are not uncommon.

All of these various changes affect the RA patient's ability to undertake physical exercise (Ekblom, 1985). For practical purposes, the patient's physical performance and functional capacity are often categorized as proposed by the ARA:

1 Complete ability to carry out all usual duties.
2 Adequate ability to carry out normal activities despite some handicap, discomfort, or limitation of motion.
3 Limited ability to carry out usual occupation or self-care.
4 Incapacitated largely and totally.

For years, physical training was considered contraindicated in RA patients, at least in the acute phase of the disease, to avoid any acute activation of the joint inflammation by training (Lyngberg & Danneskiold-Samsoe, 1988). Today, strenuous, weight-bearing activities are still largely banned in acute phase, but otherwise motion and isometric muscle exercises have been found beneficial, even in acute phase.

Concerning exercise and training during remissions, a revolutionary change towards activity occurred in the 1980s. A patient in functional class 1 may perform any type of physical exercise (Ekblom, 1985). Exceptions in some cases may include hard physical exercise (running, racquet sports), which put a hard eccentric stress on the lower extremities. Patients in class 2 and a few in class 3 can perform most types of physical exercise during low-activity phases of the disease, such as bicycling, walking, swimming and cross-country skiing. During high-activity phases, low-load exercises (low-resistance ergometer cycling) are recommended.

Although few patients in functional class 3 can perform walking, jogging or similar types of exercise, most of them can swim and exercise on a bicycle. By definition, most patients in class 4 are not able to carry out complicated movements. However, quite a few tolerate some physical activity, for example, while suspended in water, or exercising without preset levels of intensity or frequency (Ekblom, 1985).

From the mid-1970s on it has been known that RA patients are trainable and can gain significantly increased cardiovascular (14–25%) and muscular (23–73%) performance after only 5–6 weeks of systematic training (Ekblom et al., 1975). Also positive clinical, psychological and sociological effects were observed. Therefore, exercise and strength training is an essential part of modern therapy of rheumatoid patients. If the usual advice and rule (joint pain after the training should not last more than 2 h) about monitoring the intensity of the training is taken into consideration and followed, a gradually increasing exercise programme will not increase the frequency of exacerbations of the disease.

In the other types of rheumatoid diseases, the seronegative spondylarthropathies, such as ankylosing spondylarthritis, psoriarthritis, reactive arthritides and Reiter's disease, the treatment and rehabilitation instructions follow the above-mentioned guidelines of RA.

OSTEOCHONDROSES

Osteochondroses can be defined as idiopathic disturbance in enchondral ossification of the growth centres of the bone (Siffert, 1981; Orava & Virtanen, 1982). The disturbance is related to both chondrogenesis and osteogenesis. Osteochondroses are very frequent in childhood, especially in boys, of which every second or third physically active individual may have symptoms (Orava & Saarela, 1978).

The ultimate aetiology of the osteochondroses is still mostly unknown. It is not entirely known whether the increased physical activity causes the symptoms or merely provokes them (Orava & Virtanen, 1982; Kannus et al., 1988). However, it is well known that these pains are most common during the quickest phase of growth, when the growth areas of the bone are changing from cartilaginous structures to bone through the process of ossification. During that time, repetitive overstress may cause micro-fractures, secondary hyperaemia, disordered ossification and the associated symptoms (Kannus et al., 1988).

Osteochondroses, of which more than 50 types have been described, are divided into three classes according to the type of growth area they affect: (i) articular or epiphyseal; (ii) physeal; and (iii) apophysal (Siffert, 1981).

The most common articular osteochondroses are:

1 Legg−Calvé−Perthes disease at the proximal end of the femur.

2 Köhler's disease at the navicular bone of the foot.

3 Freiberg's disease at the distal end of the 2nd, 3rd and 4th metatarsals.

4 Buschke's disease at the first cuneiform bone and Kuntscher's disease at the second cuneiform bone.

5 Panner's disease at the distal end of the humerus.

6 Kienböck's disease at the lunate bone of the hand.

Occasionally, articular osteochondrosis may also affect the proximal part of the great toe. An interesting but serious group of articular osteochondroses is osteochondritis dissecans. It is a disorder of joint surfaces in which a segment of subchondral bone becomes avascular and, with the articular cartilage covering it, may separate from the surrounding bone forming a loose body. Its aetiopathogenesis remains uncertain. The most characteristic osteochondritis dissecans lesions occur in the femoral medial condyle of the knee, femoral head of the hip, talus, patella and olecranon (Fig. 12.8).

There are only two physeal osteochondroses, which have clinical significance: (i) Blount's disease at the medial part of the proximal physis of the tibia; and (ii) Scheuermann's disease at the thoracic (and occasionally at the lumbar) spine. The former is a rare condition, but often proceeds to a significant tibia vara requiring surgical treatment (Langenskiöld & Riska, 1964). The latter is much more common, but seldom needs treatment except regular clinical controls to identify the possible development of the thoracic kyphosis.

The apophyseal osteochondroses (apophysitides) are by far the most frequent osteochondroses. The most typical apophysitides are summarized in Table 12.1 (Fig. 12.9). An apophysis is a prominent site where a tendon unites with a bone, for example, the greater tuberosity of the humerus, the tibial tubercle and the epicondyles of the elbow (Clain & Hersman, 1989). In the growing child, cartilage is interposed between tendon and bone. Hence, forces applied by the muscle−tendon unit are transmitted to the bone through an area of cartilage, which is biomechanically much less resistant to tensile forces than bone or tendon. Repetitive overload can, therefore, lead to injury at the apophysis.

According to a prospective follow-up study from Finland (Kannus et al., 1988) Osgood−Schlatter disease (traction apophysitis of the tuberositas tibiae) was the most common

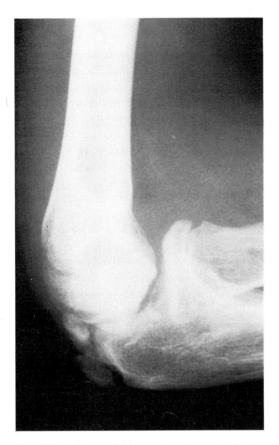

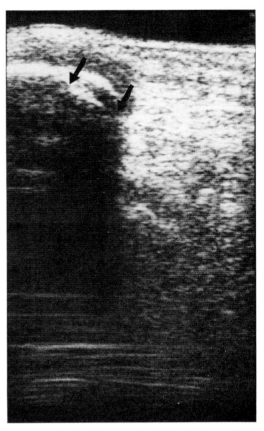

Fig. 12.8 A 13-year-old ice-hockey player who had had several months pain and extension deficit in his right elbow. The radiographs revealed a typical osteochondritis dissecans of the olecranon with two calcified fragments. The symptoms were relieved with rest and he was able to continue his career.

Fig. 12.9 An ultrasound picture from a Sinding–Larsen–Johansson disease process (traction apophysitis) at the lower pole of the patella in a 9-year-old female gymnast. The osteochondrotic focus is sclerotic and clearly separated from the surface of the patella.

athletic overuse injury in boys (18% of all injuries) and second most common in girls (13%). Sever's disease (calcaneal traction apophysitis) was the second most common osteochondrosis in both sexes (8% of all overuse injuries in boys, and 5% in girls) followed by osteochondritis dissecans of the knee and Scheuermann's disease.

In the USA, where baseball is one of the most popular sports, traction apophysis of the humeral medial epicondyle (Little League elbow) has been a great problem among young pitchers due to poor throwing biomechanics and excessive repetitive pitching (Clain & Hersman, 1989). In Finland, Finnish baseball (a modification of American baseball) produces the same types of problems. Growth disturbances, non-unions (Fig. 12.10), loose bodies, joint stiffness, flexion contracture and OA have been described as consequences of Little League elbow, and, therefore, today there is a restriction in the number of innings pitched by Little League players in one season.

In prevention of osteochondroses in children,

Table 12.1 The most common apophysitides.

Localization	Inserted tendon	Condition
Sesamoids of the great toe	Flexor hallucis longus	Wiedhoff−Greiffenstein disease
Base of the 5th metatarsal	Peroneus brevis	Iselin's disease
Navicular bone of the foot	Tibialis posterior	Os naviculare accessorius
Calcaneus	Achilles	Sever's disease
Tibial tubercle	Patella	Osgood−Schlatter disease
Lower pole of the patella	Patella	Sinding−Larsen−Johansson disease
Upper pole of the patella	Quadriceps	Mau's disease
Tuber os ischii	Hamstrings	Van Neck's disease
Symphysis	Femoral adductors	Pierson's disease
Anterior superior iliac spine	Quadriceps and sartorius	Kamm's disease
Trochanter major of the femur	Gluteal muscles and tensor fascia latae	Mandl's disease
Medial epicondyle of the humerus	Finger and wrist flexors	Little League elbow

it is of great importance that the training frequencies and intensities are supervised by parents, teachers, coaches, physicians and other medical staff. We may never break the 'slow progression principle' in training and exercise of a growing athlete. It is well known that at least 50% of all overuse injuries are caused by training errors (James *et al.*, 1978). The majority of these errors are, in turn, due to breaking this slow progression principle. This especially concerns children and adolescents (Renström, 1988).

The treatment of osteochondroses is usually very simple. All that is needed is a temporary cessation of the offending activity. Foot orthoses, anti-inflammatory medications or corticosteroid injections are seldom needed. If not properly treated in acute phase, a young athlete may suffer from serious consequences when adult. For example, children with Osgood−Schlatter disease have an increased risk in adulthood for patella alta and patellofemoral subluxation or chondromalacia problems during physical activity (Lorentzon, 1988). Therefore, supervision, protective rules, information, and education are of utmost importance in all children's sports.

AGE-RELATED MUSCULOTENDINEAL DEGENERATION

With aging, various functions of a living body gradually deteriorate. This also includes the musculoskeletal system, though not so extensively as cardiovascular functions. Regarding musculoskeletal problems, Lane *et al.* (1987) showed in a controlled study that musculoskeletal disability appeared to develop with

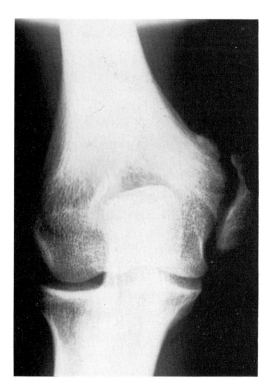

Fig. 12.10 A 16-year-old Finnish baseball player had Little Leaque elbow symptoms during several seasons when younger. Now the radiographs of his right elbow show that the medial epicondyle of the humerus is not united with the humeral bone. The patient is, however, almost asymptomatic and is able to play and pitch in the team.

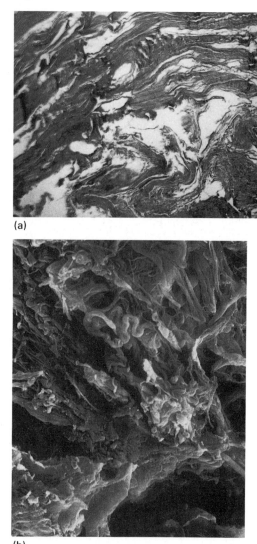

(a)

(b)

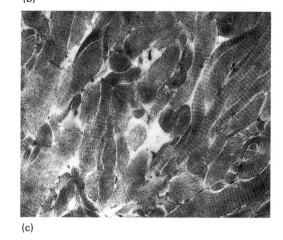

Fig. 12.11 (*Right*) Hypoxic–degenerative tendinopathy as a reason for a spontaneous Achilles tendon rupture in a 39-year-old male. (a) Fragmentation and destruction of collagen structure (van Gieson staining, ×70). (b) Disintegrated collagen fibres (scanning electron microscopy, ×1750). (c) Disintegration of collagen fibres. They vary in diameter and are often split longitudinally (van Gieson staining, ×5600).

(c)

age at a lower rate in long-distance runners aged 50–72 years than in non-running community control subjects. Runners had less physical disability, maintained more functional capacity, and had fewer physician visits per year. However, 40% had suffered from a running-related injury over the preceding year, and one-third of their physician visits were attributable to this.

The sports injury profile of elderly athletes varies from that of their younger colleagues. Kannus *et al.* (1989) showed in a 3-year prospective, controlled study that in elderly athletes the sports injuries are more frequently overuse-related than acute, and that they more commonly have a degenerative basis (OA or ligamentous or musculotendineal degeneration). For example, all shoulder problems in elderly subjects could be classified as degenerative musculotendineal diseases, while in the young controls shoulder problems were non-degenerative. The three complete Achilles tendon ruptures seen in the elderly athletes most likely had a degenerative basis (Fig. 12.11), since such injuries are extremely rare in young athletes. In a study of the veteran élite athletes competing in the World Master Championships, it was found that the most common injuries were muscle and tendon strains in the lower leg (Peterson & Renström, 1980).

Thus, musculotendineal degeneration with age is a real risk factor for sports injuries of the same (chronic inflammations, acute strains and ruptures). Prevention of sports injuries in older athletes should be concentrated on these areas. Maintenance of flexibility and neuromuscular coordination through daily stretching and calisthenics is recommended. Long warm-up and cooling-down periods should be the rule. The slow progression principle is especially suitable for elderly people. Participation in sports with smooth aerobic movements, such as walking, swimming, bicycling and rowing is encouraged.

General diseases and disorders

In injury prevention, we should always take into account that a subject may have a predisposing general disease or disorder, which may make him or her prone to sports injury. For example, a diabetic patient in a long-distance running competition needs special care, since a patient with low blood sugar levels may lose concentration and coordination capacity and hurt himself or herself. The same concerns athletes with a neurological or visual disorder. A ski-jumper or rally-driver with epilepsy needs special attention during training and competition. Poorly corrected myopia may impair the visual capacity of an athlete considerably, especially in dark or rainy conditions, making a subject prone to hitting obstacles or opponents, or losing his or her balance and falling.

Beginners are at a higher risk of an injury in many sports due to lack of specific coordination and skills necessary for successful participation. Inferior general intelligence, poor proprioception and long reaction times to a single visual stimulus have been associated with injury proneness (Taimela *et al.*, 1990). Also, many psychological (extraversion, state/trait anxiety) and psychosocial (accumulation of life stress) factors have been related to an increased risk for injuries, but in general the results have been equivocal (Lysens *et al.*, 1984).

Conclusion

Research has shown that body composition and predisposing diseases are real risk factors for sports injuries. These predisposing factors form a very complex network, and very often an injury is a result of the multidimensional interaction of these factors.

In the future, more work is needed to identify all the extrinsic and intrinsic risk factors of sports injuries. Also, the relative importance of each individual factor needs to be determined. Since many of the predisposing factors act simultaneously, a more integrated view may be needed in the future research of injury prevention.

References

Acheson, R.M. & Collant, A.B. (1975) New Haven survey of joint diseases. *Ann. Rheum. Dis.* **34**, 379–84.

Altman, R., Asch, E. & Bloch, D. (1986) Development of criteria for the classification of and reporting of osteoarthritis. *Arthr. Rheum.* **29**, 1039–49.

Bailey, D.A. & McCulloch, R.G. (1990) Bone tissue and physical activity. *Can. J. Sports Sci.* **15**, 229–39.

Beighton, P.H. & Horan, F.T. (1970) Dominant inheritance in familiar generalized articular hypermobility. *J Bone Joint Surg.* **52A**, 145–7.

Blyth, C.S. & Mueller, F.O. (1974) Football injury survey: Part I. When and where players get hurt. *Phys. Sportsmed.* **2**, 45–52.

Bray, G.A. (1985) Complications of obesity. *Ann. Int. Med.* **103**, 1052–62.

Clain, M.R. & Hersman, E.B. (1989) Overuse injuries in children and adolescents. *Phys. Sportsmed.* **17**, 111–23.

Carter, C. & Wilkinson, J. (1964) Persistent joint laxity and congenital dislocation of the hip. *J. Bone Joint Surg.* **46A**, 40–5.

Christiansen, C., Rodbro, P. & Thoger-Nielsen, C. (1975) Bone mineral content and estimated total body calcium in normal children and adolescents. *Scand. J. Clin. Lab. Invest.* **35**, 507–10.

Cooke, T.D.V. & Dwosh, I.L. (1986) Clinical features of the osteoarthritis in the elderly. *Clin. Rheum. Dis.* **12**, 155–72.

Dalsky, G.P. (1987) Exercise: Its effect on bone mineral content. *Clin. Obstet. Gynaecol.* **30**, 820–32.

Davis, M.A., Neuhaus, J.M., Ettinger, W.H. & Mueller, W.H. (1990) Body fat distribution and osteoarthritis. *Am. J. Epidemiol.* **132**, 701–7.

Ekblom, B.T. (1985) Exercise and rheumatoid arthritis. In R.P. Welsh & R.J. Shephard, (eds) *Current Therapy in Sports Medicine*, pp. 108–9. B.C. Decker Inc., Toronto.

Ekblom, B.T., Lövgren, O., Alderin, M., Fridström, M. & Sätterström, G. (1975) Effects of short-term physical training on patients with rheumatoid arthritis. A six month follow-up study. *Scand. J. Rheumatol.* **4**, 87–91.

Felson, D.T., Anderson, I.I., Naimark, A., Walker, A.M. & Meenan, R.F. (1988) Obesity and knee osteoarthritis. The Framingham study. *Ann. Int. Med.* **109**, 18–24.

Gärdsell, P., Johnell, O. & Nilsson, B.E. (1990) Bone loss in women — a longitudinal study of 15 years. *Acta Orthop. Scand.* **61**(Suppl. 237), 71.

Garrick, J.G. (1989) Anterior knee pain (chondromalacia patellae). *Phys. Sportsmed.* **17**, 75–84.

Grahame, R. (1990) The hypermobility syndrome. *Ann. Rheum. Dis.* **49**, 199–200.

Hartz, A.J., Fischer, M.E., Bril, G., Kelber, S., Rupley, D., Oken, B. & Rinn, A.F. (1986) The association of obesity with joint pain and osteoarthritis in the HANES data. *J. Chron. Dis.* **39**, 311–19.

Heinrich, C.H., Going S.B., Pamenter, R.W., Perry, C.D., Boyden, T.W. & Lohman, T.G. (1990) Bone mineral content of cyclically menstruating female resistance and endurance trained athletes. *Med. Sci. Sports Exerc.* **22**, 558–63.

Heliövaara, M. (1987) Body height, obesity and risk of herniated lumbar intervertebral disc. *Spine* **12**, 469–72.

Hinz, G. & Pohl, W. (1977) Die Bedeutung des Korpergewichtes bei degenerativen Skeletterkrankungen. (Importance of bodyweight in degenerative musculoskeletal diseases.) *Zeitschr. Orthop.* **115**, 12–18.

Jackson, D.W., Jarrett, H., Bailey, D., Kausek, J., Swanson, J. & Powell, J. (1978) Injury prediction in the young athlete: A preliminary report. *Am. J. Sports Med.* **6**, 6–14.

James, S.L., Bates, B.T. & Osternig, L.R. (1978) Injuries to runners. *Am. J. Sports Med.* **6**, 40–50.

Johnston, C.C. & Slemenda, C. (1987) Osteoporosis: an overview. *Phys. Sportsmed.* **15**, 65–8.

Kannus, P. & Järvinen, M. (1989) Posttraumatic anterior cruciate ligament insufficiency as a cause of osteoarthritis in a knee joint. *Clin. Rheumatol.* **8**, 251–60.

Kannus, P., Niittymäki, S. & Järvinen, M. (1988) Athletic overuse injuries in children. A 30-month prospective follow-up study at an outpatient sports clinic. *Clin. Pediatr.* **27**, 333–7.

Kannus, P., Niittymäki, S., Järvinen, M. & Lehto, M. (1989) Sports injuries in elderly athletes: A three-year prospective, controlled study. *Age Aging* **18**, 263–70.

Kellgren, J.H. & Lawrence, J.S. (1957) Radiological assessment of osteoarthritis. *Ann. Rheum. Dis.* **16**, 494–501.

Kujala, U.M., Kvist, M., Österman, K., Friberg, O. & Aalto, T. (1986) Factors predisposing army conscripts to knee exertion injuries incurred in a physical training program. *Clin. Orthop. Rel. Res.* **210**, 203–12.

Lane, N.E., Bloch, D.A., Wood, P.D. & Fries, J.F. (1987) Aging, long-distance running, and the development of musculoskeletal disability: A controlled study. *Am. J. Med.* **82**, 772–80.

Langenskiöld, A. & Riska, E. (1964) Tibia vara (ostechondrosis deformans tibiae). *J Bone Joint Surg* **46**, 1405–20.

Lawrence, J.S. (1975) Hypertension in relation to musculoskeletal disorders. *Ann. Rheum. Dis.* **34**, 451–6.

Leach, R.E., Baumgard, S. & Broom, J. (1973) Obesity: Its relationship to osteoarthritis of the knee. *Clin. Orthop. Rel. Res.* **93**, 271–3.

Lorentzon, R. (1988) Causes of injuries: Intrinsic factors. In A. Dirix, H.G. Knuttgen & K. Tittel (eds) *The Olympic Book of Sports Medicine*, pp. 376–90. Blackwell Scientific Publications, Oxford.

Lynberg, K. & Danneskiold-Samsoe, B. (1988) Exercise training in rheumatoid arthritis. *Scand. J. Sports Sci.* **10**, 83–7.

Lysens, R., Steverlynck, A., Auweele, Y. van den, Lefevre, J., Renson, L., Claessens, A. & Ostyn, M. (1984) The predictability of sports injuries. *Sports Med.* **1**, 6–10.

McAlindon, T. & Dieppe, P. (1989) Osteoarthritis: Definitions and criteria. *Ann. Rheum. Dis.* **48**, 531–2.

McGoey, B.V., Deitel, M., Saplys, R.J.F. & Kliman, M.E. (1990) Effect of weight loss on musculoskeletal pain in the morbidly obese. *J. Bone Joint Surg.* **72B**, 322–3.

Mazess, R.B. (1982) On ageing bone loss. *Clin. Orthop. Rel. Res.* **165**, 239–51.

Mazess, R.B. & Whedon, G.D. (1983) Immobilization and bone. *Calc. Tiss. Int.* **35**, 265–7.

Nachemson, A. (1966) The load on lumbar discs in different positions of the body. *Clin. Orthop. Rel. Res.* **45**, 107–22.

Nicholas, J.A. (1970) Injuries to the knee ligaments. Relationship of looseness and tightness in football players. *JAMA* **212**, 2236–9.

Nicholas, J.A. (1974) If we understand sports injuries we can prevent them. *Mod. Med.* **42**, 48–54.

Orava, S. & Saarela, J. (1978) Exertion injuries to young athletes. *Am. J. Sports Med.* **6**, 68–74.

Orava, S. & Virtanen, K. (1982) Osteochondrosis in athletes. *Br. J. Sports Med.* **16**, 161–8.

Pacy, P.J., Webster, J. & Garrow, J.S. (1986) Exercise and obesity. *Sports Med.* **3**, 89–113.

Peck, W.A. (1984) Osteoporosis consensus conference. *JAMA* **252**, 799–802.

Peterson, L. & Renström, P. (1980) Championships for veterans — A medical challenge (in Swedish). *Läkartidningen* **77**, 3618.

Peyron, J.G. (1989) Epidemiological aspects of osteo-arthritis. *Scand. J. Rheumatol.* **77**, 29–33.

Prior, J.C. (1990) Progesterone as a bone-trophic hormone. *Endoc. Rev.* **1**, 386–98.

Prior, J.C., Vigna, Y.M., Schechter, M.T. & Burgess, A.E. (1990) Spinal bone loss and ovulatory disturbances. *New Engl. J. Med.* **323**, 1221–7.

Renström, P. (1988) Diagnosis and management of overuse injuries. In A. Dirix, H.G. Knuttgen & K. Tittel (eds) *The Olympic Book of Sports Medicine*, Vol. I, pp. 446–8. Blackwell Scientific Publications, Oxford.

Riggs, B.L. & Melton, L.J. (1986) Involutional osteoporosis. *New Engl. J. Med.* **314**, 1676–86.

Runow, A. (1983) The dislocating patella. Etiology and prognosis in relation to generalized joint laxity and anatomy of the patellar articulation. *Acta Orthop. Scand.* **201**, 1–53.

Schoutens, A., Laurent, E. & Poortmans, J.R. (1989) Effects of inactivity and exercise on bone. *Sports Med.* **7**, 71–81.

Siffert, R.S. (1981) Classification of the osteochon-droses. *Clin. Orthop. Rel. Res.* **158**, 10–18.

Silberberg, R. (1979) Obesity and osteoarthrosis. In: R. Mancini, A. Lewis & L. Contaldo (eds) *Medical Complications of Obesity*, pp. 301–15. Academic Press, London.

Sinaki, M. (1989) Exercise and osteoporosis. *Arch. Phys. Med. Rehab.* **70**, 220–9.

Smith, E.L. & Gilligan, C. (1987) Effects of inactivity and exercise on bone. *Phys. Sports Med.* **15**, 91–100.

Steiner, M.E. (1987) Hypermobility and knee injuries. *Phys. Sportsmed.* **15**, 159–65.

Taimela, S., Kujala, U.M. & Österman, K. (1990) Intrinsic risk factors and athletic injuries. *Sports Med.* **9**, 205–15.

Virvidakis, K., Georgiou, E., Korkotsidis, A., Ntalles K. & Proukakis, C. (1990) Bone mineral content of junior competitive weightlifters. *Int. J. Sports Med.* **11**, 244–6.

Watson, A.W.S. (1981) Factors predisposing to sports injury in school boy Rugby players. *J. Sports Med. Phys. Fitness* **21**, 417–22.

Wright, D. (1979) Prevention of injuries in sport. *Physiotherapy* **55**, 114–19.

Zylstra, S., Hopkins, A., Erk, M., Hreshchyshyn, M. M. & Anbar, M. (1989) Effect of physical activity on lumbar spine and femoral neck bone densities. *Int. J. Sports Med.* **10**, 181–6.

Chapter 13

The Growing Athlete

JOHN F. MEYERS

Significant differences exist between the child and the adult athlete, and those interested in injury prevention must understand these differences. Open epiphyses and soft articular cartilage are vulnerable to injury in the growing athlete. Macrotrauma to the musculoskeletal system, which might cause ligament tears in the adult, more often cause epiphyseal damage and potential growth deformity in the child. Microtrauma or overuse training injuries can cause traction apophysitis — an injury only occurring in children.

One of the most important tools available for injury prevention is the preparticipation history and physical. This examination allows the physician to determine maturation stage and to detect physical abnormalities and muscle imbalances which would predispose the child to injury. It also allows the physician to counsel the young athlete toward an appropriate and safe sport. A safe environment is important in injury prevention. Children should compete against athletes of their own maturation stage and strength level. Protective equipment should be appropriate and fit properly. Good field and court conditions should be assured for safe competition.

Physical differences in the child and adult athlete

Cardiovascular

Children and adults differ little in their ability to perform aerobic exercise. $V_{O_{2max}}$ and anaerobic thresholds are similar in both groups. Children do expend more energy during endurance activities (Daniels et al., 1978).

Children do not perform as well anaerobically as adults. This is probably related to the child's inability to utilize glycogen as well as the adult (Bar-Or, 1983).

Children do not tolerate heat during exercise as well as adults. They produce less sweat and do not acclimatize as readily to heat as do adults (Wagner et al., 1972). Youth coaches should be educated in the signs of heat illness and heat stroke and look for them in hot and humid weather.

Endurance training has been advocated in the paediatric athlete (Ratliff, 1990). Response to training in the prepubescent athlete is similar to that in the adult. While training does not substantially improve $\dot{V}_{O_{2max}}$ in children, performance can definitely be enhanced. More studies are needed to determine why this performance improves. Endurance training seems to have its greatest effect when changes in height are greatest (Robayashi et al., 1978). Most endurance training programmes for children were modified from programmes developed through adult research. Authorities believe that paediatric programmes should be more conservative than the adult programme and that they should be fun in order to keep the athlete interested. Stress should be increased gradually so that the body will adapt to this stress and overuse injuries will not occur.

178

The skeletal system

The immature skeleton is especially vulnerable to fracture (Fig. 13.1) through the epiphyseal plate or physis, which separates the end of the bone, the epiphysis, from the metaphysis. The physis is less resistant to torsional and shear forces than the surrounding bone. Fracture through the physis usually occurs through the zone of cartilage hypertrophy. Fractures can traverse the physes, or extend back into the metaphysis or out into the epiphysis. Fractures crossing the epiphysis have a potential for growth disturbances, as do crushing injuries to the physis. If the fracture extends into the epiphysis, it often requires open reduction for anatomical restoration of the joint surface. Fractures extending into the epiphysis or crushing injuries to the physis require close long-term follow-up to check for growth disturbances.

Because children's bones are more pliable than adults, different types of fractures occur in children (Fig. 13.2). Children's bones can undergo plastic deformation or bending rather than actual breaking as a response to injury. This bending of the bone often goes unrecognized and can result in long-term deformity if not properly treated. Torus fractures can occur which involve the buckling of the metaphyseal cortex caused by a longitudinally applied force. The cortex remains intact and reduction is generally not required. These fractures should be protected for 2–3 weeks to prevent further damage to the bone. Green-stick fractures can occur in which only one cortex is broken. These tend to spring back to their prereduction deformity, and often the opposite cortex must be broken to maintain a reduction. Fractures in

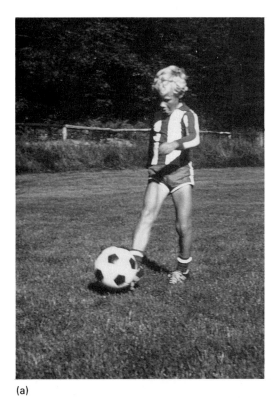

(a)

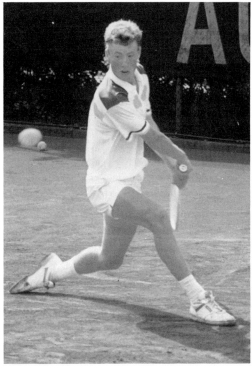

(b)

Fig. 13.1 Children (a) and adolescents (b) are active in sports. They have different tissue strength relations compared to adults, and therefore have different injury patterns. Courtesy of Dr P.A.F.H. Renström.

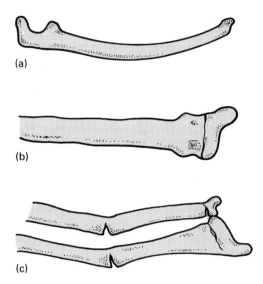

(a)

(b)

(c)

Fig. 13.2 Illustrations of (a) plastic deformation of the ulna, (b) a torus fracture of the radius, and (c) a greenstick fracture of the forearm. These fractures are unique to children.

children also differ from fractures in adults because of their potential to remodel. Growing bone has the potential to straighten deformities, especially near the ends of bone and in the plane of flexion and extension. Many fractures which would need open reduction in adults can be treated closed in children, accepting some deformity because of this remodelling potential.

Tibone (1983) has defined the differences between injuries to the shoulder girdle in children and those in adults. The joint capsule and ligaments in a child are approximately two to five times as strong as the physis. An injury to the sternoclavicular joint that would cause a dislocation in an adult, causes a fracture through the physis in a child. The epiphysis is not yet ossified, and remains in contact with the sternum. Because of the potential for remodelling, this injury can be treated closed and remodelling will occur with no residual deformity. Injuries to the distal clavicle in childhood also cause epiphyseal fractures rather than acromioclavicular dislocations. Again, these

can be treated closed because of the remodelling potential of children's bone.

The distal radius, the distal humerus and distal femur are especially susceptible to fracture in children because the collateral ligaments attach to the epiphysis rather than the metaphysis. Because the ligaments are stronger than the adjacent epiphyseal plate, fractures occur in children rather than ligament sprains which would occur in adults. It is often necessary to obtain X-rays while stressing across the joint to make this diagnosis in the child.

The muscular system

Controversy exists over the efficacy and safety of strength training in the prepubescent athlete. In 1988, the American Orthopedic Society for Sports Medicine held a conference intended to answer questions about muscular training in the child (Cahill, 1988). Participants included sports medicine physicians, athletic trainers, exercise physiologists and educators. Their findings were based on a review of the current literature and experience of the participants.

The conference came to the following conclusions on certain questions assessing the benefits of strength training in the prepubescent.

1 *Does strength training increase muscle strength?* The panel felt that while most of the existent scientific literature stated that strength training was ineffective, three recent studies indicated that strength gains are possible in the prepubescent child.

2 *Does strength training improve flexibility?* The panel felt that there was no evidence that strength training decreases flexibility or causes one to become muscle bound. They felt that a strength training programme which incorporated a full range of movement and simultaneous stretching exercises could increase flexibility.

3 *Can strength training increase motor performance?* The participants agreed, based on the literature and coaching experience, that strength training can increase muscle performance. Literature supports that strength training can increase vertical jump ability, but does not increase speed.

4 *Can strength training protect against injury?* The panel agreed that strength training does increase strength and range of motion, thereby helping to protect against injury. Strength training and conditioning in high-school football players has been shown to decrease dramatically the number of knee injuries in that sport (Cahill & Griffith, 1978).

5 *Does strength training increase muscle endurance?* The panel felt that there was a strong interrelationship between muscle strength and endurance. They felt there was a carry-over between anaerobic and aerobic conditioning.

The conference also addressed questions regarding the risks of strength training.

1 *Does strength training have the potential to cause injury to bone growth tissue?* The panel found no evidence to substantiate growth plate injuries caused from strength training. Acute injuries, however, are possible because of accidents and training errors.

2 *Does strength training have the potential to cause acute and chronic joint injury?* The participants thought that this question was unanswered. No good studies exist to show that strength training can cause damage to joints, but they agreed there was a potential for such damage, and proper supervision would greatly decrease that potential.

3 *Does strength training have the potential to cause acute and chronic musculoskeletal injuries?* The panel felt that there was a potential for acute and chronic musculoskeletal injuries, but that these were dose related, and a proper programme could prevent such injuries.

In summary, the conference decided that strength training could be beneficial and safe for young athletes. They pointed out that any programme should be carefully monitored and supervised by someone with expertise in strength training. Competitive weightlifting and maximum lifts should be avoided in the prepubescent athlete. Companies should be encouraged to develop progressive resistive machines for use in the smaller child.

Injuries unique to the child athlete

Traction apophysitis

The apophysis is the site of growth cartilage where the musculotendinous unit attaches to bone. The apophysis may be injured by direct trauma, forceful muscle contraction which leads to an avulsion, or microtrauma leading to irritation of the apophysis. Compounding the vulnerability of these sites is that during growth spurts bone grows faster than tendons and ligaments. This leads to decreased flexibility and increased stresses on the apophysis (Micheli *et al.*, 1986). Prevention of these injuries is directed toward decreasing the stress of overuse, maintaining flexibility about the joints, and using protected padding when indicated.

The most common traction apophysitis is Osgood–Schlatter disease (Osgood, 1903), which is an injury of the tibial tubercle. This growth apophysis is injured by partial avulsion from repetitive traction of the patellar ligament on the tibial tubercle. Healing occurs with excess bone formation and leads to an increase in the size of the tibial tubercle. A free bony fragment often develops in the distal patellar ligament (Ogden & Southwick, 1976). Osgood–Schlatter disease usually occurs in 13–14 year old males and 10–11 year old females. Complaints are of aching pain in the tibial tubercle aggravated by an increase in activity and by direct trauma to the tubercle. Treatment consists of stretching the often tight quadriceps muscle, icing the tibial tubercle, and nonsteroidal anti-inflammatories, such as aspirin. Relative rest is prescribed during symptomatic periods. Foam knee pads help decrease direct trauma to the tubercle. The athlete and the parents should be reassured that this is a self-limited disease and will become quiescent after the growth centre closes.

Sinding–Larsen–Johansson syndrome (Medler & Lyne, 1978) is analogous to Osgood–Schlatter disease, but occurs at the origin of the patellar ligament on the distal patella. The treatment and preventive measures for this disease are the same as for Osgood–Schlatter disease.

Sever's disease (Sever, 1912) is an injury to the apophysis of the os calcis. Symptoms consist of posterior heel pain usually associated with a growth spurt or increased sports activities. Physical findings include tenderness over the posterior aspect of the calcaneus and a tight heel cord. Biomechanical abnormalities of the foot are often associated with Sever's disease (Micheli, 1987). Treatment consists of stretching the tight gastrocnemius–soleus complex, heel cups and heel lifts. Orthotics may be prescribed if biomechanical abnormalities of the foot are present.

Traction apophysitis is also seen about the pelvis. The apophyses of the anterosuperior iliac spine, the antero-inferior iliac spine, and the hamstring insertion on the ischium are the common sites of involvement. Actual avulsions can occur during forceful jumping and sprinting. As in the other apophysites, treatment consists of stretching, ice and relative rest. Even with frank avulsions, surgery is not indicated. The avulsion is treated by protective weight-bearing with crutches, stretching and strengthening. Return to sports can be expected in approximately 6 weeks.

Apophysitis of the medial epicondyle of the elbow occurs in throwing athletes. Valgus forces generated across the elbow during the acceleration phase of pitching cause distraction on the medial side of the elbow. The injury to the apophysis varies with the age of the athlete. In the child, traction results in hypertrophy of the medial epicondyle, tears of the flexor pronator muscle group, and fragmentation of the epicondyle. In the stronger adolescent, actual avulsion fractures of the epicondyle occur. If these fractures are displaced, they should be treated surgically. Prevention of these elbow injuries consists of teaching proper throwing techniques (Albright et al., 1978; Pappas, 1982) and limited exposure to throwing (Torg et al., 1972).

Osteochondrosis dissecans

Osteochondrosis dissecans in young athletes occurs most frequently in the knee, ankle and elbow. Most investigators now feel that it is caused by trauma. This entity represents an articular fracture or an interruption to the blood supply of a portion of the epiphysis. A separate fragment of bone develops with a margin of fibrous tissue between the fragment and the rest of the epiphysis. Treated properly, many of these injuries will heal. Failure of treatment can result in a separation of the fragment and resultant intra-articular loose bodies.

Osteochondrosis dissecans of the knee occurs most often on the lateral aspect of the medial femoral condyle, but can also occur centrally on the lateral femoral condyle and on the patella or trochlear groove (Mubarak & Carroll, 1981). The common age of onset is 11–14 years of age. Conservative treatment of a non-displaced fragment in a child with open physes is usually successful (Hughston et al., 1984). Casting or non-weight-bearing with crutches is prescribed until healing is evident on X-ray. Treatment in cases of partial separation or in patients with closed physes is surgical. Drilling of the fragment, pinning, screw fixation and bone grafting can often be accomplished arthroscopically. With complete detachment of the fragment, the loose bodies should be removed from the joint. Even with large articular defects, these patients do surprisingly well (Ewing & Voto, 1988).

Osteochondrosis dissecans of the elbow occurs most often in the throwing athlete and the gymnast. As with medial epicondylitis, the valgus force across the elbow appears to be the cause (Meyers, 1990). This valgus force creates distraction of the medial elbow and compression of the lateral elbow with bony injury to the capitellum and radial head. Osteochondrosis dissecans occurs in the 13–17 year age group. It should not be confused with Panner's disease (Panner, 1927), which occurs before 11 years of age and is a benign self-limiting process characterized by fragmentation of the entire ossific centre of the capitellum. This heals with conservative treatment and loose bodies are not formed. With osteochondrosis dissecans, avascular necrosis of the anterolateral capitellum occurs. This is often complicated by breakdown of bone and loose body formation. If conservative treatment fails, good results have been reported with excision of the loose fragments and curettage of the base (McManama *et al.*, 1985). As with medial epicondylitis, prevention requires emphasis of proper throwing technique and limited exposure to throwing.

Osteochondrosis dissecans of the ankle is an osteochondral fracture of the talus, resulting from an inversion injury to the ankle. This entity should be suspected in ankle sprains which remain symptomatic after proper treatment. Undisplaced or incomplete lesions can be treated conservatively (Berndt & Harty, 1959). With persistent symptoms or displacement of the fragment, good results can be obtained by arthroscopic removal of the fragments and drilling of the base (Baker *et al.*, 1986). Lateral lesions of the talus have a poorer prognosis and usually require surgery.

The preparticipation physical examination

The preparticipation physical examination offers the physician the greatest opportunity for injury prevention. It allows identification of predisposing conditions which may render the young athlete more susceptible to injury. These conditions include diseases, muscular imbalance, weakness, lack of flexibility and delayed maturation. The preparticipation physical allows the physician to guide the athlete in correcting these deficiencies and in choosing a safe sport for his or her participation. The examination should be performed well prior to the onset of the season to allow time for strengthening and increase in flexibility, if indicated. This examination is also important because it is often the young athlete's introduction into the sports medicine system.

In the past, many of these examinations have been perfunctory and performed mainly to satisfy legal requirements. While examinations may find only 1–3% of athletes suffering from conditions which exclude them from sports (McKeag, 1985), many non-excluding conditions, if corrected, can help prevent future injury. As we learn more about the relationships of strength, flexibility and conditioning to injury, the importance of a thorough preparticipation physical examination increases.

The Virginia High School League has adopted a new expanded preparticipation evaluation following a 2-year pilot programme (Perriello *et al.*, 1989) (Fig. 13.3). For efficiency, the authors recommend a seven-point examination method.

1 Check in/check out.
2 Height/weight/urinalysis/blood.
3 Vision/hearing.
4 Blood pressure/pulse.
5 Head, ears, eyes, nose and throat/heart/lungs/maturation/body fat.
6 Orthopaedic examination.
7 Review of history and findings with the athlete.
Points 5, 6 and 7 require physicians. All other points can be covered by coaches, trainers and nurses. We have successfully used this system and can examine 30–35 athletes per hour using four physicians.

The history portion was designed to indicate specific high-risk factors. It is completed by the athlete and his or her parents prior to the examination. The physician can scan this form during the physical examination to identify specific systems requiring more careful examination. The history form is then reviewed with the athlete during the final counselling with a physician at point 7.

The Tanner maturation stage (Table 13.1) is

Fig. 13.3 (*Over page*) (a) Pre-participation evaluation history. (b) Pre-participation evaluation physical examination. Adapted with permission from the Virginia High School League.

Pre-participation evaluation
Part IV – History

(To be completed and signed by parent/guardian and examining physician)

Name_____ Date_____

Sex_____ Age_____Grade_____

This form should be completed by parent and athlete prior to time of physical examination and should be taken with physical examination form for review by the physician during the examination.

	Yes	No
1 Have you ever had any of the following?		
heart murmur	_____	_____
high blood pressure	_____	_____
other heart problems	_____	_____
broken bones	_____	_____
weak joints – ankles, knees	_____	_____
concussion	_____	_____
operation	_____	_____
seizures or epilepsy	_____	_____
2 Have you ever fainted or passed out?	_____	_____
3 Have you ever been knocked out?	_____	_____
4 Have you ever been hospitalized?	_____	_____
5 Have you ever had to stop running 1/4 to 1/2 mile for chest pain, or shortness of breath?	_____	_____
6 Have you had significant allergies?		
hay fever	_____	_____
asthma	_____	_____
bee stings	_____	_____
poison ivy	_____	_____
foods	_____	_____
medicine	_____	_____
7 Do you take any medicine regularly?	_____	_____
8 Have you had any illnesses lasting a week or more such as mononucleosis, etc.?	_____	_____
9 Have you had any blood disorders, including sickle cell trait, anemia, etc.?	_____	_____
10 Has any family member had a heart attack or other heart problems before age 50?	_____	_____
11 DATE OF LAST TETANUS IMMUNIZATION	_____	_____

Please explain any yes answers from above

_____
_____
_____
_____

Signature of parent or guardian_____ Date_____
I have reviewed this information with the student and/or his parents.

Signature of examining physician_____, MD* Date_____
*Doctor of Medicine or Doctor of Osteopathy

(a)

Pre-participation evaluation

Part V – Physical examination

(To be completed and signed by examining physician)

Name _____ School _____

Height _____ Weight _____ Sex _____ Age _____ Grade _____

Tanner stage or maturation index_____ BP_____

Percent body fat_____ Pulse (rest)_____

(Exercise)_____

(Recovery)_____

Vision _____ Orthopaedic:_____
Audiogram_____ Cervical spine/neck_____
Eyes_____ Back _____
Ears_____ Shoulders_____
Nose_____ Arm/elbow/wrist_____
Throat_____ Knees_____
Teeth_____ Ankles _____
Skin _____ Menstrual history_____
Heart _____ Urine_____
Lungs _____ Haemoglobin_____
Abdomen_____ and/or iron stores_____
Genitalia _____
Peripheral pulses _____

- -

I have examined the person herein described, reviewed his/her medical history form and make the following recommendations for his/her participation in athletics.

1 Full participation_____

2 No participation_____

   Reason _____

3 Requires additional evaluation_____

4 Comments _____

_____

_____

_____

Physician signature _____ , MD   Date _____

Physician name (print)_____

Address _____

_____

City/zip code _____

Telephone_____

(b)

Table 13.1 Maturity staging guidelines. From Tanner (1962).
(a) Boys.

Stage	Pubic hair	Penis	Testis
1	None	Preadolescent	—
2	Slight, long, slight pigmentation	Slight enlargement	Enlarged scrotum, pink slight ruga
3	Darker, starts to curl, small amount	Longer	Larger
4	Coarse, curly, adult type, but less quantity	Increase in glans size and breadth of penis	Larger, scrotum darker
5	Adult, spread to inner thighs	Adult	Adult

(b) Girls.

Stage	Pubic hair	Breasts
1	Preadolescent (none)	Preadolescent (no germinal button)
2	Sparse, lightly pigmented, straight medial border of labia	Breast and papilla elevated as small mound; areolar diameter increased
3	Darker, beginning to curl, increased	Breast and areola enlarged; no contour separation
4	Coarse, curly, abundant, but less than adult	Areola and papilla form secondary mound
5	Adult female triangle and spread to medial surface	Mature, nipple projects, areola part of general breast contour

included for several reasons. A study in New York State (Hafner *et al.*, 1982) suggested lower injury rates when the athletes in contact and collision sports were matched by maturity level rather than chronological age. The incidence of epiphyseal injuries peaks during periods of most rapid growth (Larson, 1973) (Tanner stages 3 and 4 for females, and stages 2 and 3 for males). Consideration should be given to avoiding collision sports and intense training during these stages. Finally, maturation staging can help predict eventual height, and guide children into the appropriate sport; for example, a female with a height potential of 1.8 m (5 ft 11 in) would be better suited to volleyball or basketball than gymnastics. Support for the psychological value of matching athletes by maturity level (Caine & Vrockhoff, 1987) is based on their probability of success and enjoyment in competing with others of similar athletic potential.

Percent body fat can be measured quickly and economically using skinfold fat calipers (Jackson & Pollock, 1985). Body fat greater than 20% in boys and 25% in girls is reason for concern (Perriello *et al.*, 1989). It is also helpful in counselling athletes in weight-specific sports, such as wrestling.

The exercise pulse test is performed by taking a resting pulse, performing 2 min of jumping jacks, then measuring the pulse immediately after and again after 1 min of recovery. A rise greater than 95 beat·min^{-1} or a drop after 1 min of recovery of less than two-thirds of the rise raises concern about the fitness of the subject (Perriello *et al.*, 1989).

The musculoskeletal examination includes observation for deformity, strength and flexibility testing, and in-depth examination of joints mentioned in the history. Strength testing is generally performed by manual muscle testing, but this is an imprecise measurement at best. Strength and flexibility screening can be done prior to the musculoskeletal examination by a coach or trainer. Strength can be assessed by sit-ups, pull-ups, push-ups and vertical leap. Initial studies (Kibler et al., 1989) using isokinetic testing and dynamometers have led to sport-specific examinations and recommendations. These studies, while worthwhile, are probably too expensive and time consuming for general application. Simple tests for flexibility include the Apley scratch test for shoulder flexibility, sit and reach test for lower extremity and back flexibility, straight leg raising for hamstring flexibility testing, and the stair heel drop for Achilles flexibility (Rooks & Micheli, 1988). Deficits picked up during this screening examination should be further investigated by the physician.

Point 7 in the list allows the physician time to explain the findings of the evaluation to the young athlete. Negative findings can preclude an athlete from certain sports. The American Academy of Pediatrics has guidelines to help determine fitness for participation (Table 13.2). These are only guidelines, and the physician must determine what is best and safest for an individual athlete. Specific recommendations to correct deficiencies found in the physical examination can be made at this time, and forwarded to coaches and parents. Approval for non-contact sports may be given if maturation level or physical condition indicates that contact or collision sports would be dangerous to the athlete.

This comprehensive examination is given every other year. A screening interval evaluation (Fig. 13.4) is used between these examinations. Positive findings will trigger the more comprehensive evaluation.

Epidemiology

Epidemiological studies are important in injury prevention because they can identify injuries which occur with specific sports at various ages, and can tell us if injury prevention measures, such as taping, bracing and stretching, actually work. Epidemiological studies are more difficult to perform in youth sports than in interscholastic sports because volunteer coaches and administrators have less time to devote to, and generally are not well trained in, injury detection and treatment. Also, athletic trainers are not generally available to youth sports programmes. Tabulation of injuries is usually based on insurance claims, doctors visits, and time lost from practice and competition. These methods identify major injuries, but overuse injuries and 'minor injuries' which may have long-term significance are often missed.

Two epidemiological studies are particularly relevant to paediatric sports medicine. Goldberg et al. (1984) studied injuries in youth football, and Sullivan et al. (1980) studied injuries in youth soccer. Both studies showed that the injury rate increases with age (Fig. 13.5). Many of these injuries are caused by collisions. The force of collisions increases as the mass and the velocity of the players increase with age. These studies should reassure parents that youth sports are safe for their child. There is no data which shows that ordinary youth sports is any more dangerous than free play (Godshall, 1975). Another soccer study by Backous et al. (1988) confirmed increasing injury rates with age, and also showed that taller, weak male athletes were more often injured.

Good epidemiological studies are needed to assess the efficacy of injury-prevention measures, such as warm-up, stretching, strengthening programmes, protective equipment and the value of a comprehensive physical examination.

Environment and equipment

The sports environment

A safe sports environment is a major factor in injury prevention. Playing fields should be even and well maintained with no obstacles such as posts and benches near the sidelines of fields and the edges of courts. Fields, balls, bats and other sports equipment should be sized down to fit the young athlete. Breakaway bases should

Table 13.2 Disqualifying conditions for sports participation. From American Medical Association (1979).

Conditions	Collision*	Contact†	Non-contact‡	Other§
General				
Acute infections				
respiratory, genitourinary, infectious mononucleosis, hepatitis, active rheumatic fever, active tuberculosis	X	X	X	X
Obvious physical immaturity in comparison with other competitors	X	X		
Haemorrhagic disease				
haemophilia, purpura, and other serious bleeding tendencies	X	X	X	
Diabetes, inadequately controlled	X	X	X	
Diabetes, controlled	‖	‖	‖	‖
Jaundice	X	X	X	X
Eyes				
Absence or loss of function of one eye	X	X		
Respiratory				
Tuberculosis (active or symptomatic)	X	X	X	X
Severe pulmonary insufficiency	X	X	X	X
Cardiovascular				
Mitral stenosis, aortic stenosis, aortic insufficiency, coarctation of aorta, cyanotic heart disease, recent carditis of any aetiology	X	X	X	X
Hypertension on organic basis	X	X	X	X
Previous heart surgery for congenital or acquired heart disease	¶	¶	¶	¶
Liver				
Enlarged	X	X		
Skin				
Boils, impetigo, and herpes simplex gladiatorum	X	X		
Spleen				
Enlarged	X	X		
Hernia				
Inguinal or femoral hernia	X	X	X	
Musculoskeletal				
Symptomatic abnormalities or inflammations	X	X	X	X
Functional inadequacy of the musculoskeletal system, congenital or acquired, incompatible with the contact or skill demands of the sport	X	X	X	
Neurological				
History or symptoms of previous serious head trauma or repeated concussions	X			
Controlled convulsive disorder	**	**	**	**
Convulsive disorder not moderately well controlled by medication	X			
Previous surgery on head	X	X		

Table 13.2 *Continued*

Conditions	Collision*	Contact†	Non-contact‡	Other§
Renal				
Absence of one kidney	X	X		
Renal disease	X	X	X	X
Genitalia				
Absence of one testicle	††	††	††	††
Undescended testicle	††	††	††	††

* Football, Rugby, hockey, lacrosse, etc.
† Baseball, soccer, basketball, wrestling, etc.
‡ Cross-country, track, tennis, crew, swimming, etc.
§ Bowling, golf, archery, field events, etc.
‖ No exclusions.
¶ Each patient should be judged on an individual basis in conjunction with a cardiologist and surgeon.
** Each patient should be judged on an individual basis. It is probably better to encourage a young boy or girl to participate in a non-contact sport rather than a contact sport. However, if a patient has a desire to play a contact sport and this is deemed a major ameliorating factor in his or her adjustment to school associates, serious consideration should be given to letting him or her participate if the seizures are moderately well controlled or the patient is under good medical management.
†† The Committee approves the concept of contact sports participation for youths with only one testicle or with undescended testicle(s), except in specific instances such as inguinal canal undescended testicle(s), following appropriate medical evaluation. Athletes, parents and school authorities should be fully informed that participation in contact sports for youths with only one testicle carries a slight injury risk to the remaining healthy testicle. Fertility may be adversely affected following injury, but the chance of injury to descended testicle(s) are rare, and injury risk can be substantially minimized with an athletic supporter and protective device.

be used in baseball to prevent ankle injuries (Hale, 1979). Gymnastics equipment must be strong and secure and frequently inspected. Mats in wrestling should be disinfected to prevent skin infections. Ill-fitting shoes are the cause of blisters and foot and ankle injuries. Shoes should not be purchased for the athlete to grow into. The athlete should use shoes designed for the sport in which he or she is participating.

Protective equipment

Well-maintained, properly fitted protective equipment should be available for appropriate contact and collision sports. Helmets should be used to prevent head injury in football, ice hockey, lacrosse, field hockey, baseball, batting and bicycle riding. While helmets have decreased serious head injuries in football, neck injuries have increased because of improper tackling techniques (Torg *et al.*, 1979). It is incumbent on coaches to prohibit dangerous tackling and blocking techniques in which the head is used to transmit force (spearing). Mouth and facial injuries can be decreased by using mouth guards and face masks. Mouth guards must be comfortable and fit well, or the players will not wear them. They should be used for football, ice hockey, field hockey, lacrosse and Rugby, and possibly for baseball, basketball, wrestling and soccer. Athletic cups should be used for appropriate sports.

The greatest controversy exists over the use of knee braces in football. The so-called prophylactic knee brace consists of a laterally applied

Pre-participation evaluation
Interim evaluation

This form is to be used if the comprehensive physical form has been completed within the pre-ceeding 24 months and no significant change in health status has occurred. It should be carefully filled out by student and parent.

Name_____ Date_____

Sex _____Age_____ Grade_____

Height _____Weight_____ BP _____

Date of last completed check up on record in school file_____

Recommendation at last comprehensive physical:_____

	Yes	No
Since the above physical evaluation have you experienced any of the following:		
high blood pressure	_____	_____
broken bones	_____	_____
concussion	_____	_____
fainted or passed out	_____	_____
severe sprain or strain of joint	_____	_____
significant illness like mono	_____	_____
severe allergic reaction	_____	_____
other illness or accident resulting in missing 3 or more days of school or practice	_____	_____
problems with eating or sleeping	_____	_____

Explain any 'yes' answers:_____
_____
_____
_____
_____
_____

This is an accurate representation of my child's interval history to the best of my knowledge.

Signature_____ Date _____
        (parent or guardian)

Reviewed by:

Coach _____ AD _____Physician _____

Recommendation:

Full participation_____ Limited participation in_____

No participation in_____ Need full physical_____

Need other additional evaluation _____

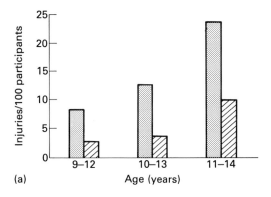

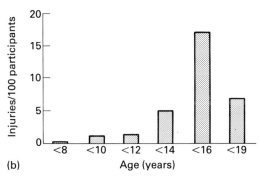

Fig. 13.5 Injury rates in (a) youth football and (b) youth soccer, showing a parallel increase with age. Adapted from the *Pediatric Athlete* with permission from the American Academy of Orthopaedic Surgeons. ▨, all injuries; ▨ significant injuries.

hinged support designed to protect the knee from medial collateral ligament injury. Citing studies by France *et al.* (1987), Teitz *et al.* (1987), Grace *et al.* (1988), and the American Academy of Pediatrics (Committee on Sports Medicine, 1990) recommend that lateral unidirectional knee braces not be considered standard equipment for football players because of lack of efficacy and the potential of actually causing harm.

Fig. 13.4 (*Opposite*) Pre-participation interim evaluation. Adapted with permission from the Virginia High School League.

Coaching

Coaches have the responsibility to teach safe techniques and prohibit dangerous play from their players. Coaching clinics must emphasize these factors to their volunteer youth coaches. Coaches should also be knowledgeable of injury prevention and first aid techniques. Little League Baseball Inc. has taken the lead in this area. They have developed a programme for the prevention and emergency management of Little League baseball and softball injuries (Little League Baseball Inc., 1989). This programme consists of text, videotape and a test which is administered by volunteers of the American Orthopedic Society of Sports Medicine. The programme is available throughout the USA to all Little League coaches prior to every season. This programme may serve as a model for other youth sports programmes.

Finally, the coach should make the sport fun for the players. Most children who quit sports cite the lack of fun as a reason. The beneficial aspects of sports and exercise throughout a lifetime can be lost if the initial athletic experience is a discouraging one.

Conclusion

Physicians can play a significant role in injury prevention in paediatric athletes. One must understand the difference in the physiology of the child and the adult, and the potential for different types of injuries in children. Training, both in strength and endurance, is possible in the young athlete, and is safe if properly supervised. Training appears to play a role in injury prevention. The preparticipation physical examination should be thorough and identify correctable risk factors, such as weakness, inflexibility, poor physical conditioning and maturation level. When these factors are identified, the physician can offer guidance in correcting them, and direct the athletes into a sport which is safe for them.

Playing conditions, protective equipment and proper coaching are all important in injury prevention. The sports medicine physician should take an active role in supervising and correcting deficiencies in these areas.

Youth sports are generally safe and beneficial when the above criteria are met. The physician should be an advocate of early sport participation as an enjoyable first experience that can lead to a long-term commitment to sports and exercise.

References

Albright, J.A., Jokl, P., Shaw, R. et al. (1978) Clinical study of baseball pitchers: Correlation of injury to the throwing arm with method of delivery. Am. J. Sports Med. 6, 15–21.

American Medical Association (1979) Medical Evaluation of the Athlete: A Guide. Pamphlet No. OP 209, Sports. AMA, Chicago.

Backous, D.D., Friedl, K.E., Smith, N.J., Parr, T.J. & Carpine Jr, W.D. (1988) Soccer injuries and their relation to physical maturity. Am. J. Dis. Child. 142, 839–42.

Baker, C.L., Andrew, J.R. & Ryan, J.B. (1986) Arthroscopic treatment of transchondral talar dome fractures. J. Arthrosc. Rel. Surg. 2(2), 82–7.

Bar-Or, O. (1983) Pediatric Sports Medicine for the Practitioner: From Physiologic Principles to Clinical Applications. Springer-Verlag, New York.

Berndt, A.L. & Harty, M. (1959) Transchondral fractures (osteochondritis dissecans) of the talus. J. Bone Joint Surg. 41(A), 988–1020.

Cahill, B.R. (ed) (1988) Proceedings of the Conference on Strength Training and the Prepubescent. American Orthopedic Society for Sports Medicine, Chicago.

Cahill, B.R. & Griffith, E.H. (1978) Effect of preseason conditioning on the incidence and severity of high school football knee injuries. Am. J. Sports Med. 6(4), 180–4.

Caine, D.J. & Vrockhoff, J. (1987) Maturity assessment: A viable preventive measure against physical and psychological insult to the young athlete? Phys. Sportsmed. 15, 67–80.

Committee on Sports Medicine, American Academy of Pediatrics (1990) Knee brace use by athletes. Pediatrics 85(2), 228.

Daniels, J., Oldridge, N., Nagle, F. et al. (1978) Differences and changes in $\dot{V}O_2$ among young runners 10 to 18 years of age. Med. Sci. Sports 10, 200–3.

Ewing, J.W. & Voto, S.J. (1988) Arthroscopic surgical management of osteochondritis dissecans of the knee. J. Arthrosc. Rel. Surg. 4(1), 37–40.

France, E.P., Paulos, L.E., Jayaraman, G. & Rosenberg, T.D. (1987) Biomechanics of lateral knee bracing, II:

Impact response of the braced knee. Am. J. Sports Med. 15, 430–8.

Godshall, R.W. (1975) Junior league football: Risks versus benefits. Am. J. Sports Med. 3, 139–44.

Goldberg, B., Rosenthal, P.P. & Nicholas, J.A. (1984) Injuries in youth football. Phys. Sportsmed. 12, 122–32.

Grace, T.G., Skipper, B.J., Newberry, J.C. et al. (1988) Prophylactic knee braces and injury to the lower extremity. J. Bone Joint Surg. 70(A), 422–7.

Hafner, J.K., Scott, S.E., Veras, O. et al. (1982) Interscholastic athletes: Method for selection and classification of athletes. N. Y. J. Med. 82, 1449–59.

Hale, C.J. (1979) Protective equipment for baseball. Phys. Sportsmed. 7, 59–63.

Hughston, J.C., Hergenroeder, P.T. & Courtenay, B.G. (1984) Osteochondritis dissecans of the femoral condyles. J. Bone Joint Surg. 66(A), 1340–8.

Jackson, A.S. & Pollock, M.L. (1985) Practical assessment of body composition. Phys. Sportsmed. 13, 76–90.

Kibler, W.B., Chandler, T.J., Uhl, T. & Maddux, R.E. (1989) A musculoskeletal approach to the preparticipation physical examination: Preventing injury and improving performance. Am. J. Sports Med. 17(4), 525–31.

Larson, R.L. (1973) Epiphyseal injuries in the adolescent athlete. Orthop. Clin. N. Am. 4, 839–51.

Little League Baseball Incorporated (1989) Prevention and Emergency Management of Little League Baseball and Softball Injuries. Little League Baseball Inc., Williamsport, Pennsylvania.

McKeag, D.B. (1985) Preseason physical examination for the prevention of sports injuries. Sports Med. 2, 413–31.

McManama Jr, G.B., Micheli, L.J., Berry, M.V. et al. (1985) The surgical treatment of osteochondritis of the capitellum. Am. J. Sports Med. 13, 11–21.

Medler, R.C. & Lyne, E.D. (1978) Sinding–Larsen–Johansson disease: Its etiology and natural history. J. Bone Joint Surg. 60(A), 1113–16.

Meyers, J.F. (1990) Injuries to the shoulder girdle and elbow. In J.A. Sullivan & W.A. Grana (eds) The Pediatric Athlete, pp. 145–53. American Academy of Orthopaedic Surgeons, Illinois.

Micheli, L.J. (1987) The traction apophysitises. Clin. Sport Med. 6(2), 399–404.

Micheli, L.J., Stater, J.A., Woods, E. & Gerbino, P. (1986) Patella alta and the adolescent growth spurt. Clin. Orthop. 213, 159–62.

Mubarak, S.J. & Carroll, N.C. (1981) Juvenile osteochondritis dissecans of the knee: Etiology. Clin. Orthop. 157, 200–11.

Ogden, J.A. & Southwick, W.O. (1976) Osgood–Schlatter's disease and tibial tubercle development. Clin. Orthop. Rel. Res. 116, 180–9.

Osgood, R.B. (1903) Lesions of the tibial tubercle occurring during adolescence. *Boston Med. J.* **148**, 114–17.

Panner, H.J. (1927) An affection of the capitellum humeri resembling Calve–Perthes' disease of the hip. *Acta Radiol.* **8**, 617–18.

Pappas, A.M. (1982) Elbow problems associated with baseball during childhood and adolescence. *Clin. Orthop.* **164**, 30–41.

Perriello Jr, V.A., Benjamin, J.T., Dickens, M.D., Ford, R.F., Gleason, C.H., Hawkes, D.L., Machen, C.W. *et al.* (1989) New medical standards for Virginia's high school athletes. *Virginia Med.* **116**(9), 359–67.

Ratliff, R.A. (1990) Endurance training of the pediatric athlete. In J.A. Sullivan & W.A. Grana (eds) *The Pediatric Athlete*, pp. 7–15. American Academy of Orthopaedic Surgeons, Illinois.

Robayashi, K., Kitamura, K., Miura, M. *et al.* (1978) Aerobic power as related to body growth and training in Japanese boys: A longitudinal study. *J. Appl. Phys.* **44**, 666–72.

Rooks, D.S. & Micheli, L.J. (1988) Musculoskeletal assessment and training: The young athlete. *Clin. Sports Med.* **7**(3), 641–77.

Sever, J.W. (1912) Apophysitis of the os calcis. *N. Y. Med. J.* **95**, 1025–9.

Sullivan, J.A., Gross, R.H., Grana, W.A. *et al.* (1980) Evaluation of injuries in youth soccer. *Am. J. Sports Med.* **8**, 325–7.

Tanner, J.M. (1962) *Growth at Adolescence*, 2nd edn, pp. 28–39. Blackwell Scientific Publications, Oxford.

Teitz, C.C., Hermanson, B.K., Kronmal, R.A. *et al.* (1987) Evaluation of the use of braces to prevent injury to the knee in collegiate football players. *J. Bone Joint Surg.* **69**(A), 2–9.

Tibone, J.E. (1983) Shoulder problems of adolescents. *Clin. Sports Med.* **2**, 423–6.

Torg, J.S., Pollack, H. & Sweterlisch, P. (1972) The effect of competitive pitching on the shoulders and elbows of preadolescent baseball players. *Pediatrics* **49**, 267–72.

Torg, J.S., Truex Jr, R., Quedenfeld, T.C. *et al.* (1979) The national football head and neck injury registry: Report and conclusions. *JAMA* **241**, 1477–9.

Wagner, J.A., Robinson, S, Tzankoff, S.P. *et al.* (1972) Heat tolerance and acclimatization to work in the heat in relation to age. *J. Appl. Physiol.* **33**, 616–22.

Chapter 14

The Female Athlete

LETHA Y. GRIFFIN

The number of women in Canada and the USA who are involved in both recreational and competitive athletics has grown significantly since the passage of Title IX of the Educational Amendments of 1972 (Burke, 1982). The latter prohibits discrimination on the basis of sex in any educational institution receiving federal funds. When women began entering the athletic arena in increasing numbers, it was felt by many involved in the prevention, evaluation and treatment of athletic injuries, that we would see a marked increase in injury rates over those traditionally seen in male athletes. Furthermore, it was felt that the types of injuries seen in females might differ significantly from those reported in male athletes in the same sports.

Initial evidence seemed to support the first of these suppositions, i.e. that we would see an increase in the number of injuries occurring (Kosek, 1973; Eisenberg & Allen, 1978). Not only did studies in the 1970s report an increase in the number of injuries, but also time lost from sport activity in female athletes when compared to their male counterparts (Protzman, 1979). This increase in injury rate and time lost from sport led many to propose that females were physiologically inferior on a genetic basis, and therefore, unable to handle the stress of competitive athletics.

Importance of conditioning in preventing injuries

Later injury studies like those reported by

Clarke and Buckley (1980), Whiteside (1980), and Garrick and Requa (1978) did, in fact, demonstrate that injuries were more sport-specific than sex-specific. When the early investigations on injury rates were reviewed, it was apparent that the increase in the number of injuries was probably related more to inadequate prevention, primarily the lack of adequate conditioning programmes, than to a true genetic predisposition to injury (Eisenberg & Allen, 1978; Lenz, 1979; Rose, 1981). As conditioning programmes became incorporated into women's sport programmes in the 1970s, injury rates decreased (Cox, 1979; Kowal, 1980).

Although at one time there was concern over the possibility of weight-training programmes resulting in the development of muscle-bound female athletes, it is now known that muscle mass potential is a genetically determined, androgenically controlled trait (Mayhew & Gross, 1974; Moulds et al., 1979). Weight-training only maximizes that genetic potential (Wilmore, 1974). Appropriate weight-training regimens should be incorporated into the conditioning programmes essential to all women's sport programmes (O'Shea & Wegner, 1981; Cinque, 1990). Conditioning helps to increase strength and flexibility and decrease the risk of injury (Stone, 1988).

Conditioning programmes should emphasize off-season aerobic conditioning, preseason strengthening and in-season sport-specific skill development. Although the conditioning programmes traditionally used for male athletes

194

can be adapted for use by female athletes, it is important to recognize the anatomical and physiological differences between the sexes that affect performance. The following few paragraphs will review some of these differences. As these differences are enumerated, one must realize that data presented is for the 'typical' male and female; however, the overlapping ranges of these parameters make the reality of such individual differences less definitive than they may seem initially. It should also be understood that these differences are presented not to define male and female sport dominions, but rather to encourage recognition of the inherent genetic strengths and weaknesses of each athlete, so that this knowledge can be used to maximize conditioning and performance.

Anatomically, women tend to have smaller bones and less articular surfaces (Klafs & Lyon, 1978). Females have shorter legs, reflecting 51.2% of their total height, as compared to 56% in males (Klafs & Lyon, 1978). In general, men have a heavier, larger, more rugged structure, which affords them a mechanical and structural advantage in athletic activities. This advantage is enhanced by the longer bones in males, which act as greater levers producing more force in sports requiring striking, hitting and kicking (Hoffman *et al.*, 1979).

Females have narrower shoulders, wider pelvises and a greater valgus angulation at the knees than males (Thomas, 1979; Hale, 1984) (Fig. 14.1). Some experts believe the increased incidence of overuse syndromes involving the hip and knee in women (especially in the unconditioned state) is directly related to the greater varus angle of the hips and the greater valgus angle of the knees (Haycock & Gillette, 1976; Powers, 1980). As a result of her wider pelvis and shorter lower extremities, the female has a lower centre of gravity, measured at only 56.1% of her height, as compared to 56.7% in the male (American Academy of Orthopaedic Surgeons, 1991). This lower centre of gravity gives the female a distinct advantage in balance sports such as gymnastics, where the male

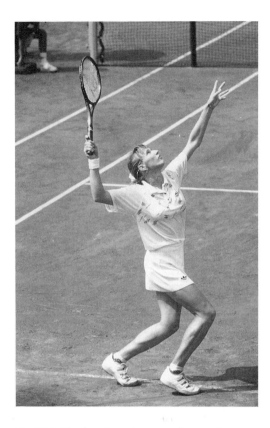

Fig. 14.1 The female anatomy predisposes to injuries different to those found in males. Courtesy of Dr P.A.F.H. Renström.

must widen his stance to obtain the same degree of balance. Hence, the balance beam, which is one of the four major events of women's gymnastic competition, is not even included in male gymnastic competition (Fig. 14.2).

For the same body weight, conditioned females have smaller heart sizes, lower diastolic and systolic blood pressures, and smaller lungs and thoracic cavities than equally trained male athletes (Thomas, 1979; Powers, 1980). These differences decrease female effectiveness in both anaerobic (burst) and aerobic (endurance) activities when compared to males. Training can and does enhance one's maximal oxygen consumption, and thus, one's aerobic capacity, but the baseline is genetically determined.

Maximal oxygen consumption (termed

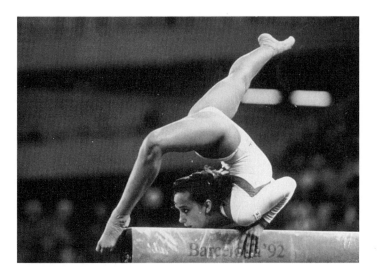

Fig. 14.2 The female anatomy allows women to carry out specific motions unsuited for males. Courtesy of the IOC archives.

$\dot{V}_{O_{2max}}$) reflects the body's ability to maximally extract oxygen from the environment and utilize it for aerobic metabolism. $\dot{V}_{O_{2max}}$ measures the lung's ability to extract oxygen, the heart's ability to deliver the oxygen to the muscle, and the muscle's ability to maximally assimilate oxygen in energy pathways (O'Toole & Douglas, 1988).

The smaller heart size, stroke volume, and lung and muscle mass of the female mean that she will have a lower baseline $\dot{V}_{O_{2max}}$ upon which to build her aerobic capacity when compared with a male of the same weight and conditioned state. Yet again, it is important to recognize the continuum for each gender when describing anatomical and physiological parameters. Indeed, some females on the upper spectrum of the $\dot{V}_{O_{2max}}$ capacity have a greater genetic baseline than some males on the lower end of the masculine profile.

The average college female is approximately 25% fat per body weight, whereas the average college male is about 15% fat per body weight (Higdon & Higdon, 1967). Studies analysing body fat in conditioned athletes have demonstrated great variability among athletes participating in different sports (Wilmore & Brown, 1974; Butts, 1982). If one looks at track athletes, the average conditioned female is about 10–15% fat, while the conditioned male is generally less than 7%. Female swimmers have

approximately 10% body fat, whereas male swimmers have approximately 8% body fat (Wells, 1985).

In addition to her greater percentage of body fat, the female has less muscle mass per body weight (23%) than an equally trained male (49%) of the same body weight (Klafs & Lyon, 1978); thus, it is more difficult for her to achieve the same power and speed. The female's increased percentage of body fat per body weight is still a disadvantage even if she is matched to a male of equal muscle mass, since the female must use the same muscle mass to 'energize' her extra body fat. If the male is made to perform in a weighted vest, the weight being equal to the excess body fat of the female, his $\dot{V}_{O_{2max}}$ is lowered to her range.

Fat does, however, insulate and give one buoyancy (Fahey, 1988), an advantage for women swimmers, especially in natural water. Fat may also provide energy support when glycogen is depleted, an advantage in endurance events such as marathons and ultramarathons (Ullyot, 1976).

It used to be thought that females were more prone to heat exhaustion than males, and that they needed higher core body temperatures before increasing their sudorific response (Dili et al., 1973). However, recent evidence has demonstrated that equally trained and conditioned males and females are similar in their thermal regulation (Nunnaley, 1978; Ferstle, 1982; Haymes, 1984).

Basal metabolic rate is lower in females (Roy & Irvin, 1983), and therefore, for the same amount of activity the female needs fewer calories. This fact is important to keep in mind when planning training tables and pregame meals for female athletes. One must plan a nutritionally balanced diet with fewer total calories than for the male athletes (Haymes, 1980). This fact, although it seems so obvious now, was overlooked when females first entered the military academies. The diet of the cadets was not altered for the women, and they gained weight eating the high-calorie foods provided for the male cadets to maintain their base body weight during this time of intense physical effort. The academies learned that they had to provide nutritional meals with fewer total calories — lean meats, fewer sauces, more fruits and vegetables — for their female cadets (Anderson, 1979).

Coordination and dexterity are difficult parameters to measure, but they do not appear to differ markedly between the sexes.

Injury-specific prevention programmes in women

Despite the establishment of what appears to be adequate off-season, in-season and pre-season conditioning programmes for women, there still seems to be an increased incidence of some injuries. Studying these injuries is important, as understanding their mechanism of occurrence may provide insights into preventing these injuries in the future.

Patella pain

Patella pain, or pain behind the kneecap, is a very common complaint in women athletes (Hunter, 1984). The onset of pain may develop from direct trauma to the patella or from the performance of repetitive knee flexion—extension activities. Decreasing the symptoms of the athlete with retropatellar pain is fre-

quently a difficult task for the physician and therapist.

Hamstring stretching and quadriceps strengthening exercises are the basis of any therapy programme (Percy & Strother, 1985). As in most acute inflammatory processes, icing following activity may be helpful. Physicians may also prescribe various braces, shoe orthotics or oral anti-inflammatory medications. Muscle-stimulating units to enhance the strength of the vastus medialis obliquus have also been used with some success.

If an athlete is identified in the preseason physical examination as having laterally tracking, laterally sitting patellas with some retropatellar irritability, prevention techniques emphasizing vastus medialis obliquus development should be instituted in the off-season and preseason conditioning periods.

Moreover, stair climbing, deep squats and full arc extension exercises, especially utilizing heavy weights, should be eliminated from the athlete's conditioning programme. In athletes with significant foot pronation which increases dynamic lateral patella tracking, consideration for arch supports can be given. Women prone to patella pain should be cautioned to avoid sitting with their knees acutely flexed and their feet tucked up under their buttocks (Hunter-Griffin, 1988).

Shoulder pain

Shoulder pain in female athletes, particularly in swimmers and softball players, is usually due to either subluxation or impingement. The athlete with shoulder subluxation complains of pain in the anterior region of her shoulder when her shoulder is placed in a position of external rotation, abduction and extension. In this position, she subluxes her humeral head against her anterior shoulder capsule, stretching the capsular tissue and causing pain. With impingement, because of a weak rotator cuff, the female athlete elevates the humerus superiorly in the glenoid with deltoid contraction, as seen with overhead motions such as throwing, tennis serves and the swim crawl. This motion causes pinching of the tissue (tendons and bursa) between the acromion and the upwardly migrated humeral head, resulting in inflammation and pain, hence the development of tendonitis and bursitis. The pain can be reproduced by applying a downward pressure on the acromion while elevating the humerus in a forward flexed manner.

Shoulder subluxation and shoulder impingement can occur together. The combination may result from inadequate stabilization of the humeral head in the glenoid secondary to weakness of the rotator cuff.

Preventive techniques for shoulder subluxation and shoulder impingement emphasize strengthening programmes for the rotator cuff and shoulder muscles while avoiding repetitive overhead activities. When instituting upper extremity strengthening programmes, it is important to first strengthen the rotator cuff muscles prior to beginning exercises emphasizing the power abductors, extenders and flexors of the shoulder, i.e. the deltoid, pectoralis and trapezius muscles. Rubber tubing exercises or exercises done prone or on one's side (Figs 14.3 & 14.4) are all adequate ways to strengthen the cuff muscles.

Low back pain

Low back pain in female athletes may be associated with a defect in the posterior elements of the spine known as spondylolysis. This defect occurs four times more often in female gym-

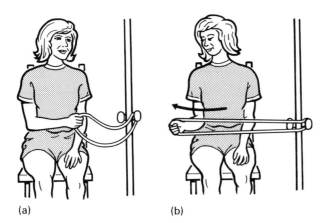

Fig. 14.3 Shoulder lateral rotation (resistive) exercise. (a) Sit next to a door with a circle of tubing hooked on the doorknob. Hold the tubing in the far hand with the elbow bent; then move the hand away from the body, keeping the elbow by the body (b). Hold for a predetermined number of counts and repeat a set number of times. From Schneider & Cecil (1989).

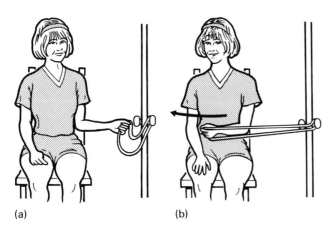

Fig. 14.4 Shoulder medial rotation (resistive) exercise. (a) Sit next to a door with a circle of tubing hooked on the doorknob. Hold the tubing in the near hand with the elbow bent; then move the hand to the stomach, keeping the elbow by the body (b). Hold for a predetermined number of counts and repeat a set lumber of times. From Schneider & Cecil (1989).

nasts than in the normal population (Jackson et al., 1976). Evaluation by the team physician is needed to determine whether this defect represents an acute stress fracture or a chronic injury in the athlete. If it represents an acute stress fracture, prolonged rest is recommended. In the case of chronic spondylolysis, rest during the acute phase with gradual return to activity is usually prescribed. Non-steroidal anti-inflammatories, muscle relaxants, ice massage and other physical therapy modalities may be helpful. Women participating in sports that require repetitive flexion–extension movements of the lumbar spine should be instructed in preseason abdominal and paravertebral muscle strengthening programmes, such as described in Figs 14.5 & 14.6.

Stress fractures

Stress fractures have been reported to occur in greater numbers in female athletes than in males (Protzman & Griffis, 1977). This increased

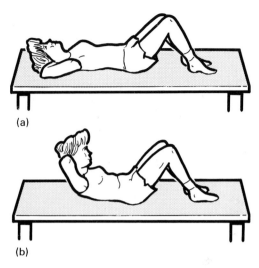

(a)

(b)

Fig. 14.6 Trunk flexion (partial sit up) exercise. (a) Lie on the back with the knees bent and feet flat. Put hands behind the neck and curl the head and chest (b). Raise the shoulder blades only. Do not bring the elbow together or pick feet up. Hold for a predetermined number of counts and repeat a set number of times. From Schneider & Cecil (1989).

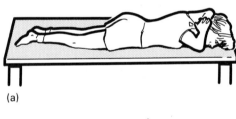

(a)

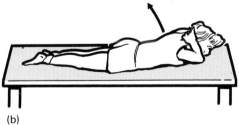

(b)

Fig. 14.5 Trunk extension (active) exercise. (a) Lie on the stomach with the hands clasped behind the lower neck. Tuck chin in and raise the chest off the mat (b). Hold for a predetermined number of counts and repeat a set number of times. From Schneider & Cecil (1989).

frequency may represent a lack of proper conditioning and training techniques rather than a genetic predisposition to injury. Stress fractures occur when the rate of normal bone breakdown from activity is greater than the rate of bone formation (repair). If an athlete has not conditioned slowly and sensibly for her sport, she will not have given her bone time to increase in cortical thickness to meet the mechanical demands of the sport.

Bunions, hammer toes and metatarsalgia

Perhaps because of shoe styles, foot problems seem to be more common in females than in male athletes (Potera, 1986). Bunions occur more frequently in feet that have a varus 1st metatarsal. This leads to a valgus phalanx from the pull of the flexor tendon and resultant medial flare of the 1st metatarsal head (Fig. 14.7). If the athlete is not careful with the fit of her shoewear, her shoe will rub the flare of the 1st metatarsal head, causing inflammation and

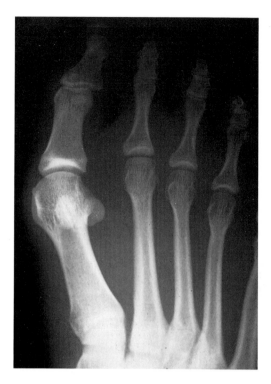

Fig. 14.7 Hallux valgus deformity (big toe).

swelling of the bursa overlying the bone with resultant pain.

The best treatment for foot problems is prevention. Bunions can be prevented by buying shoes that are wide enough and hammer toes can be prevented by buying shoes that are long enough.

If despite proper shoewear, inflammation occurs in the bursa overlying the flare of the 1st metatarsal head medially, pads and orthotics can be used to try to alter stresses to this area and allow healing.

Preventing common medical problems

Iron-deficiency anaemia

Iron is the metal contained in the haemoglobin molecule of the red blood cells and is necessary for oxygen transport. A normal iron level is especially important in athletes, where maximal oxygen carrying capacity is needed for maximal energy output (Haymes, 1973; Pate, 1983). Iron may also act as a catalyst in removing the lactate that is formed during aerobic exercise. This role of iron has not yet been clearly defined, but it is known that women who are iron deficient and yet not anaemic have increased lactate levels with submaximal exercise when compared to women with normal levels (Nilson, 1983).

Iron supplementation in the menstruating athletic female is advised if her diet does not contain 18 mg of iron, the recommended daily allowance (Pate *et al.*, 1979). Foods high in iron include liver, oysters, beef, turkey, dried apricots and prune juice.

Multivitamins plus iron generally have approximately 12 mg of iron, and may be used as a dietary iron supplement. If increased amounts of iron are needed to replenish deficient iron stores in the anaemic athlete, ferrous sulphate (in amounts providing 200–400 mg of elemental iron each day) is recommended. Ferrous sulphate should not be given in excess, as it can be toxic.

Vaginitis

Some women are more prone to recurrent vaginitis than others. Vaginitis may be caused by yeast and may be precipitated by a change in the normal vaginal flora by the use of oral antibiotics or by the sexually transmitted diseases such as trichomonas, chlamydia and herpes. Athletes prone to develop yeast vaginitis may be candidates for prophylactic treatment with vaginal suppositories if they are put on broad-spectrum antibiotics for treatment of other infections. Douching while taking oral antibiotics may also be helpful.

Urinary tract infections

Urinary tract infections are more common in women than in men. In women prone to urinary tract infections, attention should be given to adequate hydration. Fluid intake should be regularly encouraged, especially during travel when normal intake habits may be altered.

Psychological considerations in preventing injury

Sports medicine professionals must be attuned to the psychological needs, as well as the physiological needs of the female athlete. Injury is frequently precipitated by lack of confidence. Moreover, recurrent subjective complaints in an athlete with no real objective findings may indicate a psychologically troubled athlete, perhaps one who has grown tired of her sport and wishes a sanctioned pathway to retirement. It is sometimes easier for the athlete to state that she is medically unable to play rather than to admit to parents, friends and coach that she is no longer interested in competing.

In addition, the athletic female may become depressed because she feels she is not living up to the image expected of her as a female in society. Independence, fortitude, aggressiveness, achievement and the desire to win have traditionally been thought of as masculine qualities, and yet these characteristics are important in the development of the successful athletic competitor. Society's attitudes are slowly evolving, but many people still think of these traits as gender-specific. Because the teenage years are critical years for sexual identity, many talented women athletes are unable to resolve these conflicting issues, and they may choose instead to drop out of sport programmes during this time.

Conclusion

Over the last several decades, as we have seen increasing numbers of women participating in sports, we have seen a greater emphasis placed on the prevention of injuries by the use of proper equipment, as well as by the institution of adequate conditioning programmes. Continued attention to these areas, as well as to other methods of injury prevention will allow female athletes to participate more safely and effectively in sport activities.

References

American Academy of Orthopaedic Surgeons (1991) The female athlete. In American Academy of Orthopaedic Surgeons (eds) *Athletic Training and Sports Medicine*, 2nd edn, pp. 921–32. American Academy of Orthopaedic Surgeons, Park Ridge, Illinois.

Anderson, J. (1979) Women's sports and fitness programs of the US Military Academy. *Phys. Sportsmed.* 7(4), 72–8.

Burke, P. (1982) The effect of current sports legislation on women in Canada and the USA. — Title IX. In R. Howell (ed) *Her Story in Sport: A Historical Anthology of Women in Sports*, pp. 330–42. Leisure Press, West Point, New York.

Butts, N. (1982) Physiological profile of high school female cross country runners. *Phys. Sportsmed.* 10(11), 103–11.

Cinque, C. (1990) Women's strength training. Lifting the limits of aging. *Phys. Sportsmed.* 18(8), 123–7.

Clarke, K. & Buckley, W. (1980) Women's injuries in collegiate sports. *Am. J. Sports Med.* 8(3), 187–91.

Cox, J. (1979) Women in sports: The Naval Academy experience. *Am. J. Sports Med.* 7(6), 355–7.

Dill, D., Yousef, M. & Nelson, J. (1973) Responses of men and women to two-hour walks in desert heat. *J. Appl. Psychol.* 35, 231–5.

Eisenberg, I. & Allen, W. (1978) Injuries in a women's varsity athletic program. *Phys. Sportsmed.* 6(3), 112–16.

Fahey, T. (1988) Endurance training. In M. Shangold & G. Mirkin (eds) *Women and Exercise: Physiology and Sports Medicine*, pp. 65–78. FA Davis Co., Philadelphia.

Ferstle, J. (1982) Christine Wells: Asking the right questions. *Phys. Sportsmed.* 10(7), 157–60.

Garrick, J. & Requa, R. (1978) Girls' sports injuries in high school athletics. *JAMA* 239, 2245–8.

Hale, R. (1984) Factors important to women engaged in vigorous physical activity. In R. Strauss (ed) *Sports Medicine*, pp. 250–69. WB Saunders, Philadelphia.

Haycock, C. & Gillette, J. (1976) Susceptibility of women athletes to injury. Myths vs. reality. *JAMA* 236(2), 163–5.

Haymes, E. (1973) Iron deficiency and the active woman. In *American Alliance for Health, Physical Education and Recreation Research Report*, Vol. 2, pp. 91–7. American Alliance for Health, Physical Education and Recreation, Reston, Virginia.

Haymes, E. (1980) Iron supplementation. In G. Stull (ed) *Encyclopedia of Physical Education, Fitness, and Sports*, Vol. 2, pp. 335–44. Brighton, Salt Lake City.

Haymes, E. (1984) Physiological response of female athletes to heat stress: A review. *Phys. Sportsmed.* **12**(3), 45–59.

Higdon, R. & Higdon, H. (1967) What sports for girls? *Today's Health*, **10**, 21.

Hoffman, T., Stauffer, R. & Jackson, A. (1979) Sex differences in strength. *Am. J. Sports Med.* **7**(4), 265–7.

Hunter, L. (1984) Women's athletics: The orthopaedic surgeon's viewpoint. *Clin. Sports Med.* **3**(4), 809–27.

Hunter-Griffin, L. (1988) Orthopaedic concerns. In M. Shangold & G. Mirkin (eds) *Women and Exercise: Physiology and Sports Medicine*, pp. 195–219. FA Davis Co., Philadelphia.

Jackson, D., Wiltse, L. & Cirincrone, R. (1976) Spondylolysis in the female gymnast. *Clin. Orthop. Rel. Res.* **117**, 68–73.

Klafs, C. & Lyon, J. (1978) *The Female Athlete*, 2nd edn, pp. 15–23. CV Mosby, St Louis.

Kosek, S. (1973) Nature and incidence of traumatic injury to women in sports. In *Proceedings, National Sports Safety Congress*, pp. 50–2. Cincinnati.

Kowal, D. (1980) Nature and causes of injuries in women resulting from an endurance training program. *Am. J. Sports Med.* **8**(4), 265–9.

Lenz, H. (1979) Women's sports and fitness programs at the US Naval Academy. *Phys. Sportsmed.* **7**(4), 42–50.

Mayhew, J. & Gross, P. (1974) Body composition changes in young women with high resistance weight training. *Res. Q.* **45**(4), 433–40.

Moulds, B., Carter, D., Coleman, J. *et al.* (1979) Physical responses of a women's basketball team to a pre-season conditioning program. In J. Terands (ed) *Science in Sports*. Academic Publishers, Delmar.

Nilson, K. & Schoene, R. (1983) Iron repletion decreases maximal exercise lactate concentration in female athletes with minimal iron deficiency anemia. *J. Lab. Clin. Med.* **102**, 306–12.

Nunnaley, S. (1978) Physiological response of female athletes to thermal stress: A review. *Med. Sci. Sports* **10**(4), 250–5.

O'Shea, J. & Wegner, J. (1981) Power weight training and the female athlete. *Phys. Sportsmed.* **9**(6), 109–20.

O'Toole, M. & Douglas, P. (1988) Fitness: Definition and development. In M. Shangold & G. Mirkin (eds) *Women and Exercise: Physiology and Sports Medicine*, pp. 3–22. FA Davis Co., Philadelphia.

Pate, R. (1983) Sports anemia: A review of the current research literature. *Phys. Sportsmed.* **11**(2), 115–26.

Pate, R., Maguire, M. & Wyk, J. (1979) Dietary iron supplementation in women athletes. *Phys. Sportsmed.* **7**(9), 81–6.

Percy, E. & Strother, R. (1985) Patellalgia. *Phys. Sportsmed.* **13**(7), 43–59.

Potera, C. (1986) Women in sports: The price of participation. *Phys. Sportsmed.* **14**, 149–53.

Powers, J. (1980) Knee. In *The Athlete's Knee: Surgical Repair and Reconstruction*, AAOS Symposium IX. CV Mosby, St Louis.

Protzman, R. (1979) Physiologic performance of women compared to men. Observations of cadets at the United States Military Academy. *Am. J. Sports Med.* **7**(3), 191–4.

Protzman, R. & Griffis, C. (1977) Stress fractures in men and women undergoing military training. *J. Bone Joint Surg.* **59A**, 825.

Rose, C. (1981) Injuries in women's field hockey: A four-year study. *Phys. Sportsmed.* **9**(3), 97–100.

Roy, S. & Irvin, R. (1983) *Sports Medicine*, pp. 457–67. Prentice-Hall, Englewood Cliffs, New Jersey.

Stone, J. (1988) Conditioning and rehabilitation of athletes. In J. Puhl, C. Brown & R. Voy (eds) *Sport Science Perspectives for Women*, pp. 67–84. Human Kinetics, Illinois.

Schneider, J. & Cecil, J. (1989) *Progressive Individualized Exercises*. Communication Skill Builders, Tucson, Arizona.

Thomas, C. (1979) Factors important to women participants in vigorous athletics. In R. Strauss (ed) *Sports Medicine and Physiology*. WB Saunders, Philadelphia.

Ullyot, J. (1976) *Women's Running*. Anderson World Publications, Mountain View, California.

Wells, C. (1985) *Women, Sport and Performance*. Human Kinetics, Illinois.

Whiteside, P. (1980) Men's and women's injuries in comparable sports. *Phys. Sportsmed.* **8**(3), 130–40.

Wilmore, J. (1974) Alterations in strength, body composition and anthropometric measurements consequent to a 10-week weight training program. *Med. Sci. Sports* **6**, 133–8.

Wilmore, J. & Brown, C. (1974) Physiological profile of women distance runners. *Med. Sci. Sports Exerc.* **6**(3), 178–81.

Part 3b

Sport-Related Factors in Injury Prevention

Chapter 15

Training Errors

JACK E. TAUNTON

Aetiological factors associated with running injuries can be divided into intrinsic and extrinsic elements. The intrinsic factors involve alignment abnormalities of the pelvis, knee, tibia and feet. In addition, leg length discrepancy and strength–flexibility imbalances or deficiencies are also well-recognized intrinsic aetiological factors. Extrinsic factors include training errors, the effects of various running surfaces and terrain, plus poor or improperly selected shoes. James *et al.* (1978) were among the first to relate errors in training, often stated as 'too much too soon', as a major aetiological factor in the genesis of running injuries. Brody's excellent symposia on running injuries (1980) stated that training errors are the most frequent cause of running injuries. These errors appear to overwhelm the body's natural ability to adapt. Sheehan (1990), in a recent editorial, described the athletes suffering an overuse injury as individuals who are 'dedicating their leisure time to doing quite unremarkable things for a remarkable amount of time'.

James *et al.* (1978) attributed some 60% of running injuries to a training error. Brody (1980) stated that 60% of runners will, at some time, sustain a significant injury that requires them to stop training. He felt that novice runners are too enthusiastic but are in poor physical condition and are injured when they run excessively in a short period of time. On the other hand, the experienced competitive runners experience annoying overuse injuries when they race too much or incorporate intense interval training along with increasing mileage. This chapter will investigate the various training errors that have been associated with running injuries, and discuss safe exercise training principles.

Training errors

Clement *et al.* (1981) have shown that specific training errors include:
1 Persistent high-intensity training without alternate easy days.
2 Sudden increases in training mileage.
3 Sudden increases in intensity without allowing the supporting structures of the lower extremities sufficient time to adapt to the increased work load.
4 A single severe training or competitive session such as a 10-km race or a marathon.
5 Repetitive hill running.
Brody (1980) would add to this list:
6 Inadequate warm-up.

As previously mentioned, James *et al.* (1978) found that 60% of 232 injuries were attributable to training errors. More recently, Lysholm and Wiklander (1987) reported errors in training as responsible for 72% of the 65 injuries in runners training at a high level.

Specific injuries and training errors

Clement *et al.* (1981) reported a 2-year retrospective study of 1650 running patients with a total of 1819 injuries. Aetiological factors were analysed along with alignment features, shoes and specific injuries. The knee was the most common injury site, accounting for 41.7% of all injuries. The least injured areas were the lower back and upper leg, accounting for 3.7 and 3.6% of all injuries, respectively. Patellofemoral pain syndrome was the most common single diagnosis which accounted for 25.8% of the total injuries. A total of 468 cases of patellofemoral pain syndrome were seen.

Interestingly, the running mileage performed overall was not as high as we originally felt might be seen. On average, the men ran 27 miles·week^{-1} (43 km·week^{-1}) prior to their injury and the women ran 19 miles·week^{-1} (30.5 km·week^{-1}). Koplan et al. (1982) and Marti et al. (1988) have shown a linear relationship between weekly training mileage and running injuries. Marti et al. (1988) found that increased weekly training mileage led not only to an increased incidence in running injuries but also to an increased total number of medical consultations. There was also a significant correlation between running injury incidence and what was described as a competitive motive for running. They hypothesized that running injuries could be prevented if total weekly mileage was divided into several shorter sessions as described by Pollock et al. (1977). This was studied in a subgroup of runners who had similar weekly running distances but ran this mileage in two, three or four weekly training sessions. Analysis, however, showed no significant differences in the incidence of running injuries. Lysholm and Wiklander (1987) have reported a significant relationship between the injury rate in a given month and the distance run in the previous month.

With our original retrospective study (Clement et al., 1981) we found that of the 468 cases of patellofemoral pain, 57 cases (12%) were attributed to a sudden increase in mileage and 30 cases (6%) followed a single severe session. The second most common injury, accounting for 13.2% of the total, was tibial stress syndrome. This amounted to 239 cases of which 27 occurred following a sudden increase

in mileage. Achilles peritendonitis was the third most common problem with 109 cases (6%). A sudden increase in mileage was seen as a single aetiological factor in 13 patients and a further 11 patients developed their Achilles peritendonitis after a single severe training session. We found that for the top 10 most common injuries, training errors often precipitated injuries if associated with significant malalignment or strength−flexibility imbalances. As an example, plantar fasciitis which was seen in 105 cases, was associated with moderate to severe excessive foot pronation in 48 cases, rigid pes cavus feet in 11 cases and in 14 cases of gastrocnemius−soleus insufficiency. On its own, without biomechanical factors or muscular imbalances, a sudden increase in mileage resulted in 12 cases of plantar fasciitis.

The intensity and volume of training appears to be related to specific injuries seen in different running groups. Macintyre et al. (1991) showed that in the higher mileage marathon runners, iliotibial band friction syndrome (ITBFS) was the most frequent injury, with recreational runners having a higher frequency of patellofemoral pain syndrome. The competitive middle-distance runners who utilized more intense interval training twice or three times per week, had a higher frequency of Achilles tendonitis and tibial stress fracture.

Taunton et al. (1981) studied 62 runners treated for lower extremity stress fractures. A combination of errors in training and changes in footwear accounted for 44% of the stress fractures. In all patients there was some degree of malalignment of the lower extremity. Twenty-four of the 62 runners ran in excess of 50 km·week^{-1}. The intensity of the running programme was recognized as a major initiating feature of the stress fracture with 27% of the cases following a rapid commencement of training; 10% followed a single severe training session, 8% followed a rapid increase in mileage, and 6% after a sudden exposure to hill running. We proposed that training errors, leading to stress overload (Fig. 15.1), result in local muscular fatigue, decreasing the muscular

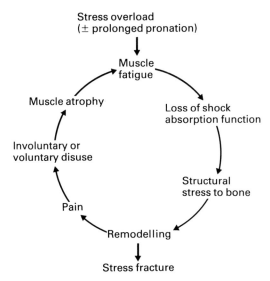

Stress overload
(± prolonged pronation)

Muscle fatigue

Muscle atrophy

Loss of shock absorption function

Involuntary or voluntary disuse

Structural stress to bone

Pain

Remodelling

Stress fracture

Fig. 15.1 Theoretical aetiology of stress fractures. From Taunton *et al*. (1981).

function of shock absorption and hence more structural stress to bone. This then initiates more osteoclastic bone remodelling and if rest and recovery by osteoblastic activity is not permitted to balance the osteoclastic remodelling then a stress fracture will occur. Similarly, patellofemoral pain syndrome can be seen with stress overload of the quadriceps, particularly vastus medialis, resulting in greater lateral patellar translation and shear stress. In both of these situations a cycle of overload, muscular fatigue and pain, followed by involuntary or voluntary disuse leading to muscular atrophy, can occur.

Empirically, alternate day training and small increases of 10% per weekly mileage appears to allow recovery to prevent the development of muscular fatigue. However, the adaptive process is very individual depending upon age, gender, previous muscular development and nutritional status, among other factors. Individuals who have well-developed cardiovascular systems from cycling or swimming have been known to develop tibial stress fractures quite quickly when exposed to an off-season running programme. It is possible that their lower

extremity musculature or bony architecture is not sufficient to withstand the repetitive impact from running.

In a much larger series of 320 stress fractures in athletes that we studied, Matheson *et al*. (1987) identified training errors in only 22.4% of all stress fractures and these errors were equally common in all sites of stress fracture. An analysis of variance revealed no significant difference in weekly mileage between the sites of stress fractures. The early reports on stress fractures and, in fact, some of the most extensive clinical surveys of stress fractures were in military recruits (Gilbert & Johnson, 1966). Comparison with our large series on very active athletes revealed some interesting differences from the military studies. In the athletes, the most common site of injury was the tibia, whereas in the marching soldier the most common site was the calcaneus or metatarsals. The differences between the sites and the frequency of stress fractures in the athletes and military recruits could be related to the fitness of the athlete and the type of exercise involved. The stress fracture frequency in untrained recruits results from a vigorous progressive training programme, over a short period of time, which overcomes the osseous system resulting in insufficient time for bone remodelling.

Lombardo and Benson (1982) showed that the loading rate to the osseous system is more important than the absolute load in the development of femoral neck stress fractures. In addition, the fitter athlete has trained over a period of months to years allowing adaptive changes to occur to the osseous system. The athletes in this study were generally of a high calibre and had a lower frequency of training errors and, in addition, the athletes trained on a variety of surfaces and used running shoes whereas the military recruits marched on hard surfaces in less forgiving combat boots.

Rubin and Lanyou (1987) showed that a new loading regimen must last longer than 2 weeks before the bone responds with increased strength. The strength of the bone increased only after 14 days but the muscle strength increased sooner and overtraining could occur with an imbalance of muscle strain against the relatively weaker bone. In addition, if the stress to the bone is increased with daily increases in training, a stress fracture can occur as the bone strength has not increased during this period. Adaptation for running follows a principle of progressive overload which requires a delicate balance of the components of intensity, duration, frequency and progression. To allow adaptation of the soft osseous tissues, modern training programmes now incorporate elements of cross-training utilizing cycling, swimming or pool running, for the serious runner.

Age as a factor

Age is another important consideration with the application of exercise training. Both the younger athlete's and the older masters runner's training programmes must be modified in terms of the progression of time, frequency of intense workouts, and number of rest days.

High-intensity workouts with more eccentric training can produce more traction apophysitis injuries at the calcaneus and tibial tubercle in the adolescent runner (Micheli, 1987). Clement et al. (1981) reported sudden increases in mileage as important aetiological factors for the development of traction apophysitis. Garrick (1988) states that overuse injuries in the paediatric population are the greatest challenge but also offer the greatest opportunity to change behaviour. He states that, in the paediatric age group, overuse injuries are usually the result of training errors. Hence overuse injuries lend themselves more readily to change and ultimately, prevention.

Marti et al. (1988) showed that middle-aged runners with high weekly training mileage were particularly prone to muscle strains of the thigh and calf and also Achilles tendonitis. These injuries resulted in greater disability and time off running, than with the younger runners. They did show, however, that the overall incidence of running injuries was decreased in this age group, possibly related to a long-term adaptive process from training but with reduced regenerative capacity and hence the longer time to recovery.

Prospective studies

Putting these results from retrospective studies to the stronger rigours of prospective analysis, Walter et al. (1989) studied 1680 runners who participated in two community road race events that included both a longer and a shorter race. Participants completed a questionnaire covering training, running environment, use of stretching, warm-up and cool-down exercises, characteristics of shoes and previous injury status, among other factors. All participants were then followed by telephone interview at 4, 8 and 12 months.

During the follow-up period, 48% of the runners experienced at least one injury and of these 54% were new injuries. Competitive runners had a substantially increased risk of new injuries as compared to the fitness runners. Risk of new injury was also seen with running more than 40 miles·week^{-1} (65 km·week^{-1}), increasing daily mileage on running days, length of the longest run during the week, number of running days per week, and running year round. The increased risk of these factors was similar for men and women. Interestingly, runners who never warmed up had less risk than those who did. Runners who sometimes stretched were reported to be at higher risk than those who usually, or never, stretched. A previous injury was highly predictive for developing a new injury. Factors such as pace, running surface, hill running or intense training had no apparent effect on the risk of new injury. Interestingly, injury rates were similar in all sex and age groups and were unrelated to years of running experience.

Recently, also, Macera et al. (1989) investigated, by questionnaire, 583 habitual runners and then followed them for 12 months. During this 12-month follow-up, 52% of men and 49% of women reported at least one injury which interrupted their training or caused them to seek medical advice. The most important predictor of injury in men was running 64 km or more per week. Other predictors were an injury in the preceding year and having been a runner for less than 3 years. With the multiple logistic regression analysis utilized in this study, the only predictor of injury that was statistically significant for the female runners was running more than two-thirds of the time on concrete.

These studies confirmed the earlier reports of training errors. Jacobs and Berson (1986) specifically investigated what training factors were associated with running injuries by randomly sampling entrants to a 10-km road race, by questionnaire. There were 451 respondents, 355 men and 96 women, with a non-response rate of 12.7%. Of the respondents, 47% had sustained a running-related injury in the previous 2 years. Their results showed that injured runners differed significantly from non-injured runners in that they ran more miles and more days per week and at a faster pace. In addition, the injured runners ran more races in a year and did not participate in other sports. Similar to the later report of Walter *et al.* (1989), the injured runners stretched before running as compared to the non-injured runners. There was no correlation with injury regarding running surfaces, running hills, sprints or intervals.

Stretching and warm-up

As Jacobs and Berson stated (1986), the topic of stretching before and after training is controversial. In most coaching and training reports, such as Davis (1982), the beneficial reports of flexibility and warm-up are presented. Stretching is beneficial if performed properly, but some stretching drills can be dangerous, especially if done with bouncing ballistic thrust. Medial meniscal injuries have been seen with the hurdler stretch done with the knee in valgus and with the hip internally rotated as in the hurdler position rather than with the plantar surface of the foot placed against the medial

aspect of the opposite leg and the hip in external rotation. Valgus stress injury to the medial collateral ligament can also occur with a ballistic bounce stretch of the adductor during the groin stretch with weighting on the medial aspect of the foot rather than on a flat foot. In addition, stretching can cause an injury if done too vigorously when the muscle is not warmed up such as first thing in the morning, especially in older runners. We recommend a gentle warm-up of 5–10 min to increase the core temperature such that light perspiration occurs and then to commence a stretching programme before and after the workout. Static long sustained stretches of 30–60 s, as outlined by Stewart (1980) and Clement (1982) are recommended. The major muscles to be stretched are the prime movers in running: the gluteals, hamstrings and gastrocnemius–soleus, in addition to the quadriceps, iliopsoas, hip flexors and paralumbars.

Although these studies have identified a positive correlation of injury with stretching, this does not necessarily imply cause and effect, but as Jacobs and Berson suggest (1986) it may just indicate that runners who are injured stretch because of their injury. Blair (1985) did not find any association between stretching habits and the incidence of injury. As Powell *et al.* (1986) state in their article on an epidemiological perspective on the causes of running injuries, more studies are needed in this area. They feel, and correctly so, that the issue is whether those who stretch, weight-train for lower extremity strengthening, warm-up or cool-down, are less likely to be injured in the future than those who do not.

Summary

In the history of an injury, one must obtain training history which includes length of runs, distance covered, intensity and terrain whether it be flat, hills, uneven, cross-country, trails or roads. Also, inquire about the frequency of intense interval training with the length and number of repetitions plus rest phase. The number of runs per week and days of rest is also of importance, as is frequency of racing and intensity of runs following races.

Exercise training principles

To prevent running injuries, Clement (1982) has suggested that exercise should be viewed as a pharmacological agent, and dosage, frequency, host response, side-effects and sensitivities must be considered in the design of an exercise programme. As he states, exercise has potent physiological effects on the musculoskeletal and cardiovascular systems but exercise must be respected as a therapeutic modality. The greatest adaptations in achieving fitness occur in the enzyme and fueling capacities within the muscle cells. The most common site of breakdown in exercise programmes is within the musculoskeletal system, not in the cardiovascular system. The enzymes of the aerobic and anaerobic metabolism need to be challenged and increase with training. In addition, the tensile strength of tendons and the density of bone are increased, as we know, as an adaptation to the stress of exercise. As mentioned, it is the method of applying this stress of exercise that is usually responsible for the overuse injury.

Elements of the programme

The elements of a running training programme include:
1 Long slow endurance distance runs in excess of 1 h.
2 Pace and tempo runs of repetitions of 3–10 min.
3 Aerobic intervals of 5–15 min.
4 Anaerobic intervals of 0.5–4 min.
The adaptation to the specific type of training is seen within the muscle. Strength increase is seen with greater recruitment of motor units. This adaptation occurs partly by improved innervation of the muscle fibres within the motor unit and in part by increases in the concentration of metabolic enzymes within the

muscle cells. The ratio of slow twitch to fast twitch fibres appears to be fixed at birth but by exposure to endurance training some fast twitch fibres can function more aerobically. Specific exercise programmes then enhance enzymatic changes in response to the stress in relationship to the aerobic to anaerobic ratio. Training is that specific, such that long slow distance prepares one for an endurance event, and speed in running short distance is improved only by similar specific training to enhance motor unit recruitment and anaerobic metabolism.

Overload and adaptation

The application of an exercise stimulus follows a basic principle of overload. The exercise load temporarily produces fatigue and reduces the work potential. During recovery and adaptation over time the work potential recovers to a new level of supercompensation. New exercise loads can then be applied resulting in a higher peak of supercompensation, however, rest must occur to allow this ideal level of adaptation (Fig. 15.2).

If full recovery does not occur, the work

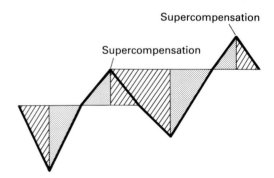

Fig. 15.2 An ideal training programme, allowing recovery and adaption. The exercise load provides a stimulus which evokes a response of a temporary reduction in work potential due to fatigue. Recovery and adaptation leads to supercompensation. A further stimulus applied at the peak of supercompensation leads to a new peak of supercompensation at an even higher work potential. From Clement (1981) ▨, fatigue; ▧, recovery and adaptation.

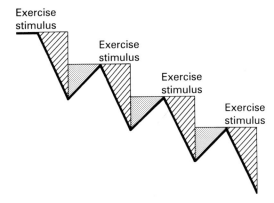

Fig. 15.3 A training programme which fails to allow recovery time. If insufficient recovery and adaptation time are allowed after the stimulus and before the next stimulus, the second fatigue effect lowers the work potential. The effect of applying this exercise load before full recovery and supercompensation is a continuing decrease in work potential. From Clement (1982). ▨, fatigue; ▨, recovery.

potential is never permitted to recover let alone reach the level of supercompensation (Fig. 15.3). With subsequent days of exercise loading the work potential progressively drops until profound fatigue or an injury occurs forcing a termination in training.

Clement (1982) points out that proper exercise management employs an easy–hard microcycle in training programmes. He feels that recovery from training sessions is closer to 48 than 24 h. As a result, full training loads should be applied no more than two or, maximally, three times per week. Novice runners should run on alternate days, allowing 1 day of recovery and adaptation between runs. The progression is such that the load is increased moderately for 3

consecutive training days then the intensity or load is reduced by one level before an increase in load occurs (Fig. 15.4). This microcycle is then fitted within a larger macrocycle measured in weeks. The total volume is progressively increased over 3 weeks adding 10% per week, then reducing the total work load on the fourth week before another 3-week cycle of progressive load. Another variation of this concept is shown in Fig. 15.5.

It must be remembered that when athletes enter into a group training programme they must progress at their own rate. The adaptation to training is a very individual process and so often the new runners will sacrifice their adaptive process within the group training and hence ignore the basic principles of progressive resistance training. As we have discussed, the fatigue of the muscle system leads to reduction in

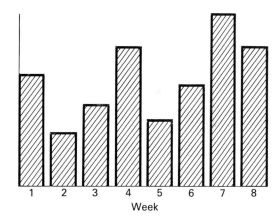

Fig. 15.5 Macrocycle in training programmes. The total workload in week 1 is reduced to 50% in week 2, increased to 75% in week 3, and further increased to 125% in week 4. From Clement (1981).

Fig. 15.4 Microcycle in training programmes. Full training loads should be applied at maximum three times per week. The load is increased moderately for 3 consecutive training days then reduced by one level before a further increase in load occurs. From Clement (1981).

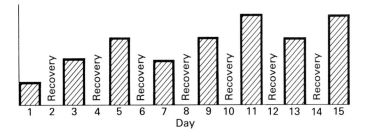

shock absorption and the potential of micro-trauma to tendon, muscle or bone with continued training.

Conclusion

This discussion of training errors must be considered in conjunction with the other chapters, discussing the effects of running surfaces and various terrains plus the contribution of the shoe, to complete an understanding of the extrinsic factors associated with running injuries.

References

Blair, S.N. (1985) Risk factors and running injuries. *Med. Sci. Sports Exerc.* **17**(2), xii.

Brody, D.M. (1980) Running injuries. *Clin. Symp.* **32**(4), 1–36.

Clement, D.B. (1982) The practical application of exercise training principles in family medicine. *Can. Fam. Phys.* **28**, 929–32.

Clement, D.B., Taunton, J.E., Smart, G.W. & Nicol, K.L. (1981) A survey of overuse running injuries. *Phys. Sports Med.* **9**(5), 47–58.

Davis, V.G. (1982) Flexibility conditioning for running. In R. D'Ambrosia & D. Drez (eds) *Prevention and Treatment of Running Injuries.* Charles B. Slack Inc., New Jersey.

Garrick, J.G. (1988) Epidemiology of sports injuries in the pediatric athlete. In J.A. Sullivan & W.A. Grava (eds) *The Pediatric Athlete.* American Academy Orthopedic Surgery Seminar, Illinois.

Gilbert, R.S. & Johnson, H.A. (1966) Stress fractures in military recruits. A review of 12 years experience. *Milit. Med.* **137**, 716–21.

Jacobs, S.J. & Berson, B.L. (1986) Injuries to runners: A study of entrants to a 10 000 meter race. *Am. J. Sports Med.* **14**(2), 151–5.

James, S.L., Bates, B.T. & Osternig, L.R. (1978) Injuries to runners. *Am. J. Sports Med.* **6**, 40–50.

Koplan, J.P., Powell, K.E., Sikes, P.K., Shirley, R.W. & Campbell, C.C. (1982) An epidemiologic study of the benefits and risks of running. *JAMA* **248**(23), 3118–21.

Lombardo, S.C. & Benson, D.W. (1982) Stress fractures of the femur in runners. *Am. J. Sports Med.* **10**, 219–27.

Lysholm, J. & Wiklander, J. (1987) Injuries in runners. *Am. J. Sports Med.* **15**(2), 168–71.

Macera, C.A., Pate, R.R., Powell, K.E., Jackson, K.L., Kendrick, J.S. & Craven, T.E. (1989) Predicting lower-extremity injuries among habitual runners. *Arch. Intern. Med.* **149**, 2565–8.

Macintyre, J.G., Taunton, J.E., Clement, D.B., Lloyd-Smith, D.R., McKenzie, D.C. & Morrell, R.W. (1991) Running injuries: A clinical study of 4173 cases. *Clin. J. Sports Med.* **1**(2), 7–11.

Marti, B., Vader, J.P., Minder, C.E. & Abelin, T. (1988) On the epidemiology of running injuries. *Am. J. Sport Med.* **16**(3), 285–94.

Matheson, G.O., Clement, D.B., McKenzie, D.C., Taunton, J.E., Lloyd-Smith, D.R. & Macintyre, J.G. (1987) Stress fractures in athletes. A study of 320 cases. *Am. J. Sports Med.* **15**(1), 46–58.

Micheli, L.J. (1987) The traction apophysitis. *Clin. Sports Med.* **6**(2), 389–403.

Pollock, C.T., Gettman, L.K., Mileses, C.A., Bali, M.D., Durstine, L. & Johnson, R.B. (1977) Effects of frequency and duration of training on attrition and incidence of injury. *Med. Sci. Sports Exerc.* **9**, 31–6.

Powell, K.E., Kohl, H.W., Caspersen, C.J. & Blair, S.N. (1986) An epidemiological perspective on the causes of running injuries. *Phys. Sports Med.* **14**(6), 100–14.

Rubin, C.T. & Lanyou, L.E. (1987) Osteoregulatory nature of mechanical stimuli: Function as a determinant for adaptive remodelling in bone. *J. Orthop. Res.* **5**, 300–10.

Sheehan, G. (1990) Sports medicine renaissance. *Phys. Sports Med.* **18**(11), 26.

Stewart, G.W. (1980) *Everybody's Fitness Book.* Doubleday, New York.

Taunton, J.E., Clement, D.B. & Webber, D. (1981) Lower extremity stress fractures in athletes. *Phys. Sports Med.* **9**, 77–86.

Walter, S.D., Hart, L.E., McIntosh, J.M. & Sutton, J.R. (1989) The Ontario cohort study of running-related injuries. *Arch. Intern. Med.* **149**, 2561–4.

Chapter 16

Regulations and Officiating in Injury Prevention

UFFE JØRGENSEN

Rules and the way they are handled by the referees are the basic background for injury prevention in each sport. The considerations underlying the primary creation of rules in sport are the first steps by sport itself towards organized injury prevention. A central point in the different sport rules (some would like it to be the most important point) is to make the actual sport as safe as possible for the athletes. This central — and vital — point is, however, often forgotten due to different factors which will be discussed in this chapter.

A misunderstanding of the basic idea of sport can lead to the unfortunate fact that certain rules and their handling by the referee actually induce injuries and prevent adequate treatment. A main purpose of this chapter is to highlight this fact so that sport injuries can be adequately treated and unnecessary injuries avoided.

History of the rules

Rules in sports have developed as a necessity in order to settle disagreements and to make the same sport possible at different places. The basic considerations have been to create an optimal frame for the sport and then add restrictions concerning safety. This has primarily been handled in the rules by giving the referee the possibility of using penalties for fouls, and making specific rules concerning compulsory equipment.

In the oldest sports, the background for the creation of the primary rules must primarily have been practical considerations, and the protection of the athlete, if considered, was based on assumptions or experience.

In younger sports (e.g. team handball and basketball) the creators of the rules have had the chance to learn from older sports with similarities (e.g. soccer) and introduce new aspects such as free substitution and rules concerning the degree of direct contact with an opponent. The rules concerning the safety of the athlete are initially based on assumptions. Modifications with time should be a natural occurrence, as in the rules concerning traffic and cars, where changes are introduced when risk factors are identified, mostly by statistics. When first created, sports were conservative with regard to changes in the rules, and if changes did appear it was most often for reasons other than safety of the athlete (like the number of steps the soccer goalkeeper is allowed to take, modifications in the offside rule, etc.).

Rule changes

Some changes have been introduced in various sports over time. The motivation for a change is generated with different interests in mind (Table 16.1).

To increase public interest in the sport. Examples of this in international soccer include the newest changes in the offside rule which could increase the number of goals, and serious con-

213

Table 16.1 The background for changes in rules over time.

1 To increase public interest in the sport

2 Economic considerations

3 Administrative considerations

4 Injury prevention

5 The role of sports medicine research

siderations over increasing the size of the goal itself. An example of a national change in the soccer rules with the purpose of increasing public interest in the game is from an Arab community where a sheikh abandoned offside and reduced the number of players from 11 to nine!

Economic considerations. An increased public interest will of course have economic implications. Television coverage and commercials are almost integrated with sports like baseball and American football. The television coverage of important sporting events often makes changes necessary concerning when different events can be held.

Administrative considerations. The national soccer rules in the lower series in Denmark concerning 'warnings' (yellow cards) was changed from a central registration with accumulation of warnings, to the yellow card meaning that the player is sent off for 10 min (Fig. 16.1). The reason was that this would reduce the costs of a central registration! The Gentofte Hospital had tried to study the effect of that change, based on the hypothesis that a direct punishment of the player and team could reduce the number of wild tackles and thereby prevent some of the serious knee injuries. However, the soccer association could not be persuaded to participate in this scientific study — but when they realized that money could be saved in the administration, they introduced the rule change without a test of the scientific validity.

Injury prevention. From the medical point of view, this is constantly used as a reason for changing rules in different sports. The basis for a change can be sport-specific research which points out typical injuries and/or certain risk factors. Examples are epidemiological studies on ice hockey which showed a very large

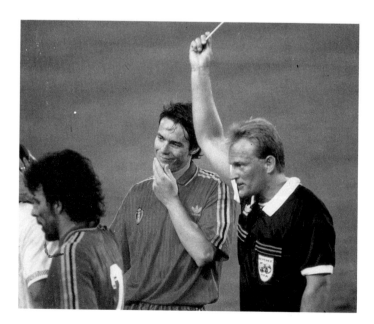

Fig. 16.1 A modification of the rules so that a warning (yellow card) in soccer results in some minutes out of the game could have an injury-preventive effect.

number of facial, head and eye injuries; this lead to a change in the ice hockey rules towards compulsory use of helmets with face guards. Following this ruling, a reduction in the number of head, and particularly eye, injuries was seen (Pashby, 1979; Vinger, 1980). More often, however, rule changes are based on personal experience and assumptions rather than on scientific data (e.g. the constant changes of rules in motor sports with regard to motor power and aerodynamics).

The role of sports medicine research. Until the 1990s, there has been too little research on injury prevention. The most solid basis for changes should be statistically significant evidence. Numerous studies have been published on injury epidemiology and several authors identify rules as causal factors in the development of sports injuries (Ekstrand, 1982; Bourgoin & Pasquis, 1983; Jørgensen, 1989).

A reason as to why sports medicine research does not have as great an influence as it should have, could be lack of communication between sports officials and scientists. Another factor could be low administrative priority of the handing of the results of sport-specific research.

Injury aetiology: rules and referees

Studies of sport-injury aetiology have revealed several points where rules and referees have had an influence on injury risk. Examples of causal factors include:

1 Failure to apply the rules strictly by the referee (Bourgoin & Pasquis, 1983).
2 Not allowing free substitution in soccer (Jørgensen, 1989).
3 Foul play (Ekstrand, 1982; Bruce *et al.*, 1984; Watson, 1984).
4 Rules concerning tackles in soccer and American football (Torg *et al.*, 1979; Ekstrand, 1982).
5 Rules concerning the status of equipment, such as ski-bindings.
6 Rules concerning compulsory protective

equipment. An adverse effect can, however, be a shift in the injury pattern as in American football where the introduction of helmets with face protection (a net) increased the number of neck injuries (Tator & Edmonds, 1984).
7 A lack of rules concerning the limits of performance can produce life-threatening conditions as seen in long-lasting events.
8 A lack of specific rules concerning the quality of sports accommodation with special respect to the floor/ground, focusing on such factors as irregularities, shock absorption and friction (Bierner, 1978; Snook, 1985).
9 Limited rules concerning the quality of sports equipment as, for instance, the release limit for ski-bindings.

Injury severity and frequency: rules and referees

In badminton, treatment of an injury during a match is not allowed. This seems to be an old-fashioned rule, not taking into consideration the development in sports medical treatment. The rule in this way often 'forces' a player to continue, with the risk of a more serious injury. The rule should be changed so that adequate investigation and a minor short treatment should be allowed.

However, if injuries seem to be more serious or are seen to handicap the player, rules in all sports should, as in boxing, have a possibility for 'technical knock-out', so that, for instance, a soccer player could be sent off the field in order not to worsen an injury. In principle injured players should not be allowed to play. However, in practice this would be very difficult to handle — it would demand not only changes in rules, but also changes in attitude of both athlete and trainer.

Referees, unfortunately, sometimes do not use their right to allow treatment of an injured athlete in sports where this is allowed. The reason is most often misjudgement or an assumption of simulation by the athlete. The rules could be changed in order to take the responsibility away from the referee and give the athlete the benefit of the doubt. Allowing simulation is an acceptable side-effect because it is better than having an injured athlete suffer from a judgement by a non-medically competent referee.

The speed and power limits set by the rules are directly proportional to the degree of injury. A reasonable limit should be based on constant monitoring and sport-specific research. In fighting sports, rules determine the degree of freedom to attack different parts of the body. Curiously enough, one of the most vulnerable areas — the face — is an area which a fighter is allowed to hit!

Interpretation of rules

The role of the referee is in most sports a very influential one, and is vulnerable to human fallibility. A referee with an 'international style' often allows more leeway, which also means a greater injury risk for the athletes. This is a fact that is widely accepted, although in basic sport terms it is wrong.

The watching crowd can influence a referee to avoid using penalties against the home team, thereby increasing the risk for injuries for both teams (Ekstrand, 1982).

The influence of the press is also a factor for a referee when choosing to use a hard or soft line. This is also a factor that can influence the injury risk.

Economic influence has been described as another determining factor for the referees decision towards a one-sided soft line, which again increases injury risk. However, society has its own laws to deal with that very unsporting attitude.

Specific aspects of rules

Equipment. In most sports, there are a set of rules concerning the equipment. They allow the sport to be played, and to make it as fair and safe as possible. Equipment-based injuries are often seen in areas where the rules do not take important risk factors into consideration, such as the shoe/floor interaction. Rules on standards for these factors could decrease such friction-based injuries as falls due to slipping or twists due to high friction.

Contact/non-contact sport. The degree and nature of allowed contact is crucial for the development of injuries and are possibly influenced by rules and their application. Non-contact injuries are more difficult to prevent, however they could be influenced by rules concerning the shoe/floor interface.

Penalty for fouls. Penalties provide the possibility for the referee to keep the game within the rules. However, the penalty laid down in the rules is often insufficient. In team handball and ice hockey, violent players and their team can be directly punished by a player being sent off the playing field for a limited cool-off period after which players re-enter the game. In soccer, however, there is not the same possibility; players are just warned not to do the foul again (Figs 16.2 & 16.3). This often results in serious injuries (Ekstrand, 1982). A modification in the rules so that a yellow card results in some minutes out of the game could have a positive effect, as seen in sports with more up-to-date rules.

Another penalty for an injury-producing 'assault' that has been discussed by some athletes, is that the injury-provoking player — the 'attacker' — should be out of the game for as long as the other player is injured!

Free substitution. Free substitution (Fig. 16.4) provides the possibility of taking injured players out of the game. This should be possible and allowed in all team sports. No increased injury risks have been reported among substitutes.

Score system. The only score systems that are influenced by injuries and fouls are the fighting

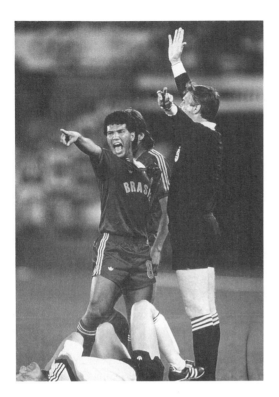

Fig. 16.2 The referee must be firm as protests are common. Courtesy of the IOC archives.

sports, where injury means a lost game and a foul can result in disqualification. One could consider changing the score in favour of the team with the injured player as a punishment for deliberate fouls resulting in serious injuries.

Treatment of sports injuries: rules and referees

The rules determine the possibilities of treating injuries developed during competition in different sports. An exact diagnosis and an adequate acute treatment is decisive for the severity and duration of an injury and should therefore be allowed in all sports where it is practically possible.

Treatments such as bracing brings up another problem of whether this should be allowed in competition or not. Here, a dialogue between rule makers, referees organizations, manufacturers and doctors is desirable. The rules in most sports leaves the decision to the referee. The referee then has to judge whether the brace could be dangerous for the opponent or not. This responsibility should be moved from the referee to the rules based on expert judgement.

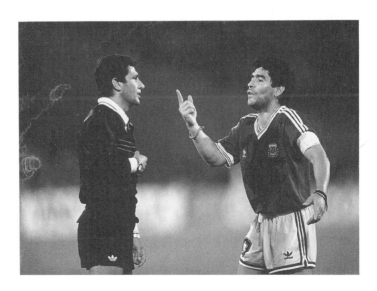

Fig. 16.3 Arguments between players and referees should be avoided. Courtesy of the IOC archives.

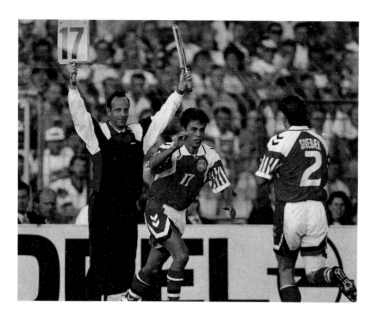

Fig. 16.4 Free substitution provides the possibility to take injured players out of the game and has been shown to reduce the duration of minor injuries (Jørgensen, 1989).

Injury prevention: rules and referees

The following are possible ways to reduce injury frequency and severity through rules.

1 For the referees to apply the rules more strictly.

2 To modify or change the rules in a more safe direction.

3 To make protective equipment compulsory.

A basis for change is, however, dependent on knowledge of injury aetiology and the possible effects of a change.

Stricter application of the rules. No research has yet been published on the possible injury-preventive effect of a stricter application of the rules. The proposals based on assumptions from referees and researchers, based on an identified injury aetiology, recommend stricter application of the rules as a possibility for preventing certain injuries (Bourgoin & Pasquis, 1983; Bruce *et al.*, 1984; Jørgensen, 1989).

Rule modifications. With respect to rule changes or modifications there is evidence of a preventive effect.

1 In American football, the banning of spear tackles has had a preventive effect on head and neck injuries according to Torg *et al.* (1979).

2 In ice hockey, the banning of high sticking and body checks from behind reduced the number of eye and head injuries according to Tator and Edmonds (1984) and Vinger (1980).

3 In karate, the banning of round-house kicks and spinning back kicks have been reported to have an injury-preventive effect (McLatchie, 1981).

4 In soccer, the first intervention study on the effect of rule changes in sports was performed by the author (Jørgensen, 1989). Free substitution was, in two comparable groups, shown to reduce the duration of minor injuries.

Protective equipment has been shown to be effective by several authors, and by changes in the rules it can be made compulsory.

1 In boxing, helmets have been shown to be effective (Schmidt-Olsen *et al.*, 1990).

2 In American football and ice hockey, helmets with face guards have been reported to reduce the number of head and facial injuries (Torg *et al.*, 1979; Vinger, 1981).

Conclusion

Rules and referees most certainly influence injury prevention and treatment. There are several points in the present rules of different sports which need to be revised. Future changes need to be based on sport-specific research including the testing (in intervention studies) of good ideas concerning safety of the athlete.

References

Bierner, K. (1978) Sportsunfalle, epidemiologie und prevention (Sports accidents, epidemiology and prevention). *Hefte Unfallheilkunde* **130**, 374−81.

Bourgoin, J.L. & Pasquis, P. (1983) Traumatologie du hockey zur grazon (Traumatology in hockey on grass). *Med. Sport* **57**, 24−8.

Bruce, D.A., Schut, C. & Sutton, L.M. (1984) Brain and cervical spine injuries occurring during organized sports activities in children and adolescents. *Primary Care* **11**, 175−94.

Ekstrand, J. (1982) *Soccer injuries and their prevention.* Thesis, Linkoping University Medical Dissertation No. 130, Linkoping, Sweden.

Jørgensen, U. (1989) Free substitution in soccer. *Nitz* **3**, 155−8.

McLatchie, G.R., Davis, J.E. & Caulley, H. (1980) Injuries in karate. *J. Trauma* **20**, 56−8.

Pashby, T.J. (1979) Eye injuries in Canadian amateur hockey. *Am. J. Sports Med.* **7**, 254−7.

Schmidt-Olsen, S., Jensen, S.K. & Mortensen, V. (1990) Amateur boxing in Denmark. The effect of some preventive measures. *Am. J. Sports Med.* **18**, 98−100.

Snook, G.A. (1985) A review of women collegiate gymnastics. *Clin. Sports Med.* **4**, 31−7.

Tator, C.H. & Edmonds, V. (1984) National survey of spinal injuries in hockey players. *Can. Med. Assoc. J.* **130**, 875−80.

Torg, J.S., Truex, R., Quedenfield, T.G. *et al.* (1979) The national football head and neck injury registry *J. Am. Med. Assoc.* **241**, 1477−9.

Vinger, P.F. (1980) Sports related eye injury. A preventable problem. *Surv. Ophthalmol.* **25**, 47−51.

Watson, A.W.S. (1984) Sports injuries during one academic year in 6799 Irish school children. *Am. J. Sports Med.* **12**, 65−71.

PART 4

GENERAL PREVENTION ACTIVITIES

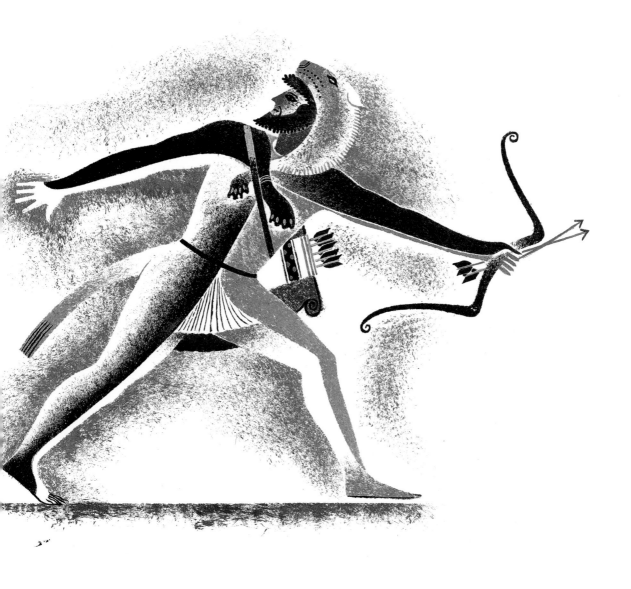

Chapter 17

Sport-Specific Screening and Testing

W. BEN KIBLER AND T. JEFF CHANDLER

The evaluation process of athletes is becoming an advanced science. More sophisticated equipment allows physicians and scientists to measure aspects of sports performance that have been previously difficult to measure. The volume of scientific and medical information available on élite and recreational athletes in specific sports is increasing. This information can be used to better characterize these sports and athletes in terms of both performance and injury prevention.

An injury to an athlete can be physically and psychologically devastating, leading to a decrease in performance as well as an impaired health status. Many types of injuries are associated with sports performance. In some instances, these injuries can be related to risk factors that may increase the chance of a particular injury in a sport. It may be possible, through proper identification and modification of risk factors, to eliminate or reduce the severity of many sport-related injuries.

Just as certain injuries can be associated with a particular sport, profiles of athletes are also sport specific. By examining sport-specific athletic profiles and correlating these profiles with risk factors and injuries, and by determining the modifiability of these risk factors, a decrease in injury risk may be possible. The purpose of this chapter is to discuss a musculoskeletal approach to athletic testing and screening for the purposes of improving athletic performance and reducing the risk of musculoskeletal injuries.

Sport-specific demands

Each sport exerts specific demands on parts of the body. These demands may be thought of as a spectrum from microtrauma to macrotrauma. Long-distance running stresses predominantly the lower extremities by the frequent but long-term application of low-intensity loads. This requires extremities to undergo repeated eccentric muscle contractions which may cause repetitive microtrauma to the muscles involved (Taimela *et al.*, 1989). Eccentric muscle contractions have been shown to create more tension in the muscle than concentric or static contractions (Armstrong, 1990). These eccentric contractions can exert a high tensile load on the musculoskeletal system, which may cause maladaptations to occur both in terms of strength of the muscles and range of motion of the joint.

These tensive loads extend across a continuum from absolute overloads where supranormal forces act on normal anatomy, to relative overloads where normal forces act on abnormal anatomy. Factors such as inflexibility, muscle weakness and strenuous exercise contribute to the overload process (see Fig. 19.2).

At the other end of the spectrum, the collision/contact sport of football places primarily macrotrauma forces on many areas of the body of the athlete as well as position-specific microtrauma in certain anatomical areas. In the middle of the spectrum, tennis places mainly microtrauma forces on the shoulder, elbow and lower body, with occasional macrotrauma involved. By examining the injuries that occur in all sports, and by classifying these injuries as traumatic, resulting primarily from macro-traumatic forces, or overload, resulting primarily from repetitive microtraumatic forces, we can better understand the role of testing in the prevention of these injuries.

Traumatic injuries may not be preventable, but the severity of such injuries may be lessened by modifying appropriate risk factors. These risk factors can be identified by proper preparticipation screening. The forces involved in injuries caused by high-velocity collisions certainly may result in musculoskeletal injury. These injuries result from forces that are applied to the musculoskeletal system such that the force exceeds the tensile or compressive strength of the musculoskeletal structures. The exact relationship between strength or flexibility and prevention of macrotrauma injuries remains unclear. Nicholas (1970) reported an increased likelihood of traumatic knee ligament rupture with increased 'looseness' of the knee. Strengthening exercises were suggested for those players with 'loose' knees to decrease the chance of knee ligament injuries. However, subsequent studies have shown no relationship between ligamentous laxity and injuries (Kalenak & Morehouse, 1975; Grana & Moretz, 1978).

Musculotendinous overload injuries secondary to repetitive microtrauma overload are common in sports and may be the most preventable type of injuries. Those overload injuries with gradual onset may be preceded by clinically measurable adaptations to the musculoskeletal system in terms of loss of strength, muscle imbalance and inflexibility (Kibler et al., 1988; Kibler, 1990a). Many of these injuries have contributing factors such as performing at too high an absolute load, or performing excessive repetitions of a normal load (Micheli, 1982; Renström & Johnson, 1985). These injuries may be related to a negative feedback overload vicious circle (see Fig. 19.3). In this concept, overload causes adaptations in strength or flexibility which result in functional biomechanical deficits. These deficits, while not overtly symptomatic, result in functional adaptations that decrease performance, cause inefficiency in performance, or may increase injury risk. These adaptations can be identified by a proper preparticipation examination.

Flexibility adaptations and related injuries

With intense participation and as a result of sport-specific demands, inflexibilities and muscle weaknesses may worsen as scar tissue forms, interfering with the ability of the muscle to contract efficiently and move through a normal range of motion. Pain may lessen the intensity and frequency with which the athlete uses his or her muscles, and this becomes an additional factor adding to muscle weakness. The athlete is now in the negative feedback vicious cycle consisting of inflexibilities, muscle weakness and further injury with continued use. Due to these clinical and subclinical adaptations of the body to tensile overload, efficient biomechanical movement patterns become difficult, usually leading to a change in movement patterns and an increase in muscle firing necessary to perform at a high level, potentially decreasing the skill level at which an activity is performed. This cycle continues until participation in the sport is no longer possible, the athlete no longer experiences success at his or her sport, and/or overt injury occurs.

Several studies have reported sport-specific adaptations in terms of joint range of motion in participation in specific sports. Ice-hockey players demonstrated significant differences in hip abduction by position (Agne et al., 1987). Goalies demonstrated greater hip flexibility than the forwards and the defence players. Flexibility was generally fair with a number of players demonstrating poor low back flexibility. It was suggested that hockey players should perform much more regular stretching in order to prevent injuries.

In baseball, Gurry et al. (1985) reported that catchers demonstrated greater gastrocnemius flexibility and trunk flexion and the least amount of trunk rotation, while pitchers showed the least flexibility in the hamstrings and the greatest hip extension, internal and external rotation. The outfielders showed the least flexibility in the gastrocnemius muscles, hip extension, and shoulder internal and external rotation. Professional baseball pitchers have been shown to demonstrate a decrease in internal rotation flexibility of the dominant arm, along with an increase in external rotation flexibility when compared to the dominant arm of position players (Brown et al., 1988). In lacrosse, Jackson and Nyland (1990) reported that overall upper body and lower body flexibility in club players was average, with areas of tightness in the hamstrings and quadriceps muscle groups.

The frequency of muscle tightness and injuries in senior division soccer players (mean age 24.6 years) was reported by Ekstrand and Gillquist (1982). Soccer players were generally less flexible than a group of age-matched non-playing controls. All measurements were performed on the lower body and included hip flexion with the knee straight, hip extension, hip abduction, knee flexion lying prone, and ankle dorsiflexion with the knee straight. This may be due to running and kicking (Hershman, 1984). This tightness may lead to hamstring strain and further injury. Similar results were reported by Kibler and Chandler (1993) in that quadriceps were tighter in young soccer players than tennis players or non-playing controls.

Strength adaptations and related injuries

Many studies demonstrate that strength training improves muscle strength (Atha, 1980). The role of this improved strength in the prevention of injuries has been previously discussed. Stone (1990) concluded in a review of the literature of the effect of conditioning on injuries that conditioning, particularly strength training, reduces injuries among athletes. Possible mechanisms by which this might occur have also been identified. Garrett demonstrated that maximally stimulated muscle absorbs significantly more energy prior to failure than sub-maximally or non-stimulated muscle (Garrett et al., 1987; Garrett & Tidball, 1987). Resistive training has also been shown to strengthen other structures around a joint such as ligaments and tendons that may be a factor in injury prevention (Adams, 1966; Tipton et al., 1970, 1975; Turto et al., 1974; Laurent et al., 1978; Kovanen et al., 1980, 1984; Staff, 1982).

Adaptations in the muscular system in terms of strength may actually be deleterious to both performance and injury potential. Muscle imbalance and muscle weakness have been demonstrated in athletes participating in athletic activities. Muscle strength adaptations have been reported throughout the scientific literature (Parker, 1983; Ivey et al., 1985; Alderink & Kuck, 1986; Cook et al., 1987; Kibler, 1990a; Knapik et al., 1991; McMaster et al., 1991; Chandler et al., 1992; Kibler & Chandler, 1993). Muscle damage does occur with intense muscle contraction (Armstrong, 1990) or with tensile overload (Garrett, 1990). As mentioned previously, eccentric exercise has been shown to produce considerably more damage to skeletal muscle than other types of exercise (Talag, 1973; Armstrong et al., 1983; Lieber & Friden, 1988). This damage may be a factor in loss of strength as it is in loss of flexibility. However, no clinical study has documented the exact correlation of muscle strength loss with muscle damage.

Muscle balance between the agonist and antagonist muscles that cross a joint has been suggested as a possible cause of sport-related injury (Grace et al., 1984; Grace, 1985). It may be that overtraining is a factor in the creation of these muscle imbalances. Swimmers often develop strength imbalances between the secondary muscles and the prime movers, often leading to shoulder problems (Brown et al., 1988). In swimmers tested on a Cybex II isokinetic dynamometer, the ratio of external rotation muscular endurance to internal rotation muscular endurance was less than 40% in swimmers with shoulder pain compared to a ratio of greater than 70% in swimmers without shoulder pain (Fleck & Falkel, 1986). It is yet to be demonstrated whether or not the weakness is due to the pain, or if the weakness precedes and is contributory to the pain.

In swimmers, Dominguez (1978) found a significant decrease in shoulder pain in age group swimmers after they began resistance training. There was evidence presented in this study to support the opinion that lack of strength training was related to the development of shoulder pain. Hawkins and Kennedy (1980) utilized isokinetic exercises to increase the strength and endurance of the shoulder muscles in swimmers and other upper body athletes. These exercises reduced the incidence of shoulder problems in athletes. Falkel (1990) demonstrated that weakness of the external rotators was present in swimmers with shoulder pain, compared to swimmers with no pain and in controls. A conditioning programme designed to improve strength of the external rotators resulted in significantly reducing shoulder pain in these swimmers.

An imbalance of shoulder external/internal rotation strength has also been reported in tennis players (Chandler et al., 1991), water polo players (McMaster et al., 1991) and baseball pitchers (Hinton, 1988). Imbalances in the isokinetic strength of the shoulder musculature in élite water polo players were reported by McMaster et al. (1991). Imbalances in the rotator cuff force couples of adduction/abduction and external/internal rotation were demonstrated. The adductors in the water polo players had gained in strength compared to the abductors, resulting in an adduction/abduction strength ratio of about 2:1. The internal rotators had increased in strength relative to the external rotators, resulting in a decrease in the external/internal strength ratio to about 0.6:1. The muscle imbalances demonstrated were more apparent at a test speed of $30°·s^{-1}$. Ivey et al. (1985) showed no significant differences between the dominant and non-dominant shoulder in external/internal rotation strength in baseball players as measured on a Cybex isokinetic dynamometer. A trend of increased strength in the dominant arm was also observed.

Muscle balance of the hamstrings and quadriceps may be important to prevent overload injury. The quadriceps provide the force for knee extension, while the hamstring must act to decelerate the tibia during knee extension, absorbing the energy developed by the quadriceps (Garrett et al., 1984). If the quadriceps is relatively stronger or the hamstring relatively weaker, a hamstring strain could result. The athlete with a 10% or greater difference between the quadriceps or hamstrings compared to the contralateral side is felt to have a greater risk of musculotendinous injury (Safran et al., 1989). Also, an athlete with a hamstring strength of less than 60% of the quadriceps is felt to be at risk of muscle strain injury.

Heiser et al. (1984), in a restrospective study of hamstring injuries in a college football team, reported that by eliminating muscle imbalances, hamstring injuries fell from an incidence rate of 7.7% with a 31.7% recurrence rate to a rate of 1.1% and no recurrences. It was concluded that isokinetic evaluation of muscle imbalances followed by a strengthening programme designed to correct identified imbalances could prevent hamstring strains. Also, rehabilitation programmes that utilize isokinetic criteria of muscle balance and return to normal strength significantly reduce the chance of reinjury. However, Grace et al. (1984) failed to show a relationship between muscle imbalances of the thigh and injuries to the knee in 172 high-school football players.

Agne et al. (1987) noted no significant differences in strength measurements via Cybex testing among the various positions in ice-hockey players. In runners with plantar fasciitis, weakness of the plantar flexors of the foot have been demonstrated as a predisposing factor (Kibler et al., 1991).

Adaptations and injuries to the skeletal system

Forces occurring to the body in athletic participation may injure the skeletal system (Falch, 1982; Jones, 1989). By the 1980s, as many as

10% of the injuries seen in sports medicine practices were stress fractures (MacBryde, 1985). The skeletal system may respond to these stresses with calcium deposition and resorption along the lines of stress. If calcium resorption outpaces deposition, stress fractures may occur. The potential causes of stress fractures can be related to muscle strength imbalances, inflexibilities, muscle weakness or abnormal mechanical loads on the bone. Weak muscles may be unable to dissipate either absolute or relative force overloads, causing those forces to be transferred to the skeletal system. Fatigued muscles, as might be readily exhibited in an overtrained state, may react in the same manner as weak muscles, increasing the forces on the skeletal system and producing a stress reaction. Muscle strength imbalances may modify the forces on the skeletal system in a similar manner and may cause an abnormal stress to the skeletal system producing a stress reaction.

Inflexibilities of the surrounding muscle groups may also be a factor in stress fractures. By altering the biomechanical pattern of the normal activity, these muscular adaptations may cause stresses to be placed on bone that in a repetitive overload situation might develop into a stress reaction. Other mechanical stresses, such as bony malalignment, improper shoes, abnormal stress due to running surfaces, or injury to other body parts, may also increase the bony load and predispose to stress fracture.

Conditioning may be important in the prevention of stress fractures. In a study of nationally competitive male athletes, those athletes who had the greatest strain placed on the lower limbs had the highest bone mineral content (Nilsson & Westlin, 1971). Two groups of controls for this study consisted of 24 age-matched physically active males and 15 age-matched sedentary males. The physically active controls had significantly more bone mineral than the sedentary controls. The competitive athletes had more bone mineral than the controls as a single group. In a study such as this, the possibility exists that the subjects with the greatest bone density chose to be more active in sports.

Bone mass of the humerus in tennis players has been shown to be significantly greater in the dominant arm compared to the non-dominant arm (Jones *et al.*, 1977). Montoye *et al.* (1980) also demonstrated that both bone width and mineral content of the dominant ulna, radius and humerus were significantly greater than in the non-dominant side of 61 senior male tennis players. In young male baseball players, the bone mineral content of the humerus but not the ulna and radius was significantly greater on the dominant compared to the non-dominant side (Watson, 1974). Because of the lack of control groups or very small control groups, no definitive conclusions can be drawn regarding bone density in the dominant compared to the non-dominant arms in these studies, as 'handedness' may be an important factor.

Sport-specific musculoskeletal profiling

Anatomical adaptations have been shown to occur that are both activity specific and sports specific. To best document these changes, the profiling examination must also be sports specific.

Because each sport has specific characteristics for both success in that sport and reduced injury risk, the profiling of each sport should focus on different areas depending on the demands placed on the body by the sport. 'Anatomical demands' refers to loads or forces placed on the anatomical structures. Throwing sports will exhibit an increased focus on the strength, endurance, muscle balance and range of motion of the back, shoulder and elbow joints. Jumping sports will include an increased focus on the hip, knee and ankle musculature in terms of strength, power and range of motion. Running sports will exhibit a different focus depending upon the intensity of the activity. Short-distance high-intensity running sports may focus more on the strength and power of the leg musculature and bony alignment of the lower limb, while long-distance lower intensity activities may focus more on muscular endurance, cardiorespiratory endurance and limb alignment.

Loads placed on the musculoskeletal system may be generally classified as tensile or compressive. Tensile loads are greatest in the musculature that undergoes an eccentric contraction. Several studies have been discussed that indicate a decreased range of motion in musculature used eccentrically and repetitively in sporting activities. This decreased range of motion is a measurable phenomena and should be included as part of a profiling system (Kibler, 1990b).

The metabolic demands of a sport can also be identified. These are demands on the energy-generating systems in the body. In profiling metabolic characteristics, data can be collected on aerobic fitness level, anaerobic capacity and anaerobic power. Relative to aerobic fitness, tests of both maximal and submaximal aerobic fitness can be included. Field tests such as runs for time or distance or a step test can be included. Fibre typing can be used as a measure of the capacity of the muscular system to perform aerobically or anaerobically. Muscle fibre type has been used to profile athletes in certain sports. Nygaard and Nielson (1978) showed that swimmer's show fewer type II muscle fibres in the upper body than a control group, thus supporting the belief that swimming training methods selectively utilize slow twitch muscle fibres. Not only should profiling be specific to each sport, but also within each sport athletes may play specific roles that require completely different demands on their respective musculoskeletal systems which may be reflected in the data obtained.

For instance, an American football team may be divided into groups: linemen, tight ends, linebackers, offensive running backs and quarterbacks, and defensive backs and wide receivers. The group of linemen may show greater upper body tightness than other positions (Gleim, 1984) and may demonstrate a negative correlation between total leg strength and flexibility. Body fat was correlated directly to time in the 45-yard dash, thus the slower players demonstrated a higher percentage of body fat and were also linemen.

Testing formats

The evaluation of sports-specific adaptations or sports-specific preparedness with a sports-specific examination is best accomplished in a preseason fitness examination. The most efficient and most commonly used method for collecting data in this examination is a station testing format (Hershman, 1984; Kibler, 1990b) where athletes move from one testing area to the next. Organization and prior planning are keys to an efficient use of space, equipment, testing personnel and the athlete's time. An alternative to the station method is the straight line format where athletes must enter at one station and proceed to the next (Kibler, 1990b). The straight line method, however, leaves some stations idle, thus wasting time. With the station format, all of the stations can be collecting data at the same time. This reduces the amount of time it takes an athlete to complete the evaluation. The advantages of the straight line format are that the sequence of testing events can be controlled so that each athlete is able to complete each test with the same degree of fatigue or amount of rest as the other athletes. By controlling the order of testing, the results should be more reproducible, making comparisons between athletes as well as comparison of an individual athlete from one year to the next more accurate.

After relevant sport-specific fitness parameters have been chosen, space, personnel and equipment for testing must be chosen. This can keep wasted time to a minimum, thus avoiding confusion, sloppy data collection, bottlenecks and aggravation for all involved parties. Large numbers of athletes can thus be tested in a relatively short amount of time. Examinations can be performed in gymnasiums, sports medicine centres or by individual physicians on a one on one basis. Sports medicine centres have the advantage of being better equipped to measure clinical data such as Cybex evaluations, urinalysis and blood analysis in a short period of time. The clinical setting is suited to private evaluation of the athlete in examination rooms. These rooms should be clearly marked and separated such that a smooth flow of traffic is possible, providing curtains as necessary for privacy. The gymnasium provides several advantages and disadvantages compared to the clinical format. There is generally plenty of space to handle large numbers of athletes comfortably. There is, however, a lack of private examination rooms and specialized equipment found in the clinical setting. There are several advantages of the individual examination of athletes. The opportunity exists for a more thorough medical evaluation, but the amount of testing that can be done depends on the equipment available to the physician. This method is costly in terms of the amount of time the physician has to spend with each athlete. In both the straight line and the station format, athletes may carry testing cards with them from station to station (Thompson et al., 1982). The data cards are then seen by appropriate personnel at each station.

The orthopaedic evaluation is important to detect incompletely rehabilitated injuries, as well as predispositions to injury due to weakness and inflexibility. Pathology may be identified via 'break-point strength testing' (Hershman, 1984), strength tests with weights or machines using an 'X' repetition maximum, or with isokinetic testing. Generalized weakness in the ipsilateral limb or trunk may be due to isolated pathology in an adjacent limb (Nicholas, 1970). Strength testing of 'suspect' limbs may give an early indication of pathology. For instance, the duck walk is difficult to perform with knee pathology (Hershman, 1984) or hopping may show dysfunction in the hip abductor musculature (Nicholas, 1970). Other measurements may be taken of leg length, gait, spine alignment, tibial shape, elbow and ankle range of movement, and Achilles tendon tenderness.

A line of authority must be established with the doctor usually in charge (Kibler, 1990b). However, physical therapists, exercise physiologists, athletic trainers or nurses may also be responsible if they are more intimately involved in the preparticipation fitness evaluation.

A model for musculoskeletal testing of athletes

Profiling of the sport or activity in terms of demands on the athlete is an important component of a profiling system. A model for testing athletes has been developed based on the sports characterization system developed by Kibler (1990b) that rates a variety of sports in terms of the requirements of the sport relative to different muscle parameters. Muscle tissue has five measurable characteristics that are basic to all athletic activity: (i) flexibility; (ii) strength; (iii) power; (iv) anaerobic endurance; and (v) aerobic endurance. Flexibility is the ability of a muscle–tendon unit to lengthen through a full range of motion without undue stress to the muscle–tendon complex and surrounding joint structures. Strength is the ability of the muscle to exert force. Power is the ability of a muscle to exert force in a short time period. Anaerobic endurance is the ability of the muscle to perform repeated short intense bouts of work. Aerobic endurance is the ability of the muscle to work repeatedly at low intensities for long periods of time. All muscular activities during sport are related to a combination of these basic parameters in the characterization process.

Each parameter can be given a relative value of importance for a particular sport or activity in terms of performance and injury prevention. A rating scale was developed (Kibler, 1990b) (Table 17.1) that ranks each parameter's relative importance in a variety of sports. It should be noted that there is a degree of subjectivity with the assignment of values for each sport, but this system will provide some uniformity for looking at each sport and quantifying the differences in each sport. Notice also that sports

Table 17.1 Use of a rating system of importance of fitness variables to a sport or function within a sport.

Sport or function	Flexibility	Strength	Speed	Endurance	
				Anaerobic	Aerobic
Football	2	4	4	4	2
Basketball	3	3	4	4	4
Tennis	3	3	4	4	4
Baseball	3	3	3	3	2
pitching	4	3	2	4	4
Running	3	2	2	2	4
Sprinting	4	3	4	4	2

1, Variable is needed at a minimal level.
2, Variable is needed at a certain level, usually for injury prevention.
3, Variable is synergistic to best performance of sport or sporting function.
4, Variable is essential to best performance of sport or sporting function.

can exhibit 'position specific' characteristics. The rating scale provides information to the athlete in a variety of areas; the demands of the sport, the characteristics of the athlete important to performance in a sport, and guidelines for the areas of necessary improvement.

Kibler (1990b) has recommended a battery of tests that focus on the musculoskeletal system that relate to these five parameters of muscle function. These tests provide objective data that is reproducible, and can be used in mass preparticipation testing settings. Not all of the tests should be used in each examination. Only the tests that are appropriate for generating sport-specific information should be used for each examination. Table 17.2 lists the tests, and the personnel and equipment necessary for each. Table 17.3 lists the recommended tests for each sport.

Registration or check-in should include a medical history, questionnaire and basic anthropometric data collection such as height and weight. The medical history should include both personal and family history.

The flexibility station may include measurements of the lower back (sit and reach) quadriceps, hamstrings, gastrocnemius, iliotibial band, dominant shoulder internal and external rotation, forearm pronation/supination and wrist flexion/extension. Tests for muscular strength and endurance should include sit-ups, push-ups, vertical jump, leg or shoulder strength and endurance which can be measured by an isokinetic testing device. Power can be measured via the vertical jump, medicine-ball push, or with isokinetic testing (Figs 17.1–17.8).

Aerobic endurance can be measured via a number of methods including a submaximal or maximal stress test on a cycle ergometer or treadmill, a step test, or a 1.6–3.2-km (1–2 mile) run. Anaerobic endurance, including speed and agility, may be measured via jumping jacks for 1 min, 18-m (20-yard) dash, shuttle run or hexagon drill, and sit-ups and push-ups in 1 min. Body fat can be measured either via hydrostatic weighing or skinfolds. The skinfold method is generally chosen for mass screenings, with hydrostatic weighing being used only for special situations.

The final station should be the check-out. This is an opportunity for the physician to pull everything together and council the athlete in an appropriate manner. Testing data can be compared to norm tables related to age and gender, recommendations can be made for correction of any deficits or for a proper conditioning programme, medical history may be related to data collection, and a sport-specific plan of

Table 17.2 Tests which can be used in the preparticipation examination, giving personnel and equipment needed.

Parameter and test	Equipment	Personnel
Flexibility		
Sit-and-reach exam of lower back	Sit-and-reach box	Trainer or therapist
Goniometric exam of the following:	Goniometer	Trainer or therapist
shoulder internal/external rotation		
shoulder flexion/extension		
elbow flexion/extension		
wrist flexion/extension		
hip flexion/extension		
hip internal/external rotation		
knee flexion (quadriceps flexibility)		
knee extension (hamstring flexibility)		
iliotibial band flexibility		
gastrocnemius flexibility		
Strength		
Sit-ups	Watch, mat	Clerical
Push-ups	Mat	Clerical
Handgrip strength	Dynamometer	Clerical
One repetition squat	Squat bench and weights	Trainer or therapist
Dips	Dip bench	Clerical
Cybex exam peak torque	Cybex	Trainer or therapist
Power		
Cybex exam time to peak torque	Cybex	Trainer or therapist
Vertical jump	Open area, chalk, tape measure or yardstick	Clerical
Medicine-ball throw	Medicine ball, tape measure	Clerical
Anaerobic endurance		
Jumping jacks in 1 min	Watch	Clerical
40- or 20-yard dash	Tape, tape measure, stopwatch	Clerical
Shuttle run	Five tennis balls, stopwatch, tape	Clerical
Hexagon drill	Goniometer, tape, ruler, stopwatch	Clerical
Sit-ups in 1 min	Watch, mat	Clerical
Aerobic endurance		
Step test	Step test box, stopwatch, metronome	Clerical
Timed mile run	Stopwatch	Coaches
Submaximal treadmill or bicycle stress test	Treadmill or bicycle ergometer	Physician, physiologist

Table 17.3 Recommended tests for each sport.

Parameter and test	Football	Basketball	Baseball	Tennis	Swimming	Long-distance running	Sprinting	Golf	Soccer	Volleyball	Cheerleading
Flexibility											
Sit-and-reach	X		X	X	X	X	X	X	X	X	X
Shoulder internal/external rotation			X	X	X			X	X	X	X
Shoulder flexion/extension		X	X	X	X		X	X	X	X	X
Elbow flexion/extension			X	X	X			X		X	
Wrist flexion/extension			X	X	X			X		X	
Hip flexion/extension		X	X	X		X	X		X	X	X
Hip internal/external rotation		X	X	X			X		X	X	X
Knee flexion (quadriceps flexibility)	X	X	X	X	X	X	X	X	X	X	X
Knee extension (hamstring flexibility)	X	X	X	X	X	X	X	X	X	X	X
Iliotibial band	X	X	X			X	X			X	X
Gastrocnemius	X	X	X	X		X	X		X	X	X
Strength											
Sit-ups	X	X	X	X	X	X	X	X	X	X	X
Push-ups	X	X		X	X			X	X	X	X
Handgrip dynamometer	X	X	X	X	X	X	X	X	X	X	
One repetition squat	X										
Dips	X	X			X						
Cybex exam peak torque	X	X	X	X	X	X	X	X	X	X	X
Power											
Cybex exam time to peak torque	X	X	X	X	X	X	X	X	X	X	X
Vertical jump	X	X	X	X			X	X	X	X	X
Medicine-ball throw	X	X		X			X	X	X	X	X
Anaerobic endurance											
Jumping jacks in 1 min			X		X	X	X	X	X	X	X
40- or 20-yard dash	X	X					X				
Shuttle run			X	X			X		X	X	
Hexagon drill			X	X			X		X	X	
Sit-ups in 1 min	X	X	X	X	X	X	X	X	X	X	
Aerobic endurance											
Step test	X	X	X	X	X	X		X	X	X	
Timed mile run				X		X	X	X	X	X	
Submaximal treadmill or bicycle stress test	X	X			X	X	X	X			X

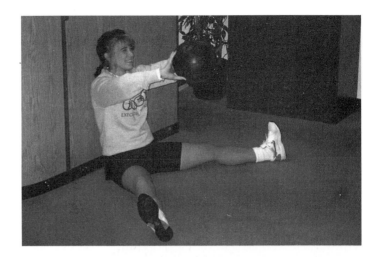

Fig. 17.1 Medicine-ball push.

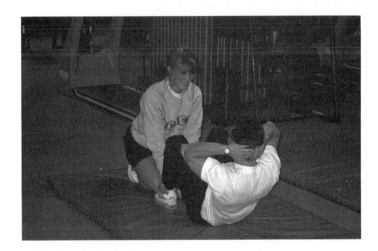

Fig. 17.2 Sit-ups.

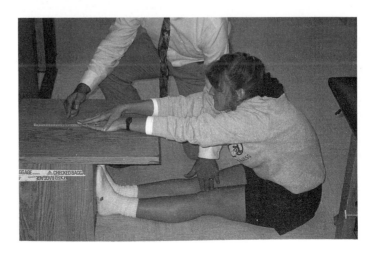

Fig. 17.3 Sit-and-reach.

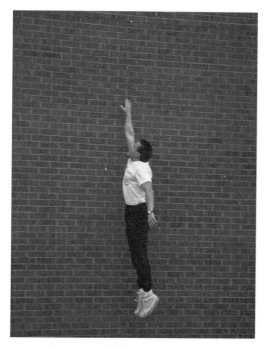

Fig. 17.4 Vertical jump.

action may then be initiated for training or therapy. These results and plan of action may be reviewed with the coach and/or the parent so that any problems or deficiencies may be worked out with the athlete.

Results

Data have been collected on a number of athletes in a number of sports utilizing the above format. In a study that demonstrates the sport-specific musculoskeletal adaptations imposed by the demands of the sport, Kibler *et al.* (1989) tested 1478 male and 629 female athletes in strength and flexibility. The subjects were divided into upper body and lower body, and into males and females, depending on the primary area of tensile load in their respective sports. The results showed that males were significantly stronger than the females in all parameters tested, but the females were significantly more flexible than the males in all muscle groups tested. In addition, the athletes were

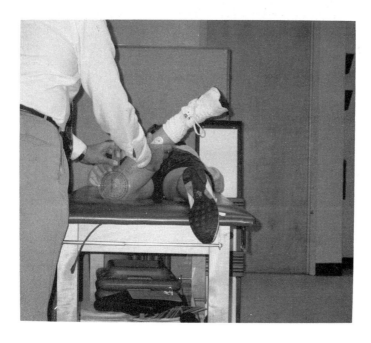

Fig. 17.5 Hip external rotation roll.

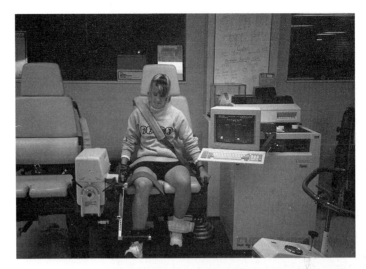

Fig. 17.6 Knee flexion/extension (Cybex).

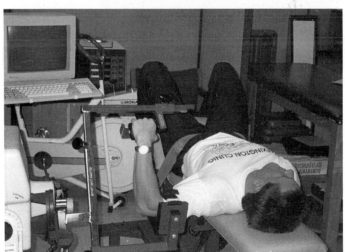

Fig. 17.7 Shoulder internal rotation/external rotation (Cybex).

divided into upper-body and lower-body athletes. Although there is an overlap in this classification, lower-body athletes were classified as those athletes whose primary sport involved tensile loads primarily to the lower body; and upper-body athletes were those athletes whose primary sport involved tensile loads primarily to the upper body. Lower-body athletes, both males and females, tended to be less flexible in the lower body measurements than upper-body athletes. Females, although more flexible in general showed a tendency toward inflexibility in those muscle groups that were placed under tensile load in the sport or activity. Upper-body athletes demonstrated a decrease in shoulder internal rotation and an increase in shoulder external rotation in both the dominant and non-dominant arms. All athletes tended to show tightness in the muscle groups corresponding to areas of tensile loads applied during a sport.

Tennis has been evaluated in depth utilizing

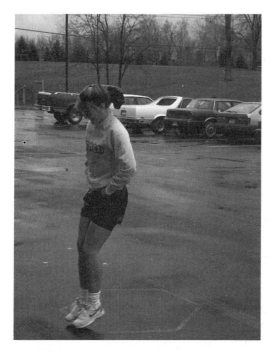

Fig. 17.8 Hexagon agility test.

Table 17.4 Specific tests used in the tennis examination.

Parameter and test	Tennis
Flexibility	
Sit-and-reach	×
Shoulder internal/external rotation	×
Shoulder flexion/extension	×
Elbow flexion/extension	×
Wrist flexion/extension	×
Hip flexion/extension	×
Hip internal/external rotation	×
Knee flexion (quadriceps flexibility)	×
Knee extension (hamstring flexibility)	×
Iliotibial band	×
Gastrocnemius	×
Strength	
Sit-ups	×
Push-ups	×
Handgrip dynamometer	×
One repetition squat	
Dips	
Cybex exam peak torque	×
Power	
Cybex exam time to peak torque	×
Vertical jump	×
Medicine-ball throw	×
Anaerobic endurance	
Jumping jacks in 1 min	
40- or 20-yard dash	×
Shuttle run	×
Hexagon drill	×
Sit-ups in 1 min	×
Aerobic endurance	
Step test	×
Timed mile run	
Submaximal treadmill or bicycle stress test	

the proposed model. Table 17.4 shows the specific tests used in the tennis examination; Fig. 17.9 shows a completed copy of the examination.

Flexibility adaptations in tennis can be observed and may be related to the use patterns of dominant versus non-dominant limbs used in playing the sport, much like that of other throwing sports (Chandler *et al.*, 1990). The repetitive demands of tennis place the shoulder under maximum stress. Chandler *et al.* (1990) found that flexibility differences in tennis players were related to the musculoskeletal demands imposed by the sport. Tennis players were significantly tighter in the sit and reach and dominant and non-dominant shoulder internal rotation, but more flexible than non-tennis players in dominant and non-dominant external rotation.

Chandler *et al.* (1991) demonstrated that college level tennis players increase the strength of the shoulder musculature in internal rotation, without subsequent strengthening of the external rotator muscle group, creating a functional muscle imbalance that may predispose the athlete to injury. Using the non-domi-

Name JOHN		Age 16 Sex M Date 17-11-92		
Dominant hand Ⓡ L		Sport TENNIS		
Year/age		1992/16		
Height		68 W		
Weight		145 lbs		
Blood pressure		117/78		
Resting pulse		72		
% body fat		12.7		
Low back (box)		-2 cm		
Hamstring	R	53		
	L	58		
Gastrocnemius	R	5		
	L	6		
Quadriceps	R	125		
	L	130		
IT band	R	5		
	L	7		
Hip I.R.	R	43		
	L	38		
Hip E.R.	R	41		
	L	37		
Hip flexion	R	0		
	L	0		
Shoulder I.R.	R	36		
	L	48		
Shoulder E.R.	R	98		
	L	94		
Forearm pronation	R	79		
	L	91		
Forearm supination	R	83		
	L	96		
Wrist flexion	R	81		
	L	90		
Wrist extension	R	90		
	L	90		
Sit-ups (1 min)		53		
Push-ups (1 min)		40		
Grip strength	R	85		
	L	80		
Vertical jump		15.5		
CR endurance		51.63		
Hexagon		10.86		
20-yard dash		2.81		
5-point agility		16.90		
Medicine ball		230.0 IN		

Fig. 17.9 A completed fitness evaluation sheet for a highly ranked junior tennis player. Courtesy of the Lexington Clinic Sports Medicine Center. E.R., external rotation; I.R., internal rotation.

nant arm as a control, these tennis players demonstrated significantly greater strength in internal rotation in peak torque at $60° \cdot s^{-1}$, peak torque at $300° \cdot s^{-1}$, average power at $60° \cdot s^{-1}$, and average power at $300° \cdot s^{-1}$. In external rotation, the tennis players were significantly stronger on only one of the four measurements, peak torque at $300° \cdot s^{-1}$. By increasing the strength of the internal rotator muscle groups without subsequent strengthening of the external rotators, a muscle imbalance is created that may predispose the athlete to overload injury.

Kibler (1989) found that aerobic and anaerobic endurance were above average in tennis players.

Analysis of the metabolic demands of tennis show that even though tennis players run long cumulative distances over long cumulative times, tennis is basically an anaerobic sport. The average tennis point lasts between 2.3 and 14.6 s, depending on the surface, sex or skill level. The average work/rest ratio is about $1:2.6$ to $1:4.8$.

Thus, the profile that develops in an average high-intensity tennis player shows good points and bad points in relation to the demands of the sport. The high aerobic and anaerobic capacity of the player indicates a good ability to respond to the metabolic demands of the sport. However, the inflexibility and strength findings indicate additional risk factors for injuries and decreased performance. These can be corrected to provide optimum prevention of injuries. Only by testing for these sport-specific characteristics can this prevention be done.

Conclusion

Collected data from preparticipation examinations is the starting point, not only for injury prevention, but also the road to maximizing athletic performance. Negative information which would disqualify an athlete from participation is not obtained frequently, only approximately 1–5% of the time (Rice, 1979; Tennant

et al., 1981). The occurrence of negative information is generally associated with injury or other pathology such as hypertension, diabetes, cardiovascular disease, gross obesity, unstable joints and incompletely healed fractures.

Positive information, such as joint inflexibilities, muscle imbalances and inadequate rehabilitation are much more frequently observed and can be used to reduce injury risk to the musculoskeletal system of the athlete. Inflexibility and muscle weakness may indicate that the athlete's musculoskeletal system has sustained microtrauma in the past due to inabilities to tolerate past physical activities (Kibler, 1990b). The incidence of finding this type of injury varies between sports, but can be seen in a good profiling examination in as high as 75% of the athletes. Reproducibility of the preparticipation fitness evaluation is obviously important, as is validity of the results. Data acquisition must be comprehensive, efficient, accurate, and must be related to gender-related and age-related norms. Tests should be chosen based on the demands of the sport, and should provide an adequate general physical examination. In addition, acquired data must be related to the athlete in a practical and understandable manner.

The information obtained during a preparticipation fitness evaluation can be shared with the athlete and all other relevant parties such as the parent, coach, exercise physiologist, nurse, physical therapist or team physician. This sharing of information can be done only if informed consent is given and proper release forms have been signed. If rehabilitation is needed, it should be done using a multidisciplinary approach that includes all the members of the sports medicine team. If this information is to be valuable to the athlete and coach, it must provide a basis for rehabilitation if necessary, and a plan for conditioning the athlete to reach maximal athletic potential.

A system of profiling should be employed for both the sport and the athlete. In this manner, demands specific to the sport may be understood, and the individual athlete's preparedness to respond to the demands may be identified. These two factors interact at the 'critical point' (see Fig. 19.1) to determine athletic performance and injury risk. Most sports medicine investigators look at the results of the interaction. Use of this model allows a look at the factors that may favourably affect the results of the interaction.

References

Adams, A. (1966) Effect of exercise upon ligaments and tendons. *Med. Sci. Sports* 7(3), 165–75.

Agne, J.C., Casal, D.C., Leon, A.S., McNally, C., Baxter, T.L. & Serfass, R.C. (1987) Professional ice hockey players: Physiology, anthropometric, and musculoskeletal characteristics. *Arch. Phys. Med. Rehab.* 69(3), 188–92.

Alderink, G.J. & Kuck, D.J. (1986) Isokinetic shoulder strength of high school and college-aged pitchers. *J. Orthop. Sports Phys. Ther.* 7, 163–72.

Armstrong, R.B. (1990) Initial events in exercise-induced muscular injury. *Med. Sci. Sports Exerc.* 22(4), 429–35.

Armstrong, R.B., Ogilvie, R.W. & Schwane, J.A. (1983) Eccentric exercise-induced injury to rat skeletal muscle. *J. Appl. Physiol.* 54, 80–93.

Atha, J. (1980) Strengthening muscle. *Exerc. Sport Sci. Rev.* 9, 1–73.

Bender, J.A., Pierson, J.K., Kaplan, H.M. & Johnson, A.J. (1964) Factors affecting the occurrence of knee injuries. *J. Assoc. Phys. Ment. Rehab.* 18, 130–5.

Brown, L.P., Niehues, S.L., Harrah, A. *et al.* (1988) Upper extremity range of motion and isokinetic strength of internal and external shoulder rotations in major league baseball players. *Am. J. Sports Med.* 16, 577–85.

Chandler, T.J., Kibler, W.B., Kiser, A.M. & Wooten, B.P. (1992) Shoulder strength, power, and endurance in college tennis players. *Am. J. Sports Med.* 20(4), 455–7.

Chandler, T.J., Kibler, W.B., Uhl, T.L., Wooten, B., Kiser, A. & Stone, E. (1990) Flexibility comparisons of junior élite tennis players to other athletes. *Am. J. Sports Med.* 18(2), 134–6.

Cook, E.E., Gray, V.L., Savinar-Nogue, E. & Medeiros, J. (1987) Shoulder antagonistic strength ratios: A comparison between college-level baseball pitchers and nonpitchers. *J. Orthop. Sports Phys. Ther.* 8(9), 451–61.

Dominguez, R.H. (1978) Shoulder pain in age group swimmers. In B. Eriksson & B. Furberg (eds) *Swimming Medicine*, Vol. IV, pp. 105–9. University Park Press, Baltimore.

Ekstrand, J. & Gillquist, J. (1982) The frequency of muscle tightness and injuries in soccer players. *Am. J. Sports Med.* 10(2), 75–8.

Falch, J.A. (1982) The effect of physical activity on the skeleton. *Scand. J. Soc. Med.* 29(Suppl.), 55–8.

Falkel, J.E. (1990) Swimming injuries. In B. Sanders (ed) *Sports Physical Therapy*, pp. 477–504. Appleton & Lang, Connecticut.

Fleck, S.J. & Falkel, J.E. (1986) Value of resistance training for the reduction of sports injuries. *Sports Med.* 3, 61–8.

Garrett, W.E. (1990) Muscle strain injuries: Clinical and basic aspects. *Med. Sci. Sports Exerc.* 22(4), 436–43.

Garrett, W.E., Califf, J.C. & Bassett, F.H. (1984) Histochemical correlates of hamstring injuries. *Am. J. Sports Med.* 12(2), 98–103.

Garrett, W.E., Safran, M.R., Seaber, A.V., Glisson, R.R. & Ribbeck, B.M. (1987) Biomechanical comparison of stimulated and nonstimulated skeletal muscle pulled to failure. *Am. J. Sports Med.* 15(5), 448–54.

Garrett, W.E. & Tidball, J. (1987) Myotendinous junction: Structure, function and failure. In S.L. Woo & J.A. Buckwalter (eds) *Injury and Repair of Musculoskeletal Soft Tissues.* American Academy of Orthopaedic Surgeons and National Institute of Arthritis and Musculoskeletal and Skin Diseases, Chicago.

Gleim, G.W. (1984) The profiling of professional football players. *Clin. Sports Med.* 3(1), 185–97.

Grace, T.G. (1985) Muscle imbalance extremity injury: A perplexing relationship. *Sports Med.* 2, 77–82.

Grace, T.G., Sweetser, E.R., Nelson, M.A., Ydens, L.R. & Skipper, B.F. (1984) Isokinetic muscle imbalance and knee joint injuries. *J. Bone Joint Surg.* 66A, 734–40.

Grana, W.A. & Moretz, J.A. (1978) Ligamentous laxity in secondary school athletes. *JAMA* 240(18), 1975–6.

Gurry, M., Pappas, A., Michaels, J., Maher, P., Shakman, A., Goldberg, R. & Rippe, J. (1985) A comprehensive preseason fitness evaluation for professional baseball players. *Phys. Sports Med.* 13(6), 63–74.

Hawkins, R.J. & Kennedy, J.C. (1980) Impingement syndrome in athletes. *Am. J. Sports Med.* 8, 151–8.

Heiser, T.M., Weber, J., Sullivan, G., Clare, P. & Jacobs, P.P. (1984) Prophylaxis and management of hamstring muscle injuries in intercollegiate football. *Am. J. Sports Med.* 12, 368–70.

Hershman, E. (1984) The profile for prevention of musculoskeletal injury. *Clin. Sports Med.* 3(1), 65–84.

Hinton, R.Y. (1988) Isokinetic evaluation of shoulder rotational strength in high school baseball pitchers. *Am. J. Sports Med.* 16(3), 274–9.

Ivey, F.M., Calhoun, J.H., Rusche, K. & Biershenk, J. (1985) Isokinetic testing of the shoulder strength: Normal values. *Arch. Phys. Med. Rehab.* **66**, 384–6.

Jackson, D.L. & Nyland, J. (1990) Club lacrosse: A physiological and injury profile. *Ann. Sports Med.* **5**, 114–17.

Jones, H.H., Priest, J.D., Hayes, W.C., Tichenor, C.C. & Nagel, D.A. (1977) Humeral hypertrophy in response to exercise. *J. Bone Joint Surg.* **59A**, 204–8.

Kalenak, A. & Morehouse, C.A. (1975) Knee stability and knee ligament injuries. *JAMA* **243**, 1143–5.

Kibler, W.B. (1990a) Clinical aspects of muscle injury. *Med. Sci. Sports Exerc.* **22**(4), 450–2.

Kibler, W.B. (1990b) *The Sport Preparticipation Fitness Examination.* Human Kinetics, Illinois.

Kibler, W.B. & Chandler, T.J. (1993) Musculoskeletal adaptations and injuries associated with intense participation in youth sports. In B. Cahill (ed) *The Effect of Intensive Training on Prepubescent Athletes in Sports.* American Academy of Orthopaedic Surgeons, Chicago (in press).

Kibler, W.B., Chandler, T.J., Uhl, T. & Maddux, R.E. (1989) A musculoskeletal approach to the preparticipation physical examination, preventing injury and improving performance. *Am. J. Sports Med.* **17**(4), 525–31.

Kibler, W.B., Goldberg, C. & Chandler, T.J. (1991) Functional biomechanical deficits in running athletes with plantar fasciitis. *Am. J. Sports Med.* **19**(1), 66–71.

Kibler, W.B., McQueen, C. & Uhl, T. (1988) Fitness evaluations and fitness findings in competitive junior tennis players. *Clin. Sports Med.* **7**(2), 403–16.

Knapik, J.J., Bauman, C.L., Jones, B.H., Harris, J.M. & Vaughn, L. (1991) Preseason strength and flexibility imbalances associated with athletic injuries in female collegiate athletes. *Am. J. Sports Med.* **19**(1), 76–81.

Kovanen, V., Suominen, H. & Heikkinen, E. (1980) Connective tissue of fast and slow skeletal muscle in rats — Effects of endurance training. *Acta Phys. Scand.* **108**, 173–80.

Kovanen, V., Suominen, H. & Heikkinen, E. (1984) Collagen of slow and fast twitch muscle fibers in different types of rat skeletal muscle. *Eur. J. App. Physiol.* **52**, 235–43.

Laurent, G.J., Sparrow, M.P., Bates, P.C. & Milward, D.J. (1978) Collagen content and turnover in cardiac and skeletal muscles of the adult fowl and the changes during stretch-induced growth. *Biochem. J.* **176**, 419–27.

Lieber, R.L. & Friden, J. (1988) Selective damage of fast glycolytic muscle fibers with eccentric contraction of the rabbit tibialis anterior. *Acta Physiol. Scand.* **133**, 587–8.

MacBryde, A.M. (1985) Stress fractures in runners. *Clin. Sports Med.* **4**, 737–52.

McMaster, W.C., Long, S.C. & Caiozzo, V.J. (1991) Isokinetic torque imbalances in the rotator cuff of the élite water polo player. *Am. J. Sports Med.* **19**(1), 72–5.

Micheli, L.J. (1982) Upper-extremity injuries: Overuse injuries in the recreational adult. In R.C. Cantu (ed) *The Exercising Adult*, pp. 121–8. Collamore Press, Massachusetts.

Montoye, H.J., Smith, E.L., Fardon, D.F. & Howley, E.T. (1980) Bone mineral in senior tennis players. *Scand. J. Sports Sci.* **2**, 26–32.

Nicholas, J.A. (1970) Injuries to knee ligaments: Relationship to looseness and tightness in football players. *JAMA* **212**(13), 2236–9.

Nilsson, B.E. & Westlin, N.E. (1971) Bone density in athletes. *Clin. Orthop. Rel. Res.* **77**, 179–82.

Nygaard, E. & Nielson, E. (1978) Skeletal muscle fiber capillerization in extreme endurance training in man. In B. Eriksson & B. Furberg (eds) *Swimming Medicine*, Vol. IV, pp. 282–93. University Park Press, Baltimore.

Ogilvie, R.W., Armstrong, R.B., Baird, K.E. & Bottoms, C.L. (1988) Lesions in the rat soleus muscle following eccentrically-biased exercise. *Am. J. Anat.* **182**, 335–46.

Parker, M.G., Ruhling, R.O., Holt, D., Bauman, E. & Drayna, M. (1988) Descriptive analysis of quadriceps and hamstrings muscle torque in high school football players. *J. Orthop. Sports Phys. Ther.* **5**, 2–6.

Renström, P. & Johnson, R.J. (1985) Overuse injuries in sports. *Sports Med.* **2**, 316–33.

Rice, S.G. (1979) Sports medicine. *JCE Pediatr*, **21**, 13–34.

Safran, M.R., Seaber, A.V. & Garrett, W.E. (1989) Warm-up and muscular injury prevention. *Sports Med.* **8**(4), 239–49.

Staff, P.H. (1982) The effect of physical activity on joints, cartilage, tendons, and ligaments. *Scand. J. Soc. Med.* **29** (Suppl.), 59–63.

Stone, M.H. (1990) Muscle conditioning and muscle injuries. *Med. Sci. Sports Exerc.* **22**(4), 457–62.

Taimela, S., Kujala, U.M. & Osterman, K. (1989) *Individual characteristics are related to musculoskeletal injuries* (Abstract). Paavo Nurmi Congress, Turku, Finland, Aug. 28 to Sept. 1.

Talag, T.S. (1973) Residual muscular soreness as influenced by concentric, eccentric, and static contractions. *Res. Q.* **44**, 458–69.

Tennant, F.S., Sorenson, K. & Day, C.M. (1981) Benefits of preparticipation sports examinations. *J. Fam. Pract.* **13**(2), 287–8.

Thompson, T.R., Andrish, J.T. & Bergfeld, J.A. (1982) A prospective study of preparticipation sports examinations of 2670 young athletes: Methods and results. *Clev. Clin. Q.* **49**, 225–33.

Tipton, C.M., James, S.L., Mergner, W. & Tcheng, T. (1970) Influence of exercise on strength of medial collateral knee ligaments of dogs. *Am. J. Physiol.* **218**(3), 894–902.

Tipton, C.M., Matthes, R.D., Maynard, J.A. & Carey, R.A. (1975) The influence of physical activity on ligaments and tendons. *Med. Sci. Sports* **7**(3), 165–75.

Turto, H., Lindy, S. & Halme, J. (1974) Protocollagen proline hydroxylase activity in work-induced hypertrophy of rat muscle. *Am. J. Physiol.* **226**, 63–5.

Watson, R.C. (1974) *Bone growth and physical activity in young males*. International Conference on Bone Mineral Measurements. US Department of Health, Education, and Welfare, Publication No. NIH 75–683, 380–5.

Chapter 18

Warming Up and Cooling Down

THOMAS M. BEST AND WILLIAM E. GARRETT Jr

The field of sports medicine has experienced a rapid growth in knowledge about the diagnosis and treatment of athletic injuries. Despite the fact that warming up and cooling down appear to provide numerous physiological and mechanical benefits, there has been surprisingly little research carried out to support these theories. Although warming up and cooling down form an integral part of athletic performance almost universally, experimental and clinical evidence are lacking to conclude that they aid in injury prevention.

Effects of heat

Connective tissue

It has been difficult to reach a consensus about the effects of temperature on the mechanical properties of soft tissues. Several authors have reported that the stress–strain and relaxation behaviour of tendons and ligaments is unaffected by alteration of temperature within the physiological range (Rigby et al., 1958; Dorlot et al., 1980). In contrast, others have shown a temperature dependence of the mechanical properties of tendons and ligaments. Walker et al. (1976) demonstrated that the elastic modulus was decreased and the hysteresis energy increased in canine Achilles and patellar tendons when the temperature was increased from 23 to 49°C. Woo et al. (1987) reported similar findings on the viscoelastic properties of the canine medial collateral ligament and found

that the cyclic load relaxation behaviour plateaued at a higher value at lower temperatures. Furthermore, the tensile load at a predetermined ligament strain level was inversely related to temperature.

Skeletal muscle

A considerable amount of work has been done on the thermal effects on skeletal muscle. This may be an important consideration since superficial muscles in particular are capable of wide fluctuations in temperature in response to extreme ambient conditions (Saltin & Hermansen, 1966; Pugh, 1967; Saltin et al., 1970). Intramuscular temperature can be altered in response to a number of conditions typically classified as either passive warming, e.g. sauna baths or heat packs, or active warming, e.g. exercise.

Studies on the contractile function of muscle have demonstrated little change in maximum isometric force in response to increases in temperature (Close & Hoh, 1968; Edwards et al., 1972; Ranatunga, 1982). On the other hand, the kinetics of tension development can be influenced by temperature. Hill (1938) found that increasing the temperature of muscle improved its contractile speed. Other studies have reported that time to peak tension is decreased when temperature is increased (Close & Hoh, 1968; Petrofsky & Lind, 1981). In humans, Davies and Young (1983) found that increasing muscle temperature by 3.1°C caused a decrease in both contraction time and one-half relaxation time by 7 and 22%, respectively. Twitch and tetanic tensions were not affected. In contrast, a decrease in intramuscular temperature by 8.4°C resulted in an increase in both contraction time (38%) and one-half relaxation time (93%). Taken together, these studies suggest that the relaxation rather than force development properties of muscle can be affected by temperature. Activation of skeletal muscle is known to increase its temperature from the heat of activation, from elastic energy and from the thermoelastic heat that is produced after the contraction ends (Hill, 1938, 1961). This warming effect of contraction lasts up to 0.5 h after the contraction (Hill, 1950). The effects of temperature on the neural activity of muscle have also been studied. Heating of a muscle reduces the activity of the γ nerve fibres and the sensitivity of the muscle spindles to stretch (Kulund & Tottossy, 1983). Furthermore, nerve conduction velocity increases at higher temperatures (Hill, 1927). This may be particularly important to individuals engaged in activities requiring rapid movement of body parts. Finally, data exists to suggest that the fatigue properties of muscle can be affected by temperature. Petrofsky and Lind (1981) found that maximum voluntary contractions and isometric endurance time in forearm muscles decreased at water temperatures below 20°C. In order to perform dynamic exercise in muscle cooled from 35 to 29°C, Blomstrand et al. (1986) speculated that more fast twitch fibres might be recruited. The greater participation of fast twitch glycolytic fibres could contribute to the higher rates of lactate production and shorter endurance times often noted with exercise in cold weather.

The general feeling is that muscle strain injuries are more common in cold weather and cold athletes; however, epidemiological studies are not available to confirm this clinical suspicion. The general consensus is that cold muscles are relatively stiff and that this stiffness predisposes to muscle injury (Brewer, 1960; Ekstrand & Gillquist, 1983). A recent laboratory study has provided support for this theory demonstrating that a decrease in muscle temperature results in an increase in stiffness and load developed by the injured muscle (Noonan et al., 1991). This thermally dependent increase in tissue elasticity has been shown in other tissues (Lehmann et al., 1970; Warren et al., 1971). Perhaps more convincing is the evidence that alterations in muscle temperature can lead to an improvement in athletic performance. Although muscle temperature primarily affects contractile speed and not maximum isometric force development, studies have reported an increase in peak power production (4% per °C) in activities such as cycling and the vertical jump (Sargeant, 1983). In a separate study, temperature increases in the vastus lateralis from 30.4 to 38.5°C resulted in a 44% increase in vertical jump and 32% increase in maximum cycling power (Bergh & Ekblom, 1979a).

Physiological effects

The systemic physiological effects of warm-up have been well studied. Physical activity creates a demand for increased blood flow to the contracting muscles to meet oxygen delivery requirements and to the skin to meet the heat transfer requirements of the temperature regulatory system. A large proportion of the energy released by the working muscles takes the form of heat, and this must be dissipated through the skin. Intensive exercise such as marathon running can result in heat production in the contracting muscles on the order of 15–18 times the basal metabolic rate. A heat production of this magnitutde is sufficient to raise the body core temperature of an average-sized individual by 1°C every 5 min if no temperature regulatory mechanisms are activated (Nadel et al., 1977). Warm-up results in an increase in both circulation and respiration and these effects help to promote heat transfer via increased cutaneous circulation to the skin surface where it can be dissipated primarily by the evaporation of sweat.

Martin et al. (1975) studied the effects of

warm-up on metabolic responses in strenuous exercise, and found that warm-up contributes to greater oxygen consumption thereby reducing the contribution from anaerobic metabolism. This in turn leads to a lower concentration of blood lactate. A study by Bergh and Ekblom (1979a) supports this finding. Although work time was not increased at the highest muscle temperature, blood lactate was considerably reduced in subjects performing a warm-up before their exercise. Some evidence exists that physical work capacity can be increased following warm-up (Asmussen & Böje, 1945). Subjects engaged in a 30-min warm-up were able to complete a 9300 Nm bicycle ride in much less time than when no warm-up was included.

On a cellular level, higher temperatures result in a more rapid and complete dissociation of oxygen from haemoglobin (Barcroft & King, 1909) and the release of oxygen from myoglobin is also increased (Asmussen & Böje, 1945). Åstrand and Rodahl (1977) claim warm-up to be beneficial because the increased temperature resulting from work allows for a higher metabolic process in the cells. They state that for each increase of 1°C, the metabolic rate of the cells increases by approximately 13%.

Several authors have suggested that warm-up makes an individual less susceptible to myocardial ischaemia at the onset of vigorous exercise (Bergh & Ekblom, 1979b; Kulund & Tottossy, 1983). Studies conducted by Barnard et al. (1973a,b) in normal asymptomatic men have demonstrated electrocardiogram changes of subendocardial ischaemia in 70% of the subjects who performed vigorous treadmill exercise for 10–15 s without prior warm-up. These changes could be decreased or diminished if a period of warm-up was performed prior to the strenuous exercise.

Effects of stretching

Connective tissues

Much research has been performed to develop

an understanding about the mechanics of soft tissues. We know from experimental and clinical studies that biological tissues are viscoelastic and that the time-dependent and history-dependent behaviour of these collagenous structures reflects the complex interaction of the collagen fibres and the surrounding protein matrix. Therefore, ligaments and tendons are often referred to as biphasic structures where the two phases are the collagen and ground substance. These two phases have strikingly different properties and together, help to explain much of the observed mechanical behaviour of soft tissues. The viscoelastic behaviour of ligaments and tendons provides relevant clinical and physiological significance. Stress relaxation (a reduction in load with time under a fixed deformation; Fig. 18.1a) and creep

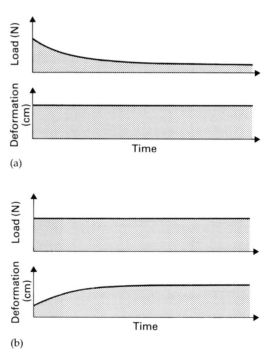

Fig. 18.1 (a) Load relaxation behaviour of a viscoelastic material. Note that the measured force falls off when the tissue is held at a constant length. (b) Creep behaviour of a viscoelastic material. Note that there is an increase in the length of the tissue when it is held at a constant load (force).

(an increase in length under constant loading; Fig. 18.1b) can both take place during exercise. For example, cyclic loading of the soft tissues to a fixed displacement that occurs during repetitive activities such as jogging and swimming can produce stress relaxation in the tissues and therefore a reduction in load at a given length. The increased ligamentous laxity seen post-exercise is an example of the creep properties of the tissue. The non-linear mechanical properties of these tissues is also important (Fig. 18.2). It is felt that the majority of human motion occurs in the toe region of the stress–strain curve where large increases in strain result in a small increase in stress. This helps to protect the musculoskeletal system during periods of high loading of the joints.

Skeletal muscle

Traditionally, it has been felt that all stretching techniques are based on a neurophysiological phenomenon involving the stretch reflex (Beaulieu, 1981; Prentice, 1983). Recent studies have challenged this concept and suggest that the changes brought about by stretching may be independent of reflex effects. Experiments on

rabbit muscle have demonstrated that changes in the load-deflection properties of passively stretched muscle can occur independently of innervation to the muscle (Taylor et al., 1990). Effects of anaesthesia and possible central nervous system depression could not be ruled out in this study. Another recent study has supported the idea that mechanical changes brought about by stretching can occur independently of nervous activity (Cole et al., 1991).

The effects of muscular activity may be totally different from the viscoelastic effects associated with stretching. Studies to evaluate these changes in failure properties of muscle held isometrically and stimulated for one single tetanic contraction lasting 10–15 s have been performed (Safran et al., 1988). This contraction was accompanied by a temperature rise of 1°C within the muscle. A single contraction did lead to changes in muscle failure properties as more stretch was possible prior to failure and more force was produced.

Injury prevention

Laboratory studies have demonstrated that the mechanical properties of connective tissues can be altered in response to loading and temperature variations which can bring about changes in joint range of motion (Woo et al., 1990). Based on these studies and the systemic benefits outlined above, it appears that an optimal routine would start with a warm-up to increase body temperature, followed by a stretching routine to enhance tissue extensibility.

Warm-up

Warming up is a term which can include light exercise, stretching and even psychological preparation. These programmes are usually individualized to the athlete and his or her sport and typically provide a subjective sensation of 'being ready' to perform. Warm-up regimens are usually classified by the following categories (Williford et al., 1986):

1 Passive warm-up – increases in body tem-

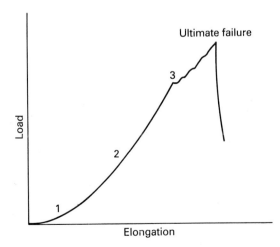

Fig. 18.2 Typical load–elongation behaviour in uniaxial tension. Note that the 'toe region' (1) is followed by a relatively linear region of constant stiffness (2), and then specimen failure (3).

perature by some external means, e.g. heating pads, steam baths or hot showers.

2 General warm-up – an increase in body temperature through active movement of the major muscle groups, e.g. jogging, callisthenics, etc. (Fig. 18.3).

3 Specific warm-up – an increase in body temperature by performing activities that involve the same movements as those involved in the actual exercise.

Williford *et al.* (1986) attempted to provide empirical evidence for warming up followed by stretching with the hypothesis that the combination of the two would increase joint flexibility. 51 subjects were studied and it was concluded that static stretching 2 days a week for 9 weeks resulted in increased flexibility, however warming the muscles prior to stretching with 5 min of jogging did not result in further significant increases in flexibility. As appropriately pointed out by the authors, this does not mean that some form of warm-up would not result in further increases in flexibility.

The optimal type of warm-up has long been debated. Conclusive evidence exists to show that passive warming, e.g. sauna baths and hot showers, are not as effective as active processes (Asmussen & Böje, 1945). In another study,

Högberg and Ljunggren (1947) compared the effect of warm-up in the form of running combined with calisthenics versus the effect of heating the body passively in a sauna bath for a period of 20 min prior to exercise. They found that the beneficial effects on performance of passively elevating the body temperature by such a bath was much less than that of elevating the body temperature by a warm-up through physical exercise. This is perhaps due to the fact that exercise to increase the body temperature results in a temperature increase due to both an alteration of metabolic processes as well as a change in the mechanical properties of the tissues. Long-distance runners in particular often spend little time stretching before a run and often use the first few minutes of their run to 'warm-up'. The role of massage before exercise to aid in preparation for the event has been very much challenged (DeVries, 1959; Wiktorsson-Möller *et al.*, 1983). It has been suggested that the effects of warm-up will persist for 45–80 min (Åstrand & Rodahl, 1977). This would of course depend largely on the activity level of the individual as well as the environmental conditions. An increase in rectal temperature of 1–2°C is felt to be sufficient for achievement of the temperature-related benefits of warm-up (DeVries, 1980). The simple

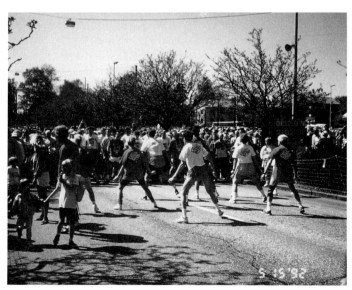

Fig. 18.3 A thorough warm-up is essential in any sports activity to avoid injury. This figure shows people encouraging participants in a half-marathon race to join in warm-up exercises. Courtesy of Dr P.A.F.H. Renström.

observance of a light to mild sweat in normal ambient conditions has been suggested as a reliable indicator of the appropriate elevation in body temperature (Saltin & Harmansen, 1966). Studies have not confirmed if these criteria do in fact result in the appropriate changes in body temperature and physiological adaptations.

It is felt that the muscles most frequently torn because of inadequate warm-up are those antagonistic to the strong contracting muscles (Morehouse & Miller, 1976). When unprepared, these antagonistic muscles relax slowly and incompletely, thus retarding free movement and hindering accurate coordinations. Adequate warm-up before exercise is often cited as a way to prevent these muscle strain injuries (Krejci & Koch, 1979; Wiktorsson-Möller et al., 1983). Based on the information currently available, it seems reasonable to accept that warm-up prior to exercise, particularly before exhaustive exercise, will help to reduce the incidence and severity of musculoskeletal injuries. Although the mechanism for this protection against injury is unknown, it is likely the result of both mechanical and physiological adaptations within the body.

Effects of stretching

There are three basic stretching techniques:
1 Ballistic — which makes use of repetitive bouncing motions.
2 Static — where the muscle is stretched usually to the point of discomfort and held at that point for a period of time.
3 Proprioceptive neuromuscular facilitation (PNF) — which uses alternating contractions and stretches of the muscle.

In the early 1900s, Sherrington (1906) defined the basic concepts of muscle facilitation and inhibition. Some of the concepts have formed the basis for specific PNF techniques. These methods are carried out with the belief that the prestretch contraction will cause the Golgi tendon organ to fire and relax the muscle. The muscle spindle and Golgi tendon organ are

receptors sensitive to stretch and change in muscle length. Each of the stretching techniques mentioned produces different responses in the stretch reflex. Although structured stretching protocols are used extensively for both preparation for competition and rehabilitation of injury, the preferred method of stretching still remains unknown. Despite the lack of consensus on the most effective way to stretch, the current thinking is that ballistic stretching can be dangerous and that static and PNF techniques are more effective. Ballistic stretching is characterized by repetitious bouncing movements where the muscles are rapidly lengthened and immediately returned to resting length. The inhibitory effects of stretch reflex on ballistic stretching are frequently mentioned as a reason for the reduced efficacy of this technique (Beaulieu, 1981). Also, there has been some debate about the placement of stretching exercises, i.e. before, during or after a bout of exercise. One study (Cornelius et al., 1988) concluded that the placement of stretching exercises in an exercise programme was not significant.

Studies comparing the effectiveness of various stretching techniques on improving flexibility have provided inconclusive evidence at best. Cureton (1941) was one of the first to suggest that improved flexibility could increase the strength and elasticity of the musculotendinous structures. A number of authors have found that stretching leads to an increase in joint range of motion (DeVries, 1962; Sadu et al., 1982; Wiktorsson-Möller et al., 1983; Wallin et al., 1985). One interesting study performed by Toft et al. (1989) found that passive tension was decreased in subjects placed on a 3-week stretching programme of their ankle dorsiflexors. There was no correlation between flexibility and the short-term effects of stretching, nor flexibility and the long-term effects of stretching.

Muscles have a natural tendency to contract and shorten. It is thus not surprising that stretching is commonly prescribed to decrease the incidence of musculotendinous injuries,

increase flexibility, improve athletic performance and reduce muscle soreness following
training (DeVries, 1961; Nicholas, 1970;
Schultz, 1979; Corbin & Noble, 1980; Glick,
1980; Ekstrand & Gillquist, 1983). Most athletes
routinely practice stretching largely because it
is felt to prevent muscle injury (Beaulieu, 1981;
Wiktorsson-Möller et al., 1983; Hubley et al.,
1984). Ekstrand and Gillquist (1982) have reported that 67% of soccer players had one or
several tight muscles in the lower extremity
and furthermore that hamstring strains were
more common in teams not using special flexibility exercises for these muscles (Ekstrand
& Gillquist, 1983). In a more general study,
Wiktorsson-Möller et al. (1983) evaluated the
effects of general warm-up (bicycle ergometer
for 15 min), massage (6–15 min) and stretching
on range of movement (ROM) and strength
(isokinetic analysis) in eight male volunteers.
Ankle dorsiflexion was increased by massage
or warm-up whereas stretching increased ROM
for all motions tested. The overall conclusion
was that stretching was the superior way to
increase flexibility, i.e. the effect of contract–
relax stretching is superior to the effect of massage and general warming up. A further study
showed that a 15-min contract–relax stretch
programme could increase ROM in the lower
extremities for 90 min. It would seem therefore
that, based on this and other studies, stretching
and warm-up can help to reduce the severity of
injuries. Data are still lacking, both from the
laboratory and clinical studies to show that
these procedures can possibly prevent injury.

The effects of stretching on delayed-onset
muscle soreness (DOMS) remain unknown at
this time. In one study (Buroker & Schwane,
1989), a programme of static stretching following 30 min of stepping to induce DOMS did
not alleviate the symptoms either immediately
postexercise or chronically. On the other hand,
DeVries (1961) found a reduction in muscle
soreness after exercise. Different stretching protocols and methods for producing DOMS make
comparison between these studies difficult.

Cooling down

It is a common practice of those who engage in
regular physical exercise not only to warm up
but also to warm down, or cool down following
their activity. Relatively little epidemiological
data exists, however one study (Ekstrand et al.,
1983a) concluded that the addition of a cool-
down period reduced the incidence of injuries.

The physiological benefits of a cool-down
period have been documented. Removal of lactic acid after exercise may be important during
athletic competition since lactic acid has been
shown to inhibit the rate of glycolysis (Karlsson
et al., 1972). Lactate can be removed from blood
and muscle most rapidly following heavy to
maximal exercise by performing light continuous aerobic activity (Bonen & Belcastro,
1976). In untrained subjects the optimal rate of
blood lactate removal occurs at an oxygen consumption ($\dot{V}o_2$) between 30 and 45% $\dot{V}o_{2max}$
(Belcastro & Bonen, 1975). With trained subjects, lactate removal is optimal at exercise intensities between 50 and 65% $\dot{V}o_{2max}$ (Gisolfi
et al., 1966). These effects may be related to the
action of the muscle pumps which prevent
blood from pooling in the extremities, particularly the legs.

It would appear that a cool-down period
would be advantageous, particularly following
exhaustive exercise. Specific cooling down procedures or activities are not as yet available.
However, it would seem that a period of light
continuous exercise in combination with
stretching would provide for optimal recovery.

Conclusion

The need for prevention of injuries is well
recognized by all personnel involved in the
field of sports medicine yet research regarding
the effects of warming up and cooling down
has not confirmed our clinical suspicions. The
effects of warm-up prior to exercise, particularly
exhaustive exercise, are well documented.
Along with the physiological adaptations, it
appears that the mechanical properties of soft

tissues can be altered resulting in increased tissue extensibility and joint ROM. These adaptations would seem favourable to injury prevention as well as improvement of performance. Despite the majority of the scientific literature supporting these ideas, studies to date have failed to demonstrate a clear advantage of these techniques. Although there are indications that training programmes employing adequate stretching and warm-up can help decrease the incidence of muscle injuries, these training programmes have employed a number of confounding variables and the individual effect of single factors has not been determined.

A variety of warm-up techniques have been used; active or passive, formal or specific, and general. It appears that most athletes and coaches today favour specific warm-up because this type of activity allows for rehearsal of the event as well as the benefits of the warm-up. Regardless of the type of warm-up, the intensity and duration should be specific to the individual's needs and consideration should be given to environmental factors which could possibly alter the temperature response and temperature regulating mechanisms.

In summary, it appears that warm-up and cool-down may perhaps be more important in aiding athletic performance rather than injury prevention. Since warm-up is highly individualized and dependent on many factors, the need to perform well-controlled clinical and experimental studies becomes evident and hopefully challenging to those interested in this topic. As further studies become available, our abilities to treat and reduce the incidence of these injuries will hopefully improve.

References

Asmussen, E. & Böje, O. (1945) Body temperature and capacity for work. *Acta Physiol. Scand.* **10**, 1–22.

Åstrand, P.-O., Cuddy, T.E., Saltin, B. & Stenberg, J. (1964) Cardiac output during submaximal and maximal work. *J. Appl. Physiol.* **19**, 268–74.

Åstrand, P.-O. & Rodahl, K. (1977) *Textbook of Work Physiology*, 3rd edn. McGraw-Hill, New York.

Barcroft, H. & King, W.O.R. (1909) The effect of temperature on the dissociation curve of blood. *J. Physiol.* **39**, 374–84.

Barnard, R.J., Gardner, G.W., Diaco, N.V., MacAlpin, R.N. & Kattus, A.A. (1973a) Cardiovascular responses to sudden strenuous exercise-heart rate, blood pressure, and ECG. *J. Appl. Physiol.* **34**, 833–7.

Barnard, R.J., MacAlpin, R., Kattus, A.A. & Buckberg, G.D. (1973b) Ischemic responses to sudden strenuous exercise in healthy men. *Circulation* **48**, 936–42.

Beaulieu, J.E. (1981) Developing a stretching program. *Phys. Sporstmed.* **9**(11), 59–65.

Belcastro, A.N. & Bonen, A. (1975) Lactic acid removal rates during controlled and uncontrolled recovery exercise. *J. Appl. Physiol.* **39**(6), 932–6.

Bergh, U. & Ekblom, B. (1979a) Influence of muscle temperature on maximal muscle strength and power output in human skeletal muscles. *Acta Physiol. Scand.* **107**, 33–7.

Bergh, U. & Ekblom, B. (1979b) Physical performance and peak aerobic power at different body temperatures. *J. Appl. Physiol.* **46**(5), 885–9.

Blomstrand, E., Kaijser, L., Martinsson, A., Bergh, U. & Ekblom, B. (1986) Temperature-induced changes in metabolic and hormonal responses to intensive dynamic exercise. *Acta Physiol. Scand.* **127**, 477–84.

Bonen, A. & Belcastro, A.N. (1976) Comparison of self-selected recovery methods on lactic acid removal rates. *Med. Sci. Sports Exerc.* **8**(3), 176–8.

Brewer, B.J. (1960) Mechanism of injury to the musculotendinous unit. *American Academy of Orthopaedic Surgeons Instructional Lectures*, No. 17, pp. 354–8. CV Mosby, St Louis.

Buroker, K.C. & Schwane, J.A. (1989) Does postexercise static stretching alleviate delayed muscle soreness? *Phys. Sportsmed.* **17**(6), 65–83.

Close, R. & Hoh, J.F.Y. (1968) Influence of temperature on isometric contractions of rat skeletal muscle. *Nature* **217**, 1179–80.

Cole, E., Malone, T., Seaber, A.V. & Garrett Jr, W.E. (1991) *Passive muscle stretch and the viscoelastic response*. Presented at the American Orthopaedic Society for Sports Medicine Annual Meeting, Orlando, Florida, July 8–11, 1991.

Corbin, C.B. & Noble, L. (1980) Flexibility: A major component of physical fitness. *J. Phys. Educ. Rec.* **51**, 23–60.

Cornelius, W.L., Hagemann, R.W. & Jackson, A.W. (1988) A study on placement of stretching within a workout. *J. Sports Med. Phys. Fitness* **28**(3), 234–6.

Cureton, T.K. (1941) Flexibility as an aspect of physical fitness. *Res. Q.* **12**(Suppl.), 381–94.

Davies, C.T.M. & Young, K. (1983) Effect of temperature on the contractile properties and muscle power of triceps surae in humans. *J. Appl. Physiol.* **55**, 191–5.

DeBruyn-Prevost, P. (1980) The effects of various warming up intensities and durations upon some physiologic variables during exercise corresponding to the WC10. *Eur. J. Appl. Physiol.* **43**, 93–100.

DeVries, H.A. (1959) Effects of various warming up procedures on 100 yard times of competitive swimmers. *Res. Q.* **30**, 11–22.

DeVries, H.A. (1961) Prevention of muscular distress after exercise. *Res. Q.* **32**, 177–85.

DeVries, H.A. (1962) Evaluation of static stretching procedures for improvement of flexibility. *Res. Q.* **33**, 222–9.

DeVries, H.A. (1980) *Physiology of Exercise for Physical Education and Athletes.* William C. Brown, Dubuque.

Dorlot, J.M., Sidi, A.B., Gremblay, G.M. & Drouin, G. (1980) Load elongation behavior of the canine anterior cruciate ligament. *J. Biomech. Eng.* **102**, 190–3.

Edwards, R.H.T., Harris, R.C., Hultman, E., Kaijser, L., Koh, D. & Nordesjo, L.O. (1972) Effect of temperature on muscle energy, metabolism, and endurance during successive isometric contractions, sustained to fatigue, of the quadriceps muscle in man. *J. Physiol.* **220**, 335–52.

Ekstrand, J. & Gillquist, J. (1982) The frequency of muscle tightness and injuries in soccer players. *Am. J. Sports Med.* **10**, 75–8.

Ekstrand, J. & Gillquist, J. (1983) The avoidability of soccer injuries. *Int. J. Sports Med.* **4**, 124–8.

Ekstrand, J., Gillquist, J. & Liljedahl, S.O. (1983a) Prevention of soccer injuries: Supervision by doctor and physiotherapist. *Am. J. Sports Med.* **11**, 116–20.

Ekstrand, J., Gillquist, J., Möller, M., Oberg, B. & Liljedahl, S.O. (1983b) Incidence of soccer injuries and their relation to training and team success. *Am. J. Sports Med.* **11**, 63–7.

Gisolfi, C., Robinson, S. & Turrell, E.S. (1966) Effects of aerobic work performed during recovery from exhausting work. *J. Appl. Physiol.* **21**, 1767–72.

Glick, J.M. (1980) Muscle strains: Prevention and treatment. *Phys. Sportsmed.* **8**(11), 73–7.

Hill, A.V. (1927) *Living Machinery.* Harcourt, Brace, and World, New York.

Hill, A.V. (1938) Heat of shortening and dynamic constants of muscle. *Proc. Roy. Soc.* **126B**, 136–95.

Hill, A.V. (1950) The dimensions of animals and their muscular dynamics. *Sci. Prog.* **38**, 209–30.

Hill, A.V. (1961) The heat produced by a muscle after the last shock of a tetanus. *J. Physiol.* **159**, 518–45.

Högberg, P. & Ljunggren, O. (1947) Uppvärmningens inverkan pa löpprestationerna (The effect of warm

up on running performance). *Svensk Idrott* **40**.

Hubley, C.L., Kozey, J.W. & Stanish, W.D. (1984) The effects of static stretching exercises on range of motion at the hip joint. *J. Orthop. Sports Phys. Ther.* **5**, 104–9.

Karlsson, J., Nordesjo, L.O., Jorfeldt, L. & Saltin, B. (1972) Muscle lactate, ATP, and CP levels during exercise after physical training in man. *J. Appl. Physiol.* **33**, 199–203.

Krejci, V. & Koch, P. (1979) *Muscle and Tendon Injuries in Athletes.* Year Book Medical Publishers, Illinois.

Kulund, D.N. & Tottossy, M. (1983) Warm up, strength and power. *Clin. N. Am.* **14**(2), 427–48.

Lehmann, J.F., Masock, A.J., Warren, C.G. & Koblanski, J.N. (1970) Effect of therapeutic temperatures on tendon extensibility. *Arch. Phys. Med. Rehab.* **51**, 481–7.

Martin, B.J., Robinson, S., Wiegman, D.L. & Aulick, L.H. (1975) Effect of warm-up on metabolic responses to strenuous exercise. *Med. Sci. Sports Exerc.* **7**(2), 146–9.

Morehouse, L.E. & Miller, A.T. (1976) *Physiology of Exercise*, 7th edn. CV Mosby, St Louis.

Nadel, E.R., Wenger, C.B., Roberts, M.F., Stolwijk, J.A.J. & Cafarelli, E. (1977) Physiological defenses against hyperthermia of exercise. *Ann. N. Y. Acad. Sci.* **301**, 98–109.

Nicholas, J.A. (1970) Injuries to knee ligaments. Relationship to looseness and tightness in football players. *J. Am. Med. Assoc.* **212**, 2236–9.

Noonan, T.J., Best, T.M., Seaber, A.V. & Garrett Jr, W.E. (1991) Thermal effects on skeletal muscle tensile behavior. *Am. J. Sports Med.* **19**.

Petrofsky, J.S. & Lind, A.R. (1981) The influence of temperature on the isometric characteristics of fast and slow muscle in the cat. *Pflügers Arch.* **389**, 139–44.

Prentice, W.E. (1983) A comparison of static stretching and PNF stretching for improving hip joint flexibility. *Athletic Training* **18**, 56–9.

Pugh, L.G.C.E. (1967) Cold stress and muscular exercise, with special reference to accidental hypothermia. *Br. Med. J.* **2**, 333–7.

Ranatunga, K.W. (1982) Temperature-dependence of shortening velocity and rate of isometric tension development in rat skeletal muscle. *J. Physiol.* **329**, 465–83.

Rigby B., Hirai, N., Spikes, J. & Eyring, H. (1958) The mechanical properties of rat tail tendon. *J. Gen. Physiol.* **43**, 265–83.

Sadu, S.P., Wortman, M. & Blanke, D. (1982) Flexibility training: Ballistic, static or proprioceptive neuromuscular facilitation. *Arch. Phys. Med. Rehab.* **63**, 261–3.

Safran, M.R., Garrett Jr, W.E., Seaber, A.V., Glisson, R.R. & Ribbeck, B.M. (1988) The role of warm up in muscular injury prevention. *Am. J. Sports Med.* **16**(2), 123−9.

Saltin, B., Gagge, A.P. & Stolwijk, J.A.J. (1970) Body temperatures and sweating during thermal transients caused by exercise. *J. Appl. Phys.* **28**(3), 318−27.

Saltin, B. & Hermansen, L. (1966) Esophageal, rectal and muscle temperature during exercise. *J. Appl. Phys.* **21**, 1757−62.

Sargeant, A.J. (1983) Effect of muscle temperature on maximal short-term power output in man. *J. Physiol.* **341**, 35P.

Schultz, P. (1979) Flexibility: Day of the static stretch. *Phys. Sportsmed.* **7**, 109−17.

Sherrington, C.S. (1906) *The Integrative Action of the Nervous System.* Yale University Press, New Haven.

Taylor, D.C., Dalton, J.D., Seaber, A.V. & Garrett Jr, W.E. (1990) Viscoelastic properties of muscle−tendon units. The biomechanical effects of stretching. *Am. J. Sports Med.* **18**(3), 300−9.

Toft, E., Espersen, G.T., Kålund, S., Sinkjaer, T. & Hornemann, B.C. (1989) Passive tension of the ankle before and after stretching. *Am. J. Sports Med.* **17**(4), 489−94.

Walker, P.S., Amstutz, H.C. & Rubinfeld, M. (1976) Canine tendon studies II. Biomechanical evaluation of normal and regrown canine tendons. *J. Biomed. Mat. Res.* **10**, 61−76.

Wallin, D., Ekblom, B., Grahn, R. *et al.* (1985) Improvement of muscle flexibility. A comparison between two techniques. *Am. J. Sports Med.* **13**, 263−8.

Warren, C.G., Lehmann, J.F. & Koblanski, J.N. (1971) Elongation of rat tail tendon: effect of load and temperature. *Arch. Phys. Med. Rehab.* **51**, 465−74.

Wiktorsson-Möller, M., Öberg, B., Ekstrand, J. & Gillquist, J. (1983) Effects of warming up, massage, and stretching on range of motion and muscle strength in the lower extremity. *Am. J. Sports Med.* **11**(4), 249−52.

Williford, H.N., East, J.B., Smith, F.H. & Burry, L.A. (1986) Evaluation of warm-up for improvement in flexibility. *Am. J. Sports Med.* **14**(4), 316−19.

Woo, S.L.-Y., Lee, T.Q., Gomez, M.A., Sato, S. & Feld, F.P. (1987) Temperature dependent behavior of the canine medial collateral ligament. *J. Biomech. Eng.* **109**, 68−71.

Woo, S.L.-Y., Young, E.P. & Kwan, M.K. (1990) Fundamental studies in knee ligament mechanics. In D. Daniel (ed) *Knee Ligaments: Structure, Function, Injury, and Repair*, pp. 115−34. Raven Press, New York.

Wright, V. & Johns, R.J. (1961) Quantitative and qualitative analyses of joint stiffness in normal subjects and in patients with connective tissue disorders. *Rheum. Dis.* **20**, 36−46.

Chapter 19

Muscle Training in Injury Prevention

T. JEFF CHANDLER AND W. BEN KIBLER

Resistance training is often used in athletic conditioning programmes to improve athletic fitness. Although it is often claimed that muscle strength will reduce injuries, specific studies that indicate an actual decrease in the injury rate with resistive training are lacking (Stone, 1990). Studies are available that show possible mechanisms by which muscle strength may be a factor in injury prevention. Differences may exist in the mechanisms of injury prevention in traumatic and overload injuries. The purpose of this chapter is to review the studies that have explored changes in injury patterns with resistive training as well at those studies that indicate possible mechanisms by which increased strength might be a factor in injury prevention of both traumatic and overload injuries.

Effects of strength training on anatomical structures

Studies that show strength increases with resistive training are numerous. A consistent finding of resistive research over the past 40 years is that resistive training results in increased muscular strength (Atha, 1981). There are several ways in which increased muscular strength may be important in injury prevention which have been reported (Fleck & Falkel, 1986). Garrett et al. (1987) demonstrated that maximally stimulated muscle absorbs significantly more energy prior to failure than submaximally or non-stimulated muscle. Both

tetanically stimulated and wave summation contracted muscle required a greater force to tear than non-stimulated control muscles. There was no statistical difference in force to failure between muscles stimulated at 16 and 64 Hz. This may indicate that a stronger muscle may absorb more energy than a weak muscle before reaching the point of muscle strain.

In addition to strengthening muscle tissue to absorb loads, resistive training has also been shown to strengthen other structures around a joint that may be a factor in injury prevention. Tendons and ligaments demonstrate increased thickness, weight and strength in response to physical activity (Tipton et al., 1970; Staff, 1982). Adams (1966) reported the effects of exercise on ligament strengths in rats. It was determined that exercised rats experienced a significant increase in ligament strength. Also, rats who were forced to exercise on an uneven treadmill had significantly stronger ligaments than the group of rats who exercised on an even treadmill. Tipton et al. (1970) demonstrated that trained dogs had significantly higher collagen contents than non-trained and immobilized dogs, and that the trained group had the largest diameters of fibre bundles and the immobilized group had the smallest diameters. These animals were exercised for 6 weeks on a motor-driven treadmill, with 3 days·week^{-1} devoted to endurance sessions and 3 days·week^{-1} devoted to sprint training. Tipton et al. (1975) tested the effect of sprint training on ligament strength in rats. Although no significant improvement in bone—ligament junction strength was found, marked increases were demonstrated in ligament weight and weight to length ratios. Sprint training is metabolically similar to resistive training and is more likely to produce strength gains than endurance training.

Ligaments have been shown to have faster healing rates if physical activity is performed as a part of the rehabilitation process (Tipton et al., 1975; Staff, 1982). This is important in preventing reinjury after the symptomatic healing of the original injury. Long-term exercise leads to increased collagen turnover and hypertrophy of ligaments (Shankman, 1989). The microtrauma resulting from exercise may lead to eventual ligament healing and increased fibre strength. In response to specific exercises, collagen fibres align in a direction parallel to load forces (Shankman, 1989).

Multicomponent systems within the joint complex are also improved by resistance training. Tipton et al. (1975) outlined several important properties of these muscle—tendon—bone and bone—ligament—bone units. In a bone—ligament—bone preparation stressed to failure, separation occurs at the junction of the ligament to the bone. In a musculotendinous unit stressed to failure, separation will occur at the muscle—tendon junction. If a muscle—tendon—bone preparation is utilized, failure is likely to occur at the tendon—bone junction, although some failures will occur at the muscle—tendon junction. Junction strength, or the force necessary to separate a ligament or tendon from bone, was shown to increase with activity and decrease with immobilization.

Joint cartilage functions to reduce friction and cushion shock at the joint, thereby reducing injury. Joint cartilage has no vascularization, receiving nutrients and oxygen from synovial fluid. It may be that physical activity, including resistive training, is partly responsible for supplying the metabolic requirements of this tissue by pumping synovial fluid during periods of joint compression followed by decompression (Staff, 1982).

The connective tissue sheaths that surround the entire muscle (epimysium), groups of muscle fibres (perimysium), and individual muscle cells (endomysium) play a major role in the tensile strength and passive elasticity of muscle tissue. Endurance training in animal models has demonstrated no change in the total amount of collagen in these connective tissue sheaths (Kovanen et al., 1980, 1984). Increased enzyme activity in the slow twitch muscles suggested that the metabolism of collagen in these muscle fibres may be accelerated by endurance training. This could potentially lead to a loss of collagen content in the endurance-trained muscle, and could be related to various overtraining and/or overload injury syndromes. Turto et al. (1974) demonstrated increases in collagen content of the plantaris muscle in rats by sectioning the gastrocnemius, thus increasing the load on the plantaris muscle. Laurent et al. (1978) demonstrated an increase in collagen content in the anterior wing muscle of young male chickens by attaching a weight to the wing. It appears that hypertrophy induced by resistive training may increase collagen content and therefore the tensile strength of the muscle, and protect against the possible decrease in collagen content associated with endurance training.

The effect of physical activity, and specifically resistive training, on bone density may affect the injury rate to bone tissue in both fractures and overload-related stresses. Localized bone loss with immobilization does occur (Falch, 1982; Krolner et al., 1982). Studies from space indicate that activation of the antigravity muscles may play an important role in the prevention of bone mineral loss (Vogel & Whittle, 1976).

In a study of nationally competitive male athletes, those athletes who had the greatest strain placed on the lower limbs had the highest bone mineral content (Nilsson & Westlin, 1971). Two groups of controls for this study consisted of 24 age-matched physically active males and 15 age-matched sedentary males. The physically active controls had significantly more bone mineral than the sedentary controls. The competitive athletes had more bone mineral than the controls as a single group. In a study such as this, the possibility exists that the subjects with the greatest bone density chose to be more active in sports.

Bone mass of the humerus in tennis players has been shown to be significantly greater in the dominant arm compared to the non-dominant arm (Jones *et al.*, 1977). Montoye *et al.* (1980) also demonstrated that both bone width and mineral content of the dominant ulna, radius and humerus were significantly greater than in the non-dominant side of 61 senior male tennis players. In young male baseball players, the bone mineral content of the humerus but not the ulna and radius was significantly greater on the dominant compared to the non-dominant side (Watson, 1974). Due to the lack of control groups or very small control groups, no definitive conclusions can be drawn regarding bone density in the dominant compared to the non-dominant arms in these studies.

At the cellular level, loading the joint is important in the maintenance of the bone matrix. The spectrum of the load, both in terms of intensity and velocity, may be important to maximize cellular function. Bone has been shown to respond positively to higher strain rates (Lanyon, 1987). In terms of ligaments, Noyes *et al.* (1974) demonstrated that speed of loading is a factor in injuries. Bone−ligament preparations tested at a higher loading rate failed at a higher maximum load and strain. It may be that the speed of loading also affects the adaptation process of muscles and tendons, allowing them to better withstand higher forces without injury.

Muscle strength and the prevention of specific injuries

The concept of sport specificity is becoming increasingly more important to athletes in terms of performance and injury prevention. Intense participation in sport carries with it certain risks of injury. As a precursor to injury, certain musculoskeletal adaptations may occur in terms of strength, flexibility and muscle balance. Each athlete enters a sport with a quantifiable musculoskeletal base in terms of strength, flexibility and muscle balance. The demands of the sport may also be observed. A critical point occurs where the demands of the sport meet the musculoskeletal base of the athlete (Fig. 19.1). If the musculoskeletal base is adequate for the specific sport, there will be a decreased chance of overload injuries. If the musculoskeletal base is exceptional for the specific sport, improved performance may well be the result, assuming an adequate skill level in the sport or activity. If the musculoskeletal base is inadequate for the sport, overload injury, fatigue and decreased performance may well be the result. As the season progresses, injury and decreased performance become more likely. Each sport has unique demands, and each sport should be analysed in terms of these demands.

Little has been reported in the scientific literature on the role of muscle strengthening exercises and prevention of athletic injuries. Hejna and Rosenberg (1982) studied the effect

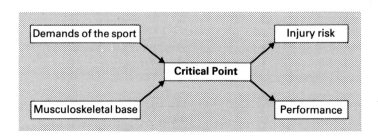

Fig. 19.1 The interaction of the demands of the sport with the musculoskeletal base of the athlete.

of variable resistance training on injury rate and time lost to rehabilitation in high school male and female athletes from a variety of sports. The injury rate of all athletes who used resistive training was 26.2%, compared to 72.4% for all athletes who did not use resistive training. The rehabilitation ratio (a ratio of time lost to rehabilitation due to injury per number of athletes in a group) was 4.82 days for the control group versus 2.02 days for the resistance training group. In the male athletes versus the female athletes, the males had an injury rate of 37% compared to an injury rate of 17.5% for the females. Injured males lost an average of 2.55 days of training or competition due to injury compared to 1.98 days for the injured females.

Muscle balance between the agonist and antagonist muscles that cross a joint have been suggested as possible causes of sports-related injuries (Grace, 1985). In swimmers tested on a Cybex II isokinetic dynamometer, the ratio of external rotation muscular endurance to internal rotation muscular endurance was less than 40% in swimmers with shoulder pain compared to a ratio of greater than 70% in swimmers without shoulder pain (Fleck & Falkel, 1986; Falkel, 1990). A pertinent question must be whether or not the weakness is due to the pain, or if the weakness precedes and is contributory to the pain.

Muscle balance of the hamstrings and quadriceps may be important to prevent injury. The quadriceps provide the force for knee extension, while the hamstring must act to decelerate the tibia during knee extension, absorbing the energy developed by the quadriceps (Garrett et al., 1984). If the quadricep is relatively stronger or the hamstring relatively weaker, a hamstring strain could result. The athlete with a 10% or greater difference between the quadriceps or hamstrings compared to the contralateral side is felt to have a greater risk of musculotendinous injury (Safran et al., 1989). Also, an athlete with a hamstring strength of less than 60% of the quadricep is felt to be at risk of muscle strain injury.

Heiser et al. (1984), in a retrospective study of hamstring injuries in a college football team, reported that by eliminating muscle imbalances, hamstring injuries fell from an incidence rate of 7.7% with a 31.7% recurrence rate to a rate of 1.1% and no recurrences. It was concluded that isokinetic evaluation of muscle imbalances followed by a strengthening programme designed to correct identified imbalances could prevent hamstring strains. Also, rehabilitation programmes that utilize isokinetic criteria of muscle balance and return to normal strength significantly reduce the chance of reinjury. However, Grace et al. (1984) failed to show a relationship between muscle imbalances of the thigh and injuries to the knee in 172 high-school football players.

Injuries in soccer players have been shown to be related to strength, range of motion and degree of rehabilitation (Ekstrand & Gillquist, 1983). 28% of the moderate and major knee injuries reported in 180 male soccer players were attributed to inadequate rehabilitation with persistent muscle weakness. Soccer players sustaining non-collision knee injuries had reduced knee extension strength in the injured leg compared to non-injured players. No significant change in the hamstring to quadricep ratio was found in the knee injury group compared to the non-injured players. The soccer players were less flexible than a control group in hip abduction, hip extension, knee flexion and ankle dorsiflexion. 27% of the players who sustained muscle rupture or tendinitis in the lower extremity had significant muscle tightness, with the remainder demonstrating normal flexibility. All 13 athletes with hip adductor rupture or tendinitis demonstrated decresed hip abduction range of motion (ROM). No significant difference in ROM was found between players with hamstring strains compared to the other athletes.

Recently, both muscle imbalances and flexibility deficits have been associated with increased injuries in athletic populations (Chandler et al., 1990, 1992). Knapik (1991) reported on the incidence of injuries in female collegiate athletes participating in one of eight varsity sports. On isokinetic testing, these athletes demonstrated an increase in the incidence of lower extremity injury if they had a right knee flexor 15% stronger than the left knee flexor at $180° \cdot s^{-1}$, or a knee flexor to knee extensor ratio of less than 0.75 at $180° \cdot s^{-1}$. The incidence of injury also increased if the right hip extensor was 15% more flexible than the left hip extensor. In club lacrosse players, Jackson and Nyland (1990) reported that all overuse injuries except one occurred in athletes who demonstrated a muscle imbalance, inflexibility, or both on the preparticipation physical examination.

In terms of flexibility, junior élite tennis players have been shown to be tighter in sit-and-reach and dominant and non-dominant shoulder internal rotation than athletes in other sports (Chandler *et al.*, 1990). The players were also significantly more flexible in dominant and non-dominant shoulder external rotation (Table 19.1). Shoulder muscle strength imbalances have also been identified in college tennis players (Chandler *et al.*, 1992) (Table 19.2).

In a review of tennis injuries, Kuland *et al.* (1979) indicated that resistance training exercises were effective in preventing pain from 'tennis shoulder' as described by Priest and Nagel (1976). Kuland *et al.* also stated that strength and flexibility exercises for the wrist

Table 19.1 Flexibility imbalances in tennis players and other athletes. Adapted from Chandler *et al.* (1990).

	Tennis players	Other athletes
Dominant shoulder (IR)	65°	74°
Non-dominant shoulder (IR)	76°	82°
Dominant shoulder (ER)	110°	96°
Non-dominant shoulder (ER)	103°	94°
Lower back	2.3 cm	6.2 cm

ER, external rotation; IR, internal rotation

Table 19.2 Isókinetic strength imbalances in shoulder rotation strength in junior élite tennis players ($60° \cdot s^{-1}$, in N·m (ft lbs)). Adapted from Chandler *et al.* (1992).

	Dominant shoulder	Non-dominant shoulder
IR peak torque	40.7 (29.9)	32.4 (23.8)
ER peak torque	24.9 (18.3)	23.5 (17.3)
IR : ER peak torque ratio	82.3 (60.5)	95.6 (70.3)

ER, external rotation; IR, internal rotation.

extensors and flexors were effective in the prevention of tennis elbow pain.

In swimmers, Dominguez (1978) found a significant decrease in shoulder pain in age group swimmers after they began resistance training. There was evidence presented in this study to support the opinion that lack of strength training was related to the development of shoulder pain. Hawkins and Kennedy (1980) utilized isokinetic exercises to increase the strength and endurance of the shoulder muscles in swimmers and other upper-body athletes. These athletes experienced a reduced incidence of shoulder pain. Falkel (1990) demonstrated that weakness of the external rotators was present in swimmers with shoulder pain, compared to swimmers with no pain and in controls. A conditioning programme designed to improve strength of the external rotators resulted in significantly reduced shoulder pain in these swimmers.

The effect of muscle strengthening exercises on joint stability has been reported in the literature. As mentioned earlier, strength training has an effect on the ligament strength as well as the ligament–bone junction strength, which would likely have a positive effect on injury prevention. Also, increasing the strength of muscles as dynamic stabilizers would likely play an important role. Early research on the role of joint looseness and injuries suggested that joint looseness increased injury risk. In football players, a preseason conditioning programme was shown to decrease both the incidence and severity of high-school football knee injuries (Cahill & Griffith, 1978). Nicholas (1970) reported an increased likelihood of knee ligament rupture with increased looseness of the knee. Strengthening exercises were suggested for those players with loose knees to decrease the chance of knee ligament injuries. Subsequent studies have shown no relationship between ligamentous laxity and injuries (Kalenak & Morehouse, 1975; Grana & Moretz, 1978). Although it has been previously believed that exercises such as the squat may stretch knee ligaments and increase the chance of knee ligament injuries (Klein, 1961), recent research has demonstrated that the squat and the leg press exercise is not detrimental to knee ligament stability (Chandler *et al.*, 1989; Lutz *et al.*, 1991).

Discussion

Injuries are and always will be a part of sports. The prevention of traumatic injuries is difficult, as the forces involved are often high. High-force traumatic injuries may be lessened in severity with muscle strength, but likely cannot be prevented.

Musculotendinous overload injuries are common in sports and may be the most preventable type of injuries. Many of these injuries are related to performing at too high an absolute load, or performing excessive repetitions of a normal load. An absolute tensile overload describes a situation where there has been too great a force applied to the musculotendinous unit, while relative tensile overload describes the situation in which there is a decreased ability of the musculotendinous unit to withstand the applied force (Fig. 19.2).

If participation continues, inflexibilities and muscle weaknesses may worsen as scar tissue forms, interfering with the ability of the muscle to contract efficiently and move through a normal ROM. Pain may lessen the intensity and frequency with which the athlete uses his or her muscles, and this becomes an additional factor adding to muscle weakness. The athlete is now in a cycle consisting of inflexibilities, muscle weakness and further injury (Fig. 19.3). Due to these clinical and subclinical adaptations of the body to tensile overload, efficient biomechanical movement patterns become difficult, usually leading to a change in movement patterns and decreasing the skill with which an activity is performed. These substitute actions may be subconscious on the part of the athlete to avoid pain, or because they lack the strength, endurance or flexibility to perform the movement. Specific examples include the baseball pitcher who has unintentionally altered the throwing motion used in order to accommodate for pain, weakness and or inflexibilities; the runner with plantar fasciitis who decreases his or her stance time due to pain; and the bench presser who alters his or her bar position to accommodate for pain. The tight weak muscle is now more susceptible to continued tensile overload. This cycle continues until eventually participation in the sport is no longer possible, the athlete no longer experiences success at his or her sport, or overt injury occurs.

Ideally, the overload injury cycle is one that

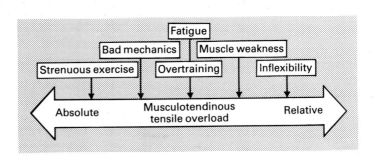

Fig. 19.2 Potential causes of tensile overload injuries to soft tissue.

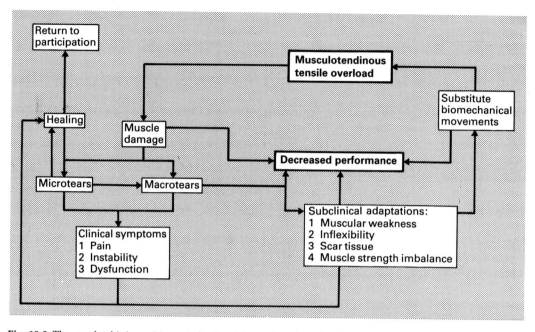

Fig. 19.3 The overload injury vicious circle. Possible results of overload injuries to the musculotendinous unit.

can be avoided with proper strength and flexibility of the muscular system prior to participating in a sport or activity. Proper resistive training for strength and muscular balance will prepare the musculoskeletal base for the sporting demands. The preparticipation evaluation (Kibler *et al.*, 1989) can potentially reduce injuries by identifying deficits in muscle strength and flexibility that can be corrected prior to the sport season. This evaluation ideally should be performed at least 1 month prior to the beginning of the season to allow the athlete time to correct any strength and flexibility deficits that might increase his or her chances of injuries.

The strength component of this examination may consist of field tests (sit-ups, push-ups, vertical jump, medicine ball push, etc.) weight-lifting tests (1, 5 or 10 RM (repetitions maximum) max. in certain lifts), or more advanced isokinetic tests of strength, power and endurance.

The concept of rehabilitation is important in the prevention of overload injuries (as mentioned previously in Table 19.2). Tennis players

have been shown to be weak in external rotation strength of the shoulder and exhibit a muscle imbalance (Chandler *et al.*, 1991). Water polo players have been shown to exhibit muscle imbalances in both shoulder internal/external rotation and shoulder adduction/abduction (McMaster *et al.*, 1991). In baseball pitchers, several studies have demonstrated muscle strength imbalances in the pitching shoulder (Alderink & Kuck, 1986; Cook *et al.*, 1987; Hinton, 1988). Alderink and Kuck (1986) reported that the pitching shoulder was significantly weaker than on the non-dominant side on isokinetic testing at speeds of 210 and $300° \cdot s^{-1}$. Cook *et al.* (1987) reported significant differences in strength ratios in college-level pitchers at 180 and $300° \cdot s^{-1}$ when the throwing arm was compared to the non-throwing arm. Also, a comparison of the shoulder strength ratios between pitchers and non-pitchers on the dominant arm was statistically significant with the pitchers demonstrating a lower strength ratio in both flexion/extension and internal/external rotation at all test speeds.

Hinton (1988) demonstrated no increase in external rotation strength in the throwing arm of high school pitchers as well as significantly lower external/internal strength ratios compared to the non-dominant arm.

Similar strength imbalances have been demonstrated in the lower body. Kibler *et al.* (1991) reported a significant decrease in the isokinetic strength of the plantar flexors of the ankle in patients with plantar fasciitis compared to both the unaffected foot and to controls (Table 19.3). Parker *et al.* (1983) reported different hamstring to quadricep ratios between athletes and non-athletes.

As sport-specific research identifies muscle strength imbalances specific to a particular sport, we can prescribe strengthening exercises for these athletes to correct these deficits and hopefully prevent many injuries occurring, and lessening the severity of other injuries. Using rehabilitation exercises prior to injury, it may be possible to prevent certain overload injuries that are common to a sport or activity.

No strength and conditioning programme will be successful in preventing injuries if general principles of conditioning are not followed. These principles must also be applied to practice and participation in all athletic activities. Violation of these principles can cause injury, even if the muscles are flexible, strong and properly balanced. Warm-up should be performed prior to activity to reduce the chances of injury (Safran *et al.*, 1989). Proper selection of training load in terms of frequency, intensity and duration is essential to the prevention of injuries, both during conditioning exercises and during specific activities.

Conclusion

The bulk of the evidence presented supports the concept that muscle-strengthening exercises are effective in preventing injuries. Muscles appear to react at the cellular and whole muscle level to resistance training so that there is an increased ability to absorb the loads generated during physical activity. In addition, fascia, ligaments, tendons and bone that have been subjected to various amounts and types of exercise including resistive training also show measurable increases in load-absorbing ability. Evaluation of muscle strength in a preparticipation evaluation is important to identify muscular strength, balance and flexibility deficits that have been demonstrated to occur and that appear to predispose the athlete to injury. Preseason conditioning programmes and in-season strength maintenance programmes are also important to prevent detraining and therefore reduce injuries. Prevention of traumatic injuries by muscle strengthening may be effective only when the magnitude of the trauma is both below a certain level and predictable. Prevention of overload injuries with muscle strengthening is promising. The rate of overload injuries caused by a workload in excess of the strength of the muscle can probably be decreased with appropriate strengthening exercises.

Table 19.3 Strength and flexibility imbalances in runners with and without plantar fasciitis (PF). Measurements given in newton metres (N·m) and foot pounds (ft lb). Adapted from Kibler *et al.* (1989).

	Controls	PF injured	PF uninjured
Total dynamic range of motion	63°	52°	38°
Isokinetic peak torque ($60°·s^{-1}$)	89.5 (65.8)	79.0 (58.1)	59.7 (43.9)
Isokinetic peak torque ($180°·s^{-1}$)	37.9 (27.9)	39.0 (28.7)	27.2 (20.0)

References

Adams, A. (1966) Effect of exercise upon ligamentous strength. *Res. Q.* **37**(2), 163–7.

Alderink, G.J. & Kuck, D.J. (1986) Isokinetic shoulder strength of high school and college-aged pitchers. *J. Orthop. Sports Phys. Ther.* **7**, 163–72.

Atha, J. (1981) Strengthening muscle. *Exerc. Sport Sci. Rev.* **9**, 1–73.

Cahill, B.R. & Griffith, E.H. (1978) Effect of preseason conditioning on the incidence and severity of high school football knee injuries. *Am. J. Sports Med.* **6**(4), 180–4.

Chandler, T.J., Kibler, W.B., Kiser, A.M. & Wooten, B.P. (1992) Shoulder strength, power, and endurance in college tennis players. *Am. J. Sports Med.* **20**(4), 455–7.

Chandler, T.J., Kibler, W.B., Uhl, T.L., Wooten, B., Kiser, A. & Stone, E. (1990) Flexibility comparisons of junior élite tennis players to other athletes. *Am. J. Sports Med.* **18**(2), 134–6.

Chandler, T.J., Wilson, G.D. & Stone, M.H. (1989) The effect of the squat exercise on knee stability. *Med. Sci. Sports Exerc.* **21**(3), 299–303.

Cook, E.E., Gray, V.L., Savinar-Nogue, E. & Medeiros, J. (1987) Shoulder antagonistic strength ratios: A comparison between college-level baseball pitchers and nonpitchers. *J. Orthop. Sports Phys. Ther.* **8**(9), 451–61.

Dominguez, R.H. (1978) Shoulder pain in age group swimmers. In B. Eriksson & B. Furberg (eds) *Swimming Medicine*, Vol. IV, pp. 105–9. University Park Press, Baltimore.

Ekstrand, J. & Gillquist, J. (1983) The avoidability of soccer injuries. *Int. J. Sports Med.* **4**, 124–8.

Falch, J.A. (1982) The effect of physical activity on the skeleton. *Scand. J. Soc. Med.* **29**(Suppl.), 55–8.

Falkel, J.E. (1990) Swimming injuries. In B. Sanders (ed) *Sports Physical Therapy*, pp. 477–504. Appleton & Lang, Connecticut.

Fleck, S.J. & Falkel, J.E. (1986) Value of resistance training for the reduction of sports injuries. *Sports Med.* **3**, 61–8.

Garrett, W.E., Califf, J.C. & Bassett, F.H. (1984) Histochemical correlates of hamstring injuries. *Am. J. Sports Med.* **12**(2), 98–103.

Garrett, W.E., Safran, M.R., Seaber, A.V., Blisson, R.R. & Ribbeck, B.M. (1987) Biomechanical comparison of stimulated and nonstimulated skeletal muscle pulled to failure. *Am. J. Sports Med.* **15**(5), 448–54.

Grace, T.G. (1985) Muscle imbalance extremity injury: A perplexing relationship. *Sports Med.* **2**, 77–82.

Grace, T.G., Sweetser, E.R., Nelson, M.A., Ydens, L.R. & Skipper, B.F. (1984) Isokinetic muscle imbalance and knee joint injuries. *J. Bone Joint Surg.* **66A**, 734–40.

Grana, W.A. & Moretz, A.J. (1978) Ligamentous laxity in secondary school athletes. *J. Am. Med. Assoc.* **200**(18), 1975–6.

Hawkins, R.J. & Kennedy, J.C. (1980) Impingement syndrome in athletes. *Am. J. Sports Med.* **8**, 151–8.

Heiser, T.M., Weber, J., Sullivan, G., Clare, P. & Jacobs, P.P. (1984) Prophylaxis and management of hamstring muscle injuries in intercollegiate football. *Am. J. Sports Med.* **12**, 368–70.

Hejna, W.F. & Rosenberg, A. (1982) The prevention of sports injuries in high school students through strength training. *Natl. Strength Cond. Ass. J.* **4**, 28–31.

Hinton, R.Y. (1988) Isokinetic evaluation of shoulder rotational strength in high school baseball pitchers. *Am. J. Sports Med.* **16**(3), 274–9.

Jackson, D.L. & Nyland, K. (1990) Club lacrosse: A physiological and injury profile. *Ann. Sports Med.* **5**, 114–17.

Jones, H.H., Priest, J.D., Hayes, W.C., Tichenor, C.C. & Nagel, D.A. (1977) Humeral hypertrophy in response to exercise. *J. Bone Joint Surg.* **59A**, 204–8.

Kalenak, A. & Morehouse, C.A. (1975) Knee stability and knee ligament injuries. *J. Am. Med. Assoc.* **234**(11), 1143–5.

Kibler, W.B., Chandler, T.J., Uhl, T. & Maddux, R.E. (1989) A musculoskeletal approach to the preparticipation physical examination, preventing injury and improving performance. *Am. J. Sports Med.* **17**(4), 525–31.

Kibler, W.B., Goldberg, C. & Chandler, T.J. (1991) Functional biomechanical deficits in running athletes with plantar fasciitis. *Am. J. Sports Med.* **19**(1), 66–71.

Klein, K.K. (1961) The deep squat exercise as utilized in weight training for athletes and its effect on the ligaments of the knee. *J. Assoc. Phys. Ment. Rehab.* **15**, 6–11.

Knapik, J.J., Bauman, C.L., Jones, B.H., Harris, J.M. & Vaughn, L. (1991) Preseason strength and flexibility imbalances associated with athletic injuries in female collegiate athletes. *Am. J. Sports Med.* **19**(1), 76–81.

Kovanen, V., Suominen, H. & Heikkinen, E. (1980) Connective tissue of fast and slow skeletal muscle in rats – effects of endurance training. *Acta Physiol. Scand.* **108**, 173–80.

Kovanen, V., Suominen, H. & Heikkinen, E. (1984) Collagen of slow and fast twitch muscle fibers in different types of rat skeletal muscle. *Eur. J. Appl. Physiol.* **52**, 235–43.

Krolner, B., Tondevold, E., Toft, B., Berthelsen, B. & Nielsen, P.S. (1982) Bone mass of the axial and appendicular skeleton in women with Colles' fracture: Its relation to physical activity. *Clin. Physiol.* **2**, 147–57.

Kuland, D.N., McCue, F.C., Rockwell, D.A. & Gieck, J.A. (1979) Tennis injuries: Prevention and treatment. *Am. J. Sports Med.* **7**, 249–53.

Lanyon, L.E. (1987) Functional strain in bone tissue as an objective and controlling stimulus for adaptive bone remodeling. *J. Biomech.* **2**, 1083–93.

Laurent, G.J., Sparrow, M.P., Bates, P.C. & Milward, D.J. (1978) Collagen content and turnover in cardiac and skeletal muscles of the adult fowl and the changes during stretch-induced growth. *Biochem. J.* **176**, 419–27.

Lutz, G.E., Palmitier, R.A., An, K.N. & Chao, E.Y.S. (1991) Closed kinetic chain exercises for athletes after reconstruction of the anterior cruciate ligament (Abstract). *Med. Sci. Sports Exerc.* **23** (Suppl. 4), S69.

McMaster, W.C., Long, S.C. & Caiozzo, V.J. (1991) Isokinetic torque imbalances in the rotator cuff of the élite water polo player. *Am. J. Sports Med.* **19**(1), 72–5.

Montoye, H.J., Smith, E.L., Fardon, D.F. & Howley, E.T. (1980) Bone mineral in senior tennis players. *Scand. J. Sports Sci.* **2**, 26–32.

Nicholas, J.A. (1970) Injuries to knee ligaments. *J. Am. Med. Assoc.* **212**(13), 2236–9.

Nilsson, B.E. & Westlin, N.E. (1971) Bone density in athletes. *Clin. Orthop. Rel. Res.* **77**, 179–82.

Noyes, F.R., Delucas, J.L. & Torvick, P.J. (1974) Biomechanics of anterior cruciate ligament failure: An analysis of strain rate sensitivity and mechanisms of failure in primates. *J. Bone Joint Surg.* **56A**(2), 236–53.

Parker, M.G., Ruhling, R.O., Holt, D., Bauman, E. & Drayna, M. (1983) Descriptive analysis of quad-

riceps and hamstrings muscle torque in high school football players. *J. Orthop. Sports Phys. Ther.* **5**, 2–6.

Priest, J.D. & Nagle, D.A. (1976) Tennis shoulder. *Am. J. Sports Med.* **4**, 28–42.

Safran, M.R., Seaber, A.V. & Garrett, W.E. (1989) Warm-up and muscular injury prevention. *Sports Med.* **8**(4), 239–49.

Shankman, G. (1989) Training guidelines for strengthening the injured knee: Basic concepts for the strength coach. *Natl. Strength Cond. Ass.* **11**(4), 32–42.

Staff, P.H. (1982) The effect of physical activity on joints, cartilage, tendons, and ligaments. *Scand. J. Soc. Med.* **29** (Suppl.), 59–63.

Stone, M.H. (1990) Muscle conditioning and muscle injuries. *Med. Sci. Sports Exerc.* **22**(4), 457–62.

Tipton, C.M., James, S.L., Mergner, W. & Tcheng, T. (1970) Influence of exercise on strength of medial collateral knee ligaments of dogs. *Am. J. Physiol.* **218**(3), 894–902.

Tipton, C.M., Matthes, R.D., Maynard, J.A. & Carey, R.A. (1975) The influence of physical activity on ligaments and tendons. *Med. Sci. Sports* **7**, 165–75.

Turto, H., Lindy, S. & Halme, J. (1974) Protocollagen proline hydroxylase activity in work-induced hypertrophy of rat muscle. *Am. J. Physiol.* **226**, 63–5.

Vogel, J.M. & Whittle, M.W. (1976) Bone mineral content changes in the Skylab astronauts. *Am. J. Roentgenol.* **126**(6), 1296–7.

Watson, R.C. (1974) *Bone growth and physical activity in young males*. International Conference on Bone Mineral Measurements. US Department of Health, Education, and Welfare, Publication No. NIH 75-683, 380–5.

Chapter 20

Flexibility in Injury Prevention

WILLIAM D. STANISH AND STEVE F. McVICAR

Stretching exercises are often performed as a warm-up prior to participation in many exercise-related activities. Reasons for stretching relate to beliefs that stretching will increase flexibility, decrease the incidence of muscle–tendinous injuries, improve athletic performance and/or prevent muscle soreness (Schultz, 1979; Corbin & Mable, 1980; Beaulieu, 1981; Anderson et al., 1984). While evidence indicates that stretching can increase flexibility, there is concern as to what stretching techniques or procedures should be used for optimal gains in flexibility (DeVries, 1962; Schultz, 1979; Corbin & Mable, 1980; Beaulieu, 1981; Anderson et al., 1984; Williford & Smith, 1985). Although stretching exercises can be very beneficial to athletes, adding them to conditioning programmes has not always had positive results. Many teams and individual athletes have had an increase in muscle injuries, and runners claim an increase in muscle–tendinous injuries as a result of stretching (Osler, 1978; Benjamin & Roth, 1979; Fixx, 1980).

The theoretical basis for stretching is fairly well defined, but the epidemiological and scientific evidence to support flexibility training is somewhat scanty. This chapter reviews the clinical and scientific evidence available to show how and why flexibility exercises can be used to enhance athletic performance and prevent sports injuries.

Physiology of flexibility without injury

The muscle at rest can be clinically appreciated as a soft tissue with a constant desire to shorten. Athletic activities producing muscle hypertrophy will predictably produce transient, and sometimes permanent muscle contracture, coupled with the subjective feeling of tightness. It has been our experience that if contraction is allowed to persist, the contracted soft tissue, muscle and tendon will be susceptible to injury when flexibility is demanded in the athletic challenge. Stolov and Thompson (1979) demonstrated that there is adaptive shortening of the tissue if it remains in a shortened position. There is also evidence which supports the theory that the muscle–tendon unit is less likely to break down if its inherent characteristics of elasticity are consistently trained through stretching exercises.

Tendon injuries occur far more frequently than intrinsic muscle injuries. Cross-sectioning of the tendon reveals progressively smaller subunits decreasing in diameter from the tendon bundle to the fibril, microfibril and, the smallest subunit, trophocollagen. The tendon fascicle is composed of many fibres, and in the unstretched condition, it has a pleated, wavy appearance that disappears when the fascicle is stretched. Experimentally, when a tendon is stretched, the resultant stress (i.e. the load over a cross-sectioned area) follows (Fig. 20.1).

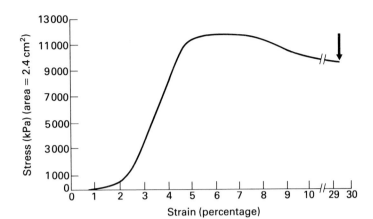

Fig. 20.1 Tendon normal stress—strain curve for the tendon. A 30% strain level was reached before the specimen failed. The measured strain rates were: 0–4%, 18%·mm^{-1}; 4–10% 34%·mm^{-1}.

Initial elongation occurs with little increase in load. This is associated with wavy collagen fibres straightening out. As the fibres become orientated to the direction of loading, there is an increase in tissue stiffness, and the stress versus strain relationship becomes linear. Following this point, there is progressive tissue failure and damage begins to occur.

Maintaining a fixed length in connective tissue results in relaxation of the tissue, and less force is required to stay at that same length. Conversely, if the force is constant, the tissue elongates, a process called creep. These properties depend on sustaining the mechanical disturbance. Rapid application of force to collagenous tissues results in increased stiffness. More force is required to achieve the same elongation that is possible when less force is used at slower rates of stretching. Thus, the ideal way to elongate these tissues is to apply force more slowly and maintain it (Kottke *et al.*, 1966).

The quality of the elastic compliance of a muscle—tendon unit is proportional to the ratio of muscle to tendon in the contractural unit. For example, experiments with dogs have demonstrated the higher level of elasticity in the sartorius, which is principally muscle along its entire length, with very little tendon, in contrast with the gastrocnemius, which has a long tendinous component. Clinically there are greater numbers of tendon injuries than intrinsic muscle breakdowns, suggesting that muscle, with its superior inherent compliance, is less likely than tendon to be disrupted under comparable stress.

The muscle—tendon unit contains two basic components: (i) a contractile or active element; and (ii) a non-contractile or passive element. The active component results from cross-bridge interaction between the contractile proteins, actin and myosin within the muscle fibres. The non-contractile components include connective tissue elements within and around the muscle, the perimysium, epimysium and endomysium; the sarcolemma; associated tendons and their insertions; and connections between the sarcolemma and the tendon (Borg & Caulfield, 1980; Moore, 1983; Garrett & Fidball, 1988) (Fig. 20.2). To understand the physiology of flexibility, both neurophysiological and mechanical aspects of muscle control and behaviour must be examined.

Understanding the myotatic reflexes, the stretch reflex and the inverse stretch reflex, is important because they play a crucial role in the development of greater flexibility (DeVries, 1974). There are two types of muscle fibre, the intrafusal and extrafusal. The extrafusal fibres are innervated by α motor neurones and are the main 'motor' of the muscle. The intrafusal fibres are part of the muscle spindles, and sensory elements within the muscle that signal both length change and rate of change of length,

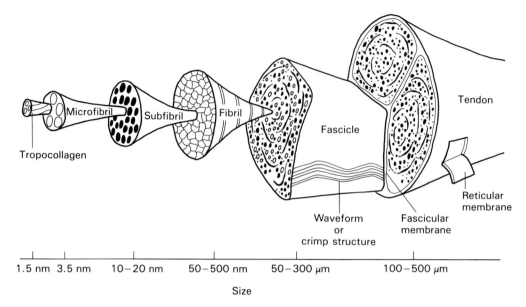

Fig. 20.2 The hierarchical organization of the tendon, showing the various stages from molecule to tendon. With permission from Curwin & Stanish (1984).

innervated by γ-motor neurones (Fig. 20.3). Afferent signals from receptors in the muscle spindles travel to the central nervous system via IA and II sensory nerves (Boyd, 1981) (Fig. 20.4).

Whenever a muscle is stretched, the stretch reflex mechanism fires and protects it from being overstretched. Stretching of muscle lengthens intrafusal and extrafusal muscle fibres. The consequent deformation of sensory end organs within the spindles results in the firing of the stretch reflex, which contracts the stretched muscle. Contraction relieves the stretch on the muscle spindles, as both the extrafusal and intrafusal fibres are in parallel position to each other and therefore decreases the activity of the receptors within the spindles. The stretch reflex is sensitive to both phasic (jerky) and static (maintained) stretching. The amount and rate of the contraction elicited from the stretch reflex are proportional to the amount and rate of the stretching. If a muscle is stretched quickly, the resulting contraction is likely to be more forceful than if the muscle is stretched gently and slowly.

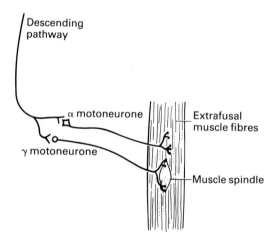

Fig. 20.3 Muscle spindle innervation.

Although the stretch reflex only responds to stretching, the inverse stretch reflex responds to both stretching and contracting. The sensory receptors believed to be associated with this response are located in the Golgi tendon organ. These receptors, the Golgi tendon organs, are located near the myotendinous junction and send afferent signals along Ib sensory organs

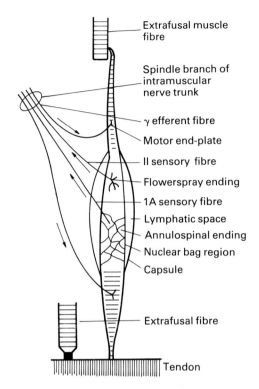

Extrafusal muscle fibre

Spindle branch of intramuscular nerve trunk

γ efferent fibre

Motor end-plate

II sensory fibre

Flowerspray ending

1A sensory fibre

Lymphatic space

Annulospinal ending

Nuclear bag region

Capsule

Extrafusal fibre

Tendon

Fig. 20.4 Muscle spindle. With permission from Stanish (1982).

(Bistevins & Awad, 1981). The inverse stretch reflex prevents overstressing the muscle tissue caused by too much tension from active contraction or overstretching.

The Golgi tendon organ is very sensitive to tension caused by active contraction. When the muscle contracts, the Golgi tendon organ discharges to inhibit the contraction and relax the active muscle (the agonist). They also depolarize α motor neurones to the opposite muscle (the antagonist) and facilitate contraction.

The Golgi tendon organ's response to stretching is also inhibitory in nature. The inverse stretch reflex has a higher threshold to stretch than the stretch reflex (DeVries, 1974). When sufficient force is achieved to reach the threshold of the tendon organ, the inverse stretch reflex will inhibit the muscle under stretch in an attempt to relax the muscle tension. This may explain the phenomenon that is familiar

to people who are experienced in the use of stretching exercises: when a subject assumes and sustains a stretching position that develops considerable tension in the muscle, a point is reached where the tension dissipates and the muscle can be stretched even further.

Proper use of the stretch reflexes results in less tension in the stretched muscle. The more relaxed a muscle is, the less likely it is to be injured during the stretch. Yogis, gymnasts and dancers have discovered from experience that the more relaxed stretching techniques are the safest way to increase flexibility (Beaulieu, 1980). Knowledge of the myotatic reflexes is important in understanding the advantages or disadvantages of the different stretching techniques and will enable a person to select the best technique.

Physiology of flexibility with injury

Indirect muscle injuries caused by excessive force or stress on a muscle include strains, muscle pulls and muscle tears. These injuries occur frequently in sports and result in lost training time or withdrawal from competition (Ethnyre & Abraham, 1986; Lysholm & Wiklander, 1987). Overstretching the muscle–tendon unit causes injury, yet the nature, location and healing of such injuries are still unclear. The general clinical thought is that torn muscle fibres are replaced by scar (connective tissue) that must not be allowed to heal in the shortened position, or muscle extensibility will be lost. However, new evidence suggests that muscle regeneration may be possible (Appell et al., 1988).

Complete muscle–tendon unit tears occur almost exclusively at tissue junctions (Kvist & Jarvinen, 1982; Garrett & Fidball, 1986; Nikolaou et al., 1987; Garrett et al., 1988). When a muscle is pulled to failure, rupture occurs through the muscle fibrous near the myotendinous junction (Garrett et al., 1988). If the muscle is active and pulled to failure, then injury occurs at the same location, but more energy is absorbed by the muscle before failure

(Garrett *et al.*, 1987) (Fig. 20.5). Elongation and failure is the same in both cases (Fig. 20.6). This implies that a stiffer muscle may be more resistant to injury, because more energy is absorbed at a given amount of elongation before injury is produced.

The exact site of muscle rupture has not yet been examined thoroughly. Nikolaou *et al.* (1987) show that muscle fibres near the myotendinous junction are the site of injury and that fibres a few millimetres long can still be attached to the tendon at failure. Sarcomeres in this region of the muscle are stiffer and less extensible than those in other parts of the muscle (Garrett & Fidball, 1988). However, it is

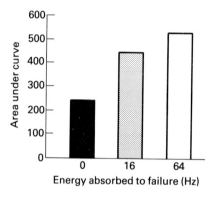

Fig. 20.5 The energy absorbed by passive (0 Hz), slightly contracted (16 Hz), and maximally contracted (64 Hz) skeletal muscle while being pulled to failure. Adapted with permission from Garrett *et al.* (1987).

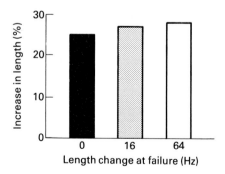

Fig. 20.6 The changes in length by passive (0 Hz), slightly contracted (16 Hz), and maximally contracted (64 Hz) skeletal muscle pulled to failure. Adapted with permission from Garrett *et al.* (1987).

not clear how this finding relates to the fact that stiffer muscles overall may be more able to resist injury.

Although studies of complete ruptures help clarify the mechanism of muscle injury, incomplete tears are more commonly seen. Nikolaou *et al.* (1987) produced this type of injury in rabbit anterior tibial muscles by stretching the muscle to 80% of its maximum isometric tension. Initially, fibre disruption and haemorrhage were present. During the next 4 days, a cellular inflammatory response occurred, and scar tissue was present by the seventh day. Also by this time, the muscle had regained normal tension production. This is similar to the pattern of force reduction and recovery after eccentric muscle injury (Horswill *et al.*, 1988).

Unlimited physical activity early in healing may reinjure the tissue, causing the formation of more scar tissue. This would increase the barrier to regenerating muscle fibres (Lehto *et al.*, 1985), yet exercise can also enhance softtissue healing (Vailas *et al.*, 1981). Immobilization, on the other hand, increases joint stiffness (Akeson *et al.*, 1973; Butler *et al.*, 1978) and decreases muscle strength by reducing the number of sarcomeres in series (Gossman *et al.*, 1982; Baker & Matsumoto, 1988). This creates a major problem in rehabilitation because the ideal combination of rest and exercise for optimal recovery has not been determined. Few animal studies have examined the effects on recovery of various stretching and flexibility protocols. Thus, the use of flexibility training in rehabilitation is determined only by the subjective complaints of the individual and the clinician's knowledge of the healing processes. Several questions about optimum rehabilitation of these injuries remain unanswered.

Factors affecting flexibility

Age and gender

Joint range of motion in muscle flexibility decreases with age (Kendall & Kendall, 1948;

Walker *et al.*, 1984). The shoulder joint's range of motion decreases approximately 15–20% between 20 and 60 years of age, and ankle motion declines by as much as 50% (Kendall & Kendall, 1948; Wallin *et al.*, 1985). This decrease can be attributed to changes in periarticular tissue, such as increasing collagen content and cross-linking, that increase tissue stiffness (Akeson *et al.*, 1973; Alnaqeeb *et al.*, 1984; Voss *et al.*, 1985). Similar changes occur in these tissues during immobilization, suggesting an accelerated aging affect. Conversely, some forms of aerobic exercise decrease cross-linking and increase glycosaminoglycan concentration, which may indicate retardation of maturation or aging (Viidik, 1979; Vailas *et al.*, 1985; Kovanen *et al.*, 1987; Curwin *et al.*, 1988).

Muscle flexibility also decreases with age, although the biochemical and ultrastructural changes that occur are largely unknown. Research has demonstrated that this flexibility can be regained with exercise programmes, 12 weeks and 25 weeks in duration (Raab *et al.*, 1988).

Females are generally more flexible than males (Boone & Azen, 1979; Kirby *et al.*, 1981), at least in younger age groups. Whether these differences are maintained throughout aging is unknown. Similarly, the quantitative responses of males and females to flexibility training programmes have received little attention, although it appears that they are equally trainable (Tanigawa, 1972).

Thermal effects

The problem with most of the stretching techniques is that effects are lost shortly after the stretching ends, indicating very little retention. This suggests that the type of deformation is mostly elastic, because the muscle returns to its original length after the stretching force is removed with little permanent deformation taking place. Two studies have shown that low static forces, applied for a long duration to heated tissue, result in a permanent deformation of the muscle–tendon unit and, in

particular, the connective tissue structures (Lehmann *et al.*, 1970; Warren *et al.*, 1976). Increased temperature has a considerable effect on collagen. Temperatures above 40°C relax collagen fibres, so that less force is required to produce deformation, or, alternatively, so that the same force produces more elongation (Lehmann *et al.*, 1970). The time required to deform collagen to failure decreases, and the force required increases, as the temperature increases. The most effective way to combine heat and deformation to achieve elongation is to apply them both simultaneously and to maintain the lengthened position after the heat is removed (Warren *et al.*, 1976; Henricson *et al.*, 1984).

These findings may be important in assessing the value of a warm-up exercise before stretching. Intramuscular temperatures may increase to 39°C with active exercise (Saltin & Hermansen, 1966), which may influence collagen behaviour. Golgi tendon organ sensitivity also increases with rising temperatures and contributes to muscle relaxation. While clinical evidence indicates that warming the connective tissue prior to stretching will increase flexibility, there is no empirical evidence to suggest that warming the joints by a warm-up exercise such as jogging and then stretching will significantly increase flexibility. Slow static stretching without warm-up exercises could possibly produce sufficient warming of the muscles to aid in increases in flexibility (Williford *et al.*, 1986). Further research is needed to investigate the relationships between warming the muscle and connective tissue and increases in flexibility.

Cold appears to have no effect on collagen, and thus does not influence the mechanical components of muscle flexibility. Cold applications decrease muscle spasticity (Miglietta, 1964; Kelly, 1969) and may decrease muscle spindle afferent activity, which may promote muscle relaxation. Combining cold and static stretching is more effective than combining heat and stretching in reducing muscle pain and electromyographic activity in an injured muscle within 24 h of injury (Prentice, 1982). Cold may be applied via ice packs, cold-water immersion or vapocoolant sprays. The effectiveness of vapocoolant sprays on flexibility is unclear; they may or may not have an effect (Halkovich *et al.*, 1981; Newton, 1985; Koury *et al.*, 1986).

Specificity of sport

Movement patterns are highly specific and there may even be task-specific groups of motor units within multifunctional muscles (Sale, 1988). Joint range of motion and muscle flexibility also show sport specificity (Ekstrand & Gillquist, 1982; Reid *et al.*, 1987). Gymnasts and ballet dancers are much more flexible in some movements than those who do not engage in these activities, but less flexible in others. Pitchers show more lateral and less medial rotation of the shoulder than other baseball players (Brown *et al.*, 1988). This may result from sport-specific training or a natural selection process whereby individuals with these characteristics excel.

Reflex activity can also be altered with train-

ing. Volleyball players can adjust their response to drop jumps from a height so that quadriceps electrical activity increases during the eccentric phase of the jump, rather than decreases as it does in normal persons (Komi, 1984; Sale, 1988).

Training techniques for improved flexibility

In healthy states

The three most popular stretching techniques used by athletes are ballistic, static and the proprioceptive neuromuscular facilitation (PNF) techniques, as described in Table 20.1. All three increase flexibility but no one technique is predominantly more effective (Riddle, 1956; Landreth, 1957; DeVries, 1962; Carr, 1971; Hartley-O'Brien, 1980). However, certain techniques involve greater risks of injury.

The ballistic stretching techniques performed by jerking or bouncing movements performed near the end of the available range of motion, together with the force of the bouncing, stretches the muscles. Quick or forceful bounc-

Table 20.1 Types of flexibility training.

Stretching method	Description
Static	Stationary position with joints maintained in a position that stretches muscle
Ballistic	Quick, bobbing movements at the end of the available range of motion, produced by limb weight or contraction of muscle groups antagonist to those being stretched
Proprioceptive neuromuscular facilitation	
contract–relax	Stretch statically at the end of range of motion; contract muscle slightly; relax as assistant gently pushes limb further
hold–relax	Same as contract–relax, but emphasize isometric contraction
contract–relax–antagonist contract	Same as contract–relax but antagonist muscles are contracted to assist in moving limb further

ing evokes a strong stretch reflex contracture against a stretch and also causes increased muscle stiffness. The tension created in the muscle during ballistic stretching is more than double that created during a slow, gentle stretch (Walker, 1961). Stretching of muscle against this amount of tension increases the chance of injury to the muscles and tendons. However, this may be beneficial in certain preparatory phases for athletic activity (Zachazewski & Reischl, 1986), because increased muscle stiffness may help prevent injury and enhance utilization of elastic energy (Thys et al., 1972).

In static stretching, the stretch position is assumed slowly and gently and held for 30–60 s. By doing so, the contraction from the stretch reflex is slow and mild. As the position is held, the tension from the stretch and stretch reflex contraction becomes strong enough to invoke the inverse stretch reflex which signals the muscle to relax and be stretched further safely (DeVries, 1974). When this happens, the athlete achieves greater flexibility. Compared to other techniques, static stretching produces the least amount of tension (Walker, 1961; Moore & Hutton, 1980) and is the safest method of improving flexibility. It should be used in athletic training, because when performed correctly, the chances of muscle or tendinous injury are very low.

The hold–relax, contract–relax and contract–relax–antagonist contract techniques are part of the PNF method first described by Voss et al. (1985) and popularized for athletes by Holt (1973). During the hold–relax and contract–relax techniques, agonist contraction causes Golgi tendon organ activity that promotes subsequent relaxation of the agonist and allows it to be stretched further. Muscle contraction also results in some extrafusal muscle fibre shortening that may decrease spindle firing even during the isometric contraction of the hold–relax technique. The contract–relax–antagonist contract technique incorporates all these features, as well as the principle of reciprocal inhibition, and may, in theory, be the most effective stretch.

Experimental evaluation of these stretching techniques shows that the contract–relax–antagonist contract method is generally superior to the contract–relax or hold–relax techniques, but the differences are quite small (Tanigawa, 1972; Thys et al., 1972; Markos, 1979; Hartley-O'Brien, 1980; Sady et al., 1982; Ethnyre & Abraham, 1986; Wood et al., 1988). Some studies found both contract–relax and hold–relax techniques to be more effective than static or ballistic stretching, but other studies found no differences (Moore & Hutton, 1980; Condon & Hutton, 1987). There is little difference between the static and ballistic methods, in terms of improvement in flexibility.

In disease states

Stretching techniques used after injury have different objectives, depending on the time elapsed after injury. During the first week after injury, gentle static stretching may be most appropriate, and the muscle–tendon unit should be maintained in a relatively lengthened position to prevent sarcomere loss (Lehto et al., 1985; Baker & Matsumoto, 1988). Active techniques including the ballistic and PNF methods are not recommended because of the potential for further injury. If muscle pain or increased reflex activity is present, perhaps caused by activation of other receptors in the muscle by chemical or pH changes, ice can be used to facilitate relaxation (Prentice, 1982).

Later in recovery, heat and stretching can be used to increase elongation of passive elements within the muscle (Wiktorsson-Moller et al., 1983), and PNF techniques can be employed to increase flexibility. Static stretching should be continued to maintain increases gained with PNF, and active exercise can begin. Ballistic exercises are not appropriate at this time. Regular measurements of muscle length, joint range of motion and strength of the affected muscle must be taken. When these are normal, controlled active movements through range and ballistic movements can be incorporated into the exercise programme.

Planning a programme

When planning a stretching programme it is important to remember that increasing flexibility is a gradual process. It will take several weeks before benefits occur. Athletes who do not begin to stretch until the beginning of a season will receive minimal benefits, if any, that season. Athletes should be encouraged to develop a year-round, daily stretching programme, but if that is not possible, they should begin to stretch at least 6 weeks before preseason training begins.

The choice of stretching methods depends on a number of factors. Static stretching is recommended because it is an easy, safe and appropriate means of maintaining flexibility. PNF methods are better for increasing flexibility and may be used when this is the primary aim. The chief drawbacks are that a partner is usually required to perform the technique correctly, and that both parties must be educated in the technique. Ballistic stretching is not recommended but it may have a place in preparation for athletic activities (Zachazewski & Reischl, 1986; Zachazewski, 1989). Table 20.2 shows a suggested preparatory routine that illustrates the appropriate use of all the stretching techniques mentioned.

Placement of the stretching routine in the workout is very important. Stretching should be preceded by a mild warm-up for several reasons:

1 Stretching muscles that have not been warmed can result in injury.
2 Warming the muscles increases muscle extensibility, which results in immediate gains in flexibility.
3 Stretching after a warm-up allows the athlete to make greater gains in flexibility.

The muscle groups should be alternated throughout the stretching routine. For example, if a routine begins with a mild hamstring stretching exercise, the next exercise should be for some other muscle group. Another hamstring exercise should come later and place a little more force on the muscle than the first. Spacing the exercises will prevent the possibility of exerting too much force on a muscle at one time, thus further reducing the chances of injury.

The important points to consider for the development of a safe stretching programme are:

1 Always precede stretching exercises with a mild warm-up.
2 Use the static stretching technique.
3 Stretch before and after each workout. If

Table 20.2 Routine for athletic participation. Adapted with permission from Zachazewski (1989).

Activity	Method and purpose
General warm-up	Repetitive exercise of muscle groups to be stretched; warms up muscle and connective tissue before strain
Preparticipation stretching	Slow static stretching to elongate passive elements; ballistic stretching at the end of range of motion if there is no pain or injury
Neuromuscular warm-up	Simulate activities, slowly at first, then increasing speed under control; proprioceptive neuromuscular facilitation can be used to increase flexibility and improve motor learning
Postparticipation stretching	Static stretching while muscles are still warm; maintains flexibility and prevents muscle soreness

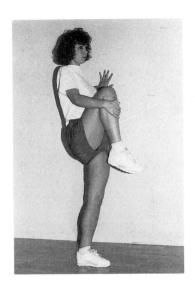 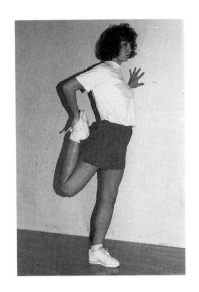

(a)   (b)

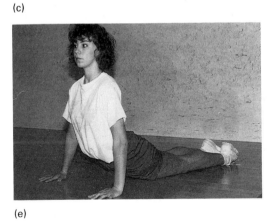 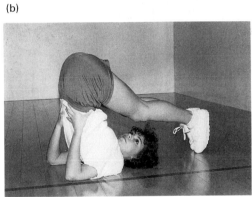

(c)   (d)

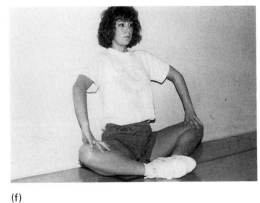

(e)   (f)

Fig. 20.7 Stretching routine.
(a) Hamstrings: pull the knee to the chest.
(b) Quadriceps: grab the foot with the hand and pull towards the buttocks.
(c) Back: rock gently back and forth 8–10 times.
(d) Back: bring legs over head.
(e) Abdomen and chest: push the upper torso back with the arms; push as far back as it will go.
(f) Groin: with the back against a wall and feet together, push down on knees.

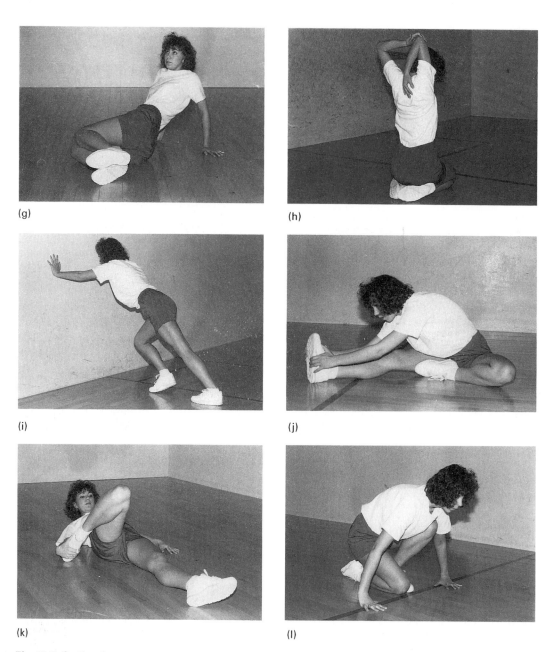

Fig. 20.7 *Continued*.
(g) Hip and sartorius: with legs together, move legs to one side.
(h) Shoulders: put elbow behind head: gently pull elbow toward the centre of the back.
(i) Lower leg: leaning on a wall, keep back foot flat and head up; slowly bend arms and lower body toward wall.
(j) Hamstrings: from position shown, grab ankle and pull body forward.
(k) Quadriceps: lie on back with knee up and leg pulled into side; slowly lower knee.
(l) Lower leg: from position shown, push left knee forward with the chest; keep toes of left foot even with knee of right leg.

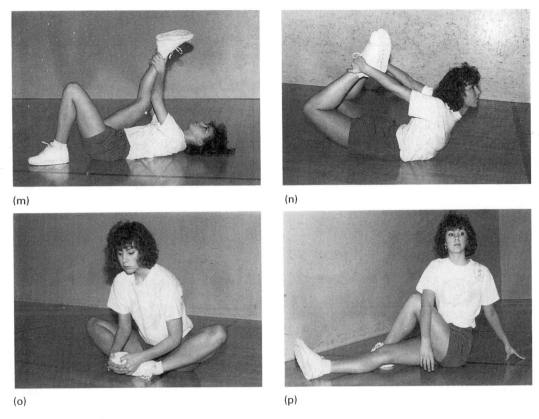

Fig. 20.7 *Continued.*
(m) Hamstrings: grab leg below the calf and pull to head.
(n) Abdomen and chest: grab both feet above the ankles; arch the back and pull the feet toward the head.
(o) Groin: put bottoms of feet together, pull heels toward groin and body forward.
(p) Hip and sartorius: cross left leg and bring right arm through as shown; push on leg with arm and twist body; turn head to the rear.

there is time for only one routine, stretching before the workout is most important. A post-workout stretching routine, however, is an excellent way to relax muscles and minimize muscle soreness.

4 Begin with mild exercises and proceed to ones of moderate difficulty.

5 Alternate exercises for muscle groups.

6 Assume a stretch position gently and hold until tightness and not pain is felt.

7 Hold the position for 30–60 s.

Regardless of the objective or the type of exercise used, the athlete's discomfort should be closely monitored, and the entire process must be totally pain-free.

There has been some speculation that over-flexibility in a joint may result in injury (Nicholas, 1970), and that stretching can lead to overflexibility. These views have not been supported in the literature. Studies show that joint laxity in healthy athletes is not a good predictor of injury (Goodshall, 1975; Grana & Morety, 1978; Jackson *et al.*, 1978). Also, athletes using mild to moderate stretching exercises have never been known to develop overflexibility in a joint. While yogis, dancers and gymnasts can develop hyperextension of the joint, which is a sign of overflexibility, through stretching, that development requires many years of intensive and advanced stretching. Most overflexibility seems to be an anatomical characteristic and not a result of stretching exercises.

As most stretching routines for athletes are sport-specific, it is impossible in this chapter to present stretching routines for all sports. Since running or jogging are very popular sports, Fig. 20.7 shows a stretching routine based on the principles discussed in this chapter. The exercises should be done in the order shown (a–p), and serious runners should do all the exercises.

If the guidelines discussed in this chapter are implemented, the result will be a safe, effective stretching programme that will lessen the chances of injury and enhance athletic performance.

References

Akeson, W.H., Woo, S.L.-Y., Amiel, D. *et al.* (1973) The connective tissue response to immobility: Biochemical changes in periarticular connective tissue of the immobilized rabbit knee. *Clin. Orthop.* **93**, 356–62.

Alnaqeeb, M.A., Alzaid, N.S. & Goldspink, G. (1984) Connective tissue changes and physical properties of developing and aging muscle. *J. Anat.* **139**, 677–89.

Anderson, B., Beaulieu, J.E., Cornelius, W.L. *et al.* (1984) Roundtable: Flexibility. *Natl. Strength Cond. Ass.* **6**, 10–73.

Appell, H.J., Frorsberg, S. & Hollmann, W. (1988) Satellite cell activation in human skeletal muscle after training: Evidence for muscle fiber neoformation. *Int. J. Sports Med.* **9**, 297–9.

Baker, J.H. & Matsumoto, D.E. (1988) Adaptation of skeletal muscle to immobilization in a shortened position. *Muscle Nerve* **11**, 231–44.

Beaulieu, J.E. (1980) *Stretching for All Sports*. Athletic Press, California.

Beaulieu, J.E. (1981) Developing a stretching program. *Phys. Sports Med.* **9**, 59–69.

Benjamin, B. & Roth, P. (1979) Warming up versus stretching. *Running Times* **34**, 15–21.

Bistevins, R. & Awad, E.A. (1981) Structure and ultrastructure of mechanoreceptors at the human musculotendinous junction. *Arch. Phys. Med. Rehab.* **62**, 74–83.

Boone, D.C. & Azen, S.P. (1979) Normal range of motion of joints in male subjects. *J. Bone Joint Surg.* **61A**, 756–9.

Borg, T.K. & Caulfield, J.B. (1980) Morphology of connective tissue in skeletal muscle. *Tissue Cell* **12**, 197–207.

Boyd, I.A. The action of the three types of intrafusal fibre in isolated cat muscle spindles on the dynamic and length sensitivities of primary and secondary sensory ending. In A. Taylor & A. Prochazka (eds) *Muscle Receptors and Movement*, pp. 17–32. Oxford University Press, New York.

Brown, L.P., Nichues, S.L., Harrah, A. *et al.* (1988) Upper extremity range of motion and isokinetic strength of the internal and external shoulder rotators in major league baseball players. *Am. J. Sports Med.* **16**, 577–85.

Butler, D.L., Grood, E.S., Moyes, F.R. *et al.* (1978) Biomechanics of ligaments and tendons. *Exerc. Sport Sci. Rev.* **6**, 125–82.

Carr, G.L. (1971) *The effects of slow stretch and proprioceptive neuromuscular facilitation — Reversal of antagonist exercises on sprinting velocity*. Thesis, Southern Illinois University.

Condon, S.M. & Hutton, R.S. (1987) Soleus muscle electromyographic activity and ankle dorsiflexion range of motion during four stretching procedures. *Phys. Ther.* **67**, 24–30.

Corbin, C.B. & Mable, L. (1980) Flexibility: A major component of physical fitness. *J. Phys. Educ. Rec.* **51**, 23–60.

Curwin, S. & Stanish, W.D. (1984) *Tendinitis: Etiology and Treatment*. Collamore Press, Lexington, Massachusetts.

Curwin, S., Vailas, A.C. & Wood, J. (1988) Immature tendon adaptation to strenuous exercise. *J. Appl. Physiol.* **65**, 2297–301.

DeVries, H.A. (1962) Evaluation of static stretching procedures for improvement of flexibility. *Res. Q.* **33**, 222–9.

DeVries, H.A. (1974) *Physiology of Exercise for Physical Education and Athletics*, 2nd edn. William C. Brown, Iowa.

Ekstrand, J. & Gillquist, J. (1982) The frequency of muscle tightness and injuries in soccer players. *Am. J. Sports Med.* **10**, 75–8.

Ethnyre, B.R. & Abraham, L.D. (1986) Gains in range of ankle dorsiflexion using three popular stretching techniques. *Am. J. Phys. Med.* **65**, 189–96.

Fixx, J. *Second Book of Running*. Random House, New York.

Garrett Jr, W.E. & Fidball, J. (1988) Myotendinous junction: Structure, function, and failure. In S.L.-Y. Woo & J.A. Buckwalter (eds) *Injury and Repair of the Musculoskeletal Soft Tissues*, pp. 171–207. American Academy of Orthopaedic Surgeons, Illinois.

Garrett Jr, W.E., Nikolaou, P.K., Ribbeck, B.M. *et al.* (1988) The effect of muscle architecture on the biomechanical failure properties of skeletal muscle under passive extension. *Am. J. Sports Med.* **16**, 7–12.

Garrett Jr, W.E., Safran, M.R., Seaber, A.V. *et al.* (1987) Biomechanical comparison of stimulated and nonstimulated skeletal muscle pulled to failure. *Am. J. Sports Med.* **15**, 448–54.

Goodshall, R.W. (1975) The predictability of athletic injuries: An eight-year study. *J. Sport Med.* **3**, 50–4.

Gossman, M.R., Sahrmann, S.A. & Rose, S.J. (1982) Review of length-associated changes in muscle: Experimental evidence and clinical implications. *Phys. Ther.* **62**, 1799–808.

Grana, W.A. & Morety, J.A. (1978) Ligamentous laxity in secondary school athletes. *JAMA* **240**, 1975–6.

Halkovich, L.R., Personius, W.J., Claamann, H.P. *et al.* (1981) Effect of fluori methane spray on passive hip flexion. *Phys. Ther.* **6**, 185–9.

Hartley-O'Brien, S.J. (1980) Six mobilization exercises for active range of hip flexion. *Res. Q.* **51**, 625–35.

Henricson, A.S., Fredriksson, K., Persson, I. *et al.* (1984) The effect of heat and stretching on the range of hip motion. *J. Orthop. Sports Phys. Ther.* **6**, 110–15.

Holt, L.E. (1973) *Scientific Stretching for Sport*. Sport Research Ltd, Halifax.

Horswill, C.A., Layman, D.K., Boileau, R.A. *et al.* (1988) Excretion of 3-methylhisticline and hydroxyproline following acute weight-training exercise. *Int. J. Sports Med.* **9**, 245–8.

Jackson, D.W., Jarrett, H., Bailey, D. *et al.* (1978) Injury prediction in the young athlete. *Am. J. Sports Med.* **6**, 6–14.

Kelly, M. (1969) Effectiveness of a cryotherapy technique on spasticity. *Phys. Ther.* **49**, 349–53.

Kendall, H.O. & Kendall, F.P. (1948) Normal flexibility according to age groups. *J. Bone Joint Surg.* **30A**, 690–4.

Kirby, R.L., Simms, F.C., Symington, V.J. *et al.* (1981) Flexibility and musculoskeletal symptomatology in female gymnasts and age-matched controls. *Am. J. Sports Med.* **9**, 160–4.

Komi, P.V. (1984) Physiological and biomechanical correlates of muscle function: Effects of muscle structure and stretch-shortening cycle on force and speed. *Exerc. Sports Sci. Rev.* **12**, 81–121.

Kottke, F.J., Pauley, D.J. & Ptak, R.A. (1966) The rationale for prolonged stretching for correction of shortening of connective tissue. *Arch. Phys. Med.* **47**, 345–52.

Koury, S., Mamary, M., Kagan, R. *et al.* (1986) Effect of fluori-methane spray on hamstring extensibility during 'contract/reflex' and active stretching (Abstract). *Phys. Ther.* **66**, 806.

Kovanen, V., Suominen, H. & Peltonen, L. (1987) Effects of aging and life-long physical training on collagen in slow and fast skeletal muscle in rats: A morphometric and immuno-histochemical study. *Cell Tissue Res.* **248**, 247–55.

Kvist, M. & Jarvinen, M. (1982) Clinical, histochemical and biomechanical features in repair of muscle and tendon injuries. *Int. J. Sports Med.* **3**(Suppl. 1), 12–14.

Landreth, W.G.A. (1957) *A comparative study of two methods for improving range of movement*. Thesis, University of California, Los Angeles.

Lehmann, J.F., Masock, A.J., Warren, C.G. & Hoblanski, I.N. (1970) Effect of therapeutic temperatures on tendon extensibility. *Arch. Phys. Med. Rehab.* **51**, 481–7.

Lehto, M., Duance, V.C. & Restall, D. (1985) Collagen and fibronectin in a healing skeletal muscle injury: An immunohistological study of the effects of physical activity on the repair of injured gastrocnemius muscle in the rat. *J. Bone Joint Surg.* **67B**, 820–8.

Lysholm, J. & Wiklander, J. (1987) Injuries in runners. *Am. J. Sports Med.* **15**, 168–71.

Markos, P.D. (1979) Ipsilateral and contralateral effects of proprioceptive neuromuscular facilitation techniques on hip motion and electromyographic activity. *Phys. Ther.* **59**, 1366–73.

Miglietta, O. (1964) Electromyographic characteristics of clonus and influence of cold. *Arch. Phys. Med.* **45**, 508–12.

Moore, M.J. (1983) The dual connective tissue system of rat soleus muscle. *Muscle Nerve* **6**, 416–22.

Moore, M.A. & Hutton, R.S. (1980) Electromyographic investigation of muscle stretching techniques. *Med. Sci. Sports Exerc.* **12**, 322–9.

Newton, A. (1985) Effects of vapocoolants on passive hip flexion in healthy subjects. *Phys. Ther.* **65**, 1034–6.

Nicholas, J.A. (1970) Injuries to knee ligaments. Relationship to looseness and tightness in football players. *JAMA* **212**, 2236–9.

Nikolaou, P.K., MacDonald, B.L., Glisson, R.R. *et al.* (1987) Biomechanical and histological evaluation of muscle after control strain injury. *Am. J. Sports Med.* **15**, 9–14.

Osler, T. (1978) *Serious Runners Handbook*. World Publications, California.

Prentice Jr, W.E. (1982) An electromyographic analysis of the effectiveness of heat or cold and stretching for inducing relaxation in injured muscle. *J. Orthop. Sports Phys. Ther.* **3**, 133–40.

Raab, D.M., Ayre, J.C., McAdam, M. *et al.* (1988) Light resistance and stretching exercise in elderly women: Effect upon flexibility. *Arch. Phys. Med. Rehab.* **69**, 268–72.

Reid, D.C., Burnham, T.S., Saboe, L.A. *et al.* (1987) Lower extremity flexibility patterns in classical ballet dancers and their correlation to lateral hip and knee injuries. *Am. J. Sports Med.* **15**, 347–52.

Riddle, K.S. (1956) *A comparison of three methods for increasing flexibility of the trunk and hip joints.* Dissertation, University of Oregon.

Sady, S.P., Wortman, M. & Blanke, E. (1982) Flexibility training: Ballistic, static, or proprioceptive neuromuscular facilitation? *Arch. Phys. Med. Rehab.* **63**, 261–3.

Sale, D.G. (1988) Neural adaptation to resistance training. *Med. Sci. Sports Exerc.* **20**(Suppl.), S135–45.

Saltin, B. & Hermansen, L. (1966) Esophageal, rectal, and muscle temperature during exercise. *J. Appl. Physiol.* **21**, 1757–62.

Schultz, P. (1979) Flexibility: Day of the static stretch. *Phys. Sportsmed* **7**, 109–17.

Stanish, W.D. (1982) Neurophysiology of stretching. In R. D'Ambrosia & D. Drez (eds) *Prevention and Treatment of Running Injuries.* Charles B. Slack, Thorofare, New Jersey.

Stolov, W.C. & Thompson, S.C. (1979) Soleus immobilization contraction in young and old rats. *Arch. Phys. Med. Rehab.* **60**, 556–7.

Tanigawa, M.C. (1972) Comparison of the hold–relax procedure and passive mobilization on increasing muscle length. *Phys. Ther.* **52**, 725–35.

Thys, H., Traraggiana, T. & Margaria, R. (1972) Utilization of muscle elasticity in exercise. *J. Appl. Physiol.* **32**, 491–4.

Vailas, A.C., Pedrini, V.A, Pedrini-Mille, A. *et al.* (1985) Patellar tendon matrix changes associated with aging and voluntary exercise. *J. Appl. Physiol.* **58**, 1572–6.

Vailas, A.C., Tipton, C.M., Matthes, R.D. *et al.* (1981) Physical activity and its influence on the repair process of medial collateral ligaments. *Connect. Tiss. Res.* **9**, 25–31.

Viidik, A. (1979) Connective tissues: Possible implications of the temporal changes for the aging process. *Mech. Aging Dev.* **9**, 267–85.

Voss, D.E., Jonta, M.K. & Myers, B.J. (1985) *Proprioceptive Neuromuscular Facilitation: Patterns and Techniques,* 3rd edn. Harper & Row, Philadelphia.

Walker, J.M., Sue, D., Wiles-Elkousy, N. *et al.* (1984) Active mobility of the extremities in older subjects. *Phys. Ther.* **64**, 919–23.

Walker, S.M. (1961) Delay of twitch relaxation induced by stress and stress relaxation. *J. Appl. Physiol.* **16**, 801–6.

Wallin, D., Ekblom, B., Grahn, R. *et al.* (1985) Improvement of muscle flexibility: A comparison between two techniques. *Am. J. Sports Med.* **13**, 263–8.

Warren, C.G., Lehmann, J.F. & Hoblanski, J.N. (1976) Heat and stretch procedures: An evaluation using rat tail tendon. *Arch. Phys. Med. Rehab.* **57**, 122–6.

Williford, H.N., East, J.B., Smith, F.H. *et al.* (1986) Evaluation of warm-up for improvement in flexibility. *Am. J. Sports Med.* **14**, 316–19.

Williford, H.N. & Smith, J.F. (1985) A comparison of proprioceptive neuromuscular facilitation and static stretching techniques. *Am. Corr. Ther. J.* **39**, 30–3.

Wood, T.O., Cooke, P.H. & Goodship, A.E. (1988) The effect of exercise and anabolic steroids on the mechanical properties and crimp morphology of the rat tendon. *Am. J. Sports Med.* **16**, 153–8.

Wiktorsson-Moller, M., Oberg, B., Ekstrand, J. *et al.* (1983) Effects of warming up, massage, and stretching on range of motion and muscle strength in the lower extremity. *Am. J. Sports Med.* **11**, 249–52.

Zachazewski, J.E. (1989) Improving flexibility. In R.M. Scully & M.R. Barnes (eds) *Physical Therapy,* pp. 698–738. JB Lippincott, Philadelphia.

Zachazewski, J.E. & Reischl, S.R. (1986) Flexibility for the runner: Specific program consideration. *Topics Acute Care Trauma Rehab.* **1**, 9–16.

Chapter 21

Proprioception and Coordination Training in Injury Prevention

HANS TROPP, HANNU ALARANTA AND PER A.F.H. RENSTRÖM

During recent years there has been increasing attention to the fact that reduced motor skill and coordination may complicate musculoskeletal disorders. Decreased motor skill may be the effect of musculoskeletal injuries, but the question has also been raised whether decreased motor skill, coordination or postural control could be a risk factor, or a cause for musculoskeletal disorders, and if it is possible to improve this kind of dysfunction. Can improvement of motor skill and coordination be of significance in the prevention of musculoskeletal injuries?

Neurophysiological background

Two-way communication between the sensory and motor systems is essential for normal motor control. Vision is one of most important senses (visual input). Reports from the inner ear about head positions in relation to gravity and to head movements (vestibular input) is also important. The most important body sense is proprioception. Sensory organs in the tendons that anchor muscles to the bones signal how hard the muscles are pulling, and the sense organs within the muscle signals how the muscles are stretched (Fig. 21.1). This is known as proprioceptive feedback. In addition, we use kinesthetic input from receptors in the joints, and somatic input from skin sensors for touch, temperature or pain.

If there is a mismatch between the intended motor programme and the actual movements, appropriate corrections can be made by the central nervous system (CNS), even without conscious decisions. The better the programmes have been learned, the fewer the corrections that are needed. The movements become faster and smoother. In other words, they are more skilful. Motor skill, the optimal use of programmed movements, is further improved by adjusting muscle tensions to make accurately programmed movements with the greatest economy.

Motor control seems to be hierarchically organized into different levels (Nashner & Woollacott, 1979; Nashner et al., 1979, 1982) and in the execution of a voluntary movement, the nervous system is brought into operation at all these levels (Eccles, 1981).

The cerebral cortex initiates and prescribes a sequence of stereotype patterns for all voluntary movements, establishes the level of activity, and carries out in detail the interpretation of sensory information (Grillner, 1975). In 1906, Sherrington pointed out that agonist and antagonist coactivation originated from the motor cortex as a general command to perform a specific motion rather than individual control of a single muscle. Complex locomotion movements are broken down into much simpler, stereotype patterns, each of which is executed by spinal movement pattern generators.

Central programming reduces the number of motor procedures to a smaller number of centrally organized strategies, simplifies the process of adaptation, and shortens the reaction

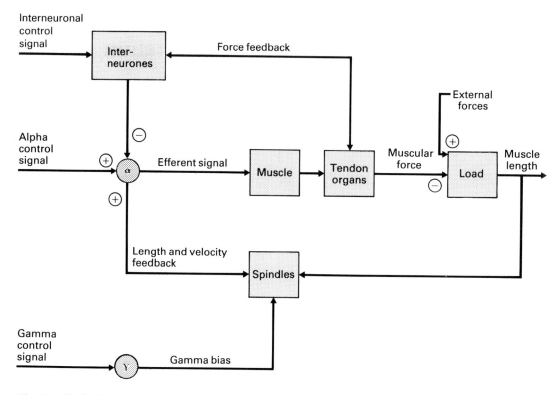

Fig. 21.1 Block diagram of muscle control system. Muscle and its load are regulated by two feedback pathways, one signalling length and velocity through spindle receptors (in parallel with muscle) and the other signalling muscular force through tendon organs (in series with muscle). The central nervous system initiates movement and modifies feedback by sending three sorts of control signals to various neurones in the spinal cord. Gamma bias edits feedback from spindles. Responses of tendon organs are not edited and, therefore, report actual muscular force. Messages from both spindles and tendon organs project to spinal neurones as shown, as well as further centrally into the brain (not shown). Excitation and inhibition are denoted by + or −. With permission from Houk (1974).

latencies (Brooks, 1979; Horak & Nashner, 1986). An example of this is to simplify two strategies earlier used to describe postural control mechanisms, i.e. ankle and hip strategies (Nashner & McCollum, 1985). By combining these two distinct strategies of different magnitude and temporal relation, a manageable number of motor behaviours is obtained.

A motor programme is a set of muscle commands that are structured before a movement begins: all allowing the entire sequence to be carried out uninfluenced by peripheral feedback (Keele, 1968). Anticipatory postural corrections associated with voluntary movement have been shown to be centrally prepro-

grammed because they are performed in a consistent pattern and come into play well before the actual movement (Bouisset & Zattara, 1987). This fact may be of importance in certain sports such as tennis.

At spinal level, there are numerous pathways for interaction (Grillner, 1975; Roberts, 1978). Inter-limb coordination is achieved by interaction of the generators of both limbs. Impairment in functional tests after an injury is often bilateral (Gauffin, 1991). Inter-limb coordination may conceal impairment if differences between limbs are found, which sometimes is the case (Odensten, 1984; Tegner et al., 1986). Training of one limb can improve performance of the contralateral, untrained limb. This is indirectly supported by a randomized and controlled training study by Kannus et al. (1992). The strength of the contralateral quadriceps was increased, although real training only was prescribed ipsilaterally. These findings underline the importance of the central motor programmes.

Even if motion is preprogrammed and works automatically after initiation, there are effective ways of adaptation based on different systems. Sensory impulses, their sources described above, are transmitted across motor neurones and activate reflex circuits at various CNS levels. Information from the higher centres, where previous experiences are stored, initiates conscious movements to bring about adjustments. Information concerning aims of motion and types of efferent signals 'the efferent copy' is available. The cerebellum can provide a comparison between the current state as reported by the peripheral receptors and the desired state as formulated by the cerebral cortex. There is a design for mechanisms which allows reprogramming movements dependent on motor memories (Roberts, 1978; Eccles, 1981).

How to evaluate proprioception and coordination?

Among clinicians active in sports medicine, there has been a growing interest in the use of kinesiology and biomechanics in the analysis of the athletes' problems. There have been many attempts to study sports activities in the field, but there are obvious difficulties in studying specific impairments and deciding upon anticipatory injuries. However, there are lots of different kinds of motor control tests available (Taimela et al., 1990; Alaranta et al., 1992).

Electromyograph (EMG) timing, balance swaying, reaction time for both auditory and visual stimuli, limb steadiness, the speed of limb movement, multi-limb coordination and different jumping and running combinations such as figure 8 trails have been used (Taimela

et al., 1990; Karlsson et al., 1992). The structure of the limb will not tell us much about the underlying dysfunction. A more useful way is to extract basic motions. It may be difficult to find basic and reproducible motion sequences necessary for kinematic studies when dealing with impairments of strenuous activities. Studies have been presented which focus on one basic motion thus emphasizing one of the functions of the joint, and this has been studied using gait analysis. The dynamics of pathological motion has been studied in anterior cruciate deficient knees by Andriacchi (1990). Other testing activities such as walking, jogging and stair-climbing can be useful. The one-leg jump, as a more potent extractor of stability demanding knee function, has been studied by Gauffin (1991).

World Health Organization classification (WHO, 1980) concerning the consequence of disease and effects of illness are: (i) loss of anatomical structure or function — impairment; (ii) decrease in terms of performance — disability; and (iii) limitations in activity — handicap.

Some injuries such as anterior cruciate and ankle joint ligament injuries have their basic effects upon disability through some of their qualities of impairment. The inability to counteract external knee load without tibia translation and the difficulties of maintaining postural equilibrium by means of ankle joint corrections, produce a large amount of disability for the athlete (Fig. 21.2). These disabilities may also have an effect on handicap, which, however, is dependent on the quality and intensity of the sports performed.

Motor ability

Beginners in a sport are at a higher risk of injury compared to non-beginners (Berson et al., 1981; Bernard et al., 1988). The novice lacks specific coordination to perform the particular type of activities safely (Taimela, 1991). A total of 38% of 991 athletes, aged 20–63 years, who entered a fitness programme experi-

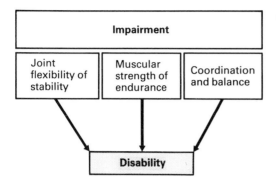

Fig. 21.2 The biomechanical components of musculoskeletal impairment affecting disability.

enced a new injury during the first 4 months (Sedgwick, 1988). Poor coordination and slow psychomotor speed may predispose for injury (Beck, 1985; Edwards, 1988).

Motor control of the knee joints

The anterior cruciate ligament is the most commonly injured ligament of the knee joint (Johnson *et al.*, 1992). A complete tear can lead to severe knee damage including articular cartilage defects, meniscus tears and secondary stretching of the capsule and ligaments, and continued functional disability.

The cruciate ligaments constitute primary restraints to anteroposterior displacement. The secondary restraints are recruited to compensate for loss of the anterior cruciate ligament. Injury to the secondary restraints makes the prognosis after rupture of the anterior cruciate ligament worse.

It is only in the last 10 years that all the mechanoreceptors or neuroreceptors such as Ruffini endings, pacinian, corpuscle, golgi tendon organs and free nerve endings have been described in the cruciate ligament of the human knee joint (Schultz *et al.*, 1984). Most receptors are located near the bone attachment. Between 1 and 2% of the total volume of the anterior cruciate ligament is neuronal tissue. These facts have led to suggestions that knee ligaments have a significant sensory function

(Schultz *et al.*, 1984; Schutte *et al.*, 1987). Mechanoreceptors have also been demonstrated in various dissections of animal knees in structures such as the medial collateral ligament (MCL) (Freeman & Wyke, 1964; Andrew, 1990) and the menisci (Kennedy *et al.*, 1982), particularly in the posterior horns (O'Connor, 1984). Andersson and Stener (1959), Stener (1959) and Peterzén and Stener (1959) earlier tested the ligament muscle reflex arch hypothesis in cats and humans. The muscle receptors could possibly contribute to position sense (Goodwin *et al.*, 1972; Roland, 1975) merely to modifying muscle tension (Guyton, 1986). Kennedy *et al.* (1982) hypothesized that knee injury leads to ligamentous laxity resulting in failure of mechanoreceptor feedback and loss of reflex muscular contractions, and contributing to repetitive injuries and clinical deterioration.

Loss of proprioceptive feedback has been shown in patients with ruptured anterior cruciate ligament, and has been suggested to contribute to progressive instability and disability of the knee (Skinner *et al.*, 1986; Barrack & Skinner, 1990). However, a secondary reflex is proposed to appear from the joint capsule or thigh muscle receptors, which is capable of causing stability in patients with anterior cruciate ligament deficiency (Solomonow *et al.*, 1987). Neuromuscular training can, to some degree, compensate for the loss of sensory input following knee ligament injuries (Ihara, 1986; Barrack & Skinner, 1990). There is an altered gait both in osteoarthritis and cruciate ligament deficient knees, shown by using biomechanical analysis of human mobility with emphasis on activity patterns and related load (Prodromos *et al.*, 1985).

Using a kinesiological approach to the problem and by means of motion analysis integrated with EMG, force plate recording and computerized biomechanical modelling, impaired performance of one-leg distance jump was found among patients with old anterior cruciate ligament rupture (Gauffin, 1991). Non-injured limb also showed impaired one-leg distance jump.

The dynamic analysis revealed adapted movement and muscular activation patterns for the injured compared to the non-injured knee at touch down after a one-legged jump. A knee model disclosed a simultaneous decrease in sagittal shear load, which was interpreted as an adaptation to avoid increased intrinsic joint movements or gross subluxations. The symptom of functional instability is due to a subluxation in the knee joint that muscle activation cannot prevent.

In a cat experiment, Johansson et al. (1991a) suggest that the secondary muscle spindle afferents are affected by stretching the anterior cruciate ligament (Fig. 21.3). This could have an afferent effect upon control of muscle stiffness through the gamma-muscle—spindle system. Without an intact anterior cruciate ligament, the knee is more prone to injury. This indicates that the joint detects the increased amount of unphysiological movements and adjusts for impaired mechanical stability not only through reflex-mediated hamstring activity, but also through a change in motor-control patterns.

Traditionally, quadriceps strength training used to be employed. The discovery that isolated quadriceps contraction increases the strain within the anterior cruciate ligament five-fold (Renström et al., 1986), together with reports that quadriceps activity might be harmful, alters the goals for rehabilitation (Paulos et al., 1981). It seems important to emphasize the co-contraction of hamstrings muscle, which must anticipate quadriceps activity. Biomechanically it would, therefore, seem important to exercise against the external forces, which create flexion of both knee and hip joints (e.g. leg press exercises).

When using dynamic analysis of motion, it is important to realize that the adaptations might be necessary for continued joint function and not be a reason for, or a negative effect caused by the injury. If this adaptation fails, the function will be deteriorated, e.g. a symptomatic, unstable knee will be the site of inflammation, cartilage injury, meniscus damage and result in a repaired knee with limping in extension.

There is still an unclear correlation between

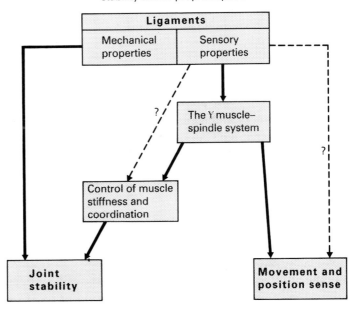

Mechanisms by which ligaments may contribute to regulation of joint stability and to proprioception

Fig. 21.3 Basic organization of how reflexes from ligamentous joint afferents may contribute to the regulation of muscle stiffness around joints, joint stability and movement and position sense. With permission from Johansson et al. (1991b).

proprioception and clinical ligament stability testing. Barrett (1991) found no relation between proprioception and tightness in contrast to Barrack and Skinner (1990) who found significant correlation with arthrometer readings and proprioceptive measurements. Corrigan *et al.* (1992) measured joint position sense and found that subjects with anterior cruciate ligament tears and greater hamstring dominance had better proprioception than those with lower values. The quadriceps atrophy seen in anterior cruciate ligament deficient knees, may be reflexly induced in order to optimize proprioception from the knee.

In prevention, it is possible to prescribe controlled use of the injured limb for simulation of reflex activities, and a sensory directed adaptation of motor programmes at the spinal level, by using previously reviewed knowledge about motor control and adaptation. Instability should be provoked in such situations so that altered muscular activation can be achieved.

Motor control of the ankle joint

Injury to the lateral ligaments of the ankle are the most common injuries in sports and active life. Residual disability has been shown after both conservative and surgical treatment. The most common disorder is called instability of which two forms are known. Mechanical instability can be defined as lack of or insufficiency of adequate stabilizing structures and mobility exceeding physiological limits; and the cause of injury is damage to the capsule ligamentous structures (Rasmussen, 1985). The more diffuse term 'functional instability' may be defined as recurrent sprains and/or a feeling of giving way of the ankle with cause unclear (Tropp *et al.*, 1985a).

Proprioceptive deficits have been demonstrated after ankle sprains (Freeman, 1965), but it is also hard to prove any effect on postural control (Gauffin, 1991). Position sense following ankle injury showed a linear trend between the degree of error and the degree of angle of movement, compared with the uninjured joint, the error being greatest for the most severely injured group of subjects (Glencross & Thornton, 1981). Loss of precision months after injury improved after training, which implies that rehabilitation involves relearning as much as physical recovery.

Mechanically unstable ankle joints cause increased reaction times in peroneus muscles due to an increase in the time taken to stretch the receptors in the elongated ligaments and capsule (Karlsson *et al.*, 1992). Thus, the proprioceptors may be intact, but are activated first at the wider angle joint.

Freeman (1965), who was the first to discuss this disability in functional terms, found functional instability in 40% of the patients who had sustained ankle lateral ligament injury. He suggested that the main cause of proprioceptive damage to the joint produces proprioceptive deficit and impaired postural control. By objective measurement of postural sway-stabilometry, it has been confirmed that ankle joint function is correlated to the ability to maintain equilibrium in single limb stance (Tropp & Odenrick, 1988). When working properly, the ankle can govern correction of posture. If this motion pattern of postural control is insufficient, equilibrium has to be maintained by movements in upper segments of the body. Impaired postural control indicates that the risk of ankle joint injury is increased even in previously uninjured soccer players. Players with previous ankle problems were also at higher injury risk (Tropp *et al.*, 1985a). Soccer players with functional instability had pathological stabilometry values, but the degree of mechanical instability was not reflected by the figures (Tropp *et al.*, 1985b). This probably means that if an ankle injury is related to defective postural control, it will lead to functional instability and renewed injury.

Postural control is hierarchically organized with stereotype patterns for rapid postural adjustment (Horak & Nashner, 1986). After an injury, a person may, therefore, learn new patterns of voluntary command to the muscles to compensate for pain, loss of muscular strength and changes in reflex sensitivity.

The nature of the instability must, however, be analysed before deciding on the form of treatment. Mechanical instability can be helped with muscle strength training, and if needed with late surgical repair of the lateral ligaments (Broström, 1966; Peterson et al., 1979; Karlsson et al., 1991). Indications for reconstructive surgery are mechanical instability and related problems such as pain due to synovitis. In cases with functional instability, there is no rational indication for surgery. Coordination training on an ankle disc improves postural control and pronator muscle strength, and reduces the feeling of giving way of the ankle (Tropp & Askling, 1988).

Ankle disc training is not only effective for symptoms caused by functional instability, but is also effective in preventing further ankle sprains (Tropp et al., 1984).

If both mechanical and functional instability are present, reconstructive surgery is often required. Karlsson et al. (1991) presented results in 100 consecutive patients with chronic lateral functional instability treated in physiotherapy, including active range of motion training, strengthening exercises and coordination with a tilt-board. In 49 patients, the results were excellent or good. The outcome was better in patients with painful functional instability or mild mechanical instability, but those with pronounced mechanical instability required reconstructive surgery. Despite physiotherapy 10−20% of the patients developed functional instability. The predictors for poor prognosis are not known, but severe mechanical instability is of importance. Nevertheless, the degree of joint laxity cannot determine whether immediate surgery is needed, and non-operative functional treatment should be tried first (Kannus & Renström 1991).

Surgery is primarily aimed at structural factors such as ligamentous laxity. Improvement in functional instability has, in spite of this, been reported probably due to limitation of subtalar motion (Sammarco & DiRaimondo, 1988) It is probably important to include ankle disc training in the postoperative programme to improve postural control and ankle joint function, and the risk for traumatic reinjury will thereby be reduced.

Functional treatment is preferred in the acute treatment of injury to the lateral ligaments of the ankles. Strapping and mobilization are preferred, although surgery is sometimes indicated in young athletes (Evans et al., 1984). Functional instability can probably be prevented after a primary injury if ankle disc training is included in the rehabilitation programme.

Analysis of the different types of residual instability is probably the best approach to understanding ankle problems in athletes and also to improving first-line treatment, rehabilitation and prevention of these common injuries.

Coordination training

Biomechanically the term 'load sharing' means that in any specific situation there are gravity, inertia and reaction forces creating a specific external load described by the net forces and torque upon the musculoskeletal system. This load is counteracted by the internal forces on musculotendinous and capsular structures, together with joint contact forces. The internal forces balance the external, but might be produced in many different ways. The anterior cruciate deficient knee, the previously injured shoulder and the mechanically unstable ankle joint demand musculotendinous stabilization forces because the injured joint has an impaired capsuloligamentous stability. The actual load sharing has to be adjusted. The initiation for that is the sensory feedback from load mechanoreceptors. This is not an on-line effect but takes place during some weeks or hours of controlled motion.

Good proprioception and coordination means that all the components of musculoskeletal fitness are in balance (Fig. 21.4). If any one of these links is poor, the whole chain may break. Beyond the specific proprioception and coordination training, the aim should also be to achieve a good balance of all the subcomponents in order to achieve musculoskeletal fitness. In prevention, training of relaxation, elasticity and flexibility may be needed and, therefore, these elements should be more prominent than the other subcomponents. Posttraumatic or postoperative rehabilitation may require more emphasis on strength, endurance and velocity in the final phase before returning to the sports arena.

There is no direct scientific evidence showing that training has any effect upon proprioception even if this is often implied (Freeman, 1965). The adaptation mechanism is active in situations which are physiological, representing basic situations that can be met by the athlete, but do not involve a direct risk of reinjury or joint damage. The anterior cruciate ligament hamstrings reflex may be so rapid that the ligament can be protected from overload damage. The joint capsule hamstring reflex, however, probably occurs after subluxation and does not prevent, but only corrects

the injury. The general increase in hamstring activation in anterior cruciate ligament deficient knees is a learnt behaviour and is therefore of value in the prevention of recurrent injuries (Solomonow *et al.*, 1989).

Anterior cruciate ligament injuries in active people should be treated operatively (Johnson *et al.*, 1992), but if the patient is willing to decrease his or her activity level, the injury can sometimes be treated conservatively. Conservative treatment is not suitable for athletes in sports activities which include cutting, jumping or deceleration such as soccer, basketball and similar activities.

The acquisition of refined skills necessitates prior learning of gross skill patterns (basic skills). Highly refined skills are modifications of basic motor patterns such as high jumping and throwing. Every athletic activity embraces basic skills. Refinements and variations of these basic skills make the difference between mediocrity and excellence (Jensen & Garth, 1979). Once a tennis player has learned the basic tennis strokes, modifications can be made, which can result in a top spin or a slice of the ball. It is suggested that the same mechanisms take place in coordination training after

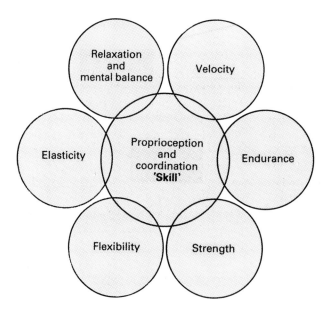

Fig. 21.4 The components of musculoskeletal fitness focused on proprioception and coordination.

an injury and at adaptational re-education of joint instability.

Several factors are related to the development of refined skills and activation factors. These include reciprocal inhibition, which means the blocking of antagonistic muscle groups. Reciprocity can, however, be impaired by anxiety and emotional involvement.

Strength and endurance are probably other important factors because refined coordination is adversely affected by the onset of fatigue. Golfers, for example, make more mistakes in the latter phases of a tournament. Ankles are sprained twice as much in the second than the first half of a soccer game (Renström *et al.*, 1977; Tropp, 1985).

Mental training gives awareness of body position, which is also determined by a variety of sensory inputs to the CNS. Mental training should not be underestimated because psychological factors are important contributing factors in sustaining injuries (Taimela, 1991).

Training of the central integration of postural control may improve the awareness of risks for injury. An orthosis or taping may improve awareness and proprioceptive joint input. Essentially, improvement in postural control involves determining the correct mechanics and practising the skill many times. The skill must

be practised correctly until the movement patterns become effective and efficient.

Mechanically unstable ankle joints will become increasingly injury prone if a coordination deficit appears. Previously uninjured and asymptomatic joints are injury prone if impaired postural control can be detected by stabilometry recording (Tropp *et al.*, 1984). The ligaments and their mechanoreceptors may guard for unphysiological motion and the symptom of instability until the joint is injured. Coordination training may thereby improve the ability to adjust for provocations and diminish the risk of injury. Tropp and Askling (1988) found that 10 min of daily coordination training over 10 weeks was adequate for functionally unstable ankles (Fig. 21.5). Until then ankle bracing or tape can be used for prevention of reinjury. Ankle disc training should be performed without bracing. Similar effects can be achieved by using trampoline, balance platforms, rope jumping and gliding boards (Fig. 21.6). For non-athletes balance training can begin with single limb stance on the floor.

For knee rehabilitation bicycle training is recommended as it includes co-contraction of quadriceps and hamstrings, and the knee is protected from sagittal shear forces. Progressively one can increase the intensity of simul-

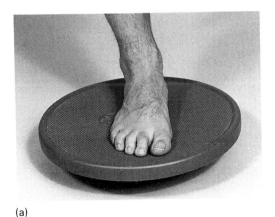

(a)

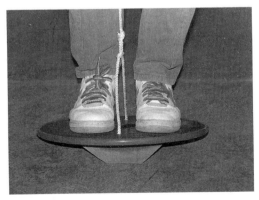

(b)

Fig. 21.5 (a) Ankle disc in coordination training. With permission from Tropp (1985). (b) Alternative technique. With permission from Kuntovalinieco, Helsinki, Finland.

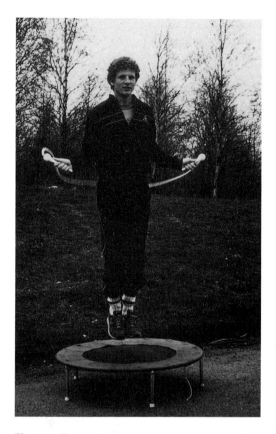

Fig. 21.6 Trampoline training in combination with rope jumping.

also as a crucial proprioceptive detector (Muller, 1983).

The length of time for training to improve postural control has not been determined, although Tropp and Askling (1988) did find that 10 weeks of ankle disc training gave optimal results with this technique (Fig. 21.7). A few trials may be enough to alter postural reactions to confined platform perturbations, but weeks or years may be necessary to alter functional postural strategies. Millions of repetitions may be needed to improve motor control, which must progress from slow velocity, low load and low arc according to Kottke (1980) (Table 21.1). Perhaps similar strategies will prove necessary for improving postural control. The most meaningful dependent variables will be functional tasks assessed over a long period of time rather than isolated, dependent variables, which, although objective and reliable, may not be representative enough of function to be meaningful.

Sport-specific training including conditioning can usually be achieved by training within the sport itself, e.g. many soccer coaches prefer training carried out on the soccer field; the same is true for tennis (Renström & Kannus,

taneous knee flexor and extensor training with progressive leg press exercises. Knee bracing has so far not shown to be of any significant value for muscular activation during fast activities. Braces have been shown to give no major stabilizing effect on the anterior cruciate ligament during higher loads (Beynnon & Renström, 1991). Theoretically a well-fitted functional brace may be contraindicated during coordination training because mechanoreceptors are not activated and adaptation does not take place.

The meniscus contains proprioceptive receptors which have a significant role in the mechanical stability of the knee. It is important to save the meniscal structure after ruptures as the meniscus works not only as a stabilizer, but

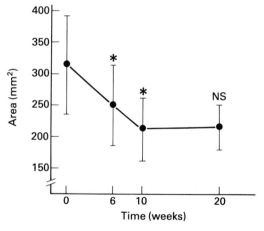

Fig. 21.7 Stabilometry results initially and after 6, 10 and 20 weeks of ankle disc training. With permission from Tropp et al. (1985b). * $P > 0.001$; NS, not significant.

Table 21.1 Training of a coordination engram. Adapted from Kottke (1980).

Introduce movement pattern into patient's repertory:
1 Set up conditions for training in which each task is consistently performed correctly
2 Desynthesize pattern to units simple enough to be consistently performed correctly

Train each individual unit by voluntary control training:
1 Instruct in and demonstrate desired performance by sensory stimulation and passive movement
2 Repeat slow, effortless precise performance of movement unit, allowing no co-contraction of muscles not in unit being trained
3 If patient shows fatigue or diminishing control, repeat the correct pattern passively and then discontinue that task for treatment session
4 Allow strength of muscular contraction to be increased only when there is no undesired co-contraction
5 Be sure that the patient can perform independently and correctly before proceeding to more advanced activity

Repetition of correct performance causes formation of engram:
1 Maintain precision by low effort and slow speed
2 Practice at speed and force which allows successful precise performance of movement unit
3 Increase speed and force only as precision can be maintained
4 Patient needs to repeat correct and precise contraction of each movement unit many times each day
5 Many thousands of repetitions are necessary to develop an engram which can be repeated precisely with speed and force

Combine movement units when they can be successfully performed into subtasks for advance practice:
1 Repetition of the linked subtasks with precision, speed and force establishing an enlarged engram
2 Increase intensity of effort during practice as performance improves. Speed and precision are improved only by practising near the peak of performance
3 Repeated maximal practice perfects the engram
4 Frequent practice at peak of performance is necessary to maintain each engram

1991). If the sport event is dangerous by nature such as boxing, free-style skiing or involves high risk of injury such as gymnastics and American football, simulating exercises should be performed before taking part in the sport itself. In free-style skiing, this involves training and jumping into a water pool.

Sport-specific training often includes all the other parts of preventive training and is therefore one of the most effective approaches to the primary prevention of sports injuries. After an injury, the sport-specific exercise programme should be the final step in rehabilitation before returning to the sports arena.

Conclusion

Proprioceptive or 'kinaesthetic' awareness is one aspect of rehabilitation obtained through exercise, education and/or sensory feedback and reorganization. Increased postural and movement accuracy increases the consistency with which activities can be performed safely. Many people with musculoskeletal dysfunctions become less aware of functional positions and movements. With improved accuracy of trunk and joint positioning, fewer muscles will be needed, thereby decreasing fatigue and stress.

Prevention of injuries will be an increasingly

important part of medicine, as the costs for treatment and rehabilitation of sports injuries are getting out of control. However, many problems remain to be solved. There is no doubt that future advances in clinical biomechanics, together with an improved understanding of acute and overuse injuries in terms of functional anatomy, kinesiology and basic neurophysiology, as well as psychology, constitute powerful tools for relevant research in the field of functional instability, performance, rehabilitation and, not least, prevention. Proprioceptive and coordination training will play an increasingly important role in the prevention of injuries.

References

Alaranta, H., Moffroid, M., Elmqvist, L.G., Held, J., Pope, M. & Renström, P. (1993) Clinical considerations of proprioceptive aspects of postural control in adults. *Crit. Rev. Phys. Med. Rehab.* (in press).

Andersson, S. & Stener, B. (1959) Experimental evaluation of the hypothesis of ligamentomuscular protective reflexes: II. A study in cat using medial collateral ligament of the knee joint. *Acta Phys. Scand.* **48**, 27–49.

Andrew, B.L. (1990) The sensory innervation of the medial ligament in the knee joint. *J. Physiol. Lond.* **123**, 241–50.

Andriacchi, T.P. (1990) Dynamics of pathological motion: applied to anterior cruciate deficient knee. *J. Biomech.* **23**(1), 99–105.

Barrack, R.L. & Skinner, H.B. (1990) The sensory function of knee ligaments. In D.M. Daniel, W.H. Akeson & J. O'Connor (eds) *Knee Ligaments, Structure, Function, Injury and Repair*, pp. 95–114. Raven Press, New York.

Barrett, D.S. (1991) Proprioception and function after anterior cruciate reconstruction. *J. Bone Joint Surg.* **73B**, 833–7.

Beck, J.L. & Day, R.W. (1985) Overuse injuries. *Clin. Sports Med.* **4**, 553–73.

Bernard, A.A., Corlett, S., Thomsen, E. *et al.* (1988) Ice skating accidents and injuries. *Injury* **19**, 191–2.

Berson, B.L., Rolnick, A.M., Ramos, C.G. & Thornton, J. (1981) An epidemiologic study of squash injuries. *Am. J. Sports Med.* **9**, 103–6.

Beynnon, B.D. & Renström, P.A. (1991) The effect of bracing and taping in sports. *Clin. Gynecol.* **80**(2), 230–8.

Bouisset, S. & Zattara, M. (1987) Biomechanical study of the anticipatory postural adjustments associated with voluntary movement. *J. Biomech.* **20**, 735–42.

Brooks, V.B. (1979) Motor programs revisited. In R.E. Talbott & D.E. Humphrey (eds) *Posture and Movement*, pp. 13–49. Raven Press, New York.

Broström, L. (1966) Sprained ankles VI. Surgical treatment of chronic ligament ruptures. *Acta Chir. Scand.* **132**, 551–65.

Corrigan, J.P., Cashman, W.F. & Brady, M.P. (1992) Proprioception in the cruciate deficient knee. *J. Bone Joint Surg.* **74B**, 247–50.

Eccles, J.C. (1981) Physiology of motor control in man. *Appl. Neurophysiol.* **44**, 5–15.

Edwards, R.H.T. (1988) Hypotheses of peripheral and central mechanisms underlying occupational muscle pain and injury. *Eur. J. Appl. Physiol.* **57**, 275–81.

Evans, G.A., Hardcastle, P. & Frenyo, A.D. (1984) Acute rupture of the lateral ligament of the ankle. *J. Bone Joint Surg.* **66B**, 209–12.

Freeman, M.A.R., Dean, M.R.E. & Hanham, I.M.F. (1965) The etiology and prevention of functional instability of the foot. *J. Bone Joint Surg.* **47B**, 678–85.

Freeman, M.A.R. (1965) Instability of the foot after injuries to the lateral ligament of the ankle. *J. Bone Joint Surg.* **47B**, 669–77.

Freeman, M.A.R. & Wyke, B.D. (1964) The innervation of the knee joint. An anatomical and histological study in the cat. *J. Anat.* **101**, 505–32.

Gauffin, H. (1991) *Knee and ankle kinesiology and ankle instability*. Medical dissertation, Linkoping, Sweden.

Gauffin, H. (1992) Altered movement and muscular activation patterns for the one-legged jump in patients with old anterior cruciate ligament rupture. *Am. J. Sports Med.* (in press).

Glencross, D. & Thornton, E. (1981) Position sense following joint injury. *Am. J. Sports Med.* **21**, 23–7.

Goodwin, G.M., McCloskey, D.I & Matthews, P.B. (1972) The persistence of appreciable kinesthesia after paralysing joint afferents but preserving muscle afferents. *Brain Res.* **37**, 326–9.

Grillner, S. (1975) Locomotion in vertebrates: central mechanisms and reflex interaction. *Physiol. Rev.* **55**, 247–304.

Guyton, A.C. (1986) *Textbook of Medical Physiology*, 7th edn. Philadelphia, WB Saunders.

Horak, F.B. & Nashner, L.M. (1986) Central programming of postural movements: Adaptation of altered support-surface configurations. *J. Neurophysiol.* **55**, 1369–81.

Houk, J.C. (1974) Feedback control of muscle: a synthesis of the peripheral mechanisms. In V.B. Mountcastle (ed) *Medical Physiology*, 13th edn. CV Mosby, St Louis.

Ihara, H. & Nakayama, A. (1986) Dynamic joint control training for knee ligament injuries. *Am. J. Sports Med.* **14**(4), 309–15.

Jensen, C.R. & Garth Fisher, A. (1979) *Scientific Basis of Athletic Conditioning*, 2nd edn, p. 216. Lea & Febiger, Philadelphia.

Johansson, H., Sjölander, P. & Sojka, P. (1991a) Receptors in the knee joint ligaments and their role in the biomechanics of the joint. *Crit. Rev. Biomed. Eng.* **18**, 341–68.

Johansson, H., Sjölander, P. & Sojka, P. (1991b) A sensory role for the cruciate ligaments. *Clin. Ortho. Related Res.* **265**, 161–75.

Johnson, R.J., Beynnon, B., Nichols, C. & Renström, P. (1992) The treatment of ACL injuries. *J. Bone Joint Surg.* **74A**, 140.

Kannus, P., Alosa, D., Cook, L. *et al.* (1992) Effect of one-legged exercise on the strength, power and endurance of the contralateral leg. A randomized, controlled study using isometric and concentric isokinetic training. *Eur. J. Appl. Physiol.* **64**, 117–26.

Kannus, P. & Renström, P. (1991) Treatment for acute tears of the lateral ligaments of the ankle. Current concepts. A review. *J. Bone Joint Surg.* **73A**(2), 305–12.

Karlsson, J., Lansinger, O. & Faxen, E. (1991) Conservative treatment of chronic lateral instability of the ankle. *Läkartidningen* **88**, 1404–7.

Karlsson, J., Peterson, L., Andreasson, G. & Högfors, C. (1992) The unstable ankle: a combined EMG and biomechanical modeling study. *Int. J. Sport Biomech.* **8**(2), 129–44.

Keele, S.W. (1968) Movement control in skilled motor performance. *Physiol. Bull.* **70**, 387–403.

Kennedy, J.C., Alexander, I.J. & Hayes, K.C. (1982) Nerve supply of the human knee and its functional importance. *Am. J. Sports Med.* **10**, 329–35.

Kottke, F.J. (1980) From reflex to skill: the training of coordination. *Arch. Phys. Med. Rehab.* **61**, 551–61.

Muller, W. (1983) *The Knee: Form, Function, and Ligament Reconstruction*. Springer-Verlag, Berlin.

Nashner, L.M., Black, F.O. & Wall, C. (1982) Adaptation to altered support and visual conditions during stance: patients with vestibular deficits. *J. Neurosci.* **5**, 536–44.

Nashner, L.M. & McCollum, G. (1985) The organization of human postural movements: a formal basis and experimental synthesis. *Behav. Brain Sci.* **8**, 135–72.

Nashner, L.M. & Woollacott, M. (1979) The organization of rapid postural adjustments of standing humans: an experimental conceptual model. In R.E. Talbott & D.R. Humphrey (eds) *Posture and Movement*. Raven Press, New York.

Nashner, L.M., Woollacott, M. & Tuma, G. (1979)

Organization of rapid responses to postural and locomotor-like perturbations of standing man. *Exp. Brain Res.* **36**, 436–76.

O'Connor, B.L. (1984) The mechanoreceptor innervation of the posterior attachments of the lateral meniscus of the dog knee joint. *J. Anat.* **138**, 15–26.

Odensten, M. (1984) *Treatment of the torn anterior cruciate ligament*. Medical Dissertation No. 177, Linköping University, Sweden.

Paulos, L., Noyes, F., Grood, E. *et al.* (1981) Knee rehabilitation after ACL reconstruction and repair. *Am. J. Sport Med.* **9**, 140–9.

Peterson, L., Althoff, B. & Renström, P. (1979) Reconstruction of the lateral ligaments of the ankle joint. In *Proceedings of the First World Congress of Sports Medicine Applied to Football*, p. 609–13. FIFA, The International Football Federation, Rome.

Peterzen, I. & Stener, B. (1959) Experimental evaluation of the hypothesis of ligamentomuscular protective reflexes. III. A study in man using the MCL of the knee joint. *Acta Phys. Scand.* **48**(Suppl.), 51–61.

Prodromos, C.C., Andriacchi, T.P. & Galante, J.O. (1985) A relationship between gait and clinical changes following high tibial osteotomy. *J. Bone Joint Surg.* **67A**, 1188–94.

Rasmussen, O. (1985) Stability of the ankle joint. *Acta Orthop. Scand.* **56**(Suppl.), 211.

Renström, P., Arms, S., Stanwyck, T. *et al.* (1986) Strain within the ACL during hamstring and quadriceps activity. *Am. J. Sports Med.* **14**, 83–7.

Renström, P. & Kannus, P. (1991) Prevention of sports injuries. In R.J. Shepard & P.-O. Åstrand (eds) *Endurance in Sport*. Blackwell Scientific Publications, Oxford.

Renström, P., Peterson, L., Edberg, B., Svenneng, J. & Olofson, B. (1977) Frekvens och art av fotbollsskador I Göteborg — riskfaktorer vid fotbollspel. (Frequency and type of football-soccer injuries in Göteborg — risk factors). *SNV PM* **846**, 39–50.

Roberts, T.D.M. (1978) *Neurophysiology of Postural Mechanisms*, 2nd edn. Butterworths, London.

Roland, P.E. (1975) Do muscular receptors in man evoke sensations of tension and kinesthesia? *Strain Technol.* **50**, 162–5.

Sammarco, G.J. & DiRaimondo, C.V. (1988) Surgical treatment of lateral ankle instability syndrome. *Am. J. Sports Med.* **16**, 501–11.

Schultz, R.A., Miller, D.C., Kerr, C.S. & Micheli L. (1984) Mechanoreceptors in human cruciate ligaments. A histologic study. *J. Bone Joint Surg.* **66A**, 1072–6.

Schutte, M.J., Dabezies, E.J., Zimny, M.L. & Happel, L.T. (1987) Neural anatomy of the human anterior cruciate ligament. *J. Bone Joint Surg.* **69A**, 243–7.

Sedgwick, A.W., Smith, D.S. & Daview, M.J. (1988)

Musculoskeletal status of men and women who entered a fitness programme. *Med. J. Aust.* **148**, 385–99.

Skinner, H.B., Wyatt, M.P., Hodgdon, J.A., Conard, D.W. & Barrack, R.L. (1986) Effect of fatigue on joint position sense of the knee. *J. Orthop. Res.* **4**, 112–18.

Solomonow, M., Baratta, R. & D'Ambrosia, R. (1989) The role of the hamstrings in the rehabilitation of the anterior cruciate ligament-deficient knee in athletes. *Sports Med.* **7**, 42–8.

Solomonow, M., Baratta, B., Zhou, B. *et al.* (1987) The synergistic action of the ACL and thigh muscles in maintaining joint stability. *Am. J. Sports Med.* **15**, 207–13.

Stener, B. (1959) Experimental evaluation of the hypothesis of ligamentomuscular protective reflexes I. A method of adequate stimulation of tension receptors in the MCL of the knee joint of the cat and studies of the innervation of the ligament. *Acta Physiol. Scand.* **48**(Suppl.), 5–26.

Taimela, S. (1991) *Individual-related characteristics and musculoskeletal injuries: with special reference to reaction time, mental ability and psychological factors.* Thesis, Turku Finland.

Taimela, S., Österman, K., Kunjale, U. *et al.* (1990) Motor ability and personality with reference to soccer injuries. *J. Sports Med. Phys. Fitness* **30**, 194–201.

Tegner, Y., Lysholm, M., Lysholm, M. & Gillquist, J. (1986) A performance test to monitor rehabilitation and for evaluation of anterior cruciate ligament injuries. *Am. J. Sports Med.* **14**, 156–9.

Tropp, H. (1985) *Functional instability of the ankle joint.* Medical dissertation, Linköping, Sweden.

Tropp, H. & Askling, C. (1988) Effects of ankle disk training on muscular strength and postural control. *Clin. Biomech.* **3**, 88–91.

Tropp, H., Askling, C. & Gillquist, J. (1985a) Prevention of ankle sprains. *Am. J. Sports Med.* **13**, 259–62.

Tropp, H., Ekstrand, J. & Gillquist, J. (1984) Stabilometry in functional instability of the ankle and its value in predicting an injury. *Med. Sci. Sports Exerc.* **16**, 64–6.

Tropp, H. & Odenrick, P. (1988) Postural control in single limb stance. *J. Orthop. Res.* **6**, 833–9.

Tropp, H., Odenrick, P. & Gillquist, J. (1985b) Stabilometry in functional and mechanical instability of the ankle joint. *Int. J. Sports Med.* **6**, 180–2.

WHO (1980) *International Classification of Impairments, Disabilities, and Handicap.* World Health Organization, Geneva.

Chapter 22

Prevention of Overtraining

MOIRA O'BRIEN

Overtraining is not a new phenomenon. The symptoms of prolonged fatigue, loss of motivation, burn out and staleness have been described in athletes for many decades (Maclaren, 1866). Overtraining is an imbalance between training and recovery (Kuipers & Keizer, 1988). It may be short or long term and is the maladaptive response to the stimulus of training as the result of an extended period of overload. It encompasses a wide range of physiological and psychological effects. When you are overtrained you are stale (the American term for overtraining) (Costill, 1986). It is now thought to be a dysfunction of the neuroendocrine system localized at hypothalamic level (Kuipers & Keizer, 1988).

Diagnosis and those at risk

Diagnosis is based on medical and training history and the typical physical and psychological symptoms. Fatigue and poor performance are often the first signs of overtraining — increase in resting heart rate, weight loss, irritability and sleep disturbance. Medical causes have to be excluded. The causes and effects of overtraining vary. Overtraining tends to occur in highly motivated athletes, in those who are training themselves, or who are coached by enthusiastic amateurs with no understanding of basic physiological principles (O'Brien, 1988; Levin, 1991). It is more likely to occur in team sports.

Factors that predispose to overtraining

Both physical and psychological factors can contribute to overtraining or staleness, the stress may be sports related or due to family, social or work commitments. Excessive physical stress may be due to too many hard sessions or competitions and inadequate monitoring. Many athletes, even though they feel tired, push themselves to do more; as they are afraid of detraining, they never taper or peak. If staleness occurs in an athlete who has kept a constant training load or has gradually increased it, another cause must be sought. Too early a return to training and competition after an infection or injury, particularly mononucleosis, may increase the risk of overtraining.

Dietary considerations

Deficient caloric intake, particularly insufficient carbohydrate and dehydration may make athletes more susceptible (Aakvaag & Opstad, 1985). When the carbohydrate intake is adequate but consists mainly of concentrated food, vitamin intake may be compromised. Prolonged exercise when hypoglycaemic may result in deterioration of physical performance, for several weeks (Kuipers & Keizer, 1988). Glycogen depletion leads to rapid fatigue and may predispose to more prolonged fatigue (Costill *et al.*, 1988).

Overtraining may be a combination of

physical and mental stress. Sleep disturbance or deprivation will aggravate the symptoms. The symptoms and signs will depend on which system the athlete uses excessively.

Training principles

During athletic training, workloads are gradually increased — the overload principle is an important part of modern training and is considered to provide the optimal stimulus for adaptation (Harre, 1982). Periodization, when short cycles of heavy training are combined with periods of recovery, results in improvement in performance. If there is a failure to improve after this form of training, it denotes overtraining. Gradually increasing training loads improves the stability of the adrenocortical system, which is reflected in lower basal levels of stress hormones such as prolactin and adrenocorticotrophic hormone (ACTH) (Viru, 1984; Keizer et al., 1987). If the load is too great, recovery is incomplete, and overtraining may result. The intensity of training seems to contribute more than the duration. When a muscle is tried, its capability to absorb shock decreases and abnormally high repetitive stresses are transmitted to bone (Nordin & Frankel, 1980). Training and performance standards should take into account the physical and psycho-

logical maturity as well as the age and experience of the athlete. In certain sports, particulary gymnastics, overtraining may manifest itself by an increase in the number of injuries, mainly of the skeletal system or a delay in the normal growth spurt.

Physiological changes

It is thought that if there is insufficient recovery, the motor units normally recruited during a particular intensity of exercise will be prematurely fatigued and more energy will be required to do the work, resulting in an increased heart rate, ventilation rate and blood lactate at a given work load (Kuipers et al., 1985). Elevated serum creatine phosphokinase (CPK) levels are found after training and competition and may be elevated for several days after a marathon (Noakes, 1986).

If the athlete's training has been regularly monitored by measuring lactate curves, using an incremental work protocol, there will be a shift of the curve to the x axis and the slope will become more vertical, if the athlete is overtrained (Fig. 22.1). Overtraining often occurs in the final preparation for important competitions and many athletes have the bitter experience of a completely wasted season. Costill et al. (1985) reduced the training of the Ball

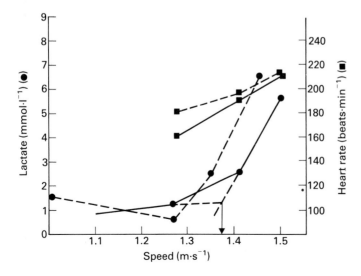

Fig. 22.1 Figure showing the lactate curve's shift to the left and becoming more vertical as a result of overtraining and an increasing heart rate.

State swimming team by half, and improved their position in the Mid-American Conference from last to third. Kirwan *et al.* (1988) studied a group of 12 comparable swimmers and doubled their normal training for 10 days; four were overworked and could not maintain the training pace and had mood disturbances. How an athlete feels is the most sensitive indicator, and the profile of mood states is a very useful method of assessment (Morgan *et al.*, 1988). Training must be individualized. Current levels of training are simply too much for some athletes. Even top-class athletes make training errors which may cause them to be overtrained. It is only in retrospect when athletes eventually stop training and discuss the problem with someone who will take the time to look at all aspects of their lifestyle, that they understand the situation but this may have cost them a season.

Warning signals

Athletes must be alerted to the warning signals of increasing resting heart rates, poor performance, delayed recovery after exercise, sleep disturbance, loss of weight and fatigue, in order to prevent it occurring again in the future. The athlete must be protected from doing too much. It is the science and art of coaching to provide the optimal amount and intensity of training without exceeding the athlete's exercise tolerance and recovery capacity.

Stress

High levels of stress are associated with increased muscle tension (Nideffer, 1981). Biofeedback is a useful method of reducing tension and stress management programmes are helpful. The cause of the stress in the athlete and how it affects the individual must be identified. Athletes should be trained in mental imagery and relaxation skills. The athlete should be prepared for the anticipated stress and helped to confront the situation. They should rehearse how they are going to deal with it (Miller *et al.*, 1990).

Sleep

Highly stressed athletes tend to have more problems with sleep (Morgan, 1979; Morris, 1982; Miller & Vaughan, 1986). As little as 20 h sleep deprivation negatively affects various parameters of mental performance (Vidacek *et al.*, 1986). This is also an important factor in mental health, as is jet lag. There is a high incidence of psychiatric admission at Heathrow Airport after long-distance flights.

Sleep is divided into two main phases, rapid eye movement (REM) and non-REM. There are four distinct phases in non-REM (Fig. 22.2), the first two are relatively light, the third and fourth stages are deep and characterized by large slow δ waves on the electroencephalogram, the fourth stage is thought to be more restful. REM sleep follows the slow-wave sleep of stage 4 and is normally repeated in cycles of 90 min. Growth hormone is secreted and peaks during slow-wave sleep (Sissin *et al.*, 1969). Growth hormone is an anabolic hormone that promotes protein synthesis and gluconeogenesis, and it is enhanced in some athletes. People with sleep disturbances have less slow-wave and REM sleep. Shapiro *et al.* (1981) found that both the quantity and quality of slow-wave sleep was increased in fit athletes after a 92-km road race and that fit lean athletes had an increased slow-wave sleep, while unfit people had no increase. Sleep is restorative. Stress can cause insomnia, and fear of not sleeping sets up a vicious cycle. Athletes should practice relaxation techniques, and a pre-sleep ritual may help. People who are sleep deprived have a lower oral temperature and feel the cold. Time to exhaustion is also decreased.

Hormones

There is also an increase in insulin resistance, and a decrease in glucose tolerance, which may be related to the effects of growth hormone.

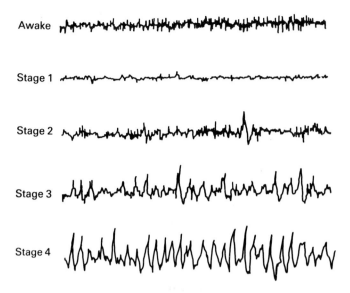

Awake

Stage 1

Stage 2

Stage 3

Stage 4

Fig. 22.2 The four stages of non-rapid eye movement sleep.

Growth hormone is also secreted during both specific and non-specific stress. Trained subjects exhibit a lower growth hormone response to psychological stress and exercise stimulus than untrained subjects (Mikulaj *et al.*, 1975; Bloom *et al.*, 1976). Conversely, trained subjects respond with a significantly higher secretion of growth hormone in insulin-induced hypoglycaemia than untrained subjects.

Excessive exercise stress leads to alterations in the neuroendocrine axis and may contribute to overtraining. Continued training when the hormonal balance is upset will further stress the system thus compromising recovery (Kuipers & Keizer, 1988).

Excessive stress in females is often associated with menstrual dysfunction, with its decreased levels of progesterone and oestrogen, and an increased incidence of osteoporosis and stress fractures. Keizer *et al.* (1987) noted that very intense exercise on consecutive days affected the normal pulsatile secretion pattern of luteinizing hormone which is necessary for a normal menstrual cycle. Prior (1987) postulates that exercise-induced amenorrhoea is a symptom of hypothalamopituitary dysfunction and a stress response to overtraining, which may also be reflected in low thyroxine levels and a decrease

in the response of thyroid-stimulating hormone to thyrotropin-releasing hormone (Barron *et al.*, 1985).

There is an increase in the level of cortisol which is a catabolic hormone and a decrease in testosterone which is anabolic, as a result of intense physical exercise. Prolonged exhaustive physical exercise in humans results in a decrease in plasma testosterone which may slump down to female levels. This is associated with a rise in the serum hormone binding gobulin and low testosterone levels (Adlercreutz *et al.*, 1986). The increase in the binding of cortisol in muscle tissue combined with the high level of cortisol may lead to greater protein catabolism (breakdown) inside the muscle cells, and may explain some of the weight loss which occurs. Weight loss can be monitored by weighing the athlete at the same time of day.

Immune system

Overtraining is associated with an increased incidence of injuries and increased infection. The hormonal changes associated with excessive training, may affect the immune system. Lewicki *et al.* (1987) found a decreased responsiveness of the non-specific immunity in conditioned cyclists compared with non-athletes. Decreased levels of C-reactive protein were found in athletes after a period of intense exercise (Liessen, 1977), and decreased levels of immunoglobulins were found in overtrained athletes (Hollmann & Hettinger, 1980; Ryan et al., 1983). There is a higher incidence of upper respiratory infection in élite athletes than in controls (Peters & Bateman, 1983; Reilly & Rothwell, 1987). Acute exercise will exacerbate intercurrent infection (Fry et al., 1991).

Sport-mediated immune responses play a major role in determining increased susceptibility to infection associated with training and competition, and may be an important factor contributing to immune suppression (Morgan et al., 1987). Psychological stress is capable of suppressing immunity (Keast et al., 1988). The immune system relies on glutamine for cell replication (Ardawi & Newsholme, 1985). Muscle is an important source. Newsholme (1990) proposes that stress may reduce the supply of glutamine from muscle in the overtrained state.

Prevention

To prevent overtraining, each athlete must be carefully monitored and his or her training must be individualized. The training must be well structured and allow adequate periods of rest; excessive training and competition must be avoided. A well-coordinated team approach that looks at all aspects of the athlete's lifestyle and how they are coping with stress is essential.

Early detection of overtraining is important, as the time required for complete recovery is proportional to the length of time they have been overtrained. Complete rest is the most effective treatment. The precipitating cause must be identified and dealt with.

Athletes should keep a training diary in which they record their training schedules, and how they felt during and after the session. Performance times, and resting and recovery heart rates should also be monitored. Weight loss, any increase in fatigue and the hours of sleep should also be noted. Female athletes should keep an accurate record of their menstrual cycle. An increase in the resting heart rate of more than five beats for no obvious reason or a flattening of the recovery heart rate curve may be an early warning sign. Psychological profiles using the profile of mood state questionnaires are extremely useful.

Fatigue and a decrease in the level of performance are the first indicators of overtraining, but at the moment there is no specific diagnostic test of overtraining. Depending on the facilities available, a battery of physiological, haematological, biochemical and immunological tests can be performed. Sports-specific tests such as time trials can be carried out during the training cycle to monitor the effects of training (Fry et al., 1991). Educating the athlete and all those involved is the most effective method of preventing overtraining.

References

Aakvaag, A. & Opstad, P.K. (1985) Hormonal responses to prolonged physical strain. Effects of caloric deficiency and sleep deprivation. In Fotherby & Pal (eds) Exercise Endocrinology, pp. 25–64. de Gruyter, Berlin.

Adlercreutz, H., Harkomen, M., Kuoppasalma, K. et al. (1986) Effect of training on plasma anabolic and catabolic steroid hormones and their response during physical exercise. Int. J. Sports Med. 7 (Suppl. 1), 27–8.

Ardawi, M.S. & Newsholme, E.A. (1985) Metabolism in lymphocytes and its importance in the immune response. Essays Biochem. 21, 1–43.

Barron, J.L., Noakes, T.D., Levy, W., Smith, C. & Millar, R.P. (1985) Hypothalamic dysfunction in over-trained athletes. J. Clin. Endocrinol. Metab. 60, 803–6.

Bloom, S.R., Johnson, R.H., Park, D.M., Rennie M.J. & Sulaman, M. (1976) Differences in metabolic and hormonal responses to exercise between racing cyclists and untrained individuals. J. Physiol. 258, 1–18.

Costill, D.L. (1986) Inside Running, pp. 123–32. Benchmark Press Inc., Indianapolis.

Costill, D.L., Flynn, M.G., Kirwan, J.P., et al. (1988) Effects of repeated days of intensified training on muscle glycogen and swimming performance. Med.

Sci. Sport Exerc. **21**, 249–54.

Costill, D.L., King, D.S., Thomas, R. & Hargreaves, M. (1985) Effects of reduced training on muscular power in swimmers. *Phys. Sports Med.* **13**, 94–101.

Fry, R.W., Morton. A.R. & Keast, D. (1991) Overtraining in athletes. An update. *Sports Med.* **12**, 32–65.

Harre, D. (1982) Principles of sports training. Introduction to theory and methods of training. Sports Verlag, Berlin.

Hollman, W. & Hettinger, T. (1980) Sports Medizin. Arbeits und Trainingsgrundlagen, pp. 549–52. F.K. Shattaeur Verlag, Stuttgart.

Keast, D., Cameron, K. & Morton, A.R. (1988) Exercise and the immune response. *Sports Med.* **5**, 248–67.

Keizer, H.A., Kuipers, H., DeHaan, J., Beckers, E. & Habets, L. (1987) Multiple hormonal responses to exercise in eumenorrheic trained and untrained women. *Int. J. Sports Med.* **8**, 139–50.

Kirwan, J.P., Costill, D.L., Flynn, M.G. *et al.* (1988) Physiological responses to successive days of intense training in competitive swimmers. *Med. Sci. Sports Exerc.* **20**, 255–9.

Kuipers, H. & Keizer, H.A. (1988) Overtraining in elite athletes. *Sports Med.* **6**, 79–92.

Kuipers, H., Verstappen, F., Keizer, H., Geurten, P. & Kranenberg, G. Van (1985) Variability of aerobic performance in the laboratory and its physiological correlates. *Int. J. Sports Med.* **6**, 197–210.

Levin, S. (1991) Overtraining causes Olympic size problems. *Phys. Sports Med.* **19**(5), 112–18.

Lewicki, R., Tchorzewski, H., Denys, A., Kowalska, M. & Golinska, A. (1987) The effect of physical exercise on some parameters of immunity in conditioned sportsmen. *Int. J. Sports Med.* **8**(5), 309–14.

Liessen, H., Dufaux, B. & Hollman, W. (1977) Modification of serum glycoproteins during the days following prolonged physical exercise and the influence of physical training. *Eur. J. Appl. Physiol.* **37**, 243–54.

Maclaren, A. (1866) *Training in Theory and Practise.* Macmillan, London.

Mikulaj, L., Komadel, L. & Vigas, M. (1975) Hormonal changes after different kinds of motor stress in trained and untrained young men. In Howald & Portman (eds) *Metabolic Adaptations to Prolonged Exercise*, Vol. 7, pp. 333–8. Birkhausen Verlag, Basle.

Miller, T.W. & Vaughan, M.P. (1986) *Psychological stresses and symptom formation in female cross country runners.* Colloquim presentation in Department of Mental Health and Behavioral Sciences, VA and University of Kentucky Medical Centre, 21 October.

Miller, T.W., Vaughan, M.P. & Miller, J.M. (1990) Clinical issues and treatment strategies in stress oriented athletes. *Sports Med.* **9**(6), 370–9.

Morgan, W.P. (1979) *Phys. Sports Med.* **7**(2), 57–70.

Morgan, W.P., Brown, D.R., Raglin, J.S., O'Connor, P.J. & Ellickson, K.A. (1987) Psychological monitoring of overtraining and staleness. *Br. J. Sports Med.* **21**(3), 107–14.

Morgan, W.P., Costill, D.L., Flynn, M.G., Raglin, J.S. & O'Connor, P.J. (1988) Mood disturbance following increased training in swimmers. *Med. Sci. Sports Exerc.* **20**, 408–14.

Morris, A.F. (1982) Sleep disturbance in athletes. *Phys. Sports Med.* **10**(9), 75–85.

Newsholme, E.A. (1990) Psychoimmunology and cellular nutrition — An alternative hypothesis. *Biol. Psychiatr.* **27**, 1–3.

Nideffer, R. (1981) *The Ethics and Practice of Applied Sports Psychology*, pp. 66–74. Movement Publications, Ithaca.

Noakes, T. (1986) *Love of Running.* Oxford University Press, Capetown.

Nordin, M. & Frankel, V.H. (1980) *Basic Biomechanics of the Skeletal System.* Lea & Febiger, Philadelphia.

O'Brien, M. (1988) Overtraining and sports psychology. In A. Dirix, H.G. Knuttgen & K. Tittel (eds) *The Olympic Book of Sports Medicine*, pp. 635–45. Blackwell Scientific Publications, Oxford.

Peters, E.M. & Bateman, E.D. (1983) Ultra marathon running and upper respiratory tract infections. An epidemiological survey. *S. Afr. Med. J.* **64**, 582–4.

Prior, J.C. (1987) Physical exercise and the neuroendocrine control of reproduction. *Clin. Endocrinol. Metab.* **1**, 299–317.

Reilly, T. & Rothwell, J. (1987) *Correlates of injury and illness in female distance runners.* British Association of Sport and Medicine, Congress University of Liverpool.

Ryan, A.J., Brown, R.L., Frederick, E.C., Falsetti, H.L. & Burke, R.E. (1983) Overtraining of athletes: A round table. *Phys. Sports Med.* **11**(6), 93–110.

Shapiro, C.M., Bortz, R., Mitchell, D. *et al.* (1981) Slow wave sleep a recovery period after exercise. *Science* **214**, 1253–4.

Sissin, J.F., Parkes, D.C., Johnson, L.C. *et al.* (1969) Effects of slow wave sleep deprivation on human growth hormone release in sleep. Preliminary study. *Life Sci.* **8**, 1299–307.

Vidacek, S., Kalenterme, L. & Radosevic Vidacek, B. (1986) Productivity on a weekly rotating shift system — circadian adjustments and sleep deprivation effects. *Ergonomics* **29**, 1583–90.

Viru, A. (1984) The mechanism of training effects; A hypothesis. *Int. J. Sports Med.* **5**, 219–27.

Chapter 23

Nutrition and Diet

PETER BRUKNER

The importance of diet in the development and maintenance of a healthy body is now well recognized. There is considerable evidence linking certain disease states with poor dietary practices. There has also been considerable interest in the relationship between diet and athletic performance. However, there has been little research into the relationship between diet and injuries.

Diet and health

Diet has been shown to be a significant factor in the development of certain disease states. Coronary atherosclerosis, hypercholesterolaemia and obesity have been linked to excessive intake of saturated fats. Excessive intake of unrefined sugars may contribute to dental caries and obesity; excess alcohol intake may lead to obesity and alcoholic liver disease. Excessive salt intake has been linked with hypertension; and certain gastrointestinal conditions such as haemorrhoids, diverticular disease and cancer of the bowel have been linked to inadequate intake of fibre.

A number of dietary guidelines have been developed to maximize good health. These vary slightly between different countries, but are basically similar. They are:
1 Eat a variety of foods every day. A variety of foods is necessary to supply the many nutrients required for good health. One should choose foods from the five basic food groups: (i) meat or meat substitute group; (ii) milk and milk products; (iii) bread and cereals; (iv) fruit and vegetables; and (v) fats.
2 Prevent and control obesity.
3 Eat less fats.
4 Eat less refined sugars.
5 Eat more complex carbohydrate and dietary fibre.
6 Limit alcohol intake.
7 Reduce salt intake.
8 Drink more water.

Nutrition and athletic performance

The relationship between nutrition and athletic performance has been studied extensively in recent years. In that time our ideas on optimum nutrition for athletes have changed considerably. The first aim of optimum nutrition is to satisfy the athletes caloric requirements. Increased energy output needs to be matched by increased caloric intake. These calories can be consumed as three main nutrients, (i) carbohydrate; (ii) fat; and (iii) protein. The average Western diet consists of approximately 40% carbohydrate, 45% fats and 15% protein. This is far from the optimum ratios for good health and athletic performance.

The training diet

An appropriate training diet is essential for the maintenance of good health and to maximize athletic performance. It may also be an important factor in the prevention of injuries. The dietary requirements of athletes in training vary greatly depending on age, gender, body size and composition, type of sport, environment and the frequency, intensity and duration of training sessions. A marathon runner's dietary needs, for instance, will be very different to those of a discus thrower; a weightlifter's needs different to those of a gymnast. However, there are some basic requirements which must be met in order to meet the goals of health maintenance and performance maximization.

The diet must provide adequate energy to meet the energy requirements of training. Protein, fat, alcohol and carbohydrates can all contribute to the total energy intake. Ideally, athletes should consume a diet high in complex carbohydrates and low in fat with adequate protein and fibre as well as sufficient fluid (Fig. 23.1).

If the body's energy requirements are not met on a daily basis by the training diet, the body is forced to mobilize its own fuel reserves. Initially these are carbohydrate (in the form of glycogen) and fat. Once these reserves are depleted, then protein is mobilized as an additional energy source. This breakdown of

protein from muscles and other organs may lead to injury. Therefore adequate energy intake is essential in the maintenance of health, performance and possibly in the prevention of injury (Inge & Brukner, 1986).

Low body weight

In many sports the maintenance of low body weight and low body fat is important. In some sports this is thought to give a competitive advantage, e.g. distance running and gymnastics, while other sports set weight limits, e.g. wrestling and boxing. Therefore some athletes are constantly battling to lower their weight, while others tend to have rapid, large fluctuations in weight as they attempt to lower their weight immediately prior to competition.

Short-term weight losses are composed mainly of water, fat, protein and glycogen (Van Itallie & Yang, 1977), while longer term energy restriction leads to a greater contribution of fat stores to the amount of weight lost. Those athletes who lose weight regularly over short periods of time may have significant losses of lean body tissue and water.

Many athletes have energy intakes well below their energy outputs. These athletes initially lose weight, but eventually maintain a relatively constant low or low−normal weight despite this difference in energy intake and expenditure without any obvious ill effect. Two factors may contribute to this phenomenon, (i) metabolic rate; and (ii) food efficiency.

It is recognized that people on low-calorie diets have a reduced metabolic rate (Bray, 1969; Welle *et al.*, 1984). Athletes with low food intake and low body weight may have an even lower metabolic rate than those on diet alone (Phinney, 1985). There is evidence that the decline in resting metabolic rate with low-calorie diets may be prevented by the addition of exercise (Stern *et al.*, 1986).

Food efficiency is defined as the ratio of weight change to ingested calories. It is an index of how much a person must eat to maintain a given weight or body composition. Food

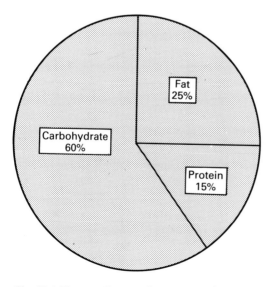

Fig. 23.1 The contribution of nutrients to total energy requirements.

efficiency increases when the calorie level necessary to sustain a 1 kg of body weight decreases (Brownell *et al.*, 1987).

The issue of food efficiency has not been addressed directly in athletes, but there is some indirect evidence (Brownell *et al.*, 1987) to support the hypothesis that food efficiency is increased in athletes with low body weights. There is presently little evidence to link low body weight with an increase in the frequency of injury, however there is evidence that sufferers of anorexia nervosa may be prone to bony injury probably through a hypo-oestrogenic effect.

The role of body composition and percentage body fat in the development of menstrual irregularities in female athletes has been studied extensively. The critical fat hypothesis (Frisch *et al.*, 1980) maintained that a specific percentage body fat is needed to initiate menarche (17%) and to sustain fertility thereafter (22%). This theory has now been abandoned, but studies confirm that the incidence of menstrual irregularities is higher in those sports characterized by low body weight such as distance running and ballet, than in those whose average body fat is higher such as swimming. It would appear that low body fat is one important contributing factor in the aetiology of menstrual irregularities, but there is no direct causal relationship.

Athletes with hypo-oestrogenic amenorrhoea and those with anorexia nervosa have both been shown to have increased incidence of reduced bone density and the athletic group shown to have an increased incidence of stress fractures.

There is some evidence of lowered testosterone in male athletes with low body weight (Wheeler *et al.*, 1984; Strauss *et al.*, 1985). Suppressed testosterone may be the parallel of menstrual dysfunction in females.

The effect of body weight patterns on general health may be considerable. Few athletes are obese, but those who are must avoid this risk factor for coronary disease, hypertension and diabetes.

There is evidence that chronic caloric restriction reduces risk for certain cancers (Ross *et al.*, 1985; Krichevsky *et al.*, 1986). Repeated bouts of weight loss may affect blood pressure (Ashley & Kannel, 1974) and renal blood flow leading to renal ischaemia and possibly hypertension (Tcheng & Tipton, 1973; Zambraski *et al.*, 1976).

The evidence linking low body weight and injury is, except for those with athletic amenorrhoea and anorexia nervosa, largely circumstantial. It would appear that athletes with low body weight and chronic caloric restriction may be susceptible to loss of protein, however the body has a number of mechanisms by which it adapts to this imbalance between caloric intake and expenditure.

Eating disorders

Low weight/low body fat is an important component of many sports including gymnastics, ballet, figure skating and distance running. Some athletes become obsessed with their weight and practice pathogenic weight control behaviour.

Serious eating disorders, such as anorexia nervosa and bulimia, may develop. It has been postulated that addiction to running may be a similar process to anorexia nervosa (Yates *et al.*, 1983), although this theory has been rejected by other researchers (Blumenthal *et al.*, 1984; Weight & Noakes, 1987).

Anorexia nervosa and bulimia may lead to dehydration and/or starvation or semistarvation which may not only affect athletic performance, but may have deleterious health effects.

There is considerable evidence that the risk of osteoporosis is increased in anorectics (Rigotti *et al.*, 1984; Brotman & Stern, 1985; Szmukler *et al.*, 1985), although those with high levels of physical activity have a greater bone density than those who were less active (Rigotti *et al.*, 1984). This decrease in bone density may increase susceptibility to stress fractures and other bony injuries.

Specific nutrients

Thus far we have looked at the overall effect of an inadequate diet on health and injury. We will now examine the role of specific nutrients and the role they may play in the development of injury. There is very little direct evidence to link nutrients, or more specifically, lack of certain nutrients, to the development of injury. However, there is considerable theoretical evidence of the important role these nutrients play in energy and muscle metabolism. Because of this involvement, the nutrients must be considered a possible aetiological factor in the development of injuries. These nutrients include carbohydrates, protein, water, calcium, potassium and certain vitamins and minerals.

Carbohydrate

Carbohydrate is stored in the liver and muscle in the form of glycogen. This storage form of carbohydrate is readily available for use by the athlete in heavy training. A heavy training session depletes the body of glycogen and an essential component of the training diet is to replenish these glycogen stores prior to the next training session. The degree and rate of muscle glycogen resynthesis is dependent on a number of factors including the extent of muscle trauma, the severity of glycogen depletion and the amount of dietary carbohydrate (Costill, 1988). The type of exercise as well as the duration and intensity of the training session will influence the rate of muscle glycogen recovery. The depletion of muscle glycogen results in a marked activation of glycogen synthetase activity (Costill, 1988) and in the absence of muscle fibre damage associated with eccentric exercise, the rate of glycogen repletion should be proportional to the dietary carbohydrate content (Costill, 1988).

The importance of the carbohydrate intake in the diets of heavily training athletes has been illustrated in a number of studies (Costill & Miller, 1980; Jacobs et al., 1982; Costill et al., 1988). In these trials athletes who fail to ingest sufficient carbohydrate to match the demands of their heavy training commitments succumb to chronic muscle glycogen depletion and fatigue (Burke & Read, 1989).

More recently, studies have shown the importance of the time factor in replenishment of muscle glycogen. The sooner carbohydrate is ingested following the completion of exercise, the more efficiently glycogen supplies are restored (Blom et al., 1987; Ivy et al., 1988).

In the case of chronic muscle glycogen depletion, the body again relies on its fat and protein stores as an alternative energy source. This may result in increased protein breakdown possibly leading to soft tissue injury.

Protein

Protein is essential for all living creatures and is involved in every process within the body. Proteins are essential components of muscle, skin, cell membranes, blood, hormones, antibodies, enzymes and genetic material. Apart from water, protein is the most abundant substance in the body comprising approximately 20% of body weight. The major depot of protein in the body is skeletal muscle.

The importance of protein and exercise has been debated for many years. Until recently most observers thought that changes in protein metabolism during exercise are non-existent or minimal at best (Lemon et al., 1984). With the use of more sophisticated procedures to study protein requirements such as nitrogen balance, urinary excretion of urea or N-methylhistidine, and radiolabelled metabolic tracers, there is now considerable evidence of increased protein utilization with exercise. It is possible to quantitate skeletal muscle protein breakdown from 3-methylhistidine excretion since the concentration of 3-methylhistidine in skeletal muscle is relatively constant (Bilmazes et al., 1978).

It would appear that in certain circumstances, athletes break down body protein to provide energy for exercise. This appears to occur both in endurance exercise of moderately high intensity and in weightlifting.

The effect of a single bout of strength exercise on protein metabolism is the subject of some confusion. Hickson *et al.* (1986) found no change in urea excretion in the 24 h following a single bout of strength exercise. Dohm *et al.* (1982), on the other hand, reported that strength exercise led to increased 24-h urea and 3-methylhistidine excretion from four male powerlifters.

The effect of a regular programme of strength exercise has also been studied by Hickson and Hinkelman (1985). They found an increase in the urinary 3-methylhistidine excretions indicating an increased rate of skeletal muscle protein catabolism. At the same time there was evidence of decreased urinary urea excretion suggestive of increased efficiency of protein metabolism. Other studies have shown an increased protein need with endurance exercise (Celejowa & Homa, 1970; Torun *et al.*, 1977). Hickson and Wolinsky (1989) hypothesize that these metabolic adaptations for exercise may have enabled accelerated remodelling of skeletal muscle tissue to accommodate the exercise stress.

The effect of endurance exercise on protein metabolism has also been studied extensively. There is ample evidence of increased protein metabolism during isolated bouts of endurance exercise. Lemon and Nagle (1981) suggest that the breakdown of protein during endurance exercise is an important contributor to total energy needs. It would appear that protein may become an important source of energy when glycogen stores become depleted. Pre-exercise glycogen levels can affect the contribution of protein to exercise caloric cost (Lemon & Mullin, 1980). This may explain some of the advantageous effects of pre-exercise carbohydrate loading practised by endurance athletes.

Gontzea *et al.* (1974), on the other hand, suggest that the increased nitrogen excretion results from increased 'oligatory' losses of protein due to the prolonged elevation in metabolism.

Dohm *et al.* (1982) suggest that the purpose of protein degradation may be to provide amino acids as precursors for glucose production in the liver enabling the endurance athlete to maintain glucose levels. They also suggest that the increased urinary excretion of 3-methylhistidine after exercise indicates that skeletal muscle is the source of the degraded protein. Lemon *et al.* (1982) also suggested that skeletal muscle was the likely source of increased leucine oxidation observed with intense exercise.

The energy provided from protein may be due to decreased protein synthesis and/or increased protein degradation (Dohm *et al.*, 1982). There is evidence that skeletal muscle is the site of the protein degradation (Lemon *et al.*, 1982).

Continued protein losses with exercise would lead eventually to a net loss of body protein. There are a number of possible mechanisms by which this may be prevented. Gontzea *et al.* (1974) suggested that there was an adaptation of protein metabolism in response to repeated endurance exercise which may prevent this loss of body protein.

After exercise there is a compensatory increase in protein synthesis to allow for an increased incorporation of amino acids into skeletal muscle protein. This is evidenced by nitrogen retention, an elevated rate of amino acid incorporation into various fractions of skeletal muscle proteins and an increased protein content of exercised muscles (Viru, 1987).

Obviously, without this compensatory increase in protein synthesis, vigorous daily exercise would be deleterious rather than conducive to the maintenance and/or growth of skeletal muscle (Paul, 1989).

There is also evidence of continued degradation of protein in muscles after activity. The increase in 3-methylhistidine following exercise may be due to the breakdown of muscle tissue that was damaged during exercise (Kasperek & Snider, 1985). However, Viru (1987) believes that the increased 3-methylhistidine levels after exercise must not be considered as an index of the prevalent breakdown of contractile proteins, but as a sign of their increased turnover.

A decrease in cell mass has been observed in adult male subjects who trained with isometric exercise while on a diet containing the recommended daily allowance for protein (Torun *et al.*, 1977). Other studies have been able to reverse an increased urea excretion (protein breakdown) with exercise by increasing the protein content of the diet (Laritcheva *et al.*, 1978). It has also been shown that total food intake is important because if insufficient energy is consumed, urea excretion increases even at a protein intake that does not produce an increased urea excretion when total food intake is greater (Laritcheva *et al.*, 1978).

It would appear that the protein requirements for athletes are considerably increased compared to those of the sedentary individual. The current recommended daily allowance of protein in the USA is $0.8 \, g \cdot kg^{-1} \cdot day^{-1}$. Various recommendations regarding the protein needs of certain groups of athletes have been made.

A study by Tarnopolsky *et al.* (1988) compared nitrogen balance of body builders and endurance athletes and recommended intakes of $1.2 \, g \cdot kg^{-1} \cdot day^{-1}$ for body builders and $1.6 \, g \cdot kg^{-1} \cdot day^{-1}$ for endurance athletes. They made the proviso that these intakes were recommended for males consuming a high energy, high carbohydrate diet and who are in steady-state training intensity.

Lemon *et al.* (1984) recommends a protein intake of approximately $1.8 \, g \cdot kg^{-1} \cdot day^{-1}$ for exercising adults and $2 \, g \cdot kg^{-1} \cdot day^{-1}$ for exercising individuals who belong to any group with elevated protein needs. The additional protein required for endurance athletes may be utilized in the repair of damaged muscle fibres and as an auxillary fuel source. For strength athletes additional protein may be required to maintain a positive nitrogen balance so that hypertrophic stimulation of resistance exercise is maximized.

In summary, it would appear that there are considerable theoretical reasons why inadequate dietary protein intake may lead to muscle injury. There is considerable evidence of skeletal muscle breakdown as a result of continued intense training, especially in the presence of inadequate carbohydrate intake, and in the case of inadequate dietary protein intake, further muscle breakdown may occur after exercise in order to liberate the amino acids required for protein synthesis. The protein requirements of athletes are increased, but are usually met by an adequate training diet. The recommended percentage of calories provided by protein in the training diet is approximately 15%. With the increased caloric requirement of exercise this percentage usually provides sufficient protein without resorting to additional protein supplementation. Certain groups however, such as vegetarians, may be more susceptible to inadequate protein intakes.

Whether a correlation exists or not between the observed protein breakdown and the development of soft tissue injury is uncertain. There is certainly some similarities between the two processes. Injury is less likely to occur with steady-state training than with one-off bouts of exercise or sudden increases in training intensity. This correlates with the theory that there is an adaptation of protein metabolism that prevents breakdown occurring in repeated bouts of steady-state exercise. Further research needs to be undertaken to determine the clinical significance of these findings.

Fluids

Water is an essential component of all cells. Exercise may lead to excessive loss of water especially in a hot environment (Fig. 23.2). Dehydration may be associated with increased core temperature and resultant heat-related injuries ranging from heat cramps to the more serious heat stroke and ultimately death. Rhabdomyolysis has also been observed with exercise in hot conditions in unacclimatized, susceptible individuals.

Hypohydration can result in compromised blood flow to working muscle (Armstrong *et al.*, 1985). Whether this compromised blood flow results in increased susceptibility to injury has not been researched. The effect of hypo-

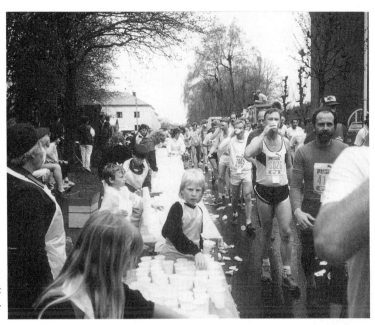

Fig. 23.2 It is essential in long-distance running to replace lost fluids. Courtesy of Dr P.A.F.H. Renström.

hydration on the amount and composition of joint fluid is uncertain.

Calcium

There has been particular interest in the role of calcium and its relationship to bone health in the light of the common occurrence of postmenopausal osteoporosis, and more recently, the discovery that athletes with hypo-oestrogenic amenorrhoea may also develop osteoporosis.

Bone mass is affected by a number of different factors, heredity (Seeman *et al.*, 1989), physical activity, dietary factors and hormonal factors. There is evidence for a strong hereditary role in the development of bone mass in women by the age of 25, independent of dietary factors. However, dietary factors, physical activity and hormonal status can modulate the genetically predetermined quantity, size and shape of bone (Pollitzer & Anderson, 1989). Regular physical activity creates loads on the skeleton that enhance or maintain its mass. Oestrogens have a similar effect on bone mass

although they operate through a different mechanism involving bone cells (Anderson, 1990).

Levels of all nutrients through adolescence and early adulthood help to fulfil the genetically predetermined potential for bone mass. Nutrients other than calcium, especially protein, phosphorous and vitamin D, also exert important effects on calcium metabolism. Adequate amounts of these nutrients along with energy are needed for the phases of bone growth and mineral consolidation in the existing skeletal tissue. Those with high nutrient intake have significantly greater bone mass than those with low nutrient intake.

In a number of animal studies, calcium deficient diets resulted in osteoporosis which was subsequently reversed by restoring calcium intake to adequate levels (Goldring & Krane, 1981; Seeman & Riggs, 1981). In humans, the evidence is less convincing, but does suggest a relationship (Nordin, 1966; Matkovic *et al.*, 1979; Heaney *et al.*, 1982).

Peak values for bone mass are attained at the age of 25 in men and approximately 35 in women. Women who consume calcium in amounts below 75% of the recommended daily allowance attain a bone mass that is, on average, below their potential peak. The importance of calcium intake in the adolescent growth years is shown by the recommended daily allowance of 1200 mg·day^{-1} compared to 800 mg·day^{-1} for a premenopausal adult female.

Every attempt should be made through adequate nutrition and physical activity to maximize the peak bone mass attained. The higher the peak bone mass, the less likely that postmenopausal bone loss will lead to osteoporosis and subsequent fractures. High calcium intake in the postmenopausal woman will not necessarily prevent bone loss, but may slow the rate of calcium loss from bone. A few studies, however, have shown a modest improvement in bone mass of treated compared to non-treated women (Recker et al., 1977; Lee et al., 1981). It would appear that additional calcium consumption by postmenopausal women is warranted. However, it is a matter of some debate what level of calcium should be recommended. A level of 1200 mg·day^{-1}, similar to that of adolescents, would appear to be reasonable. Hormone replacement should be considered in postmenopausal women.

The fact that young, thin women who exercise intensely have irregular periods, or in many cases cease to have periods altogether, has been noted for some time. Initially, this was thought to be a relatively harmless condition which could be easily reversed by a reduction of exercise or a slight increase in weight if pregnancy was required. However, Cann et al. (1984) noted a decrease in bone mineral density in this group similar to that of the postmenopausal women. Other researchers have confirmed these findings (Drinkwater et al., 1984; Lindbey et al., 1984; Cook et al., 1987). The exact mechanism of this phenomenon is not wholly understood, but there seems to be a relationship between low body fat content, intense exercise both in quality and quantity, and menstrual irregularity. An increased incidence of stress fractures has also been noted in this group

(Lindbey et al., 1984; Lloyd et al., 1986; Barrow & Saha, 1988). Hormonal studies have shown that these women are hypo-oestrogenic.

The exact role of hormone and calcium supplementation in these amenorrhoeic athletes has not yet been determined although it would seem reasonable to encourage these women to maintain a high calcium intake of at least 1200 mg·day^{-1}. Many clinicians now feel that hormone supplementation in the form of a combination of oestrogen and progesterone therapy or in the form of the oral contraceptive pill is the treatment of choice to prevent bone mineral loss and subsequent stress fractures in this group who are already at risk of stress fracture due to their high exercise level.

An interesting study performed by Myburgh et al. (1988) looked at a group of athletes with shin pain and the incidence of a number of aetiological factors, mainly biomechanical, one of which included calcium intake. This study showed a significant relationship between shin pain and low calcium intake. However, another study was unable to reproduce these results (Brukner et al., 1989).

Potassium

The effect of exercise on potassium has been reviewed by Lindinger and Sjogaard (1991). Exercise results in a release of potassium from contracting muscles which decreases the intracellular potassium concentrations of contracting muscles and increases plasma potassium concentrations during the period of activity. The magnitude of the decrease in intracellular potassium concentrations and increase in plasma concentrations is proportional to the intensity of exercise. Muscle potassium loss also continues with prolonged moderate-intensity exercise.

It is proposed that the reduction in intracellular potassium concentration, in association with the demands on cellular energy supply, contributes directly to decreases in muscle activation, i.e. muscle fatigue, at the level of the sarcolemma.

Cessation of exercise results in a rapid decrease in plasma potassium concentrations to, or below, resting levels. Potassium is removed from the plasma by both recovering muscle and non-contracting tissues. Training in all individuals results in a blunting of the exercise-increased uptake of potassium by both inactive tissues and contracting muscles.

Iron

Iron plays an essential role in exercise performance through oxygen transport by haemoglobin and myoglobin, cytochrome activity and various metabolically important enzymes. There has been considerable interest in recent years in the relationship between iron and athletic performance. While it is widely accepted that anaemia results in impaired athletic performance due to decreased oxygen transport, it is still debated whether or not iron deficiency without anaemia, as indicated by decreased body iron stores, has an effect on performance. This is theoretically possible due to the important role of iron in muscle metabolism. Iron deficiency results in a decrease in the muscle activities of myoglobin (McDonald et al., 1984), succinate dehydrogenase (Koziol et al., 1978) and cytochrome C (Hagler et al., 1981).

Researchers suggest (Ohira et al., 1983) that the increase in blood lactate common to iron deficiency may be a result of a loss in the oxidative potential of the skeletal muscles. These investigators found that the soleus muscle of iron-deficient rats had greater total lactate dehydrogenase and specifically the isozymes M_2H_2 than normal rats.

Because iron deficiency causes a reduction in the rate of oxidative metabolism without an apparent decrease in glycolysis (Finch et al., 1979), the cytosolic concentration of pyruvate, the end-product of glycolysis, would rise. This would shift the energetic equilibrium in favour of the production of lactate instead of the conversion of pyruvate to acetyl-coenzyme A and entry into the oxidative phosphorylation process of the mitochondria.

This build up of lactate may be a contributing factor to musculoskeletal injury. Iron deficiency is often present in conjunction with overuse syndromes, but this is almost certainly due to the fact that they are both common problems associated with overtraining. The incidence of iron deficiency especially among female endurance athletes is high. All athletes should be encouraged to pay close attention to their iron intake, preferably in the form of haem iron contained in red meat, as this is absorbed more readily than the non-haem forms of iron.

Zinc

Serum zinc concentrations can increase significantly during strenuous exercise. This is thought to be due to muscle leakage of zinc into the extracellular fluid following muscle damage (Karlson et al., 1968). It has been suggested (Dressendorfer & Sockolov, 1980) that a high level of constant exercise can have long-term effects on zinc metabolism. This suggestion was based on the observation that a significant number of endurance runners were characterized by low serum zinc concentrations even prior to an exercise bout. These serum zinc levels probably result from an increase in zinc losses from the body perhaps due to urine and/or sweat (Anderson & Guttman, 1988). Serum zinc levels decrease with chronic exercise (Couzy et al., 1990; Ohno et al., 1990).

Severe dietary zinc deficiency can affect muscle growth and composition. The impact of a marginal zinc deficiency on muscle growth and function is less clear (McDonald & Keen, 1988). It has been reported that changes in extracellular zinc levels influence twitch–tension relationships in muscle (van Rij et al., 1986). As yet there has been no evidence of the relationship between zinc and athletic injury.

Magnesium

It has been estimated that over 50% of the population of the USA had a dietary intake of magnesium less than the 1980 recommended daily allowance for this nutrient (Morgan *et al.*, 1985). Reduction in serum magnesium has also been noted in relation to exercise. This is thought to be a function of both sweat losses and redistribution of serum magnesium into the working muscle (McDonald & Keen, 1988).

The physiological consequences of the reduction of serum magnesium concentrations during prolonged intense exercise have not been firmly identified (McDonald & Keen, 1988). Epileptic-type convulsions (Jooste *et al.*, 1979) and carpopedal spasms (Liu *et al.*, 1983) have been reported in athletes with low serum magnesium concentrations.

The detailed effects of marginal magnesium deficiency on athletes are unknown. However, magnesium-deficient rats show a reduced endurance capacity, mild anaemia, low plasma protein and insulin concentrations and altered calcium, zinc and iron metabolism (Keen *et al.*, 1987).

Chromium

The main metabolic functions of chromium have not yet been clearly defined, but are directly related to the regulation of carbohydrate and lipid metabolism primarily by potentiating insulin action (Anderson, 1981). Exercise results in a marked mobilization of chromium from body stores. This leads to increased urinary loss of chromium. It is not known if the body adapts in some way to these increased chromium losses due to exercise (Campbell & Anderson, 1987).

Two studies have shown that chromium supplementation resulted in significant losses in body fat and increases in lean body mass in young men participating in weight-training programmes (Evans, 1989). However, Clarkson (1991) urges caution in the interpretation of these results.

Copper

Copper is an essential nutrient that has a wide variety of functions including key roles in iron metabolism, cross-linking of connective tissues, neurotransmitter and brain function, lipid metabolism and energy production (O'Dell, 1984). Copper losses through sweat may be considerable, especially for people living in warm and humid climates.

Studies investigating the effect of exercise on copper status have shown conflicting results with some studies showing an increase in serum copper levels with regular exercise (Dowdy & Burt, 1980; Lukaski *et al.*, 1983). This effect may be similar to the increase in copper levels found with stress (Keen & Hackman, 1984).

Vitamins

The relationship between vitamins and exercise is a controversial one. Many athletes take vitamin supplements in an attempt to improve performance and/or health despite minimal evidence to support their use. Vitamins are important organic substances required to perform specific metabolic functions in the body. With the exception of vitamin B, they cannot be synthesized by the body and must be obtained from the diet or synthesized by the microflora of the gastrointestinal tract (Belko, 1987). The relationship of vitamins with exercise involves their role as coenzymes in the oxidative processes of cells or in the production and protection of red blood cells. There is no doubt that vitamins are essential for the maintenance of good health and healthy tissue. The question that remains to be answered is whether deficiencies in these vitamins impairs the maintenance of healthy tissue and therefore makes the exercising athlete more susceptible to injury. To understand the possible roles of vitamins in injury prevention, it is important to examine the role of each vitamin in the different energy processes.

THIAMINE (VITAMIN B_1)

Thiamine plays an important role in energy metabolism and in the nervous system. Specifically it takes a key place in the oxidative decarboxylation of pyruvate to acetyl-coenzyme A. Thiamine deficiency has been associated with fatigue, loss of ambition and loss of efficiency during daily work (Egana *et al.*, 1942); fatigue, irritability, lack of pep, anorexia and increased leg pain during work (Barboka *et al.*, 1943).

RIBOFLAVIN (VITAMIN B₂)

Riboflavin functions as a coenzyme for a group of flavoproteins involved in biological oxidation, the most common of these is flavine adenine dinucleotide (FAD). There is a close relationship between the level of protein intake and riboflavin allowance since it has been shown that with low protein intakes, the body protein stores are catabolized and depleted of riboflavine (van der Beek, 1985). This is seen particularly in subjects consuming low-calorie or starvation diets (Consolazio *et al.*, 1971).

Physical training may increase riboflavin requirements (Belko *et al.*, 1983; Ohno *et al.*, 1988). There is some evidence that training may cause an increased retention of riboflavin in skeletal muscles (Hunter & Turkki, 1987).

NICOTINIC ACID (NIACIN, VITAMIN B₃)

Nicotinic acid is a component of two important enzymes concerned with glycolysis, fat synthesis and the intracellular respiratory mechanism of all cells. Deficiency of nicotinic acid results in pellagra, a disease characterized by muscle weakness, anorexia, diarrhoea, dermatitis, glossitis and nervous system abnormalities.

Studies have shown that nicotinic acid blocks the release of fatty acids from adipose tissue during exercise. As a result, blood glucose and muscle glycogen are relied upon to a greater extent to provide energy resulting in an increase in glycogen depletion (Bergstrom *et al.*, 1969; Pernow & Saltin, 1971; Lassers *et al.*, 1972).

VITAMIN B₆ (PYRIDOXINE)

Vitamin B₆ in the coenzyme form, pyridoxal-5-phosphate, is involved in virtually all aspects of amino acid metabolism. Vitamin B₆ requirements appear to increase when high-protein diets are consumed (Keith, 1989). Vitamin B₆ is involved in catecholamine, haemoglobin and general protein synthesis. In addition, the enzyme, glycogen phosphorylase, necessary for the breakdown of muscle glycogen, contains pyridoxal phosphate.

Borisov (1977) found low levels of 4-pyridoxic acid excretion in students at a physical culture institute and suggested that physically active students had vitamin B₆ requirements 1.5–2 times as high as the normal population. Other studies have given conflicting results.

PANTOTHENIC ACID

Pantothenic acid is a factor of vitamin-B complex whose action depends on the activity of its conjugated nucleotide form coenzyme A, the intermediate metabolite of carbohydrate and fat metabolism leading to energy release. It is contained in all animal and plant tissues and its richest source is royal jelly.

Pantothenic acid deficiency in humans is rare. Some studies have shown that exercise may decrease pantothenate status (Nijakowski, 1966; Bialecki & Nijakowski, 1967).

FOLIC ACID

Folic acid serves as a coenzyme that plays a role in protein and nucleic acid metabolism. It is also essential for the maintenance of normal red blood cell production. No studies have investigated the relationship between folic acid and exercise.

VITAMIN B₁₂ (CYANOCOBALAMIN)

This vitamin is a required nutrient for the normal functioning of all cells, particularly the cells of the haemopoietic and nervous systems.

Vitamin B_{12} functions in protein metabolism and may also be involved in fat and carbohydrate metabolism.

There is no evidence of increased vitamin B_{12} requirements with exercise. In spite of this, the use of vitamin B_{12} injections prior to competition is widespread.

ASCORBIC ACID (VITAMIN C)

Vitamin C plays a number of roles, being involved in the synthesis of collagen, in the metabolic reactions of amino acids including tyrosine, and in the synthesis of adrenaline and the glucocorticoids of the adrenal gland.

The effect of physical performance on vitamin C metabolism is unclear. In a review of the literature, Keith (1989) noted that eight out of 10 studies reported that physical activity did, in some manner, affect vitamin C metabolism. While more work is warranted in this area, the present data do indicate that strenuous exercise alters vitamin C metabolism. This may mean an increased need for the vitamin in persons performing strenuous work.

Because of its role in collagen synthesis, vitamin C may play a role in recovery from intense exercise and in injury repair.

VITAMINS A, D AND K

Vitamins A, D and K are fat soluble vitamins which are present in abundant quantities in the body and are unlikely to be affected by physical activity.

Vitamin A is necessary for normal vision, bone growth and epithelial tissue integrity. It appears to influence the membrane stability of mitochondria and lysosomes.

Vitamin D is involved in the formation of teeth and bone. Studies have shown no relationship between exercise and vitamin A or D metabolism. Vitamin K compounds are necessary for normal blood clotting.

VITAMIN E

Vitamin E is also a fat soluble vitamin. The exact role of vitamin E in body function is uncertain and is the subject of considerable controversy. The role of vitamin E is reviewed by Kagan et al. (1989).

It is thought that vitamin E may play a decisive role in the maintenance of the functional activity of muscle tissues, which is determined to a considerable extent by its stabilizing effects on the membrane structures of myocytes. The effects of vitamin E are thought to be due to the radical-scavenging activity of tocopherols. Vitamin E deficiency causes myodystrophy in animals.

Vitamin E deficiency is rarely observed in humans and the amount of this vitamin in the standard Western diet is sufficient. However, increased physical loading which activates free-radical reactions, results in an increased requirement for vitamin E. This may lead to muscle damage and may necessitate additional intake of vitamin E. However, supplementation with vitamin E did not reduce the amount of muscle damage during endurance exercise (Helgheim et al., 1979; Robertson et al., 1990).

The whole subject of oxygen free radicals and the role of antioxidants is the source of considerable debate and many experts do not accept the above hypotheses.

VITAMINS: SUMMARY

Vitamins are involved in many important bodily processes. Vitamin deficiencies are rare in Western society and the ideal training diet mentioned previously should contain well above the recommended levels of all vitamins. It is still unclear whether the vitamin requirements of athletes are increased and if so, by how much. While vitamin and mineral supplementation is widely used among athletes, there is little scientific evidence to support this. There is no clinical evidence of a direct link between vitamin deficiency and injury, although as noted, there are many theoretical reasons why this may occur.

Conclusion

The role of nutrition in the prevention of injury is largely uncertain. There are certainly a number of theoretical reasons why deficiencies of certain nutrients especially carbohydrate, protein and calcium may be a contributing factor to the development of injuries. However, considerable work needs to be done to investigate the links between the various nutrients and the development of injury in the athlete.

References

Anderson, J.J.B. (1990) Dietary calcium and bone mass through the life cycle. *Nutr. Today* Mar./Apr., 9–14.

Anderson, R.A. (1981) Nutritional role of chromium. *Sci. Total Environ.* **17**, 13–29.

Anderson, R.A. & Guttman, H.N. (1988) Trace minerals and exercise. In E.S. Horton & R.L. Terjung (eds) *Exercise, Nutrition and Energy Metabolism*, pp. 180–95. Macmillan, New York.

Armstrong, L.E., Costill, D.L. & Frisk, W.J. (1985) Influence of diuretic-induced dehydration on competitive running performance. *Med. Sci. Sports Exerc.* **17**, 456–61.

Ashley, F.W. & Kannel, W.B. (1974) Relation of weight change to changes of atherogenic traits. *J. Chron. Dis.* **27**, 103–14.

Barboka, C.H., Foltz, E.E. & Ivy, A.C. (1943) Relationship between vitamin-B complex intake and work output in trained subjects. *JAMA* **122**, 717–20.

Barrow, G. & Saha, S. (1988) Menstrual irregularity and stress fractures in collegiate female distance runners. *Am. J. Sports Med.* **16**, 209–16.

Belko, A.Z. (1987) Vitamins and exercise — An update. *Med. Sci. Sports Exerc.* **19**(5), S191–6.

Belko, A.Z., Miller, D., Haas, J.D. & Roe, D.A. (1983) Effects of exercise on riboflavin requirements of young women. *Am. J. Clin. Nutr.* **41**, 270–7.

Bergstrom, J., Hultman, E., Jorfeldt, L., Pernow, B. & Wahnen, J. (1969) Effect of nicotinic acid on physical working capacity and on metabolism of muscle. *J. Appl. Physiol.* **26**, 170–6.

Bialecki, M. & Nijakowski, F. (1967) Behavior of pantothenic acid in tissues and blood of white rats following short and prolonged physical strains. *Acta Physiol. Polon.* **18**, 33–8.

Bilmazes, C., Vany, R., Havergerg, L.N., Munro, H.N. & Young, V.R. (1978) Muscle protein breakdown rates in humans based on N-methylhistidine (3-methylhistidine) content of mixed protein in skeletal muscle and urinary output of N-methylhistidine. *Metabolism* **27**, 525–30.

Blom, P.C., Hostmark, A.T., Vaage, O., Vardal, K.R. & Machlum, S. (1987) Effect of different post-exercise sugar diets on the rate of muscle glycogen synthesis. *Med. Sci. Sports Exerc.* **19**, 491–6.

Blumenthal, J.A., O'Toole, L.C. & Chong, J.L. (1984) Is running an analogue of anorexia nervosa? An empirical study of obligatory running and anorexia nervosa. *JAMA* **252**, 520–3.

Borisov, I.M. (1977) Pyridoxine allowance of the students in a sports school. *Voprosy Pitania* **3**, 48–52.

Bray, G.A. (1969) Effect of caloric restriction on energy expenditure in obese patients. *Lancet* **ii**, 397–8.

Brotman, A.W. & Stern, T.A. (1985) Osteoporosis and pathologic fractures in anorexia nervosa. *Am. J. Psychol.* **142**, 495–6.

Brownell, K.D., Nelson Steen, S. & Wilmore, J.H. (1987) Weight regulation practices in athletes: Analysis of metabolic and health effects. *Med. Sci. Sports Exerc.* **19**(6), 546–56.

Brukner, P.D., Garden, L. & Inge, K. (1989) Relationship between shin pain and nutrition. *Proceedings 26th Annual Conference, Australian Sports Medicine Federation* (Abstract).

Burke, L.M. & Read, R.D.S. (1989) Sports nutrition. Approaching the nineties. *Sports Med.* **8**(2), 80–100.

Campbell, W.W. & Anderson, R.A. (1987) Effects of aerobic exercise and training on the trace minerals chromium, zinc and copper. *Sports Med.* **4**, 9–18.

Cann, C.E., Martin, M.C., Genant, H.K. & Jaffe, R.B. (1984) Decreased spinal mineral content in amenorrheic women. *JAMA* **215**, 626–9.

Celejowa, I. & Homa, M. (1970) Food intake, nitrogen and energy balance in Polish weightlifters during a training camp. *Nutr. Metab.* **12**, 259–74.

Clarkson, P.M. (1991) Minerals: Exercise performance and supplementation in athletes. *J. Sports Sci.* **9**, 91–116.

Consolazio, C.F., Johnson, H.L., Krzywicki, T.A., Daws, T.A. & Barnhart, R. (1971) Thiamin, riboflavin and pyridoxine excretion during acute starvation and caloric restriction. *Am. J. Clin. Nutr.* **27**, 165–78.

Cook, S.D., Harding, A.F., Thomas, K.A., Morgan, E.L., Schnurpfeil, K.M. & Haddad, R.J. (1987) Trabecular bone density and menstrual function in women runners. *Am. J. Sports Med.* **15**, 503–7.

Costill, D.L. (1988) Carbohydrates for exercise: Dietary demands for optimal performance. *Int. J. Sports*

Med. **9**, 1–18.

Costill, D.L., Flynn, M.G., Kirwan, J.P., Houmerd, J.A. & Mitchell, J.B. (1988) Effects of repeated days of intensified training on muscle glycogen and swimming performance. *Med. Sci. Sports Exerc.* **20**, 249–54.

Costill, D.L. & Miller, J.M. (1980) Nutrition for endurance sport: Carbohydrate and fluid balance. *Int. J. Sports Med.* **1**, 2–14.

Couzy, F., Lafargne, P. & Guezennec, C.Y. (1990) Zinc metabolism in the athlete: Influence of training nutrition and other factors. *Int. J. Sports Med.* **11**, 263–6.

Dohm, G.L., Williams, R.T., Kasperek, G.J. & Van Rij, A.M. (1982) Increased excretion of urea and *N*-methylhistidine by rats and humans after a bout of exercise. *J. Appl. Physiol.* **52**, 27–33.

Dowdy, R.P. & Burt, J. (1980) Effect of intensive, long term training on copper and iron nutrition in man. *Federation Proceedings; Federation of American Societies for Experimental Biology*, **39**, 786.

Dressendorfer, R.H. & Sockolov, R. (1980) Hypozincemia in runners. *Phys. Sportsmed.* **8**, 97–100.

Drinkwater, B.L., Nilson, K., Chestnut, C.H., Bremner, W.J., Shamholtz, S. & Southworth, N.B. (1984) Bone mineral content of amenorrheic and eumenorrheic athletes. *New Engl. J. Med.* **311**, 277–81.

Egana, E., Johnson, R.E., Bloomfield, R. *et al.* (1942) The effects of a diet deficient in the vitamin B-complex on sedentary man. *Am. J. Physiol.* **127**, 731–41.

Evans, G.W. (1989) The effect of chromium picolinate on insulin controlled parameters in humans. *Int. J. Biosci. Res.* **1**, 163–80.

Finch, C.A., Gollnick, P.D., Halastala, M.P., Miller, L.R., Dillmann, E. & Mackler, B. (1979) Lactic acidosis as a result of iron deficiency. *J. Clin. Invest.* **64**, 129–37.

Frisch, R.E., Wyshak, G. & Vincent, L. (1980) Delayed menarche and amenorrhea of ballet dancers. *New Engl. J. Med.* **303**, 117–19.

Goldring, S.R. & Krane, S.M. (1981) Metabolic bone disease; Osteoporosis and osteomalacia. *Disease-a-Month* **27**, 1–103.

Gontzea, I., Sutzescu, P. & Dumitrache, S. (1974). The influence of muscular activity on nitrogen balance and on the need of man for proteins. *Nutr. Rep. Int.* **10**, 35–43.

Hagler, L., Askew, E.W., Neville, J.R., Mellick, P.W., Coppes, R.I. & Lowder, J.F. (1981) Influence of dietary iron deficiency on hemoglobin, myoglobin, their respective reductases and skeletal muscle mitochondrial respiration. *Am. J. Clin. Nutr.* **34**, 2169–77.

Heaney, R.P., Gallagher, J.C., Johnston, C.C., Neer,

R., Parfitt, A.M. & Whedon, G.D. (1982) Calcium nutrition and bone health in the elderly. *Am. J. Clin. Nutr.* **36**, 986–1013.

Helgheim, I., Hetland, O., Nilsson, S., Ingjer, F. & Stromme, S.B. (1979) The effects of vitamin E on serum enzyme levels following heavy exercise. *Eur. J. Appl. Physiol.* **40**, 283–9.

Hickson, J.F. & Hinkelman, K. (1985) Exercise and protein intake effects on urinary 2-methylhistidine excretion. *Am. J. Clin. Nutr.* **41**, 246–53.

Hickson, J.F., Wolinsky, I., Rodriguez, G.P., Pivarnik, J.M., Kent, M.C. & Shier, N.W. (1986) Failure of weight training to affect urinary indices of protein metabolism in man. *Med. Sci. Sports Exerc.* **18**, 563–7.

Hickson, J.F. & Wolinsky, I. (1989) Human protein intake and metabolism in exercise and sport. In J.F. Hickson & I. Wolinsky (eds) *Nutrition in Exercise and Sport*, pp. 5–36. CRC Press, Boca Raton.

Hunter, K.L. & Turkki, P.R. (1987) Effect of exercise on riboflavine status of rats. *J. Nutr.* **117**, 298–304.

Inge, K. & Brukner, P. (1986) *Food for Sport*. William Heinemann, Melbourne.

Ivy, J.L., Katz, A.L., Cutler, C.L., Sherman, W.M. & Coyle, E.F. (1988) Muscle glycogen storage after exercise: Effect of time of carbohydrate ingestion. *J. Appl. Physiol.* **65**, 1480–5.

Jacobs, I., Westlin, N., Karslson, J., Rasmussen, M. & Houghton, B. (1982) Muscle glycogen and diet in élite soccer players. *Eur. J. Appl. Physiol.* **48**, 297–302.

Jooste, P.L., Wolfswinkel, J.M., Schoeman, J.J. & Strydom, N.B. (1979) Epileptic-type convulsions and magnesium deficiency. *Aviat. Space Environ. Med.* **50**, 734–5.

Kagan, V.E., Spirichev, V.B. & Erin, A.N. (1989) Vitamin E, physical exercise and sport. In J.F. Hickson & I. Wolinsky (eds) *Nutrition in Exercise and Sport*, pp. 255–78. CRC Press, Boca Raton.

Karlson, J., Diamant, B. & Saltin, B. (1968) Lactic dehydrogenase activity in muscle after prolonged exercise in man. *J. Appl. Physiol.* **25**, 88–91.

Kasperek, G.J. & Snider, R.D. (1985) Increased protein degradation after eccentric exercise. *Eur. J. Physiol.* **54**, 30–4.

Keen, C.L. & Hackman, R.M. (1984) Trace elements in athletic performance. In F. Katch (ed) *Sport, Health and Nutrition*, p. 51. Human Kinetics, Illinois.

Keen, C.L., Lowney, P., Gershwin, M.E., Hurley, L.S. & Stern, J.S. (1987) Dietary magnesium intake influences exercise capacity and hematologic parameters in rats. *Metabolism* **36**, 788–93.

Keith, R.E. (1989) Vitamins in sport and exercise. In J.E. Hickson, & I. Wolinsky (eds) *Nutrition in Exercise and Sport*, pp. 233–53. CRC Press, Boca Raton.

Koziol, B.J., Ohira, Y., Simpson, D.R. & Edgerton,

V.R. (1978) Biochemical skeletal muscle and hematological profiles of moderate and severely iron deficient and anemic adult rats. *J. Nutr.* **108**, 1306–14.

Krichevsky, D., Weber, M.M., Buck, C.L. & Klurfeld, D.M. (1986) Calories, fat and cancer. *Lipids* **21**, 272–4.

Laritcheva, K.A., Yalovaya, N.I., Shubin, V.I. & Smirnov, P.V. (1978) Study of energy expenditure and protein needs of top weightlifters. In J. Parizkova & V.A. Rogozkin (eds) *Nutrition, Physical Fitness, and Health*, pp. 144–63. University Park Press, Baltimore.

Lassers, B.W., Wahlqvist, M.L., Kaijser, L. & Carlson, L.A. (1972) Effect of nicotinic acid on myocardial metabolism in man at rest and during exercise. *J. Appl. Physiol.* **33**, 72–80.

Lee, C.L., Lawler, O.S. & Johnson, G.H. (1981) Effects of supplementation of diets with calcium and calcium-rich foods on bone density of elderly females with osteoporosis. *Am. J. Clin. Nutr.* **36**, 819–23.

Lemon, P.W.R. & Mullin, J.P. (1980) Effect of initial muscle glycogen levels on protein catabolism during exercise. *J. Appl. Physiol.* **48**, 624–9.

Lemon, P.W.R. & Nagle, F.J. (1981) Effects of exercise on protein and amino acid metabolism. *Med. Sci. Sports Exerc.* **13**, 141–9.

Lemon, P.W.R., Nagle, F.J., Mullin, J.P. & Benevenga, N.J. (1982) *In vivo* leucine oxidation at rest and during two intensities of exercise. *J. Appl. Physiol.* **53**, 947.

Lemon, P.W.R., Yarasheki, K.E. & Dolny, D.G. (1984) The importance of protein for athletes. *Sports Med.* **1**, 474–84.

Lindbey, J.S., Fears, W.B., Hunt, M.M., Powell, M.B., Bell, D. & Wade, C. (1984) Exercise induced amenorrhea and bone density. *Ann. Int. Med.* **101**, 647–8.

Lindinger, M.I. & Sjogaard, G. (1991) Potassium regulation during exercise and recovery. *Sports Med.* **11**, 382–401.

Liu, L., Borowski, G. & Rose, L.I. (1983) Hypomagnesemia in a tennis player. *Phys. Sportsmed.* **11**, 79–80.

Lloyd, T., Triantafyllon, S.J., Baker, E.R., Hoots, P.S., Whitside, S.A., Kalenak, A. & Stumpf, P.G. (1986) Women athletes with menstrual irregularity have increased musculoskeletal injuries. *Med. Sci. Sports Exerc.* **18**, 374–9.

Lukaski, H.C., Bolonchuk, W.W., Klevay, L.M., Milne, D.B. & Sandstead, H.H. (1983) Maximal oxygen consumption as related to magnesium, copper and zinc nutriture. *Am. J. Clin. Nutr.* **37**, 407–15.

McDonald, R., Hegenauer, J., Sucec, A. & Saltman, T. (1984) Effects of iron deficiency and exercise on myoglobin in rats. *Eur. J. Appl. Physiol.* **52**, 414–19.

McDonald, R. & Keen, D.L. (1988) Iron, zinc and magnesium nutrition and athletic performance. *Sports Med.* **5**, 171–84.

Matkovic, V., Kostial, K., Simonovic, I., Buzina, R., Brodarec, A. & Nordin, B.E. (1979) Bone status and fracture rates in two regions of Yugoslavia. *Am. J. Clin. Nutr.* **32**, 540–8.

Morgan, K.J., Stampley, G.L., Zabin, M.E. & Fischer, D.R. (1985) Magnesium and calcium dietary intakes of the U.S. population. *J. Am. Coll. Nutr.* **4**, 195–206.

Myburgh, K.H., Grobler, N. & Noakes, T.D. (1988) Factors associated with shin soreness in athletes. *Phys. Sportsmed.* **16**, 129–34.

Nijakowski, F. (1966) Assays of some vitamins of the B complex group in human blood in relation to muscular effort. *Acta Physiol. Polon.* **17**, 477–86.

Nordin, B.E. (1966) International patterns of osteoporosis. *Clin. Orthop. Rel. Res.* **45**, 17–30.

O'Dell, B.L. (1984) Copper. In *Present Knowledge in Nutrition*, 5th edn, pp. 506–18. Nutrition Foundation Inc., Washington D.C.

Ohira, Y., Chen, C., Hegenauer, J. & Saltman, P. (1983) Adaptations of lactate metabolism in iron-deficient rats. *Proceedings of the Society for Experimental Biology and Medicine*, **173**, 213–16.

Ohno, H., Sato, Y., Ishikawa, M., Yahata, T., Gasa, S., Doi, R., Yamamura, K. *et al.* (1990) Training effects on blood zinc levels in humans. *J. Sports Med. Phys. Fitness* **30**, 247–53.

Ohno, H., Yahata, T., Sato, Y., Yamamura, K. & Taniguchi, N. (1988) Physical training and fasting erythrocyte activities of free radical scavenging systems in sedentary men. *Eur. J. Appl. Physiol.* **57**, 173–6.

Paul, G.L. (1989) Dietary protein requirements of physically active individuals. *Sports Med.* **8**(3), 154–76.

Pernow, B. & Saltin, B. (1971) Availability of substrates and capacity for prolonged heavy exercise. *J. Appl. Physiol.* **37**, 416–22.

Phinney, S.D. (1985) The metabolic interaction between very low calorie diet and exercise. In G.L. Blackburn & G.A. Bray (eds) *Management of Obesity by Severe Caloric Restriction*, pp. 99–105. PSG Co., Littleton.

Pollitzer, W.S. & Anderson, J.J.B. (1989) Ethnic and genetic differences in bone mass: A review with an hereditary vs. environmental perspective. *Am. J. Clin. Nutr.* **50**, 1244–59.

Recker, R.R., Saville, P.D. & Heaney, R.P. (1977) Effect of estrogen and calcium carbonate on bone loss in postmenopausal women. *Ann. Int. Med.* **34**, 819–23.

Rigotti, N.A., Nussbaum, S.R., Herzog, D.B. & Neer,

R.M. (1984) Osteoporosis in women with anorexia nervosa. *New Engl. J. Med.* **311**, 1601–6.

Robertson, J.D., Crosbie, L., Maughan, R.J., Leiper, J.B. & Duthie, G.G. (1990) Influence of vitamin E supplementation on muscle damage following endurance exercise. *Int. J. Vit. Nutr. Res.* **60**, 171–2.

Ross, M.H., Lustbader, E.D. & Bras, G. (1985) Dietary habits and the prediction of life span of rats: A prospective test. *Am. J. Clin. Nutr.* **41**, 1332–44.

Seeman, E., Hopper, J.L., Bach, L.A., Cooper, M., Parkinson, E., McKay, J. & Jerums, G. (1989) Reduced bone mass in daughters of women with osteoporosis. *New Engl. J. Med.* **320**, 554–8.

Seeman, E. & Riggs, B.L. (1981) Dietary prevention of bone loss in the elderly. *Geriatrics* **36**, 71–9.

Stern, J.S., Schultz, C. & Mole, P. (1986) *Effect of caloric restriction and exercise on basal metabolism and thyroid hormone.* Paper presented at the 3rd International Congress of Obesity, Rome, Italy.

Strauss, R.H., Lanese, R.R. & Malarkey, W.B. (1985) Weight loss in amateur wrestlers and its effects on serum testosterone levels. *JAMA* **254**, 3337–8.

Szmukler, G., Brown, S., Darby, A. & Parsons, V. (1985) Premature loss of bone in chronic anorexia nervosa. *Br. J. Med.* **290**, 26–7.

Tarnopolsky, M.A., MacDougall, J.D. & Atkinson, S.A. (1988) Influence of protein intake and training status on nitrogen balance and lean body mass. *J. Appl. Physiol.* **64**, 187–93.

Tcheng, T.K. & Tipton, C.M. (1973) Iowa wrestling study: Anthropometric measurements and the prediction of a minimal body weight for high school wrestlers. *Med. Sci. Sports Exerc.* **5**, 1–10.

Torun, B., Scrimshaw, N.S. & Young, V.R. (1977) Effect of isometric exercises on body potassium and dietary protein requirements of young men. *Am. J. Clin. Nutr.* **30**, 1983–93.

van der Beek, E.J. (1985) Vitamins and endurance training. *Sports Med.* **2**, 175–97.

Van Itallie, T.B. & Yang, M.U. (1977) Current concepts in nutrition: Diet and weightloss. *New Engl. J. Med.* **297**, 1158–61.

van Rij, A.M., Hall, M.T., Dohm, G.L., Bray, J. & Pories, W.J. (1986) Changes in zinc metabolism following exercise in human subjects. *Biol. Trace Element Res.* **10**, 99–106.

Viru, A. (1987) Mobilization of structural proteins during exercise. *Sports Med.* **4**, 95–128.

Weight, L.M. & Noakes, T.D. (1987) Is running an analog of anorexia? A survey of the incidence of eating disorders in female distance runners. *Med. Sci. Sports Exerc.* **19**, 213.

Welle, S.L., Amatruda, J.M., Forbes, G.B. & Lockwood, D.H. (1984) Resting metabolic rate of obese women after rapid weight loss. *J. Clin. Endocrinol. Metab.* **59**, 41–4.

Wheeler, G.D., Wall, S.T. & Belcastro, A.N. (1984) Reduced serum testosterone and prolactin levels in male distance runners. *JAMA* **252**, 514–16.

Yates, A., Leekey, K. & Shisslak, C.M. (1983) Running — An analogue of anorexia? *New Engl. J. Med.* **308**, 251.

Zambraski, E.J., Foster, D.T., Gross, P.M. & Tipton, C.M. (1976) Iowa wrestling study: weight loss and urinary profile of collegiate wrestlers. *Med. Sci. Sports Exerc.* **8**, 105–8.

Chapter 24

Drugs, Medication and Doping

ANDREW PIPE

The prompt, rapid and appropriate treatment of any athletic injury is a goal of all sport medicine professionals. Given the devastating consequences of some injuries, and the magnitude of the public health problem posed by sport and recreational injuries in many societies, it is equally valid that sport medicine practitioners should be concerned with the prevention of such injuries. In 1990, injuries occurring during sport, fitness and recreational activities in the province of Ontario, Canada ranked first among *all* types of injuries recorded at an estimated cost to that society of $563 million (Ministry of Tourism and Recreation, 1991).

Most sport medicine practitioners would agree that, apart from the treatment of established illness or injury, there is little that drugs or medications can do to prevent the incidence of injury in sport. Such a broad generalization overlooks the role that is played by the use of certain medicines in the treatment of some chronic diseases. Though I know of no evidence to support the contention, it seems reasonable to assume that the appropriate management of the asthmatic or diabetic athlete, by way of example, will at the very least minimize the chances of exacerbated illness and in an indirect way reduce the risks of injury.

Conversely, there are obvious examples of the degree to which the inappropriate use of certain medications in an injured or ailing athlete can potentiate the risk of further or aggravated injury. The injudicious use of local anaesthetics to permit participation through the masking of pain is perhaps the classic illustration of such practice.

All of us have an unfortunate understanding of the role of certain drugs in increasing the risk of accident, injury and death. Alcohol is the most culpable in this respect, and plays a highly significant role in the modern epidemic of motor vehicle accidents just as it undoubtedly contributes to a large number of recreational and sporting injuries. In a similar way, a variety of mood-altering drugs, by virtue of their ability to impair judgement and coordination, undoubtedly contribute to the burgeoning sport injury statistics.

'One of the duties of the physician' observed Sir William Osler, 'is to educate the masses not to take medicines'. Sir William's advice was appropriate in the age of the nostrum and the 'cure-all'; in some sense it is equally appropriate today given that the abuse of drugs is a common societal phenomenon. Sport has not, unfortunately, escaped this contemporary problem.

In the 1970s, the International Olympic Committee (IOC) Medical Commission recognized the need to develop policies and programmes designed to counter the use of performance-enhancing drugs in amateur sport. That decision reflected a number of concerns. Paramount was the health of the athlete. It is a sad irony of modern sport that athletes, who epitomize the ultimate in physiological achievement, may be prepared to jeopardize that very quality by the degree to which they become caught up in doping practices.

Of equal concern was the well-being of sport itself; the integrity of sport is jeopardized by the extent to which drug use becomes, or appears to become, commonplace. Sport can be a powerful, positive cultural force in any society and its welfare should be a concern for all within the sporting community.

The ethical dimension of sport is too often ignored. Sport is more than a 'social time-out' where the normal standards of human behaviour can be thrown to the wind. Athletic competition requires an acceptance of common rules and regulations — without them, or in their violation, fair and equitable contest becomes impossible. This is an area of special significance for sport medicine practitioners whose conduct will hopefully mirror the desired standards of sporting and professional behaviour. Those who would participate in the provision or prescription of doping practices violate both. They contravene fundamental rules of sport at the same time as they expose their athletic patients to the risks of illness and injury that may be a consequence of the use of banned drugs.

In the subcultures of certain sports, the use of pharmaceutical products for 'recreational' or performance-enhancing purposes has, regrettably, become commonplace. The highly publicized accounts of drug use among high-performance athletes and the international scandals that have surrounded the detection of such drug use have fuelled the cynicism of many. But to believe that the use of a variety of banned substances is a practice confined only to the highest levels of sport is to engage in dangerous self-deception. In North America, there is abundant evidence to suggest that drug use in a sporting context is prevalent at the level of the high school and community level athlete (Buckley et al., 1988; Johnson et al., 1989; Killip & Stennett, 1990). It is reasonable to assume that this is no less true in other developed nations as well. Thus health-care professionals involved in virtually every level of sport should feel very specific responsibilities

to confront and combat the problem posed by such drug use.

In this respect, no one should be complacent. In the developed world, the challenge is to eliminate, to the greatest possible extent, drug use from sport; in the developing nations, the challenge is to ensure that the phenomenon does not become established as part of the sporting culture. In both environments, there can be no argument that the most appropriate way to counter the problem is through the development and implementation of effective educational initiatives.

Up to the present day, most educational endeavours have consisted of the provision and dissemination of materials which document the common anticipated or real side-effects of the substances in question. Not surprisingly this approach has been of limited success. Experience in other areas of health promotion activity has shown that young people are particularly resistant to messages which focus solely on the health consequences of certain behaviours. This may be explained, in part, by the tendency of the young to consider themselves to be 'immortal' and thus immune to the consequences of any particular practice. Educational strategies designed to deter young athletes from using drugs or other illicit approaches to performance enhancement must therefore be broadly based and include a discussion of sporting values and ethics while emphasizing that such practices are considered to be unacceptable behaviour within and by the sporting community.

Accurate information is one of the most important forces that the health professional can bring to bear on the subject of drug use in sport. All sport medicine professionals should be familiar with the commonly abused drugs in sport and have a thorough understanding of the problems associated with their use. It may very well be the case that athletes will respond more favourably to information regarding the degree to which these products and practices may impair performance or produce injury or illness that will preclude participation than they will to the recitation of the possible long-term health consequences of the use of certain drugs. Weightlifters, for instance, may find the information that anabolic steroids can produce tendon ruptures to be more relevant than the fact that the same products have been associated with the development of peliosis hepatis.

Typically, discussions of the drug–sport problem focus on those products and practices which are specifically forbidden in sport and which have been banned by the IOC. To do so is to ignore the reality that the most common drugs of abuse in society, as in sport, are alcohol and tobacco. Sport medicine practitioners should be mindful of the role they can play in addressing the problems posed by these products in both the sporting and societal context.

In some sports the use of these products has become part of the 'culture'. Baseball players are no strangers to the use of large quantities of chewing tobacco and the associated problems of leukoplakia and oral cancer. Ice-hockey players in North America (and rugby players everywhere) often view the consumption of large quantities of alcohol as part of their sport; with disastrous results when combined with the operation of motor vehicles. These examples demonstrate that there are drug–sport problems other than those associated with the use of banned products. The use of cocaine among basketball players in North America, by way of further example, has produced a number of sporting disasters in the form of the sudden death of young athletes. No one would argue that this is not a drug–sport issue.

It is interesting to consider the degree to which athletes may receive large quantities of prescription or over-the-counter medications, provided or prescribed for the treatment of symptoms or complaints that may be almost continually present in a competitive athlete. Reviewing the list of medications declared by athletes at the time of drug testing in Canada it is difficult not to be impressed by the fact that the use of daily doses of anti-inflammatory medications seems to be a feature of an athletic life. One wonders whether in our enthusiasm to assist the injured or ailing athlete we are not too liberal in our use of such medications; medications which are not without hazard. Osler's words have particular relevance to the sport medicine practitioner in this respect.

Doping and sport injury

It is at this point neither possible, nor appropriate, to provide a definitive description of the problems or side-effects associated with the array of drugs that are abused in sport. Excellent reviews of this topic are to be found elsewhere (Haupt & Rovere, 1984; Strauss, 1987; Wilson, 1988; Wadler & Hainline, 1989) of which Wadler and Hainline's textbook (1989) is perhaps the most comprehensive. More relevant is a discussion of those aspects of the use of banned drugs which are known, or might be assumed to contribute to an increased risk of injury or illness. The IOC classification of banned doping classes or methods will be followed.

Doping classes

Stimulants

The stimulants, of which the amphetamines probably serve as the best example, have been used in sport to accentuate performance, mask fatigue and facilitate weight loss. Their use, particularly in cycling, has been associated with a number of deaths. The amphetamines cause central nervous system excitation which can produce a variety of side-effects ranging from restlessness to marked, near-psychotic levels of behaviour. Such behavioural changes are conceivably counterproductive in sporting situations requiring judgement and decision-making skills, and may predispose the user or others to injury. Severe central nervous stimulation may result in the development of convulsions, collapse and death. It is important to note that such side-effects may occur at any time even after an individual has been using the drug for a prolonged period.

The central nervous system effects of the amphetamines are much like those produced by cocaine. Users of this drug report a heightened sense of arousal and alertness. Most athletes who have used cocaine probably do so for social/recreational purposes but I have been struck by the degree to which the belief has developed, in certain specific sports, that performance can be enhanced in dramatically creative ways. There is no evidence to support this concept. In fact there is substantial evidence suggesting significant deterioration of athletic performance among cocaine users.

Cocaine's ability to produce pronounced coronary vasoconstriction and to precipitate cardiac arrhythmias mark it as a particularly dangerous drug, one which has been responsible for a number of very tragic deaths among athletes (Isner, 1986). Like the amphetamines, cocaine can also produce a wide variety of behavioural changes. Athletes should understand the particularly hazardous nature of this product; a product whose use may be difficult to stamp out in certain sporting subcultures irrespective of the degree of knowledge provided for athletes. Some have suggested that there is a tendency for the use of anabolic steroids and cocaine to be related.

Narcotics

Simply put, the use of narcotic analgesics in sport to mask the pain and discomfort of injury or exertion may predispose an individual to further injury, or exacerbate existing mechanical or medical problems. Narcotics also cloud judgement which makes their use counterproductive in the strategic sense. Physicians have an important role to play in ensuring that analgesics are used judiciously and appropriately. In many respects, physicians should serve as the advocate of their athletic patients; it is their personal well-being, not their athletic interests, which should take precedence in so far as the practice of sport medicine is concerned.

Anabolic steroids

Modifications of the male hormone testos-terone, all anabolic steroids are also androgenic. Their capacity to induce muscular hypertrophy in association with high levels of training has made these compounds a commonly used banned drug. Administered in accordance with empirically, at times bizarrely, developed protocols, these powerful compounds exert an influence on a variety of target tissues and organ systems.

In the first instance, it must be recognized that many of the products sold as anabolic steroids may, as a consequence of their black-market origin, be of questionable quality. Thus athletes purchasing such products may be exposing themselves to contaminated products and their associated risks. It has also been noted that in some environments anabolic steroids and the needles used to inject them have been shared among users with catastrophic results, notably the transmission of the human immunodeficiency virus (HIV) (Sklarek, 1984).

Anabolic steroids produce certain changes in the structure and function of tendons which render them more susceptible to injury and less capable of withstanding the forces generated by hypertrophied muscle (Laseter, 1991). Young athletes who have not reached full adult height may have final growth jeopardized by the effect of anabolics on the epiphyseal growth plate (Wadler & Hainline, 1989). Avascular necrosis of the femoral head has been associated with the use of anabolic steroids (Pettine, 1991). Behavioural changes in anabolic users have been documented by some authors (Annitto & Layman, 1980; Pope & Katz, 1988), such changes have been noted to produce psychotic or near-psychotic mood states and a repertoire of impulsive, aggressive behaviour. It is quite appropriate to assume that in certain sport situations where judgement, cooperation and strategic thought are important, anabolic steroids may confer a specific disadvantage upon the user. In many sport situations it may be reasonable to speculate that impulsive, disinhibited behaviour on the part of a steroid user may result in an increased risk of injury.

There is evidence to suggest that physical and psychological dependence on anabolic steroids can occur in users (Brower *et al.*, 1990). It is well accepted that anabolic steroids can produce changes in the lipoprotein profile of a user (Hurley *et al.*, 1984; McKillop & Ballantyne, 1987) such that there is an increased likelihood of the development of cardiovascular disease. What does not seem to be as well appreciated is that there are now a number of documented instances of significant cardiovascular events occurring in young athletes (Frankle *et al.*, 1988; McNutt *et al.*, 1988; Laroche, 1990).

Notwithstanding, as noted above, that most young athletes are heedless of the concerns raised by such evidence, it is still important that sport medicine practitioners be aware of these developments in order that they might be strong advocates in their own particular sporting environment for the development of philosophies and policies designed to facilitate drug-free sport.

β-blockers

A mainstay in the treatment of a number of cardiovascular conditions, the β-blockers have been used in a number of sporting situations because of their ability to lower the heart rate, minimize tremor and reduce anxiety. These medications profoundly affect the aerobic and anaerobic exercise capacity of those taking them. This may not be a concern to those involved in events like shooting and archery, but it has been speculated that this might be of significance in increasing the risk of injury in Alpine skiing (Karlsson *et al.*, 1983). It should be recognized that these compounds can interfere with normal sleep, may produce depression and can adversely affect sexual function — all of which can be profoundly counterproductive in the competitive athlete.

Diuretics

Diuretics have been used in a variety of sporting situations in order to produce rapid weight loss or to facilitate the excretion of other banned substances on occasions when drug testing is likely or feared.

Considerable evidence has accumulated demonstrating that there is no strategic advantage to be gained by competing at an artificially attained weight level; there is strong evidence demonstrating a significant reduction in physiological performance in such instances (American College of Sports Medicine, 1976). Nonetheless, dogma and pseudoscience often hold sway in sport and bizarre practices designed to facilitate weight loss are still regrettably commonplace in some sports, particularly the combatives. The use of diuretics in such circumstances is clearly inappropriate; the changes in electrolyte levels that may result from their use may accentuate the deterioration of performance noted in association with such practices. Such manipulations may also, it seems safe to speculate, increase the likelihood of injury through changes in strength and coordination.

Peptide hormones and analogues

Many athletes have used a variety of peptide compounds such as human growth hormone (HGH) or human chorionic gonadotrophin (HCG) because of their belief that these substances have ergogenic or anabolic properties. In many instances, when purchased from black-market sources, these compounds are not in fact what they are represented to be. Thus the athlete risks problems caused by the introduction of substances that are totally unknown or potentially contaminated.

Doping methods

Blood doping

The ability of infused red blood cells to enhance aerobic performance has been recognized for some time (Gledhill, 1982). The collection, storage and reinfusion of red blood cells are processes which can only be carried out with the assistance of physicians or other health professionals. Given that there are no currently effective means of detecting this practice, it is clear that the cooperation and integrity of sport medicine practitioners is essential in order to curb this problem.

All of the problems which might be associated with the transfusion of blood products can occur in those practising blood doping. These range from the development of a superficial phlebitis at the site of blood collection or transfusion, to the full range of risks that can occur with the use of blood products. 3% of homologous transfusions are associated with immune side-effects (Wadler & Hainline, 1989). The risks of these practices cannot be understated; the development of hepatitis B or HIV infection seems a ludicrous price to pay for an attempt to enhance aerobic capacity. This is particularly relevant when one considers that on occasion athletes and their medical advisers have used uncross-matched 'donations' from friends and acquaintances in the process of blood doping!

The development of synthetic erythropoietin has presented a new opportunity for those who would artificially accentuate their aerobic capacity. This drug, the product of genetic engineering technology, is used in clinical situations to combat the anaemias that characterize many chronic diseases including those of the chronic renal disorders. There is currently no method by which the use of this product can be detected, nor is one likely to appear in the foreseeable future. At the same time, the impression has developed among some that the use of this product is simple, straightforward and without side-effect. Nothing is further from the truth. In normal clinical use erythropoietin is associated with a number of complications relating to the development of erythrocythaemia. Such problems include hypertension, congestive heart failure and stroke. Recently, reports have begun to circulate of illness and death occurring in groups of cycling athletes who, it is speculated, have been using erythropoietin. Taken in combination, such knowledge serves only to heighten concerns

about the dangers associated with this new doping practice, and underscores the need to ensure that athletes and the members of their entourage develop standards of sporting behaviour that preclude participation in doping practices.

'Blood doping', note Wadler and Hainline (1989) 'represents a particularly challenging problem for the sports community ... Blood doping is unique in that the inability to detect its use, coupled with its clear-cut ergogenic potential, demands from the individual athlete a more profound ethical and moral decision ... the athlete is left with a choice — to embrace the meaning of the essence of sport, or participate in the practice of winning at any cost. With blood doping the ethical stakes are particularly high'.

Pharmacological, chemical and physical manipulation

In an attempt to conceal evidence of doping activity, some athletes have attempted to modify the excretion of banned substances, manipulate the contents of their bladders, or otherwise camouflage the presence of banned drugs. Such practices are hazardous, particularly the 'transplantation' of urine by a process of reverse catheterization. The risk of infection in such circumstances seems so obvious as to require no mention here; while the use of diuretics to 'flush' steroids or other illicit drugs from the system poses the problems noted earlier in this chapter. All of these processes or procedures, while perhaps posing minimal risk of 'injury' in the classical sense, may result in problems which though transient are also totally unnecessary.

Classes of drugs subject to certain restrictions

Alcohol, marijuana, local anaesthetics and corticosteroids are controlled in sport by the rules of certain sport federations (for alcohol and marijuana) or according to regulations which specify the nature or route of administration (for local anaesthetics and corticosteroids). There is little that needs to be repeated here regarding the problems that can be posed for athletes by alcohol or other mood-altering drugs.

The regulations pertaining to the administration of corticosteroids were developed by the IOC (1990) because of a concern that these medications were being used 'non-therapeutically by the oral, intramuscular and even the intravenous route in some sports'. That these powerful medications, with their potential for significant side-effects, were being prescribed so indiscriminately is a sobering reminder of the responsibility of sport medicine physicians to practise in accordance with the maxim *primum non nocere* — in the first instance do no harm.

Some final thoughts

It is a particular privilege to be able to participate in the preparation and care of élite athletes. The role of the sport medicine professional is a complex one; he or she must be versed in exercise and environmental physiology, adept at the diagnosis and management of musculo-skeletal disorders, have a fundamental understanding of the relationship between exercise and a variety of medical conditions, appreciate the unique social and physical environments in which sport may take place, and at the same time be acutely aware of the rules and regulations pertaining to drug use in sport. Simultaneously the sport physician must act to minimize the hazards or risks posed by any sport so as to reduce the risk of athletic participation and competition. Some of those hazards are to be found in the practices which permeate some sporting cultures; they range from bizarre nutritional or training practices to the systematic use of performance-enhancing substances banned in sport. Such compounds, as has been noted, may predispose athletes to illness or injury.

The sports physician is uniquely placed to be an authoritative source of knowledge and counsel regarding these practices and to exercise leadership in the movement to rid sport of the problem of doping. In so doing, one acts to safeguard the health of athletes while protecting the well-being of sport.

References

American College of Sports Medicine (1976) *Position Stand: Weight Loss in Wrestlers.* American College of Sports Medicine, Indianapolis.

Annitto, W. & Layman, W. (1980) Anabolic steroids and acute schizophrenic episode. *J. Clin. Psychiatr.*, **41**, 143—4.

Brower, K., Eliopulos, G., Blow, F., Catlin, D. & Beresford, T. (1990) Evidence for physical and psychological dependence on anabolic androgenic steroids in eight weight lifters. *Am. J. Psychiatr.* **147**, 510—12.

Buckley, W., Yeesalis, C., Friedl, K., Anderson, W., Streit, A. & Wright, J. (1988) Estimated prevalence of anabolic steroid use among male high school seniors. *J. Am. Med. Assoc.* **260**, 3441—5.

Frankle, M., Eichberg, R. & Zachariah, S. (1988) Anabolic androgenic steroids and a stroke in an athlete: case report. *Arch. Phys. Med. Rehab.* **69**, 632—3.

Gledhill, N. (1982) Blood doping and related issues: a brief review. *Med. Sci. Sports Exerc.* **14**, 183—9.

Haupt, H. & Rovere, G. (1984) Anabolic steroids: a review of the literature. *Am. J. Sports Med.* **12**, 469—84.

Hurley, B., Seals, D., Hagberg, J., Goldberg, A., Ostrove, S., Holloszy, J., Wiest, W. *et al.* (1984) High-density lipoprotein cholesterol in body-builders vs. powerlifters. Negative effects of androgen use. *J. Am. Med. Assoc.* **252**, 507—13.

International Olympic Committee Medical Commission (1990) List of doping classes and methods. In *International Olympic Charter Against Doping in Sport.* IOC, Lausanne.

Isner, J. (1986) Acute cardiac events temporally related to cocaine abuse. *N. Engl. J. Med.* **315**, 1438—43.

Johnson, M., Jay, M., Shoup, B. & Rickert, V. (1989) Anabolic steroid use by male adolescents. *Pediatrics* **83**, 921—4.

Karlsson, J., Kjessel, T. & Kaiser, P. (1983) Alpine skiing and acute beta-blockade. *Int. J. Sports Med.* **4**, 190—3.

Killip, S. & Stennett, R. (1990) Use of performance enhancing substances by London secondary school students, Report 90—03, Board of Education for the City of London. London, Ontario, Canada.

Laseter, J. (1991) Anabolic steroid-induced tendon pathology: A review of the literature. *Med. Sci. Sports Exerc.* **23**, 1–3.

Laroche, G. (1990) Steroid anabolic drugs and arterial complications in an athlete — a case history. *Angiology* **41**, 964–9.

McKillop, G. & Ballantyne, D. (1987) Lipoprotein analysis in bodybuilders. *Int. J. Cardiol.* **17**, 281–8.

McNutt, R., Ferenchick, G., Kirlin, P. & Hamlin, N. (1988) Acute myocardial infarction in a 22 year old world class weight lifter using anabolic steroids. *Am. J. Cardiol.* **62**, 164.

Ministry of Tourism and Recreation (1991) *Report.* Government of Ontario, Canada.

Pettine, K. (1991) Association of anabolic steroids and avascular necrosis of femoral heads. *Am. J. Sports Med.* **19**, 96–8.

Pope, H. & Katz, D. (1988) Affective and psychotic symptoms associated with anabolic steroid use. *Am. J. Psychiatr.* **145**, 487–90.

Sklarek, H. (1984) AIDS in a bodybuilder using anabolic steroids. *N. Engl. J. Med.* **311**, 1701.

Strauss, R. (1987) *Drugs and Performance in Sports.* WB Saunders, Philadelphia.

Wadler, G. & Hainline, B. (1989) *Drugs and the Athlete.* FA Davis Co., Philadelphia.

Wilson, J. (1988) Androgen abuse by athletes. *Endocr. Rev.* **9**, 181–99.

Chapter 25

Psychological Considerations in Injury Prevention

DAVID YUKELSON AND SHANE MURPHY

The case of Julie

At 19 years of age, Julie had a promising future as an intercollegiate athlete. A swim star in high school, who had also competed on the track team, she was offered a full athletic scholarship to a large university in the southwest. After just one semester at university, however, she left college to return home to her parents. Julie told them that her college swim coach did not understand her. She was lonely at college, made few friends, and did not get along with her teammates on the swim team. Juggling intensive workouts with a heavy course load left her feeling drained and listless, and she lost the sense of fun that had always marked her swimming career. Her coach made a plea for her to 'stick it out for one more semester', but Julie went home at the Christmas break.

Julie obtained a part-time job and joined a local cycling club. After 2 months, she felt much more enthusiastic about her sporting activities. At this time, she was recruited by a local triathlon coach who knew her from high school to join a triathlon club that trained at the national level. Soon she was involved in a rigorous training programme with 10 other top-level athletes under the direction of her new coach. Because of her tremendous abilities in swimming and running, she made rapid progress and was soon winning local and regional competitions.

In late April, Julie fell off her bike during a training ride and injured her back. Although she experienced intermittent pain, she kept training and was able to maintain her 80 km·week^{-1} (50 mile·week^{-1}) running regimen. After 3 weeks, however, she began experiencing severe leg pains. When she visited her doctor, he told her that her back injury had altered her running gait, and that this had led to several stress fractures of her right tibia. He advised complete rest for 6 weeks to allow the stress fractures to heal. Julie went to her coach to discuss the doctor's findings, and the coach advised her that if she kept training she would 'train through the pain' and feel better. So Julie resumed her running, swimming and cycling training. After another 10 days, she was in such obvious pain that her father sent her back to her doctor to have a cast placed on her leg. This time, her doctor warned her that if she did not take care of herself she ran the risk of a leg fracture.

Julie told her teammates that she was miserable with her cast on. She missed daily workouts, and worried that she would not be in shape when the cast was removed. Her goal of winning Summer Nationals seemed increasingly distant. Some of her teammates tried to reassure her that she was doing the right thing, but they noticed that she did not seem to be paying attention. She spent a lot of time talking to her coach. Two weeks after the cast was put in place, she removed it in her kitchen with a knife. The next day, she reported to her coach that she was ready for training. He was surprised to see her back so quickly, but was happy for her to rejoin the team during work-outs. On the following day, Julie told her coach that her leg pain was too severe to allow her to run, and that she would prefer to cycle instead. The coach expressed disappointment that Julie was 'backing out' so soon after rejoining the team. That afternoon, Julie went on a 8-km (5-mile) cross-country run and collapsed un-conscious at the half-way point. She was found 30 min later by a teammate, and an ambulance was called.

As the case of Julie illustrates, the role of psychological factors in preventing injury and monitoring rehabilitation can play a critical role in an athlete's life. In addition to élite athletes, more and more people are becoming actively involved in various competitive sport programmes and/or recreational physical ac-tivity pursuits. Unfortunately, statistics indi-cate that as participation patterns increase, there has been a corresponding increase in the incidence of athletic injuries, as well. Despite technological advances in equipment, physical conditioning programmes, safety precautions and improved coaching techniques, the fact of the matter is that athletic injuries across all sports continue to rise (Kraus & Conroy, 1984; Bergandi, 1985).

Although many of the causal factors in sport injuries can undoubtedly be attributed to physical (e.g. overtraining, poor conditioning), environmental (e.g. weather, surface con-ditions) and/or biomechanical factors, a growing body of research indicates various psychosocial factors may play a prominent role in contributing to injury vulnerability (Anderson & Williams, 1988, in press; Smith et al., 1990b; Heil, in press). Thus, the purpose of this chapter is to provide an overview of the literature investigating psychological consider-ations and injury prediction, and to show how principles of sport psychology can be applied to the prevention of sport injury.

Sport psychology and the injured athlete

For many, athletic injury can be extremely stressful and/or emotionally devastating. Hence, much has already been written about the psychological processes injured athletes go through when recovering from injury (Rotella, 1982; Yukelson, 1986; Wiese & Weiss, 1987; Smith et al., 1990a). These authors have high-lighted common emotional reactions to injury and suggest that sports medicine practitioners be clear in their communication with athletes concerning the nature of the injury, goals and expectations, and steps involved in the rehabili-tation process. In addition, appropriate psycho-logical interventions have been advanced to help the athlete deal more effectively with the pain and frustration often experienced during rehabilitation (Yukelson, 1986; May & Sieb, 1987; Lynch, 1988; Ievleva & Orlick, 1991; Wiese et al., 1991; Heil, in press; Petitpas, in press).

With regard to prevention, a number of psychological variables have been examined as potential predictors of injury occurrence in sport. Early research in this area provided descriptive accounts of the types of athletes thought to be prone to injury and suggested that intrapersonal conflict, anxiety, depression and low self-confidence were important con-tributors to injury occurrence (Sanderson, 1977). Unfortunately, very few studies have demonstrated a reliable relationship between personality and sport injury. Some studies have reported connections between injuries in the sports of football and track and scores on factor I and factor A of Cattell's 16 PF questionnaire, with athletes scoring near the tender-minded and reserved ends of these scales being more prone to injury than their more tough-minded and outgoing peers (Jackson et al., 1978; Valiant, 1981). Other studies found no differences be-tween injured and non-injured football players on any personality dimension when using the California psychological inventory (Brown, 1971).

At present, the ability to predict incidence of

injury based on an individual's personality disposition is speculative at best. Much of the research in this area has been criticized for being atheoretical and too simplistic, often suffering conceptual, methodological and interpretive problems (Feltz, 1986; Silva & Hardy, 1991). In particular, little consideration was given to how personality factors (e.g. anxiety, self-esteem, achievement motivation, locus of control) interact with various situational variables (e.g. amount of playing time, importance of sport in the athlete's life, stressful life events in the past year, coach–athlete relationships) to influence injury outcome. The complexity of how these variables interact make predicting an individual's susceptibility for injury difficult.

Multidimensional model of stress and athletic injury

Recently, Anderson and Williams (1988) have advanced a more promising theoretical model from which to examine the interplay of stress and various psychosocial precursors to athletic injury. The model addresses potential predictor variables of athletic injury, examines how various intrapersonal and psychosocial factors interact with one another to place an athlete at greater risk of sustaining a debilitating injury, and suggests several specific interventions aimed at reducing the likelihood of injury to an athlete (Fig. 25.1).

Central to the model is an individual's stress response with its mutually influencing cognitive, affective, physiological, attentional and behavioural components. Of great interest are the cognitive appraisals, physiological reactions and attentional changes that occur during stress.

The role of stress in disease and immune system functioning has been cited extensively in the literature (Seyle, 1946, 1974; Solomon et al., 1985; Heil, in press). Increased stress levels have been shown to decrease immune system functioning, which, in turn, reduces the body's ability to cope with infection and trauma (Borysenko, 1984; Kennedy et al., 1988). Athletes, with their intense training schedules (such as Julie, the triathlete), or those who are

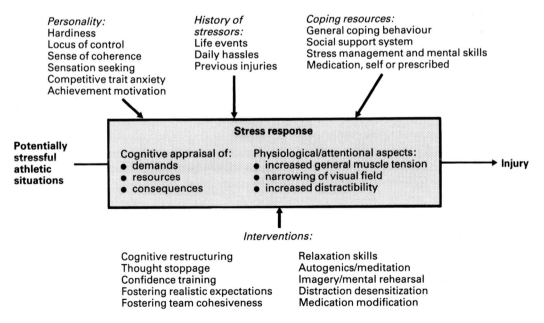

Fig. 25.1 A model of stress and athletic injury.

struggling to find and maintain a balance between work and training, are under a lot of stress and are therefore susceptible to reduced immune system functioning and increased risk of injury or illness.

The stress response is marked by a variety of psychological and physiological effects. In addition to the well-documented endocrinological and autonomic changes that occur, stress can have a disruptive influence on one's thoughts, attitudes, feelings and emotions. Fears, worries and anxieties about specific events, while disruptive in themselves, can precipitate physiological changes such as increases in generalized muscle tension, behavioural rigidity, physical fatigue and reduced motor coordination/fluidity of motion. These physiological factors may mediate the relationship between perceived psychological stress and physical injury.

Since the stress response is bidirectional in nature, an individual's autonomic, physiological and somatic reactions can reciprocally influence one's thoughts, feelings, appraisals and attentional focus. Negative thoughts and feelings evoked by stress can disrupt an individual's ability to concentrate effectively, thus leaving the athlete less vigilant to attend to salient cues in the periphery. As stress increases, it has been suggested that narrowing of the visual field occurs and relevant cues in the environment may be overlooked, thus increasing the possibility of injury occurrence (Anderson & Williams, 1988; Williams *et al.*, 1991).

It is suggested that the key mechanism underlying increased risk for injury is an individual's responsivity and resilience to stress (Anderson & Williams, in press). How an individual responds cognitively, perceptually and physiologically to stress could have a major impact on one's susceptibility for injury.

The model assumes that two of the main mechanisms behind stress–injury relationships are (i) attentional disruptions caused by negative thoughts surrounding one's preoccupation with stressful events; and (ii) increases in generalized muscle tension. Various psycho-

social factors, such as history of stressors (including stressful life events, daily hassles and previous injuries), personality disposition on the part of the athlete (e.g. trait anxiety, self-esteem, achievement motivation, locus of control, sensation-seeking tendencies and risk-taking behaviours), and general coping resources (e.g. rest and proper nutrition, stress management, mental training techniques and social support), have the potential to exacerbate or moderate the magnitude of the stress response and, thus, influence injury likelihood.

Recognizing individual differences in the way athletes perceive and respond to stress, it is hypothesized that athletes with a lot of stress in their lives will, when placed in a potentially stressful situation, be more likely to appraise the situation as stressful, exhibit greater generalized muscle tension and attentional deficits, and, subsequently, be at greater risk of becoming injured (Anderson & Williams, 1988). In accordance with Heil (in press), the risk of injury and illness to an athlete will grow as the magnitude of these psychosocial stressors increase.

Research on psychosocial moderator variables

One psychosocial factor that repeatedly shows up in conjunction with greater likelihood of injury in sport is life stress. Life events are major incidences in one's life that require adjustment (e.g. death of a family member, major injury, divorce, relocation, change in schools, changes in personal habits, etc.). These events and the adjustments that accompany them are stressful and appear to be connected with increased risk of injury and illness (Anderson & Williams, in press). In the case of Julie, she had recently experienced several major life events, including beginning and dropping out of college.

Initial interest on life stress can be traced to the work of Holmes and Rahe (1967), who developed the Social Readjustment Rating Scale (SRRS) and found that the risk for illness in navy personnel was higher for individuals with high life stress as opposed to those with low life stress. Bramwell *et al.* (1975) modified the SRRS to increase its appropriateness for athletic populations. Using the modified scale (SARRS) with intercollegiate football players, Bramwell *et al.* found that football players who experienced high life stress were more likely to incur injury than players who experienced low life stress. Similarly, Coddington and Troxell (1980) and Cryan and Alles (1983) also found a greater incidence of injury among high stress football players compared to low stress players.

Although these results suggest a possible link between injury and life event changes, the measures used in these studies have been criticized for failing to differentiate between positive and negative life event changes. Using an improved life event measure, Passer and Seese (1983) developed the Athletic Life Experiences Survey (ALES) and administered it to 104 football players from NCAA division I and II universities. They were also interested in broadening the scope of the research on stressful life events and injury by including three personality measures (e.g. trait anxiety, competitive trait anxiety and locus of control) as possible mediating factors. They reported a significant correlation between negative life changes and injury time loss for injured athletes on division II teams only. The personality variables were not found to be significant moderator variables in the life stress–injury relationship.

Interested in extending the generalizability of the relationship between life stress and athletic injury to the non-contact sport of volleyball, Williams *et al.* (1986) administered the ALES and SARRS to 179 male and female division I volleyball players from across the country. The authors were unable to replicate the findings found in previous studies with football players. In particular, no relationship was found between high and low life stress athletes and injury rate.

In contrast, Hardy and Riehl (1988) administered the ALES to 86 male and female collegiate athletes participating in baseball, softball, track and tennis. Results indicated that injury frequency could be significantly predicted by life stress scores, with athletes scoring higher on both total and negative life stress scales experiencing greater frequency of injury than their low stress counterparts. Regression analysis for gender and sport revealed that the relationship between life stress and frequency of injury was significant for females in general, and track athletes in particular. This is consistent with the research of Kerr and Minden (1988), who found that stressful life events were significantly related to both the frequency and severity of injuries in élite female gymnasts.

The life stress–injury relationship has also been demonstrated with members of the USA Alpine ski team. More specifically, May *et al.* (1985) found that skiers who had higher life stress scores, as measured by the SARRS and the ALES, reported more headaches, ear, nose and throat problems, musculoskeletal leg injuries and sleeping problems during the past year than those with lower life stress scores.

In summary, a review of the research indicates that a modest relationship exists between recent life stress, particularly negative life stress, and injury in sport. Although the use of life stress indices as a diagnostic measure to identify athletes who may be at greater risk of injury seems intuitively appealing and of clinical value, the ability to employ life stress measures as a predictive screening device to determine an athlete's potential for injury is clearly premature at this time. Both conceptual and methodological concerns still need to be addressed (Smith *et al.*, 1990b; Anderson & Williams, in press).

Many of the problems with life stress research centre around measurement issues. Several problems regarding questionnaire design and assessment need to be addressed, such as better assurances of content and construct validity, improved item weighting schemes, time frame issues such as how far one goes back in the past to assess stressful life events, distinction made between positive and negative life stress events, and the need to develop sport-specific scales for athletic populations (Anderson & Williams, 1988). In addition to modification of inventories, longitudinal studies with repeated measurements are recommended so that a pattern of changes over time can be followed and recorded.

Another problem concerning life stress research involves statistical interpretations; the positive correlations between life stress and injury occurrence have typically been very low, suggesting that major life events only account for a small proportion of the observed variance. Consequently, several researchers have suggested it may be better to assess daily hassles or microstressors in conjunction with major life events to get a better overall picture of athletes' stress and their potential for injury risk (Smith *et al.*, 1990b; Anderson & Williams, in press; Heil, in press). Daily hassles are everyday stresses and strains that cause wear and tear on one's system. Although the relationship between daily hassles and injury likelihood has not been tested empirically, research in related areas of health and illness has shown that daily hassles are better predictors of psychological distress than the measurement of life stress alone (Kanner *et al.*, 1981; Monroe, 1983; Lazarus & Folkman, 1984; Burks & Martin, 1985). In the case of Julie, learning to juggle the intensive athletic workouts with a heavy academic course load became a major source of stress and daily hassle for her, leaving her drained, listless, socially aloof and unmotivated.

Along these lines, an area of life stress that appears to have been overlooked by contemporary researchers is an athlete's ability to cope with and adapt to the demands and pressures of training and competition while keeping some sense of balance in one's personal life intact. A significant source of stress of which to be careful is overtraining and/or burn-out (Silva & Hardy, 1991). The stresses associated with overtraining or burn-out usually increase in an additive manner, often challenging the athlete's self-esteem, adaptation and personal coping skills, which in turn can possibly lead to the development of chronic injuries. Given the characteristics of overtraining and burnout (e.g. physical and emotional exhaustion, staleness, significant sleep disturbances, a sense of loss of control, and other additional psychological stress responses that indicate a negative reaction to training and competitive stress), it would seem to be highly desirable that future studies attempt to determine the correlational and causative links that may exist between the athlete's adaptation to the stress of training and the incidence of athletic injury (Silva & Hardy, 1991).

Coping skills and social support

Much of the past research on life stress and athletic injury has been conducted within a fairly simplistic, narrow scope, with little theoretical consideration given to the broad array of factors that can interact and moderate the effects of stress on injury outcome. Single moderating variables have typically been the focus of study. Researchers are just now beginning to look at ways in which certain factors within the person and environment interact to moderate or buffer an individual's responsivity to stress.

In their model of stress and athletic injury, Anderson and Williams (1988) proposed that personality factors, history of stressors and coping resources interact to influence injury outcome. Whereas personality factors are thought to influence how an individual reacts to stress, coping resources and social support systems were hypothesized as factors that may moderate or attenuate the effects of life stress on injury occurrence.

Research has shown that an athlete's coping resources and social support systems do indeed reduce the effects of stress on injury occurrence (Coddington & Troxell, 1980; Billings & Moos, 1981; Williams *et al.*, 1986; Rosenfeld *et al.*, 1989; Sarason *et al.*, 1990; Hardy *et al.*, 1991). For instance, the strongest predictor of injury occurrence among volleyball players in the Williams *et al.* (1986) study were those athletes with a low level of coping resources. Since half the items dealt with social support, the authors concluded that social support had a direct effect on athletic injury.

Smith *et al.* (1990b) also found support for the mediating effects of social support and psychological coping skills on negative life events and athletic injury among adolescents. Of particular interest was the attempt to isolate conjunctive (i.e. co-occurring) versus disjunctive (i.e. independent of one another) effects among the two moderator variables. Results provided strong evidence for a conjunctive relationship between life stress and subsequent injury in adolescents. Only athletes scoring low in both coping skills and social support exhibited a significant stress−injury relationship, with negative life events accounting for up to 30% of the injury variance. When considered separately, neither social support or coping skills were found to be significant moderator variables.

In an attempt to test specific psychosocial components of the Anderson and Williams (1988) model (i.e. history of stressors, personality variables and coping resources), a recent study found that intercollegiate track and field athletes were at increased risk for experiencing severe injuries if they possessed high levels of negative life stress and competitive anxiety, and low levels of coping resources and social support (Hanson *et al.*, 1992). Life stress scores were found to be the best predictors for both severity and frequency of injury among the athletes. Those with high levels of social support were found to be at lower risk of sustaining a severe injury than athletes with low levels of social support. Also, athletes were at increased risk for receiving multiple injuries if they had high levels of positive and negative life stress, high object loss scores (as measured on the ALES), low levels of coping resources, and a recent injury.

Intervention approaches for the prevention of injury

The literature and research discussed above suggest that several psychological variables are important to consider in the prevention of injury. These are:

1 The level of stress the athlete is experiencing.
2 The personality of the athlete.
3 The coping style and resources of the athlete.
4 The athlete's social support network.

While the sports medicine professional may not be able to intervene effectively to change the first two variables, several intervention options are available when an athlete's coping resources and social support are considered. Danish *et al.* (in press) have suggested that healthcare professionals adopt a life skills educational approach when working with athletes. Within this approach, the available coping skills of the athlete are identified, and new skills and diversification of existing skills are identified to increase the athlete's range of coping skills. A professional who educates and works with the athlete to increase his or her personal competence to deal with life events can be seen as an integral part of a forward-looking healthcare delivery system. An athlete who is personally competent has the ability to do life planning, be self-reliant and seek help and support from others. In order to promote personal competence, a number of intrapersonal psychological skills and interpersonal skills (imagery, physical relaxation, goal setting, self-talk) have been identified (Vealey, 1988; Petitpas, in press). These skills can be taught to athletes.

Goal setting

A key component of personal competence is the ability to set and attain goals (Danish *et al.*, in press). Being successful in setting and attaining one's goals increases an individual's sense of self-efficacy (Bandura, 1977) or self-control. Research has shown that using a goal-setting strategy increases productivity (Locke & Latham, 1984), and research in the sports setting has helped identify the critical components of teaching the effective use of goal setting (Weinberg *et al.*, 1990).

The team physician working with the injured athlete knows the value of having goals and striving to reach them. Some general principles have been established through research which help ensure the optimum effectiveness of a goal-setting programme (Locke & Latham, 1985). These principles are as follows.

Principle 1: Involve the athlete in setting his or her own goals. An athlete does not learn the value of goals if they are imposed on him or her. In the case of Julie, described earlier, it was clear that she was not personally invested in the goal of allowing her body sufficient time to heal from stress. A more immediate concern for her was to continue training, and so she cut the cast off her own leg.

Effective use of goals can be taught to an athlete during rehabilitation from injury. The athlete can be taught that these skills can be applied not only to the present injury, but also to other areas of life. Once the therapy regimen has been described, and appropriate outcome goals have been discussed, it is useful for the athlete to take responsibility for determining goals such as how often he or she will come to therapy, how long he or she will spend on a particular procedure, and what sort of exercises will be performed at home. The physician can be the guide during this process, helping the athlete set reasonable goals that are neither too taxing nor too easy.

Principle 2: Goals should be written down in specific, measurable terms. Research has shown that individuals will show more commitment to their goals if they are made concrete and specific, rather than vague and general. Our own experience suggests that athletes will be able to stick to their goals more easily if they write them down, for example, in a notepad. The more concrete the goal, the better. A goal such as 'I will come to the clinic for therapy 4 days a week for an hour' is better than a goal of 'I will attend therapy regularly'. Likewise, a goal that states 'I will make the 1996 Olympic team' is focused on a result rather than a process. A more effective goal specifically states what the athlete needs to do in order to achieve the desired result, e.g. 'I will work with a personal coach to draw up a training plan for the next year which will help me achieve my conditioning and technique goals'.

Principle 3: The athlete should receive regular feedback and reinforcement about his or her progress. Again, research has shown that for goal setting to be effective, the individual must be able to determine how progress is measured. If the goal is written in concrete terms, as suggested above, it is usually a simple matter to keep track of how frequently required behaviours are performed or the length of time involved. Some sort of reward system should be built into the programme by the athlete. For example, if all the goals for a week are met, the athlete will reward himself or herself by going to the movies, or engaging in some type of pleasurable activity. Although this suggestion seems simple, it is often the critical factor in determining the athlete's motivation over the long haul of training.

In addition to goal setting, a variety of psychological skills have been identified as useful in coping with stress. As discussed earlier, recent research from the field of psycho-neuroimmunology has suggested a mechanism whereby these psychological skills can prevent illness and injury. Immune system functioning is hypothesized to be adversely affected by high stress levels. If athletes can learn coping strategies which will help them deal effectively with stress, they may be able to prevent weakening of the immune system. This should make them less susceptible to the illnesses, injuries and staleness which are so common during intense periods of training.

It is therefore important that those responsible for the health care of athletes be aware of the general stress level of the athletes being seen. Athletes experiencing high stress levels may be excellent candidates for coping skills training. Often, the treating physician will become aware of an athlete who is highly stressed through seeing an athlete who is overtrained or 'burned out', or suffering from chronic injuries. A variety of emotional indicators (anxiety, frustration, depression) may accompany the overtraining or burn-out states. While rest and time away from training have been prescribed as the most appropriate treatments of chronic staleness in an athlete (Morgan *et al.*, 1987), psychoneuroimmunology research indicates that more active intervention techniques which promote coping may speed the recovery process, and may help prevent stress-related disorders. Commonly used active coping techniques described in the sport psychology literature include relaxation and imagery (Vealey, 1988).

Relaxation and thought control

A variety of interventions intended to enhance immune system functioning have been described in the psychoneuroimmunology literature (Heyman, 1989), including hypnosis, imagery and meditation. Several elements appear common to many of these interventions. The first element is the deep relaxation component. Relaxation can be taught in a variety of ways (autogenic relaxation, progressive muscle relaxation, diaphragmatic breathing, guided imagery, biofeedback), but all these approaches share the outcome of teaching the patient how to deeply relax his or her body. The second component is that some cognitive process is usually prescribed along with the relaxation. This cognitive process might be meditation, visualization or body awareness, but in some way the patient becomes actively involved in the self-healing process. The third component common to the various psychoneuroimmunological strategies is the process of self-control. The patient becomes an active participant in the treatment programme, is

given responsibility and is required to learn new skills, and is expected to improve. There is no room for the patient to be a passive recipient of the therapy. As we have suggested, engaging the patient in a goal-setting process during rehabilitation is a common strategy to promote patient involvement in therapy.

Combining these three elements suggests that athletes involved in recovery from injury, or those who wish to optimize their recovery from intense training, learn and practice a relaxation technique which has an associated cognitive element. We have had promising results, both at the Olympic Training Center in Colorado Springs and at Penn State University, using such techniques with athletes who are engaged in very demanding and intense training programmes. Further research needs to be done studying intervention results, but this promises to be a productive area for the sports medicine field. Active relaxation treatments can be employed by athletes, and taught by athletic trainers, in conjunction with more traditional therapies. In fact, they may help promote a sense of self-control in the athlete recovering from injury.

Visualization (coping rehearsal)

Imagery-based techniques have been suggested by several authors for use in injury rehabilitation and healing and in controlling pain (Jaffe, 1980; Levine, 1982; Epstein, 1989; Heil, in press). The well-known work of the Simontons (Simonton *et al.*, 1978) has popularized the use of imagery and visualization in assisting the healing process and fighting disease. Some authors have applied this approach to athletes and sports (e.g. Porter & Foster, 1986, 1990; Lynch, 1988), suggesting the use of visualization for healing sports injuries and coping with athletic pain. Utilizing imagery following deep relaxation is similar to hypnosis, so that the extensive literature on hypnosis effects is relevant in this area. Research has consistently demonstrated that hypnosis is effective in treating clinical pain, although only with hypnotic-susceptible patients (Wadden & Anderton, 1982). Surprisingly little research has been conducted on clinical uses of imagery with athletes. A number of authors have described imagery methods which are applicable in helping injured athletes (Rotella & Heyman, 1986; Yukelson, 1986; Wiese & Weiss, 1987), and, hopefully, research into such imagery applications will soon follow.

Apparently, no research investigations have yet been conducted into whether combined imagery and relaxation training interventions can actually help prevent injury and illness in athletic populations. Evidence from other areas of psychology suggests that this might be possible (Lloyd, 1987).

Visualization can also be used in combination with affirmations to promote the development of coping skills and personal competence. This approach is known as coping rehearsal or stress management (Ellis, 1973). A variety of studies have shown stress management techniques to be effective in reducing many types of anxiety, from medical and dental anxiety (Miller & Heinrich, 1984) to test anxiety (Wine, 1971). Although stress management interventions have yet to be systematically studied in the sport psychology area, those studies published to date have yielded promising results (Ziegler et al., 1982; Mace & Carroll, 1985; Crocker et al., 1988; Crocker, 1989).

Within the coping rehearsal approach, athletes rehearse their emotional response to potentially stressful situations. For example, an athlete might sit down with a sports medicine professional and list all the thoughts and feelings he or she typically experiences in a race situation. Then the subject will go back and identify those emotions that might interfere with performance, or prevent maximum effort, e.g. feeling such as intense fatigue, panic or depression (often verbalized via phrases such as 'I can't go on' or 'I'm not as good as these other competitors'). Next, the athlete and sports medicine professional devise strategies to replace these negative emotions with more ap-

propriate cognitive strategies, for example, through the use of thought-stopping, positive self-talk or self-affirmations (Porter & Foster, 1986). Affirmations that might be used in such a situation include 'I deserve to be here', 'I will run my own race and not worry about anyone else', and 'I feel fast and strong today'. Finally, the athlete rehearses a race in the imagination and sees himself or herself coping successfully, using the techniques that he or she has practiced. The goal of this intervention is for the athlete to develop and become familiar with a set of successful strategies for coping with stress (cf., Lazarus & Folkman, 1984), thereby expanding their coping resources.

Social support

A final intervention strategy to consider in the prevention of injury is to increase the level of social support of the athlete. As the literature referred to earlier indicates, social support can be an important buffer variable in the sports injury context. Athletes with higher levels of social support may suffer less injuries, and recover from injuries faster, than those with lower levels of social support. Strategies designed to increase an athlete's personal competence can also be used to teach athletes to seek more social support. Specific approaches which might be helpful in this area include social skills training (Sheperd, 1978) and assertiveness training (Alberti & Emmons, 1978; Connelly & Rotella, 1991).

For example, Julie seemed to lack the skills to accept social support from her teammates and so, although she was offered help, she was unable to utilize their support. An appropriate intervention might be to increase her assertiveness skills so that she can evaluate possible courses of action in terms of her own long-term best interests rather than relying solely on her coach's evaluations. She might need help in learning how to directly confront her coach when differences of opinion arise. Training in social skills might allow her to interact with her teammates so that she can request emotional support from them, rather than viewing them solely as competitors.

Conclusion

The relationship between psychological risk factors and athletic injury is a complicated one. A wide variety of factors interact with one another to influence injury risk. These include personality disposition on the part of the athlete, life stress, sport stress, mood states, daily hassles, overtraining, inappropriate focus of attention, low self-confidence, etc. (Anderson & Williams, 1988; Heil, in press). While the magnitude of perceived psychological stress is an important consideration, perhaps the key factor is the resourcefulness or resilience of the athlete in attenuating the stress response. Future research should focus on the cumulative effects of stress on injury risk and one's psychological skills to cope effectively. Interventions aimed at teaching athletes how to manage themselves more effectively and feel like they are in control are the key to prevention.

The approach to injury prevention suggested by psychoneuroimmunology research is complementary to the life skills model (Danish et al., in press) and the Anderson and Williams (1988) model discussed previously. Athletes under intense stress due to rigorous training demands can be encouraged to be actively involved in promoting the recovery of the immune system functioning. This, in turn, should help them avoid injury and illness and recover more quickly from training stress. Athletes should be encouraged by sports medicine professionals to expand their range of coping skills. This shifts the emphasis of consultation from simply treatment of injury to an educational approach designed to help prevent injury.

The case of Julie, although extreme, illustrates how certain attitudes and expectations can lead to self-destructive behaviour. If Julie is not helped to change, we can expect her pattern of self-injurious behaviour to continue. The research presented in this chapter suggests that Julie be referred to a professional who can help her evaluate her current coping resources and devise more effective coping strategies. Several suggestions have been made throughout this chapter for specific approaches that could be used in working with Julie. An appropriate point to begin intervention would be to examine Julie's goals. Currently, she is so focused on competition outcomes that she is unable to consider long-term goals and strategies. Teaching Julie how to cope with stress through relaxation training, imagery rehearsal and affirmations would also be appropriate. Finally, Julie might find help and support within her circle of friends and teammates if she learns the skills necessary to obtain emotional support.

References

Alberti, R.E. & Emmons, M.L. (1978) *Your Perfect Right: A Guide to Assertive Behavior*, 3rd edn. Impact Press, California.

Anderson, M.B. & Williams, J.M. (1988) A model of stress and athletic injury: Prediction and prevention. *J. Sport Exerc. Psychol.* **10**, 294–306.

Anderson, M.B. & Williams, J.M. (1993) Psychological risk factors: Injury prediction and preventative measures. In J. Heil (ed) *The Psychology of Sport Injury*. Human Kinetics, Illinois (in press).

Bandura, A. (1977) Self-efficacy: Toward a unifying theory of behavioral change. *Psychol. Rev.* **84**, 191–215.

Bergandi, T.A. (1985) Psychological variables relating to the incidence of athletic injury: A review of the literature. *Int. J. Sport Psychol.* **16**, 141–9.

Billings, A.G. & Moos, R.H. (1981) The role of coping responses and social resources in attenuating the stress of life events. *J. Behav. Med.* **4**, 139–57.

Borysenko, J. (1984) Stress, coping, and the immune system. In J.D. Matarazzo, S.M. Wiss, J.A. Herd, N.E. Miller & S.H. Weiss (eds) *Behavioral Health: A Handbook of Health Enhancement and Disease Prevention*, pp. 241–60. Wiley, New York.

Bramwell, S.T., Masuda, M., Wagner, N.N. & Holmes, T.H. (1975) Psychological factors in athletic injuries: Development and application of the social and athletic readjustment scale (SARRS). *J. Hum. Stress.* **1**, 6–20.

Brown, R.B. (1971) Personality characteristics related

to injuries in football. *Res. Q. Exerc. Sport* **42**, 133–8.

Burks, N. & Martin, B. (1985) Everyday problems and life change events: Ongoing versus acute sources of stress. *J. Hum. Stress* **11**, 27–35.

Coddington, R.D. & Troxell, J.R. (1980) The effect of emotional factors on football injury rates: A pilot study. *J. Hum. Stress* **6**, 3–5.

Connelly, D. & Rotella, R.J. (1991) The social psychology of assertive communication: Issues in teaching assertiveness skills to athletes. *Sport Psychol.* **5**, 73–87.

Crocker, P.R. (1989) A follow up of cognitive-affective stress management training. *J. Sport Exerc. Psychol.* **11**, 236–42.

Crocker, P.R., Alderman, R.B. & Smith, F.M. (1988) Cognitive-affective stress management training with high performance youth volleyball players: Effects on affect, cognition, and performance. *J. Sport Exerc. Psychol.* **10**, 448–60.

Cryan, P.O. & Alles, E.F. (1983) The relationship between stress and football injuries. *J. Sports Med. Phys. Fitness* **23**, 52–8.

Danish, S.J., Petitpas, A.J. & Hale, B.D. (1993) A developmental–educational intervention model of sport psychology. In S. Murphy (ed) *Clinical Sport Psychology*. Human Kinetics, Illinois (in press).

Ellis, A. (1973) *Humanistic Psychotherapy: The Rational–Emotive Approach*. Julian Press, New York.

Epstein, G. (1989) *Healing Visualizations: Creating Health Through Imagery*. Bantam Books, New York.

Feltz, D.L. (1986) The psychology of sport injuries. In P.F. Vinger & E.F. Hoerner (eds) *Sports Injuries: The Unthwarted Epidemic*, pp. 336–44. PSG Co., Massachusetts.

Hanson, S.J., McCullagh, P. & Tonymon, P. (1992) Personality characteristics, life stress, and coping resources in the prediction of athletic injury. *J. Sport Exerc. Psychol.* **14**, 262–72.

Hardy, C.J., Richman, J.M. & Rosenfeld, L.B. (1991) The role of social support in the life stress/injury relationship. *Sport Psychol.* **5**, 128–39.

Hardy, C.J. & Riehl, R.E. (1988) An examination of the life stress–injury relationship among non contact sport participants. *Behav. Med.* **14**, 113–18.

Heil, J. (ed) (1993) *The Psychology of Sport Injury*. Human Kinetics, Illinois (in press).

Heyman, S.R. (1989) Psychoneuroimmunology: Implications for clinical practice. In P.A. Keller & S.R. Heyman (eds) *Innovations in Clinical Practice*, Vol. 8. Professional Resource Exchange, Florida.

Holmes, T.H. & Rahe, R.H. (1967) The social readjustment rating scale. *J. Psychosom. Res.* **11**, 213–18.

Ievleva, L. & Orlick, T. (1991) Mental links to enhanced healing: An exploratory study. *Sport Psychol.* **5**, 25–40.

Jackson, D.W., Jarrett, H., Barley, D., Kausch, J., Swanson, J.J. & Powell, J.W. (1978) Injury prediction in the young athlete. *Am. J. Sports Med.* **6**, 6–14.

Jaffe, D.T. (1980) *Healing From Within*. Knopf, New York.

Kanner, A.D., Coyne, J.C., Schaefer, C. & Lazarus, R.S. (1981) Comparison of two modes of stress measurement: Daily hassles and uplifts versus major life events. *J. Behav. Med.* **4**, 1–39.

Kennedy, S., Kiecolt-Glaser, J.K. & Glaser, R. (1988) Immunologic consequences of acute and chronic stressors: Mediating role of interpersonal relationships. *Br. J. Med. Psychol.* **61**, 77–85.

Kerr, G. & Minden, H. (1988) Psychological factors related to the occurrence of athletic injuries. *J. Sport Exerc. Psychol.* **10**, 167–73.

Kraus, J.F. & Conroy, C. (1984) Mortality and morbidity from injuries in sport and recreation. *Ann. Rev. Publ. Health* **5**, 163–92.

Lazarus, R.S. & Folkman, S. (1984) *Stress, Appraisal, and Coping*. Springer-Verlag, New York.

Levine, S. (1982) *Who Dies*. Anchor Books, New York.

Lloyd, R. (1987) *Explorations in Psychoneuroimmunology*. Grune & Stratton, Florida.

Locke, E.A. & Latham, G.P. (1984) *Goal Setting: A Motivational Technique that Works*. Prentice Hall, New Jersey.

Locke, E.A. & Latham, G.P. (1985) The application of goal setting to sports. *J. Sport Psychol.* **7**, 205–22.

Lynch, G.P. (1988) Athletic injuries and the practicing sport psychologist: Practical guidelines for assisting athletes. *Sport Psychol.* **2**, 161–7.

Mace, R.D. & Carroll, D. (1985) The control of anxiety in sport: Stress innoculation training prior to abseiling. *Int. J. Sport Psychol.* **16**, 165–75.

May, J.R. & Sieb, G.E. (1987) Athletic injuries: Psychosocial factors in the onset, sequelae, rehabilitation, and prevention. In J.R. May & M.J. Asken (eds) *Sport Psychology: The Psychological Health of the Athlete*, pp. 157–85. PMA Publishing, New York.

May, J.R., Veach, T.L., Reed, M.W. & Griffey, M.S. (1985) A psychological study of health, injury, and performance in athletes on the US alpine ski team. *Phys. Sports Med.* **13**(10), 111–15.

Miller, W.H. & Heinrich, R.L. (1984) *Personal Stress Management for Medical and Dental Patients*. PSM Press, California.

Monroe, S.M. (1983) Major and minor life events as predictors of psychological distress: Further issues and findings. *J. Behav. Med.* **6**, 189–205.

Morgan, W.P., Brown, D.R., Raglin, J.S., O'Connor, P.J. & Ellickson, K.A. (1987) Psychological monitoring of overtraining and staleness. *Br. J. Sports Med.* **21**, 107–14.

Passer, M.W. & Seese, M.D. (1983) Life stress and

athletic injury: Examination of positive versus negative events and three moderator variables. *J. Hum. Stress* **9**, 11–16.

Petitpas, A.J. (1993) Psychological considerations in the care of athletic injuries. In S. Murphy (ed) *Clinical Sport Psychology.* Human Kinetics, Illinois (in press).

Porter, K. & Foster, J. (1986) *The Mental Athlete.* William C. Brown, Dubuque.

Porter, K. & Foster, J. (1990) *Visual Athletics: Visualizations for Peak Sports Performance.* William C. Brown, Dubuque.

Rosenfeld, L.B., Richman, J.M. & Hardy, C.J. (1989) Examining social support networks among athletes: Description and relationship to stress. *Sport Psychol.* **3**, 23–33.

Rotella, R.J. (1982) Psychological care of the injured athlete. In D.N. Kulund (ed) *The Injured Athlete,* pp. 213–24. Lippincott, Philadelphia.

Rotella, R.J. & Heyman, S.R. (1986) Stress, injury, and the psychological rehabilitation of athletes. In J.M. Williams (ed) *Applied Sport Psychology,* pp. 343–64. Mayfield, Palo Alto.

Sanderson, F.H. (1977) The psychology of the injury-prone athlete. *Br. J. Sports Med.* **11**, 56–7.

Sarason, I.G., Sarason, J.H. & Pierce, G.R. (1990) Social support, personality, and performance. *J. Appl. Sport Psychol.* **2**, 117–27.

Seyle, H. (1946) The general adaptation syndrome and the disease process. *J. Clin. Endocrinol.* **6**, 117–230.

Seyle, H. (1974) *Stress Without Distress.* Signet, New York.

Sheperd, G. (1978) Social skills training: The generalization problem — Some further data. *Behav. Res. Ther.* **16**, 287–8.

Silva, J.M. & Hardy, C.J. (1991) The sport psychologist. In F.O. Mueller & A. Ryan (eds) *Prevention of Athletic Injuries: The Role of The Sports Medicine Team,* pp. 114–32. F.A. Davis Co., Philadelphia.

Simonton, O.C., Mathews-Simonton, S. & Creighton, J. (1978) *Getting Well Again.* Tarcher, California.

Smith, A.M., Scott, S.G. & Wiese, D.M. (1990a) The psychological effects of sports injuries coping.

Sports Med. **6**, 352–69.

Smith, R.E., Smoll, F.L. & Ptacek, J.T. (1990b) Conjunctive moderator variables in vulnerability and resiliency research: Life stress, social support, and coping skills, and adolescent sport injuries. *J. Personality Soc. Psychol.* **55**, 360–70.

Solomon, G.F., Amkraut, A.A. & Rubin, R.T. (1985) Stress, hormones, neuroregulation, and immunity. In S.R. Burchfield (ed) *Stress: Psychological and Physiological Interactions,* pp. 99–127. Hemisphere, New York.

Valiant, P.M. (1981) Personality and injury in competitive runners. *Perceptual Motor Skills* **53**, 251–3.

Vealey, R.S. (1988) Future directions in psychological skills training. *Sport Psychol.* **2**, 318–36.

Wadden, T.A. & Anderton, C.H. (1982) The clinical use of hypnosis. *Psychol. Bull.* **91**, 215–43.

Weinberg, R., Bruya, L., Garland, H. & Jackson, A. (1990) Effects of goal difficulty and positive reinforcement on endurance performance. *J. Sport Exerc. Psychol.* **12**, 144–56.

Wiese, D.M. & Weiss, M.R. (1987) Psychological rehabilitation and physical injury: Implications for the sportsmedicine team. *Sport Psychol.* **1**, 318–30.

Wiese, D.M., Weiss, M.R. & Yukelson, D.P. (1991) Sport psychology in the training room: A survey of athletic trainers. *Sport Psychol.* **5**, 15–24.

Williams, J.M., Tonymon, P. & Anderson, M.B. (1991) Effects of stress, stressors, and coping resources on anxiety and peripheral narrowing. *J. Appl. Sport Psychol.* **3**, 126–41.

Williams, J.M., Tonymon, P. & Wadsworth, W.A. (1986) Relationship of life stress to injury in intercollegiate volleyball. *J. Hum. Stress* **12**, 38–43.

Wine, J. (1971) Test anxiety and direction of attention. *Psychol. Bull.* **76**, 92–104.

Yukelson, D.P. (1986) Psychology of sports and the injured athlete. In D.B. Bernhardt (ed) *Sports Physical Therapy.* Churchill Livingstone, New York.

Ziegler, S.G., Klinzig, J. & Williamson, K. (1982) The effects of two stress management training programs on cardiorespiratory efficiency. *J. Sport Psychol.* **4**, 280–9.

Chapter 26

General Prevention of Injuries in Sport

MERVYN J. CROSS

Sportspeople the world over, from élite athletes through to recreational players, are subject to a variety of factors that affect them in their endeavours to achieve personal goals. They must, for example, play a sport that is suited to their body type, have the necessary physical aptitude, be guided by the right coach, use the correct training methods and employ the most appropriate mental approach. Sports injuries, many of which can be directly and indirectly related to such items, are themselves a limiting factor affecting athletes in their endeavours to achieve their goals. For average players, sports injuries are at the very least a source of discomfort, frustration and disappointment. For élite athletes, they assume the proportion of a disaster, disrupting and sometimes destroying their attempts to achieve the personal life goals associated with their sports.

Prevention of sports injury is thus a topic that demands learned, in-depth discussion and research. In fact, no less a body than the World Health Organization has set as one of its major goals the reduction of sports injuries, both their number and severity, before the year 2000. In order to understand the best methods of preventing sports injuries it is essential to study the mechanisms by which such injuries occur. Much research has already been directed at defining these mechanisms, as well as at identifying the types and classifications of the sports injuries themselves. Once these mechanisms and classifications are understood, an adequate attempt can be made to reduce both the oc-

casions and the severity of sports injury through the simple act of prevention. For the purposes of this chapter, the causes of sports injuries and their prevention are broadly classified as those which are intrinsic and those which are extrinsic to the athlete.

Intrinsic mechanisms

The intrinsic mechanisms of sports injury relate to the levels of mental and physical preparedness of the athlete.

Physical factors

Athletes first of all need to choose, or be directed to choose, a sports activity appropriate to their age and body type. For instance, there are problems for the ponderous endomorph who wants to excel in ultramarathoning. It is also clear in Rugby that participants with long necks risk cervical injury by playing in certain scrum positions. Similarly, the limited musculoskeletal maturation of adolescents should preclude them from those competition and training activities that involve heavy weight-lifting. Parent, teachers, coaches and sports administrators have a serious responsibility to ensure the correct choice of sports activity and positional play as a basic method of preventing sports injury.

Athletes should also have a realistic awareness of their physical capabilities. The exuberant atmosphere of an Olympic stadium, or the

334

euphoria of a large city fun-run, can see participants exceeding their limitations, with the result that the Olympian in a semifinal may expend too much energy and unnecessarily suffer injury, while the fun runner may experience serious, even fatal, breakdown. At the same time the knowledge of one's capabilities does not rule out the possibility of exceptional performance, given adequate preparation.

Basic to any sports participation, particularly for those who have been inactive for some time or who have a problematic medical history, is the preparticipation medical screening and programme. For example, those commencing an exercise programme for the first time should undergo coronary artery disease screening (CAD) if they have a family history of premature CAD, high blood pressure, stroke, fainting or sudden death. This applies especially if the individual is over 35, overweight, smokes cigarettes and has a known history of high blood pressure, high cholesterol, diabetes, or a combination of these ailments (Cross et al., 1991). Preparticipation programmes should also exercise caution, employing a well-graduated introduction to the physical fitness elements of endurance, strength, speed, coordination and flexibility.

During the preseason, athletes should be measured for size, strength, flexibility, agility and endurance, in order to provide them with a basis for goal setting, and to establish measurements which can be used in assessing fitness after rehabilitation in the event of injury.

Athletes need also to develop the skills necessary to perform correct technique. Lifting a heavy weight incorrectly can injure the lower back or knees. In the Rugby codes, tackling with the head wrongly positioned can cause head and neck injuries. Correcting fast-bowling technique minimizes lower back stress fractures. Tennis players who hit the backhand stroke from behind their bodies or with their feet incorrectly positioned risk 'tennis elbow'. The biomechanical operation involved in each sporting manoeuvre needs to be refined so that maximum efficiency and safety are secured.

High-speed cinematographic analysis, for example, was used to help solve the problems of breast-stroker's knee and swimmer's shoulder — the resulting modifications to style were able to decrease medial ligament and patellofemoral stress and subacromial arch impingement respectively. One study, which found that the most frequent incidence of sports injury amongst schoolchildren occurred outdoors in contact versus non-contact and high jump versus low jump rate sports, suggests that preventive measures such as teaching fall technique, muscle strengthening and overall coordination exercises should be implemented in the school curriculum (Backx et al., 1991).

Athletes can experience a sudden lack of proprioception in certain injury situations, such as with shoulder abduction injuries (for example, when a Rugby player's arm is caught and wrenched in a ruck) or anterior cruciate ligament injuries (for example, when an athlete at full pace is caused to make a traumatic change in direction) (Cross & Crichton, 1987). Twisting joint injuries often cause associated damage to proprioceptive nerve endings (the sensory nerves that return positional sense to the spinal cord and brain), so that during rehabilitation the use of proprioceptive neuromuscular facilitation (PNF) techniques becomes necessary (McCloskey et al., 1983). The role that sophisticated proprioceptive training techniques might play in helping prevent such injuries in the first place is one area that merits urgent research.

Muscle tightness is a commonly overlooked factor in assessing and correcting before athletic endeavours, e.g. hamstring tightness causing knee and back pain. This is easily corrected with adequate stretching programme.

Biomechanical abnormalities, e.g. patella tendonitis in excessively tall sports people (e.g. basketball) can also predispose athletes to injury. Abnormalities such as scoliosis (curved spine), tilted pelvis (from a short leg) and excessively rotated hips can often be traced to poor coordination and control by the postural and stabilizing muscles of those areas. Appropriate exercising, assisted by stretching and strengthening programme, can lead to a more normal functioning in these areas, and so reduce the likelihood of injury.

Generalized ligamentous laxity while favouring some sports such as gymnastics can be detrimental in contact sports such as football.

Mental factors

In terms of mental preparedness, athletes and their coaches need to have a wholesome attitude to their sport, realizing that, while winning is important, the health and well-being of each athlete is paramount. There is no doubt that a wholesome mental attitude to sport in general and one's performance in particular, coupled with an athlete's alertness, intelligence and ability to make correct decisions in a crisis, play a major role in injury prevention. No more is this apparent than in the racing sports, where a car driver, bicycle rider or jockey can prejudice his or her own livelihood, and that of fellow competitors, because of a wreckless attitude and a desperate desire for victory. In the same way illegal actions, such as punching and brawling as a means of victory in contact sports, can result in fractures of the jaw, dislocations and other unnecessary injuries.

Athletes need to concentrate more on the process of their sports, and on their personal application within that process, rather than concern themselves simply with the outcome (Cross *et al.*, 1991). The end cannot justify illegal means. It is the responsibility of coaches and sports administrators to educate young sportspeople in particular in the positive values and proper ethics of their sport, so that at the very least the incidence of deliberately effected sports injury can be reduced.

Extrinsic mechanisms

The extrinsic mechanisms of sports injury refer to those factors which impinge externally on the person and performance of the athlete.

Other personnel

Coaches and other people closely associated with athletes can be responsible for overstimulating their charges before games or contests, leading to irrational performance and sometimes injury. Athletes with too high arousal levels can often experience early fatigue, thus exposing themselves to injury, or can experience distressing conditions such as hyperventilation. Coaches and athletes need to be aware that in most cases before a major performance they would be better served by a rational approach that concentrates on a game or performance plan, and is backed by a programme of thorough preparation (Cross *et al.*, 1991). Irrational crowd behaviour and stimulation can also lead to ugly incidences of injury in the sports arena, and can be prevented only by strict measures on crowd control. Referees and umpires can contribute to the stable conduct of a game by being knowledgeable, firm, fair and consistent.

Training programme design

There is no doubt that a major cause of injury to athletes is an inadequate training programme design. Adequate physical fitness is essential prior to participation in sport, as fatigued athletes have decreased skill performances which can lead to injury. The running technique of the marathoner, the tackling technique of a footballer, and the stroke technique of a swimmer or tennis player can all deteriorate with fatigue, thus increasing the possibility of injury. With today's sophisticated physiological research and communication, it should be possible for each sport to design a training programme specifically geared towards optimum performance within its discipline. Such a programme would include graduated levels of development in the acquisition of the skills specific to each sport.

An ideal training programme includes a period of warm-up and stretching, gradual increases and variation in training intensity, frequency and duration, drills specific to the sport, a time for cool-down and stretching after exercise, and adequate rest and recovery periods (Elam, 1986). The warm-up should begin with simple exercises such as callisthenics, skipping or light jogging to increase the muscle temperature, move into slow, static stretches to increase the range of movement and decrease stiffness, and conclude with light exercises specific to the task ahead, such as 'run through' at three-quarter pace for running sports, or light repetitions for those involved in weight-training. Coaches and trainers need to devise drills specific to their sport. The programme design should also take into account the varying needs of the off-season, preseason and in-season training periods, ensuring against over-training and enabling athletes to peak when appropriate and maintain a high standard of fitness for the duration of the competition season.

Environment

Sports venues intended for training and competition need to be investigated beforehand as a measure towards helping prevent injury. Grounds need to be well lit, smooth and without potholes. Swimming venues need to be checked for water depth and conditions, as well as for the presence of marine creatures that may sting or be harmful. Runners need to be wary of excessive or unaccustomed training on very hard or very soft surfaces such as concrete and sand, as this can lead to overuse injuries (Drez, 1988). Cyclists and runners should select roads that are quiet and low in fume pollution. The exercise of training runners on hills should be incorporated gradually into a training programme, as unaccustomed stresses are placed on the legs. Runners training on roads or crossing slopes need to vary the camber so as to avoid developing gait asymmetry through having a consistently discrepant leg length. Naturally, road runners and cyclists should have clothing and footwear that is easily seen, especially at night.

The weather can also be a source of danger to athletes. Rowers need to exercise caution when the weather is unpredictable, especially on occasions when they are training on wide expanses of water. Thermal injuries should also be avoided in situations where the heat generated by the body cannot be dissipated quickly enough to keep the core body temperature at its usual level of 37.6°C. Hypothermia can also occur, particularly on cold, windy days in low-intensity, long-duration athletes such as marathoners, whose fatigued bodies in the latter part of a race may not be able to generate sufficient heat to maintain core body temperature (Armstrong, 1986). Athletes can minimize thermal injuries by maintaining adequate hydration before, during and after exercise, by wearing clothing that is appropriate, and by undergoing an acclimatization process in the days prior to competition. A high level of fitness is presumed.

Clothing, footwear and other preventive measures

Training and competition clothing should be appropriate for the conditions and the nature of the sport being played. It is important in hot, humid conditions to have clothing that maximizes convective and evaporative heat loss, while in cold windy conditions, windproof and waterproof clothing is necessary. As heat loss is also great when the body is immersed in cold water, wet suits are often required by athletes engaged in water sports.

The wearing of long trousers, as in American grid iron football, or long-sleeved jerseys, as in the Rugby codes, helps prevent the abrasions, lacerations and contusions that can occur when the body comes into contact with the ground. It is also advisable before a game to place Vaseline or glycerine on the joints that are most likely to strike the surface of the playing arena. Abrasions can give rise to secondary infection, in some cases leading to septicaemia which is commonly associated with lymphadenitis. Early recognition and treatment of such injuries is important. Another use for Vaseline or talcum products is in the prevention of chafing. Distance runners, for example, can experience such discomfort, even when the fit or material of their clothing is adequate.

Athletes who spend long periods of time in the sun — for example, in sports such as cricket, rowing, snow skiing, sailing and golf — risk exposure to the harmful effects of ultraviolet radiation, and should therefore wear protective hats, sunglasses and sunscreen lotion.

Correct, suitable and safe footwear plays an important role in preventing injury, both for the athletes who take the proper precautions in selecting their shoes and those with whom they play. With regard to the latter, a loose nail in a football boot stud or a sharp stud on a boot can cause a severe laceration. In recent times referees in most football codes have been required to inspect the shoes of each player in order to eliminate the possibility of such injury.

An athlete's footwear must be able to absorb shock and provide enough stability to prevent excessive pronation (Cavanagh, 1980). For the serious athlete, this requires a regular update of shoes (every 6–12 months) as these features deteriorate with usage. The material of the midsole, while it provides much of the shock absorption, cannot be too heavy or too inflexible. Thus shoes are now designed with special gel or air inserts in the midsole in order to provide lighter, yet efficient, shock absorption qualities.

The outer sole of the shoe should have a tread pattern that provides good traction in wet and slippery conditions. At the same time racquet sports such as tennis, when sliding is involved, tend to minimize the amount of outer sole traction required. The inner sole should be comfortable, cupping the normal heel fat pad contour during landing and supporting the arch of the foot.

The toe box of the shoe should leave sufficient room for foot movement, particularly when the athlete is running down steep inclines. Too snug a fit can lead to blisters, corns, loss of toenails, and so on. Athletes competing in long-distance competitions should use shoes that have been well worn in. It is important too that the material used in manufacturing sports shoes allows the feet to breathe, thus reducing moisture and helping prevent blisters.

Pronation (rolling in of the ankle) is a natural function of weight-bearing, excessive pronation, however, is a problem often associated with lower limb overuse injuries, including plantar fasciitis (heel spur), Achilles tendinitis, shin splints and runner's knee. Running shoe design can provide greater stability and help prevent hyperpronation by including a heel counter that is firmly connected to the midsole, wedging the medial side (closer to the midline) of the midsole with materials of greater consistency than those on the lateral side (away from the midline), and using a straight, bordered last rather than a curved, moccasin-style last (Jørgensen, 1990).

Foot orthotics can also be used to correct excessive pronation at the ankle and prevent further torsional stress higher up at the shin, knee and hips (Burkett, 1985). Orthotics, which need to be individually fitted, are available in soft, medium and hard surfaces, the softer type being more comfortable for most athletes even though they provide less control.

Equipment

Many sports have introduced the use of protective equipment to help reduce the instances of sports injury. Mouth guards used in contact sports help prevent injuries to teeth, lips and jaw, as well as concussive episodes occurring from a blow to the jaw. (Morrow & Bonci, 1989). Similarly, ear plugs and goggles can help protect in salt or chlorinated water. Enclosed eye guards are also recommended for squash, where since the size of the squash ball equates with that of the eye socket, the potential for serious eye damage is heightened.

Headgear (employed, for example, by athletes such as Rugby footballers and amateur boxers, and helmets used by cyclists, grid-iron players, racing drivers and cricketers) help minimize facial and scalp lacerations, and also help protect against concussion and other dangerous unnecessary injuries. However, concussion can still result from sudden acceleration or deceleration of the brain within the skull, especially if the impact has the effect of a sudden jolt.

Footwear which is designed to extend above the ankles is often used in sports such as basketball and football, providing support in situations where sharp changes of direction occur and so helping prevent twisting ankle injuries. Skiing was a sport which had a high incidence of ankle injuries until ski boots and bindings were redesigned to address this problem. One negative side-effect is that it is now the skier's knee which is placed under greater stress.

In sports such as cricket, baseball and the contact sports, padding of certain areas of the body — shoulders, chests, forearms, hands, ribs, genitals, thighs and shins — provides some protection against injury.

The risks involved in lifting heavy weights can be minimized by regular maintenance of equipment, expert supervision of programme and technique, and working with a partner who can provide any necessary assistance.

Those involved in racquet sports, especially the young, can suffer injury from the equipment itself. A racquet that is too heavy, has string tension that is too high or too low, or a grip size that is too large or too small, can increase stress on the player's forearm and so create tendinitis problems.

The strapping and bracing of joints usually helps prevent injury and can protect already injured areas. Joints can be rendered partially or completely unstable by ligament damage; this can be further complicated if the nerve endings in the ligaments controlling joint proprioception (i.e. position sense) are affected. Strapping and bracing, therefore, can to various degrees stabilize joints in general as well as improve position sense and coordination through sensory nerve feedback. This is a controversial area, with one study suggesting that prophylactic (preventative) bracing not only

does not offer much protection for knee joint ligaments but in fact may be the cause of additional injuries in that area (Baker, 1990).

Strapping and bracing can effectively stabilize joints such as the thumb, elbow and ankle, as such joints can normally tolerate small losses in movement without affecting function. On the other hand, they are usually ineffective measures in stabilizing the knee and the shoulder for the rigours of competitive sport, limiting the function of these joints, even if assisting with proprioceptive control.

Although strapping and bracing do not necessarily weaken joints, athletes should follow appropriate rehabilitation programmes to improve strength, flexibility and proprioception (Cross et al., 1991).

Fluids, nutrition and dietary supplements

Since dehydration results in decreased skill performance, it can also result in injury. Also, dehydration is associated with thermal injuries such as hyperthermia. Fluid replacement should therefore occur, before, during and after competition and training, especially on hot, humid days. The best replacement fluid for most sports is water, as sweating decreases the dilution in the body's circulation more than it does the electrolyte stores (Wheeler, 1988). For activities longer than 60 min, a low concentration of carbohydrate (less than 12%) in the water may help prevent muscle fatigue by replenishing muscle glycogen stores. Some ultra-endurance athletes have been found to have low electrolyte levels in the blood; for these a low concentration ($200\ \text{mmol}\cdot\text{l}^{-1}$) electrolyte drink may be helpful (Murray, 1987). Electrolyte loss from exercise is normally replaced adequately in the diet.

Muscle glycogen levels need to be high before intensive competition, especially in endurance sports, in order to prevent muscle fatigue and therefore possible injury. Athletes can best derive their energy supply from a diet rich in complex carbohydrates. Sufficient quantities of vitamins, minerals and amino acids can also be obtained from a well-balanced, nutritious diet. Certain athletes, such as jockeys, ballet dancers and gymnasts, may have an inadequate diet as a result of maintaining low body weight, and therefore could require vitamin and mineral supplements.

Similarly, women athletes who develop amenorrhoea as a consequence of exercise should increase their daily calcium intake in order to help prevent osteoporosis and stress fractures. Since athletes can become anaemic because of excessive iron loss as a result of sports activity (female athletes are even more prone to iron deficiency because of blood loss from menstruation), iron tablets can help supplement and maximize the iron absorption from haemoglobin and vegetarian food sources.

Drugs

It is important that sports administrators and their sports medical personnel educate their charges in the dangers of drug abuse. Most sporting bodies have now adopted the practice of randomly drug testing athletes under their control, as a means of controlling drug abuse and so preventing injuries.

Drugs such as amphetamines, that stimulate the central and sympathetic nervous system, can first of all cause agitation, overaggression, hostility, confusion and poor judgement (Lombardo, 1986), qualities that are scarcely suited to any human activity, let alone the discipline of safe contact sport. Tragically there are many documented reports of athletes actually dying while using amphetamines. Such stimulants can cause cardiac arrhythmias, heart attack from spasm of the coronary arteries, and cardiovascular collapse, particularly in hot conditions when athletes on amphetamines, feeling no pain, overexert themselves and lose control of their core body temperature. Marijuana is another drug that can depress the central nervous system, thus causing drowsiness, and impaired mental ability, perception, information processing, orientation, balance

and muscle strength. All these factors create the potential for injury in the sports arena.

Anabolic steroids, taken by some athletes to increase their size and muscle strength, have unfortunate, irreversible side-effects. For men, these include the risk of liver damage, liver cancer, male breast development and premature baldness; women risk facial hair growth, voice deepening, baldness, amenorrhoea and clitoral enlargement; while children can be stunted in growth through premature bone growth plate closure.

Anabolic steroids also have severe local effects with muscle and tendon rupture in unusual muscles, e.g. pectoralis major rupture. Other drugs, such as narcotic analgesics, β-blockers, diuretics, peptide hormones and analogues and, by association, the masking agents used to prevent detection of banned substances, all have negative side-effects harmful to the athlete's welfare.

Travelling and touring

Management and athletes involved in travelling to away venues, especially on international tours, need to exercise discipline, informed planning and an awareness of the precautions necessary to avoid the spread of viral infection. Teams involved in travelling internationally, and to a lesser extent on long trips locally, can suffer symptoms usually described as jet lag, including exhaustion, inappropriate bowel and bladder function, lack of alertness, sleepiness, and impaired concentration, memory and physical performance (Thompson, 1987; Bellamy, 1988). The body's physiological rhythms lose synchronization, and sleep and dietary patterns can be disturbed. A variety of other factors can occur, such as stress from prolonged sitting in a dry, smoky, low pressure and slightly oxygen-deficient cabin atmosphere, emotional stress from being away from family and friends, and the problems of adapting to the social, dietary, climatic and language differences at the destination.

Team and individual managers can assist

their charges by planning their travel to allow for adequate adaptation and acclimatization upon arrival and by exercising sensible discipline so that their athletes do not overindulge in food and alcohol. Water intake can increase in order to help avoid dehydration, constipation and cramps.

A further consideration is the control of the spread of infectious viruses such as colds, influenza, gastric and febrile illnesses, in situations such as training camps, Olympic village living, and so on. Precautions, such as isolating sick individuals, providing immediate medication and ensuring that such items as towels, cups and eating utensils are not shared, should be taken. Similar measures should be taken in the manner fluids are administered to teams during training and competition.

Fitness after injury

Athletes returning after injury should successfully undergo fitness tests specific to their sports, if they wish to avoid recurrence of their injury (Cross *et al.*, 1991). They should be able to perform adequately the drills and activities appropriate to their sports (for example, swinging, throwing, bowling, pushing, jumping, sprinting, side-stepping, swerving and tackling). If preseason fitness test results are available, as recommended earlier, they can be used as a measure of recovery. Rehabilitation should address muscle wasting, joint stiffness and decreased flexibility, while fractures should not be maximally stressed until solid bony union has occurred.

In the case, for example, of an athlete returning after a cruciate ligament injury, one would need first to ensure that the muscles around the joint had restored strength and flexibility, that the joint was stable and that there was no intra-articular pathology, causing chronic effusion or pain which would interfere with its function and the rehabilitation programme. The athlete would then need to undergo a series of sport-specific exercises to train adequately proprioceptively the associated quadricep and

hamstring muscles. This would involve the athlete beginning at jogging pace, moving to gentle run-throughs, increasing to run-throughs at full pace, and then full pace sprints from a standing start. Shuttle sprinting with sudden deceleration could follow, with the athlete then moving on to figure of eight exercise running, firstly between 25-m markers, reducing gradually to a tighter 10-m marker axis of swerve. Side-stepping exercises, increasing in angle change from 45 to 90°, could conclude the training, with skills such as catching, carrying and passing a ball incorporated for variation, if appropriate to the sport. Such detail must be adhered to in order to ensure that the risk of reinjury is minimal.

Rule changes

Sometimes it is necessary for sports bodies to effect rule changes when certain factors inherent in their sport are deemed to lead to injury. The changes to the junior scrummaging rules in Rugby are a case in point, as was the decision by hockey administration to restrict the swing of the stick to below the shoulder. The distinct threat of head and spinal injuries from spear tackling has ensured that that particular technique of defence is outlawed in rugby codes. Similarly, rules relating to the removal from the arena of infectious viruses such as hepatitis and the human immuno-deficiency virus (HIV), have been widely introduced in contact sports in recent years.

It is sometimes difficult to alter the rules of a sport in order to reduce the risk of injury, without altering the nature of the sport itself. This is most obvious in boxing where the risk of punch-drunk syndrome is ever present. Some sports also increase the chance of osteoarthritic changes in later life (for example, to the elbow, wrist and fingers in boxing; to the neck and cervical spine through heading the ball in soccer; and to the shoulder in throwing sports such as baseball and cricket). The incidence of anterior cruciate ligament rupture in women's netball, through having to twist the body sharply while holding the foot fixed, is another case in point.

In a society increasingly interested in reducing the number and severity of sports injuries, pressure on sports administrators to review their rules for the sake of safety will no doubt increase.

Many factors are necessary in preparing an athlete for a specific sport in a fit and uninjured state. Preparedness predicts performance.

References

Armstrong, L.E. (1986) Signs and symptoms of heat exhaustion during strenuous exercise. *Ann. Sports Med.* **3**, 182–9.

Backx, F.J.G., Beijer, H.J.M., Bol, E. & Wietze, B.M.E. (1991) Injuries in high-risk persons and high-risk sports. *Am. J. Sports Med.* **19**(2), 124–30.

Baker, B.E. (1990) The effect of bracing on the collateral ligaments of the knee. *Clin. Sports Med.* **9**, 843–9.

Bellamy, N. (1988) The jet lag phenomenon: pathogenesis, aetiology, clinical features, and management. *Mod. Med. Australia* **8**(6), 46–55.

Burkett, L.N. (1985) Effects of shoes and foot orthotics on $\dot{V}O_2$ and selected frontal plane knee kinematics. *Med. Sci. Sports Exerc.* **17**, 158–63.

Cavanagh, P.R. (1980) *The Running Shoe Book.* Anderson World, California.

Cross, M.J. & Crichton, K.J. (1987) *Clinical Examination of the Injured Knee*, pp. 1–6. Harper & Row, Sydney.

Cross, M., Gibbs, N. & Gray, J. (1991) *The Sporting Body.* McGraw-Hill, Sydney.

Drez, D. (1988) Running. *Clin. Sports Med.* **7**, 827–33.

Elam, R. (1986) Warm-up and athletic performance. *Natl. Strength Cond. Ass.* **8**(2), 30–2.

Jørgensen, U. (1990) Body load in heel-strike running: the effect of a firm heel counter. *Am. J. Sports Med.* **18**(2), 177–81.

Lombardo, J.A. (1986) Stimulants and athletic performances. *Phys. Sports Med.* **14**(1), 85–93.

McCloskey, D.I., Cross, M.J. & Potter, E.K. (1983) Sensory effects of pulling or vibrating exposed tendons in man. *Brain* **106**, 21–37.

Morrow, R.M. & Bonci, T. (1989) A survey of oral injuries in female college and university athletes. *Athletic Training* **24**(3), 2236–7.

Murray, R. (1987) The effects of consuming carbohydrate–electrolyte beverages on gastric emptying and fluid absorption during and following exercise. *Sports Med.* **4**, 322–51.

Thompson, L.J. (1987) Disorders of circadian rhythm with air travel. *Patient Management* **9**(2), 47–64.

Wheeler, K.B. (1988) Effect of hypohydration on performance — fluid and electrolyte requirements. *Natl. Strength Cond. Ass.* **10**(5), 46–8.

Chapter 27

Principles of Health Education

VIC DAMOISEAUX AND GERJO KOK

It is generally accepted that active practice of sports will have a positive effect on health. Physical effort through the practice of sports will develop muscular strength, improve stamina and the sense of balance. Apart from this, physical effort will strengthen the skeleton and prevent the development of adipose tissue.

It has been scientifically determined that physical inactivity is a health-threatening factor. The ways of working and living in Western society make less and less of an appeal to the physical powers of people. One of the aims for stimulation of healthy positive behaviour in the World Health Organization's 1987 report *Health for All by the Year 2000* is: 'By 1995, in all Member States, there should be significant increases in positive health behaviour, such as balanced nutrition, non-smoking, appropriate physical activity and good stress management'.

From the increasing number of injuries, it seems clear that practising sports also has its negative sides. Attention to medical support and injury prevention is becoming increasingly prominent. In the recent past, numerous information campaigns have been developed in order to draw attention to the importance of sports for health and the necessity of actual participation. At the moment the attention in mass media campaigns is focused on medical support and injury prevention.

Prevention of sports injuries may involve the following.

1 Adjustment of the rules of the game and a more stringent supervision by the referee.

2 Disqualification after a sports injury until a complete recovery has been achieved.

3 Making the use of protective materials compulsory, e.g. wearing helmets, gum shields, shin protection, etc.

4 Putting uniform safety and quality demands on sport accommodation and facilities.

5 Application of warming-up and cooling-down exercises, and stretching exercises before and after the practice of sports.

6 Taping unstable joints prior to the practice of sports.

7 Educational activities, such as sports counselling and physical examinations, trainers' courses and physical training.

From the examples above it proves that prevention may involve the following.

1 Taking measures and implementing rules of conduct.

2 Making facilities available (availability of safe sport accommodation and physical examinations for this purpose.

3 Education (e.g. teaching people how to do a warm-up exercise, or how to apply tape).

Education as a component (modality) of prevention relates to a wide range of activities that are all focused on transferring information. It is important to point out that information may also be given in combination with other preventive measures. By means of information people can be taught how they are to deal with the rules of a game, or how facilities can be used optimally.

In this chapter more attention will be paid to

education as an independent activity, and it will be made clear that effective education is based on three pillars: (i) system; (ii) purpose; and (iii) method.

Health education

Health education as a preventive activity distinguishes itself from other informative activities in particular through the systematic, methodical and purposive way of dealing with the problem (Green & Kreuter, 1991). In general, all forms of information are purposive, i.e. the person giving the information has the explicit intention to effect a change in knowledge, attitude or behaviour in the recipient. The nature and extent of the change, however, may be entirely different. Sometimes an educator will settle for the fact that the public takes notice of a message; another time the educator will strain every nerve to make the public act on the message in accordance with the advice or the guidelines being given.

By means of specific methodology, health education aims at eliminating behavioural factors that threaten health and stimulate those factors that have a positive effect on the 'health behaviour' of the human being. It may be clear that incidental transfer of information will not be sufficient in health education. To change attitudes and behaviour, educational interventions that are spread over a longer period of time are applied.

The multidisciplinary character of health education contributes to the fact that interventions may consist of several methods, means and techniques.

The system of education

Influencing behaviour by means of education is based on the premise of voluntary change of behaviour. This implies that behaviour can be directed by information that fits the needs, wishes/expectations, knowledge, experiences, etc. of the target group.

It is essential to note that education presumes the possibility of motivating people to change their behaviour. It is assumed that behaviour is directed by two principles of motivation, namely the pursuits of cognitive order and of being rewarded. Cognitive order concerns the process of handling information, i.e. the message to be communicated should be composed in such a way that the receiver easily understands the information, is able to order it logically and to store it in his or her memory. The principle of being rewarded refers to the fact that the effort made to observe a communication message should be rewarding. In other words, the desired behaviour has to be attractive to the receiver and/or should offer a number of advantages.

The key to effective information is to be able to understand how behaviour is affected. The system of education includes four steps.

1 Problem analysis: What is the relation between the problem observed and the behaviour of people?

2 Behavioural determinants analysis: What kind of behaviour and whose behaviour is concerned?

3 Behavioural intervention: How can behaviour be influenced?

4 Evaluation of the intervention: What is the effectiveness of the efforts to influence?

It is obvious that in order to answer these questions meticulous research is necessary. Education presumes the solving of problems by changing knowledge, attitude or behaviour. It is therefore very important to find out whether the observed problem is related to a particular behaviour. Problem analysis provides clarity on questions such as: How serious is the problem? What is the cause of the problem? For whom is it a problem? For whom does it have consequences? and, What are the social and/or economic consequences for society as a whole or for parts of it?

The second step, analysis of the behavioural determinants, consists of research into the causes of the undesired behaviour, or the factors that obstruct the desired behaviour. The question to be answered is what motivation or motives are at the bottom of the behaviour. It should be noted that behaviour is to be interpreted in the broadest sense of the word. Behaviour not only consists of factual and visible actions, but also of factors preceding the actions or of things going on in the minds of people. Lack of knowledge, for example, can be a reason why sportsmen and sportswomen do not warm up. Analysis of behavioural determinants therefore constitutes a division of behaviour into segments.

Prior to implementation of the intervention, two important decisions have to be made on:
1 The relative importance of the determinants that cause the problem.
2 The relative changeability of the determinants. In the first decision consideration should be given to the scope and frequency of the determinant and how the determinant is related to other possible determinants (it is rarely only one determinant that causes the problem, in general it is a combination of determinants). The second decision concerns the question of whether or not the determinants can be changed into the desired direction by means of information techniques or other means. These decisions need thorough consideration of the objective of the intervention and have far-reaching consequences for the communication strategy. In order to draw a balanced conclusion, one should be well informed about the functional use of the means of communication.

Determinants of behaviour

This chapter will present more detailed information on determinants of preventive behaviour concerning injuries. Determinants of preventive behaviour can help to explain why sportspeople decide whether or not to take safety measures such as wearing protective items or adjusting their ski bindings adequately.

A model based on the sociopsychological insights of Fishbein and Ajzen (1975) and Bandura (1986) concerning attitude, social influence and self-efficacy, will serve as a basis for the explanation of behaviour. According to the model in Fig. 27.1, behaviour can be predicted by the intention to show that behaviour. The intention (i.e. the approval of or the plan to perform the behaviour) is predicted by attitude, social influence and self-efficacy. External variables that are not included in the model, such as demographic factors, are presumed to influence behaviour only through the three

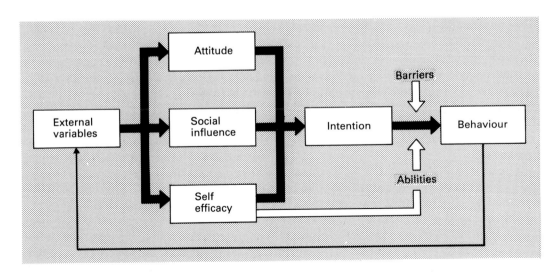

Fig. 27.1 Model of determinants of behaviour. From Kok *et al.* (1991).

determinants mentioned and through intention. Barriers can occur between intention and behaviour. Also, abilities to perform the behaviour can be lacking. Attitude, social influence and self-efficacy can be found and measured prior to the performance of the behaviour. Barriers and abilities only play a role at the moment that behaviour is being performed.

Intention as a variable is a reliable predictor of the actual behaviour. However, the theory also indicates that self-efficacy constitutes the assessment of the abilities required and (probably as a result) the possibility of overcoming barriers. This explains the direct relationship between self-efficacy and abilities.

When, finally, the behaviour is performed, this will result in feedback, which in return will influence the determinants. In the following paragraph the individual determinants will be dealt with in more detail.

Attitude is the balancing of all advantages and disadvantages that an individual links to a certain behaviour. It constitutes an evaluation of the thinking process concerning the positive or negative aspects of the behaviour to be performed. In principle, therefore, it consists of the consequences that go with this behaviour, expressed in advantages and disadvantages.

An important component of attitude is the so-called 'response-efficacy' (Bandura, 1986), which refers to the subjective assessment of the results that will be achieved when the desired behaviour is performed. For example, is carrying a gum shield sufficient to prevent injuries to the teeth? In short, response-efficacy constitutes the question an individual asks himself or herself concerning the effectiveness of observing a recommendation or prescription (Does it help?).

By measuring attitudes, predictions can be made about the way an individual thinks and feels about an object or a behaviour, and about how he or she is likely to behave. This likelihood emanates from the fact that the individual tests his or her opinion or behaviour against the standards and values of people in the direct environment or of whom he or she

esteems highly for some reason. The behaviour and the way others think about intended actions is indicative for the behaviour shown. The 'subjective standard' consists of two elements, namely 'normative beliefs' (one's view of how others, e.g. team members, judge the behaviour that might be performed), and the 'motivation to comply' (the extent of approval of the opinions of important other persons). The subjective standard is rated among the social influence, which may have restraining or stimulating effects, both directly and indirectly, on the forming of an opinion and on decision making with respect to certain behaviour. Direct and indirect social influence are two extremes of a dimension of social influence, in between which there is a variety of intermediate forms.

A positive attitude with regard to a particular behaviour and a positive influence from the social environment do not guarantee actual performance of this behaviour. As a rule, the feasibility of the behaviour will be included in the considerations that precede the actual decision to perform the behaviour. A third factor, the so-called self-efficacy (Bandura, 1986; Kok et al., 1991), is also of importance. Insight into the role of self-efficacy is especially important when analysing why the desired behaviour has not been performed. Self-efficacy is based on the earlier experiences with the behaviour (in particular on the attributes for success or failing), observation by others, persuasion by others and physiological information (e.g. nervousness).

Self-efficacy is an important determinant when the behaviour concerned costs a major effort. When the behaviour can be performed without any difficulty, and does not require any particular skills or extra work, it is useless to consider self-efficacy.

The health belief model (Janz & Becker, 1984) provides a concept that is of interest here, namely risk perception. Broadly, risk is the assessment of the possibility of becoming injured and the seriousness of the injury. Perception of risks is strongly related to the per-of an individual is constantly judged by others, ceived vulnerability for a serious injury. A strong increase of the perceived vulnerability leads to a larger preparedness to change behaviour (Cummings *et al.*, 1979).

Research (Weinstein, 1989) shows, however, that in general individuals will make mistakes in assessing the risks. One is often unrealistically optimistic about the possibility of oneself becoming a casualty of an accident. People who do estimate realistically the chance of becoming injured, will probably also show more fear for injuries. Bouter and Knipschild (1987) reach the conclusion that fear for injuries leads to a 50% decrease in the risk of getting involved in an accident. This finding joins the view of Rogers (1983), who states that a higher degree of fear results in the desired change of behaviour. It can be assumed that fear for injuries can affect the decision on whether or not preventive actions are to be taken. If so, a positive response-efficacy and a positive self-efficacy are requisites for adequate action.

In general, it can be stated that sports requiring much physical effort show a certain risk of people getting injured, while in some sports more risks are involved than in others. Hazardous behaviour during games is spontaneous and therefore hard to influence. Nevertheless, two other factors should be mentioned that can serve as an explanation of injuries, namely 'sensation seeking' and 'locus of control'. Sensation seeking is the extent to which individuals experience their needs of excitement. Individuals who have more need for excitement are more inclined to take risks (Wilde, 1988). Locus of control (Wallston & Wallston, 1984) is the individual's expectation of incidents that can happen to him or her (such as becoming injured) to be the result of his or her own behaviour (internal locus) or emanating from factors he or she cannot control, e.g. chance, coincidence or other persons (external locus).

Sensation seeking as well as locus of control are personal characteristics, which can be rated among the external variables in Fig. 27.1 because they are presumed to influence attitude,

social influence and self-efficacy. Among the external variables that can be found are knowledge, age, education and sports-specific factors such as pastime, condition and choice of sport.

The purpose of health education

In formulating an objective, a large scale of activities can be involved including information, stimulation, realization, improvement, mobilization, advice, chance, etc. Formulating an objective is no sinecure: two essential elements are overlooked all too easily.

In the first place, in general, attention is focused on the final targets, i.e. the effects that should be realized after the intervention. However, one should bear in mind that a process of change starts at an unsatisfactory situation (problem) and ends at the realization of the desired situation (solving of the problem), while passing various stages, i.e. different stages have to be completed in order to achieve the final result. In terms of health educational strategy, this means that subobjectives have to be formulated for every stage to be passed. Structuring of the objectives commonly results in specification of the objectives in the short, medium and long term. The model in Fig. 27.2, by Siero *et al.* (1989), shows the different stages that have to be passed in order to establish maintenance of behaviour.

A second essential factor in the formulation of an objective is the level of abstraction. Goals are often described on a level of abstraction that is too high, whereas translating the goals into terms of the desired, concrete result proves to be more useful. In other words, formulations like 'information in order to prevent injuries' should not be used, but instead formulations that are concrete and measurable should be made, for example '5% reduction of the number of knee injuries among soccer players in the 15–20 age range within a period of 2 years'. Rossi (1979) listed a number of aspects which might be of major importance in the operationalization of the goals.

1 The objective should denote exactly the target

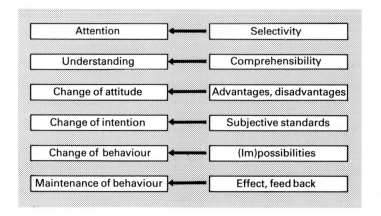

Fig. 27.2 Model of change of behaviour through education. From Siero *et al*. (1989).

group of intervention. This means detailed segmentation of the target group.

2 The objective should indicate the level on which the objective has to be realized. Is the information aiming at an increase of knowledge, change of attitude or changes of behaviour?

3 The objective should state a time limit. Delineation of time not only provides insight into the course of the information process but especially gives the opportunity to adjust the intervention or to avoid undesired side-effects.

4 The objectives should be consistent. They should be in line with each other and support each other, they should not be discordant. In realizing objectives on distinctive levels, one should bear in mind that objectives are cumulative.

5 Formulation of the objectives means playing the devil's advocate. It is important to consider critically the possible effects of an erroneous interpretation, and subsequently undesired side-effects.

6 The objectives should be realistic and feasible. Critical introspection is no luxury.

To conclude, a distinction can be made between objective of intervention and objective of communication. The objective of intervention describes the effects and the population that are aimed at, and the expected results in terms of verifiable quantities (indicators such as time and scale). An intervention can include

several objectives of communication. The objective of communication refers to the contents of the message describing which behaviour the target population is expected to perform. In the text below an example is given of the six-point route that should be followed in order to formulate an objective of communication on the basis of a problem. It also shows the difference between objectives of intervention and communication.

1 *Problem*. Treatment of, and care for, injuries has harmful consequences for society.

2 *Health problem*. The practice of skiing has harmful consequences for the well-being of the individual sportsperson.

3 *Health educational problem*. The behaviour of the sportsperson has a positive/negative effect on the prevention of injuries.

4 *Formulation of the problem*. Is it possible to influence the behaviour of the skier by means of information so as to reduce the number of injuries?

5 *Objective of intervention*. Information should lead to:

(a) increase in knowledge of security measures with respect to the gear,

(b) awareness of the danger and a positive attitude towards safety,

(c) acceptance of the security rules, and

(d) positive intention towards the use of gear.

6 *Objective of communication*. Having the ski

bindings adjusted by an expert by means of a testing device.

The method of health education

In general, it can be stated that the success of an information activity depends on the extent to which the communicator succeeds in motivating people to perform other (healthier and safer) behaviour. Motivating should be interpreted as giving people the opportunity to choose their own behaviour. In general, people prefer the kind of behaviour that is most rewarding, according to their own perception. People who choose deliberately to behave otherwise, will perform this behaviour in a better way and for a longer period. It goes without saying that information is not meant to incite different behaviour only incidentally. The point is, that the desired behaviour becomes part of the daily routine. Therefore, maintenance of behaviour is rather the target than change of behaviour. The success of an intervention, i.e. to what extent the desired targets are realized, largely depends on the quality of planning.

A model for explicit planning and evaluation of health education is presented in Fig. 27.3. In planning as well as in evaluation, five related steps to the five in Fig. 27.3 can be discriminated. These ten steps in all can be indicated by corresponding key questions. The questions are presented below and (partially) answered concerning health education among downhill skiers (Kok & Bouter, 1990).

Step 1: How serious is the problem? Most authors agree upon an incidence of 2−4 medically treated ski injuries per 1000 skier days (Eriksson & Johnson, 1980; Hauser & Gläser, 1985; Bouter, 1988).

Step 2: What behaviour is involved? Literature mentions an abundance of putative behavioural risk factors for ski injuries. However, studies adequately establishing and quantifying the aetiological role of these factors are very rare. While probably not every lower extremity equipment related (LEER) injury can be prevented by an optimal adjustment of the ski bindings, it certainly seems to be possible to lower LEER injury rates substantially by promoting proper binding adjustment procedures (Hauser, 1987).

Step 3: What are the determinants of the behaviour? A limited study of the determinants of behaviour (Rosen et al., 1982) indicated that one of the mistakes most frequently observed is that skiers readjust their bindings too much, after a fall that the skier interpreted to be due to inadvertent release. In their study, the belief that adequate adjustment can prevent injury as well as inadvertent release turned out to be an important determinant of the desirable behaviour. Furthermore, it was found that skiers are more likely to have their bindings adjusted adequately in a ski shop, when they think that experts are in favour of taking this action (Rosen et al., 1982).

Step 4: What are the options for change? Health educational intervention could stress the opinion of experts on this subject and clarify

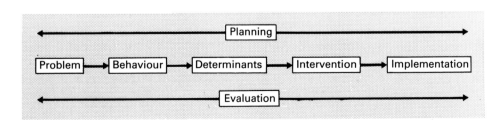

Fig. 27.3 Model of planning and evaluation of health education. From Green & Kreuter (1991).

the relationship between suboptimal adjustment and risk of injury. The core of the message should be: have your ski bindings adjusted every year in a ski shop by an expert, with the aid of a test device. A recent study (Damoiseaux *et al.*, 1990) revealed that phrasing the information in a mildly fear-arousing way, emphasizing the seriousness of the injuries and the vulnerability of the skier, was relatively effective for this purpose compared to a more neutral formulation.

Step 5: How can it be implemented? In the Dutch study mentioned above (Damoiseaux *et al.*, 1990), an audio cassette delivered by post about 1 week before the beginning of the winter sports holiday appeared to be relatively effective compared to brochures and to earlier delivery of the audio cassette.

Step 6: Was the implementation carried out as planned? This step is designed to ensure that the population of skiers risking LEER injuries was actually reached by the health educational intervention.

Step 7: Was the intervention received as planned? The central question here is whether the skiers understood the message contained in the health education intervention.

Step 8: Have the determinants of the behaviour changed? In the present example, this part of the evaluation focuses on the perceived advantages of adequate adjustment and the perception of the experts' opinion.

Step 9: Has the behaviour changed? This entails the question whether the target population would engage in optimal adjustment of the bindings more frequently.

Step 10: Has the problem been solved? This is, of course, the ultimate measure of efficacy: steps 6–9 can be considered intermediary steps. In the example, the postintervention incidence of injury, more specifically of LEER injury, will indicate the overall effectiveness of the health educational intervention. For methodological reasons this straightforward measure is often not presented, due to the relatively low incidence of the result (sports injury) (Knipschild & Bouter, 1987). This can be avoided by valid and precise knowledge of the relation between behaviour and result. In this case, behavioural change can be used as an index of decrease of the sport injury incidence at issue. This enlarges substantially the statistical efficiency of the study.

Pitfalls

Unfortunately, the ten steps mentioned above are often not given the attention they require. The most common mistake is that people jump from problem to intervention without answering the questions on planning that lie in between. Furthermore, because evaluations are rare, the ineffectiveness of such interventions remains hidden. Evaluation is necessary for testing previous decisions and for making corrections to improve the intervention. By means of careful planning, a number of possible pitfalls may be avoided. These pitfalls will be described once more by means of the ski injury example.

Pitfall 1: The development of an intervention for a problem that does not exist. In our example, ski injuries are clearly a substantial problem, especially when analysed in terms of incidence figures and severity of the injuries. However, if we had failed to carry out a thorough problem analysis, we might have developed an intervention for a type of sport that shows a very small number of injuries or relatively minor injuries.

Pitfall 2: The development of an intervention concerning behaviour, but lacking a clear relationship with the problem. Bouter (1988) showed that there is no relationship between participation in ski gymnastics and the risk of suffering an injury. So, an intervention of this kind can be successful to the extent that it shows a high participation rate, without being effective, in the sense that it does not prevent injuries from occurring. In our opinion, this possible pitfall is currently a predominant threat to effective prevention of sports injuries. Too often valid knowledge is lacking about the behavioural risk factors contributing to the aetiology of the problem at issue.

Pitfall 3: The development of an intervention that is based on a misconceived idea of the determinants of behaviour. For instance, an educational programme on warming up for downhill skiers, based on the idea that people do not know how to perform the warm-up exercises. For the majority of the participants it may be that they know very well how to do warm-up exercises, but that they refrain from doing them, because, for instance, they consider them to be ineffective or ridiculous.

Pitfall 4: The development of a wrong intervention, such as an intervention for the wrong target group. For instance, school health education with the message that children ought to wear close-fitting ski boots that are not made of thermoplastic material (Ziegler et al., 1987; Bouter, 1988). This would turn out to be ineffective, because usually the parents take the final decisions in buying ski equipment.

Pitfall 5: The development of a possibly effective intervention, but one which is not implemented correctly. For example, facilities for adequate and non-profit binding adjustments were made available to the subscribers to a ski magazine. The information about this service probably would not reach the majority of beginner skiers, who, in general, are more prone to accidents, and often have badly adjusted bindings.

Pitfall 6: Unjustified satisfaction about the intervention. This concerns the failure to evaluate the intervention thoroughly. For instance, there could be satisfaction about the large number of brochures on injury prevention that are handed out to skiers waiting at the ski lifts, but no notice is taken of the question of whether or not an actual reduction of injuries has occurred.

Conclusion

In general, education is easily put on a par with transferring information. In doing so, people expect that in due time knowledge will lead to change of behaviour. Knowledge is a necessary factor indeed, but this does not at all imply that from an increase of knowledge a change of behaviour will automatically result. In this chapter it was proposed that system, purpose and method are the foundations required to realize changes in knowledge, attitude and behaviour.

So far, prevention of sports injuries has been dominated by sports injury specialists. To be effective, these efforts should be combined with health education specialists. By means of co-operation between these two specialisms, it should be possible to achieve a reduction of sports injuries within the next 10–20 years. Health education can be an effective way of preventing sports injuries. It is important, however, to be aware of the fact that the effectiveness of health education (and health promotion) depends on the quality of planning. This implies a careful analysis of the problem, the behaviour, the determinants, the intervention and the implementation, and of the strength of the relationship between these five aspects. Concerning the prevention of most sports injuries, it seems that the stage at which particular advice is to be given to people is still to be reached. Epidemiological studies on the aetiology of sports injuries, followed by research on behavioural determinants, are necessary to fill the gaps in our knowledge.

References

Bandura, A.S. (1986) *Social Foundations of Thought and Action*. Prentice Hall, New Jersey.

Bouter, L.M. (1988) *Injury Risk in Downhill Skiing*. Results from an etiological case-control study conducted among Dutch skiers. Uitgeverij de Vrieseborch, Haarlem.

Bouter, L.M. & Knipschild, P.G. (1987) *Accident risk in downhill skiing*. Paper presented at Sport for All: Sports Injuries and their Prevention, Second Meeting of the Council of Europe Seminar, Arnhem, The Netherlands.

Bouter, L.M., Knipschild, P.G., Peij, J.A. & Volovics, A. (1988) Sensation seeking and injury risk in downhill skiing. *Personality Ind. Diff.* **9**, 667–73.

Cummings, K.M., Jette, A.M., Brock, B.M. & Haefner,

D.P. (1979) Psychological determinants of immunization behavior in a swine influenza campaign. *Medical Care* **17**, 639–49.

Damoiseaux, V.M.G., Jongh, A.M. de, Bouter, L.M. & Hospers, H.J. (1990) Designing effective health education for downhill skiers; results of a randomized intervention study. In R.J. Johnson & C.D. Mote (ed) *Skiing Trauma and Safety: 8th International Symposium*. ASTM, Philadelphia.

Eriksson, E. & Johnson, R.J. (1980) The etiology of downhill ski injuries. *Exerc. Sport Sci. Rev.* **8**, 1–17.

Fishbein, M. & Ajzen, I. (1975) *Beliefs, Attitude, Intention and Behavior: An Introduction to Theory and Research*. Addison-Wesley, Massachusetts.

Green, L.W. & Kreuter, M.W. (1991) *Health Promotion Planning: An Educational and Environmental Approach*. Mountain View, California.

Hauser, W. (1987) Experimental prospective skiing injury study (Summary). In *Proceedings of the 7th International Symposium on Skiing Trauma and Safety*. Chamonix, France.

Hauser, W. & Gläser, H. (1985) Alpine Skiünfalle und Verletzungen: Häufigkeit, Risikofaktoren, Ursachen (Injuries and accidents in downhill skiing: prevalence, risk factors and causes). *Schriftenreihe des Deutschen Skiverband* (Heft 14). Stiftung Sicherheit im Skisport des Deutschen Skiverbandes, München.

Janz, N. & Becker, M. (1984) The health belief model: a decade later. *Health Educ. O.* **11**, 1–14.

Knipschild, P.G. & Bouter, L.M. (1987) Risk factors for ski trauma: a crash course of epidemiologic methods with special reference to case-control studies (Summary). In *Proceedings of the 7th International Symposium on Skiing Trauma and Safety*. Chamonix, France.

Kok, G.J. & Bouter, L.M. (1990) On the importance of planned health education; Prevention of the injuries as an example. *Am. J. Sports Med.* **18**, 600–5.

Kok, G.J., De Vries, H., Mudde, A.N. & Strecher, V.J. (1991) Planned health education and the role of self-efficacy; Dutch Research. *Health Educ. Res.* **6**, 231–8.

Rogers, R.W. (1983) Cognitive and physiological processes in fear appeals and attitude change: A revised theory of protection motivation. In J.T. Cacioppo & R.E. Petty (eds) *Social Physiology, A Source Book*. Guilford, New York.

Rosen, J.C., Johnson, R.J., Lefebre, M.F. & Pope, M.H. (1982) Behavioral determinants of skiers' failure to adjust release bindings. *Clin. Sports Med.* **1**, 209–15.

Rossi, P.H. (1979) *Evaluation; A Systematic Approach*. Sage Publications, Beverly Hills.

Siero, S., Boon, M., Kok, G.J. & Siero, F. (1989) Modification of driving behavior in a large transport organization; A field experiment. *J. Appl. Psychol.* **74**, 417–23.

Wallston, B.S. & Wallston, K.A. (1984) Social psychological models of health behavior: An examination and integration. In A. Baum, S. Taylor & J.E. Singer (eds) *Handbook of Psychology and Health*, Vol. IV. Erlbaum, New Jersey.

Weinstein, N.D. (1989) Effects of personal experience on self-protection behavior. *Psychol. Bull.* **105**, 31–50.

Wilde, G.J. (1988) Risk homeostasis theory and traffic accidents. *Ergonomics* **31**, 441–65.

Ziegler, W.J., Jung, H., Matter, P. & Meier, P. (1987) *Risikobewust Skifahren* (Awareness of Risks of Downhill Skiing). Habegger Verlag, Derendingen.

PART 5

SPECIFIC AND PRIMARY PREVENTION ACTIVITIES

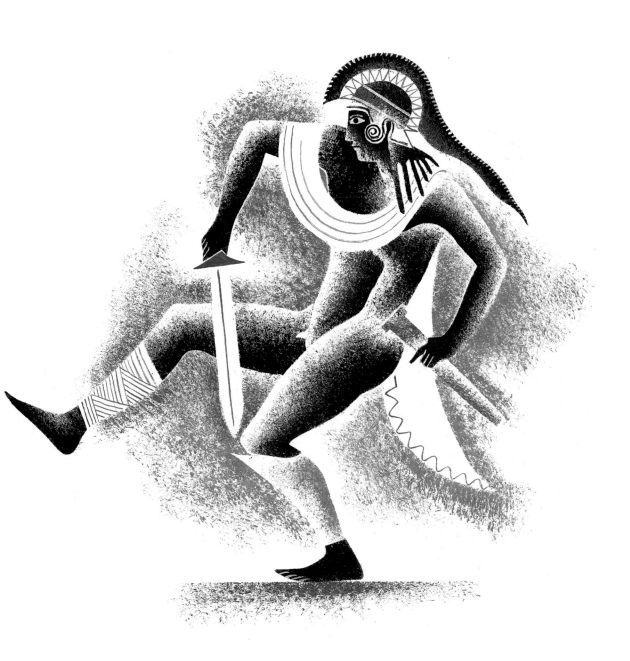

Chapter 28

Protective Equipment: Biomechanical Evaluation

PATRICK J. BISHOP

Protective equipment for sport is intended primarily to reduce the risk of injury to the wearer without creating other injury hazards to either the player or opponent and without detracting from the nature of the activity or sport being played. While the wearing of protective equipment can be, and often is, made mandatory by those governing a particular sport, the acceptability of a given piece of equipment is more often determined by such intangibles as aesthetics, comfort, fit, weight, ventilation, etc. (Fig. 28.1) However, to ensure wearers that a given piece of equipment is appropriate for use, such equipment should be evaluated by considering the injuries it is to protect against, by determining its ability to reduce and/or distribute force, and by judging its performance against appropriate tissue tolerance criteria. Such a biomechanical evaluation of protective equipment for sport is not very common; only a few protective devices are so evaluated.

A comprehensive review of this topic is given by Norman (1983) in which he considers equipment ranging from sport helmets to ski bindings. Because of the nature of this volume and its extensive review of sports injuries, this chapter will be more restricted in scope. The requirements necessary for appropriate biomechanical evaluations of protective equipment for the head and face will be updated and an overview of the difficulties encountered in protecting the cervical spine, particularly in situations of axial compressive loading, will be considered.

Requirements for biomechanical evaluation

For an appropriate biomechanical evaluation to take place, the protective device must be subjected to test conditions which simulate as nearly as possible the actual injury producing mechanism. For example, the device could be intended to provide protection in a high energy crash environment such as a bicycle accident, in a collision environment where multiple blows are common such as football or ice hockey, or where an impact from a low mass—high velocity projectile is likely such as from a baseball or ice-hockey puck. The requirements for protection in these circumstances are different as are the requirements necessary for an appropriate test simulation.

In attempting to evaluate equipment through appropriate simulations two approaches are possible. As discussed by Hodgson (1982) these include (i) an engineering approach, in which only the protective device absorbs energy and its performance is judged on kinetic or kinematic measures which may not be related to injury; or (ii) a biomechanical approach ·in which an attempt is made to subject a surrogate model that has a high level of biofidelity to a worst case impact condition and then evaluate its performance in relation to human tolerance. It is not easy to maintain both biofidelity and durability in most surrogate models and frequently other requirements, such as simplicity and reproducibility, dictate the actual test con-

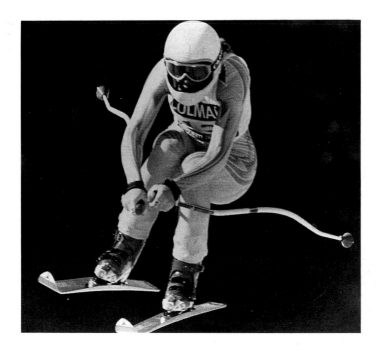

Fig. 28.1 All helmets must be well designed with regard to the needs of the wearer and the sport. Courtesy of the IOC archives.

ditions utilized. A compromise between the two approaches is often taken and the effectiveness of the protective device in reducing the risk of injury is judged by its performance both in the laboratory and in the field. To do adequate field evaluation, however, requires intensive effort in obtaining valid and reliable epidemiological measures of injury and injury reduction.

Biomechanical evaluation of head protection

A great deal of effort has been devoted to biomechanical evaluations of sport helmets. Injuries to the head are a common phenomenon and range from scalp lacerations to brain concussion with an expected outcome that varies from complete return of function to severe impairment to death.

In sport, the head must be protected against two distinct types of head injury, namely (i) focal lesions, and (ii) diffuse lesions. The focal lesions which are precipitated by the con-

tact phenomenon and linear acceleration of direct blunt trauma include skull fracture, epidural and subdural haematoma, while diffuse brain injury involves a number of axonal lesions induced by excessive angular acceleration of the head (Gennarelli, 1991).

Numerous standards exist for helmets worn by ice hockey, football and baseball players and by pedal cyclists. While these standards exist to provide at least some minimum level of safety to the wearer, they are not uniform in their approach.

Test protocols: blunt trauma

Helmet performance is usually judged in terms of the helmet's ability to withstand blunt trauma and is determined in the laboratory by subjecting an instrumented headform, fitted with the test helmet, to a gravity assisted guided fall against a firm surface. The guided fall can be conducted on a test rig with a single track (i.e. monorail) or with the aid of two or three guidewires or guiderods (Fig. 28.2).

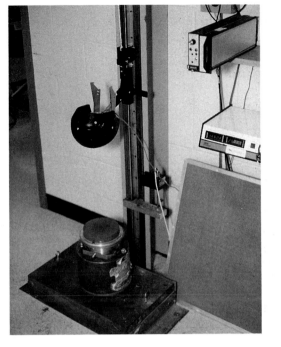

(a)

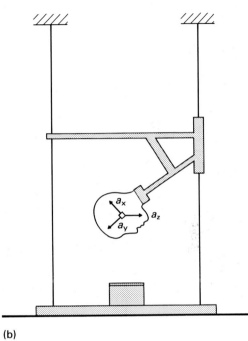

(b)

Fig. 28.2 (a) Monorail and (b) guidewire test rigs used in helmet testing.

The energy of impact varies according to the activity for which the helmet is used (e.g. ice hockey, 40 J; cycling, 80 J; etc) as does the number of impacts (e.g. 1–3) to a given location. The impact surface can be (i) padded to simulate a yielding surface such as the ground; (ii) unpadded to simulate a hard, unyielding surface such as the ice; (iii) flat to simulate a distributed impact; or (iv) curved to simulate a concentrated impact. The ability of the helmet to attenuate shock is usually determined by an accelerometer, either uniaxial or triaxial, located at the headform centre of mass. Headforms consist of skull forms made from metal (aluminium–magnesium alloy) or a rubber–epoxy combination, of complete heads fabricated from wood but without facial features, and of complete heads with facial features and with mass distribution and impedance response characteristics similar to those of the human head

(the so-called humanoid headform). Performance criteria include peak headform acceleration, the severity index (SI) or both.

That helmets are subjected to performance tests which differ in terms of headform type, pass/fail criteria, impact surface, location or frequency leads to a number of difficulties when trying to interpret the results obtained from one test protocol against those obtained from another protocol.

HEADFORMS

The problem of using different headforms is particularly acute when considering, for example, the development of international standards for head protection. The four headform types, summarized in Table 28.1, were each subjected to two successive impacts, in our laboratory, at each of six locations (front, rear,

Table 28.1 Headform characteristics and performance at 40 J.

Headform	Size*	Mass† (kg)	Peak G at 40 J	Failure criterion (G)‡
Magnesium—aluminium alloy (ASTM)	M (7¼)	5.11	396	258
Rubber—epoxy (CSA)	M (7⅛)	5.23	335	235
Wood: no facial features (SIS)	M (7¼)	4.74	323	226
Humanoid (WSU)	M (7¼)	5.95	240	168

* Hat size in brackets.
† Includes follower assembly, clamps, etc.
‡ Based on reducing headform acceleration by 30%.
ASTM, American Society for Testing and Materials; CSA, Canadian Standards Association; SIS, Swedish Standards Institute; WSU, Hodgson—Wayne State University.

right and left side, crown, right frontal boss) against a padded impact surface (modular elastomer programmer, 2.5 cm thick, Shore A hardness of 70) using a monorail drop test rig. The headforms were tested at impact energy levels of 10, 20 and 30 J and peak acceleration was recorded from the headform centre of mass using a triaxial accelerometer. The performance results were not uniform either between headforms or within headforms at different test locations (Fig. 28.3).

Peak acceleration measures for each headform at each test location were plotted against impact energy and the regression lines shown in Fig. 28.4 were drawn. From these, a 40-J impact would be expected to yield the peak acceleration for each headform shown in Table 28.1. Given these different values it is difficult

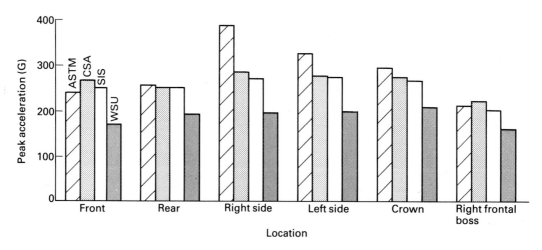

Fig. 28.3 Average peak acceleration for four different headforms (see Table 28.1) subjected to 30 J impacts at six locations. ASTM, American Society for Testing and Materials; CSA, Canadian Standards Association; SIS, Swedish Standards Institute; WSU, Hodgson—Wayne State University.

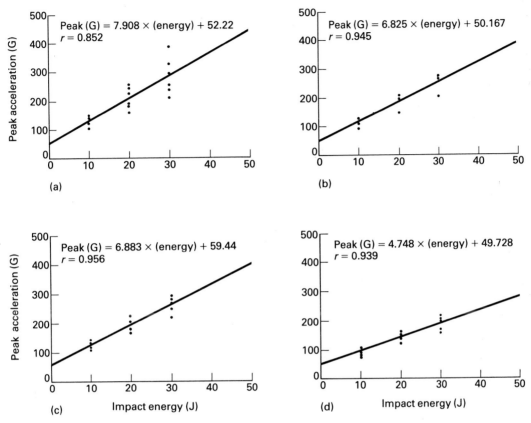

Fig. 28.4 Regression equations for peak acceleration versus impact energy for four headform types. (a) American Society for Testing and Materials; (b) Canadian Standards Association; (c) Swedish Standards Institute; (d) Hodgson–Wayne State University.

to suggest an appropriate pass/fail criterion. For example, if the requirements of a particular activity dictated that the helmet should reduce these non-helmeted peak headform accelerations by at least 30%, then the pass/fail criterion for a given helmet would also be different depending on the headform used (Table 28.1). Clearly, a universal pass/fail criterion expressed in Gs is not appropriate and any performance measure must be stated in conjunction with the headform used for testing.

FAILURE CRITERION

To determine whether a helmet provides adequate protection, it is necessary to know the level of impact at which injury occurs and to somehow translate that to the response of the skull–brain surrogate (i.e. headform). As Ommaya (1988) has indicated, it is necessary to distinguish between the terms injury criterion, which is some physical parameter that correlates well with injury severity for a given body part, and tolerance level, which must be specified by the magnitude of the load on the body which produces a specific type of injury at a specified level of severity. Where possible, human tolerance levels should be expressed in terms of gender and age.

Human tolerance can only be determined indirectly through cadaveric or animal responses to crash tests that involve impact and/

or impulsive loading. Gurdjian *et al.* (1964, 1966) have related moderate brain concussion to the presence of linear skull fracture. Given the physical differences between bone and the complex nature of the brain tissue and its vascular elements, it is likely that this relationship is only a first approximation to the presence of brain damage and that tolerance limits for both the skull and brain are needed. Functional or structural failure limits for the brain have not yet been adequately determined and brain injury is often specified in terms of the magnitude or history of mechanical parameters such as peak and average linear and angular accelerations, as well as their duration and rate of onset, intracranial pressure, force and energy applied to the cranium (Ommaya, 1988).

Linear acceleration data from human cadavers and live animal tests were used by Gurdjian *et al.* (1964, 1966) to develop the Wayne State tolerance curve (WSTC) (Fig. 28.5), which has been used to estimate the threshold values of tolerance for linear acceleration and time duration. The curve is really a boundary measure for safe and unsafe impact pulses with any point on the curve representing the same injury threshold as any other point. Severe impacts (i.e. those which produce high levels of acceleration) can be tolerated if they are short in duration while long duration impacts are tolerable if the acceleration is small (Fan, 1971).

The WSTC has been widely criticized in terms of the theory and the data on which it was based and for a detailed review of these criticisms readers are referred to the works of Versace (1971), Fan (1971) and Newman (1975).

One of the problems in interpreting the meaning of the WSTC was in the definition of the term 'effective acceleration'. Originally it was taken as a value slightly greater than half the peak (Patrick *et al.*, 1963), but later it was interpreted as the average acceleration over the entire pulse (Hodgson & Thomas, 1972).

To overcome the difficulty of determining the 'effective acceleration' in the WSTC, Gadd (1966) developed a severity index based upon a log–log plot of the WSTC which he simplified between 4 and 50 ms with a straight line approximation of the slope. This SI was represented by the integration of the acceleration–time pulse and is expressed by the equation

$$\mathrm{SI} = \int_0^t a^{2.5}\, \mathrm{d}t$$

where *a* represents the acceleration pulse, and *t* represents the pulse duration.

The SI, like the WSTC from which it was derived, is also a boundary measure. By fitting several rectangles of acceleration and time under the tolerance curve, Gadd arrived at a criterion value of 1000 which could be considered as a threshold of danger to life from an internal head injury due to frontal blows. For impacts against a yielding surface the criterion level was later increased to 1500 (Gadd, 1972). The SI has likewise been criticized, mainly because it does not represent a scaling of injury severity (Versace, 1971) but recently, Hodgson (1991) provided the risk curve of Prasad and Mertz (1985) and demonstrated how the SI could be used as an indication of injury risk in the population and how it is possible to choose a level of risk for which a helmet is to be designed for a given impact environment.

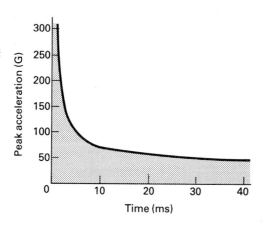

Fig. 28.5 The Wayne State tolerance curve. From Gurdjian *et al.* (1966).

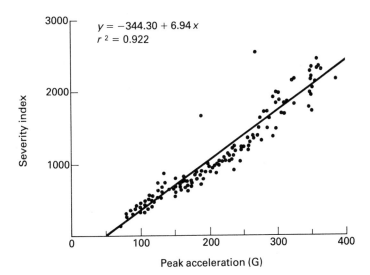

$$y = -344.30 + 6.94\,x$$
$$r^2 = 0.922$$

Fig. 28.6 Linear regression of severity index versus peak acceleration.

It is likely that the SI will also be headform dependent because it is so heavily weighted on peak acceleration. Figure 28.6 is a linear regression plot based on 162 ice hockey helmet tests conducted in our laboratory. A monorail test rig was used in conjunction with a rubberized epoxy headform (ISO size J). The impact energy was 40 J against a non-padded, flat, rigid surface. The linear regression model predicted that 92% of the variance in SI was accounted for by the peak headform acceleration. Calvano and Berger (1979) combined humanoid and metal headform data from crown impacts and showed similar results ($r = 0.97$) between SI and peak acceleration.

As stated earlier, it is not only necessary to know the level of impact at which injury occurs, but it is necessary to translate that to the response of the headform used. An SI of 1500 or greater in a humanoid headform is taken as a failure in evaluating football helmets in North America (Hodgson, 1975). While this value may be appropriate for use with a humanoid head, the use of 1500 SI as a universal measure with other headforms is questionable.

MONORAIL VERSUS GUIDEWIRE TESTS

The use of different test rigs for conducting helmet evaluations presents a number of difficulties when attempting to compare the results obtained from one system with those obtained from the other. A monorail and guidewire test system were compared in our laboratory using a rubberized epoxy headform (ISO size J) tested at three impact locations (front, crown and rear), against a non-padded, flat, rigid anvil. Three trials of each of two different hockey helmets were run with each system and impact location. The heights from which the helmeted headforms were dropped were adjusted to produce an identical impact energy of 40 J for each system. The monorail system yielded a mean peak headform acceleration over the three locations that was 31% greater than that of the guidewire system (Fig. 28.7).

This difference cannot be accounted for by differences in friction between the two systems because the energy at impact for both systems was standardized at 40 J. As suggested by the work of Calvano and Berger (1979) much of the difference is likely attributable to an eccentric loading of the headform when using the guidewire system, which results in energy dissi-

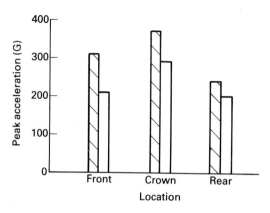

Fig. 28.7 Peak headform acceleration obtained for an ice-hockey helmet at three locations using a monorail (▨) and guidewire test rig (□).

pation through the bending of the guidewires. Some eccentricity in loading takes place in the monorail system as well, but not to the same extent, with the result that the guidewire system produces much lower peak headform acceleration values.

The differences in performance are also demonstrated by the acceleration−time curves illustrated in Fig. 28.8. Here, there is not only a greater peak acceleration for the monorail system but the acceleration−time curves generally rise to that peak sooner, giving the appearance that the monorail system produces higher frequency acceleration−time curves. It would appear that the monorail test rig is stiffer and provides a more severe test of the helmet than the guidewire system.

These test rig differences produce a dilemma, when considering which system should be used in helmet evaluation. On the one hand, the use of a system in which an appreciable amount of energy is taken up in the bending of the apparatus might allow some helmets to be accepted when they should be rejected (false positives). On the other hand, the use of a system which provides for a more severe evaluation of the helmet might lead to the development of liner materials which are too stiff for practical use

but which are necessary in order to satisfy the requirements of the impact test. The most appropriate system lies somewhere between these extremes. There is little doubt, however, that helmet results obtained on one system cannot be compared with those obtained on the other system.

Helmet liner stiffness

Most sport helmets are designed to reduce the risk of head injury by means of a firm outer shell intended to distribute the impact over a large area, and by means of a liner to absorb the energy of the blow. Consideration for the type of liner to be used in a helmet is based on the type of activity in which the helmet will be used rather than on the characteristics of the wearer. For activities where multiple blows of low to moderate intensity are common (e.g. ice hockey, football, lacrosse) helmet liners consist of medium density resilient foams. Such liners usually perform well but if they are too soft, bottoming of the liner will occur and the force of the blow will be transmitted directly to the skull. For more severe single impact collision conditions (e.g. cycling, skiing) stiffer and higher density non-rebound liners are generally used. These stiff liners require a great deal of input energy before they crush and if this energy is not available (i.e. the collision is not sufficiently severe) the impact force can again be transferred to the wearer's skull. That these two liner types perform differently was demonstrated by Bishop and Briard (1984) who compared bicycle helmets with rebound and non-rebound liners by subjecting them to two successive impacts. On the first impact the resilient, non-rebound liners yielded peak headform accelerations that were 12% lower than those from rebound liners. On the second drop, however, the rebound liners outperformed the resilient, non-rebound liners by 12%.

The stiffness characteristics needed in helmet liners are dictated not only by the collision

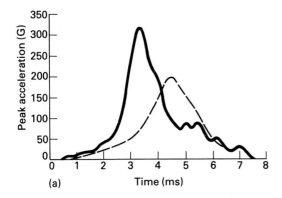

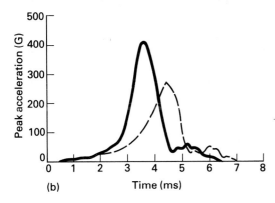

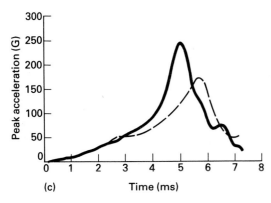

Fig. 28.8 Acceleration–time curves obtained for an ice-hockey helmet subjected to 40-J impacts at three locations using a monorail (——) and guidewire test rig (— —). (a) Front, (b) crown and (c) rear locations.

environment but by certification requirements in which helmets are tested against non-compliant surfaces at fairly high energy levels using stiff headforms. As a result, some helmets which meet certification standards may not be appropriate for all wearers. This is particularly true if helmets, certified to male characteristics, are to be used by women and/or children.

One of the first expressions of concern for the stiffness of helmet liners came from Hodgson (1983) with regards to polystyrene liners. Based upon a series of quasistatic loading tests, he noted that much of the protective capabilities of polystyrene liners could be expected to be above the level at which serious head injury would occur. Others, including Long et al. (1989) and Corner et al. (1987) have also expressed concern that polystyrene liners typically used in bicycle helmets are too stiff, particularly for children. Part of this concern is based upon the fact that while the child's head is more compliant than that of the adult, it does not tolerate trauma well (Corner et al., 1987), and the tolerance limit for moderate head injury in children is estimated to be about 80% of that of the adult (Mohan et al., 1979). We examined the data of Schneider and Nahum (1972) and noted that four adult female cadaver heads experienced definite fracture in the temporo-parietal area at an average of 3220 N compared to 3760 N for four adult male cadavers. While this data is scanty, it suggests that the female skull is less resistant to fracture than is the male skull.

Concern regarding the requirements for head protection in children has also been expressed by Lane (1986) and Corner et al. (1987) who suggest that, in addition to more research to determine the appropriate requirements for children's bicycle helmets, the liners presently used in adult helmets are too stiff. Long et al. (1989) recommend that, in addition to a 200-G maximum acceleration criterion, a localized loading test should be included in evaluating helmets. Finally, Mills (1990) analysed the protective capabilities of bicycle helmets for frontal and side impacts and concluded that the upper limit on liner thickness is about 20 mm to keep the headform acceleration below 200 G and to protect the wearer from impacts up to 6.6 m·s^{-1} into a rigid flat surface. There was no indication as to whether these characteristics applied to men, women and children or to men only.

Test protocols: concentrated trauma

While test protocols against blunt trauma are well established, the problem of determining helmet performance against concentrated or focal trauma is not. Some efforts have been made to consider the problem of a concentrated impact in bicycle and motorcycle helmet standards by including a curved anvil on which the helmet is to be dropped. However, there are few performance tests or standards for evaluating helmets for sport activities in which there is a risk of being struck with an implement travelling at high velocity (e.g. baseball, ice hockey).

The development of a protocol suitable for such conditions requires an appropriate headform and a device, such as an air cannon, to propel the ball or puck against the helmet. It is also necessary to specify an adequate performance measure that is representative of the trauma likely to be induced, and test procedures that are repeatable, reproducible and simple to use. The most appropriate measure would seem to be the force acting on the skull in response to the puck or ball impact. However, measuring that force is not trivial. Instrumenting the headform with force transducers or strain gauges capable of responding in the appropriate frequency range is costly and they tend to be frangible, thus increasing the chance of damaging the test equipment. Other problems include the number of transducers required, their location on the headform and ensuring that the impact force is directed to those locations.

One way to assess concentrated trauma is with the use of Fuji prescale film to determine

the pressure applied to the skull from either a ball or puck impact. The film consists of two separate sections, one containing a microcapsular layer of colour-forming material which generates a vivid colour when it reacts with the colour developing material on the second layer. The two layers are superimposed on each other and upon the application of pressure (e.g. from a thrown ball) a coloured mark is left on one film layer. The density of the coloured mark is proportional to the applied pressure, and is determined by means of a light densitometer.

Hodgson (1989) used this technique to evaluate baseball helmets and to examine the relationship between the applied pressure and the SI. Fuji film revealed very high pressures on the headform (greater than 630 N·cm^{-1}), due to a baseball propelled from an air cannon at 27 m·s^{-1}, but these were accompanied by SIs (determined from peak headform accelerations) which would indicate serious head injury in only a small amount (2–3%) of the population. Thus, the SI, a criterion measure intended to assess the potential risk of concussion, is not sufficiently sensitive for evaluating the potential for other types of head injury (e.g. skull fracture) associated with baseball or other such projectile impacts to the head and direct force or pressure measurements are needed.

Before the Fuji film technique can be incorporated as a test of concentrated trauma, however, a number of issues require clarification and resolution. Firstly, the values recorded from the film are really static measures. The technique does not reveal anything regarding the time history of the applied pressure and only provides an estimate of the peak pressure. Secondly, the film cannot be calibrated dynamically which presents a serious limitation when using it under dynamic conditions. Finally, there is the issue of tolerance and the appropriate performance measure for determining the helmet's acceptability. Should the performance measure be the peak pressure on the headform, the change in pressure between the outside and inside of the helmet or some other? Clearly, a great deal needs to be done before a satisfactory protocol for evaluating helmets against concentrated trauma is established.

Performance of helmets in preventing head injury

Have biomechanical evaluations of sport helmets resulted in improved head protection? Evidence that this is so comes indirectly from injury data gathered before and after the introduction of performance standards for particular sport helmets.

Head injury death in North American football players at the high school and university level has decreased dramatically since the introduction of a football helmet standard and rule changes regarding the use of the helmeted head. From a peak of about 30 head-injury deaths per year in 1968, fatalities have declined steadily, particularly since 1975–1976, to the point of one or two in 1989 (Clarke, 1991). Concussion rates in this sport have averaged about 2.5% over the last few years and would represent over 36 000 concussions annually, given the large number of people who play college and high school football (Hodgson, 1991).

Prior to the introduction of an ice-hockey helmet standard in Canada several players died from blows to the head even though they were wearing head protection (Fekete, 1968). Since the Canadian Standards Association hockey helmet standard was adopted in 1972, the risk of fatality in ice hockey has been markedly reduced (deaths are almost unheard of). However, other forms of head injury, particularly concussion, appear to be prevalent as suggested by the research summarized in Table 28.2.

It is likely that these head injury rates in ice hockey and the concussion rates for both ice hockey and football are too high and additional efforts, in the form of improved protection and rule enforcement, are needed to reduce them.

One of the difficulties associated with determining the effectiveness of bicycling helmets is that most injuries are reported for situations in which the bicycle is used for transportation or fitness training and where there are no mandatory requirements for wearing them. In a survey of bicycle-related injuries over a 5-month period at a large Canadian hospital only 2% of the patients had been wearing a helmet at the time of injury although 13% claimed they owned one for cycling (Cushman et al., 1990). In a case-control study on the effectiveness of bicycle helmets, Thompson et al. (1989) reported that only 7% of patients were wearing helmets at the time of their head injuries. Using regression analysis to control for age, gender, income, education, cycling experience and injury severity, these researchers estimated that helmeted riders had an 85% reduction in their risk of brain injury.

While the success of helmet use in reducing the risk of serious injury cannot be attributed to biomechanics alone, it seems clear that a

Table 28.2 Head injury and concussion rates in ice hockey.

Author	Year	Sample	Head injury rate (%)	Concussion rate (%)
Jørgensen et al.	1986	Danish élite	28	14
Bishop & Manton	1987	Intercollegiate	8.4	8
Gerberich et al.	1987	High school	18	12
Posch et al.	1989	Swedish élite	9 (head and neck)	NR

NR, no results.

sound biomechanical approach to helmet evaluation has resulted in improved levels of head protection.

Biomechanical evaluation of facial protection

Injuries to the face, particularly lacerations and trauma to the mouth and teeth, used to be considered hazards inherent to certain sporting activities. However, as an increasing number of catastrophic injuries to the eyes began to emerge, primarily through the work of Pashby (Pashby *et al.*, 1975; Pashby, 1977, 1979, 1985) in ice hockey and Vinger (Vinger & Toplin, 1978; Vinger, 1981) and Easterbrook (1978, 1981) in the racquet sports, it became apparent that improved facial protection was needed. Over the past 20 years efforts at reducing the risk of eye injuries has taken place through improved participant education, and biomechanical evaluation of protective facial wear has led to the development of standards to ensure that such products are safe.

Test protocols

From a biomechanical perspective, the evaluation of eye and face protectors must be conducted with a dynamic impact test using a headform with appropriate facial features. Such procedures are presently used by the Canadian Standards Association (CSA) for evaluating facial protection for ice-hockey players, and by CSA and the American Society for Testing and Materials (ASTM) for evaluating eye protectors used in the racquet sports.

When conducting dynamic impact tests, the ball or puck is propelled to strike the protectors from a device such as an air cannon. For squash and racquetball, the ball speed is 40 m·s^{-1} and the protector is struck on the front and side. For ice hockey, the puck speed is 28 m·s^{-1} for facial protectors used by forwards and defense players, and 36 m·s^{-1} for those used by goaltenders. The protector is struck from the front and side over the eye and mouth areas. The

standards for these devices specify that under impact, eye or facial contact is not permitted by either the projectile or the protector itself. Thus, the failure criterion is really a boundary measure of touch or no touch and there is no attempt to scale the potential for injury risk or injury severity.

The development and implentation of standards for facial protection requires a facially featured test headform that is durable enough to withstand the rigours of dynamic impact testing. When the CSA and ASTM standards programmes for eye protectors for the racquet sports were initiated in the mid-1980s, several apparently appropriate products were unable to meet the performance requirements because of problems with the test headform. Likewise, the CSA had difficulty in certifying face protectors for ice hockey, intended specifically for children, because of an inappropriate headform. The CSA responded by developing two facially featured headforms, one for an average 6-year-old child and one for an average 12-year-old male (18-year-old female). These two headforms incorporate soft and bony tissue measurements derived from a number of sources including dental and facial X-rays gathered over several years as well as skull sizes conforming to international standards. However, the headforms are not mass produced and they are difficult to obtain. Adult male facially featured headforms are available (e.g. Alderson headform, the Hybrid III headform, the WSU humanoid headform) but these are not completely satisfactory for evaluating facial or eye protectors and additional work is needed to produce a headform that is.

Performance of eye and facial protectors in preventing injury

ICE HOCKEY

Eye injuries in ice hockey have been documented for some time by Pashby (1977, 1979, 1985) and Pashby *et al.* (1975) who gathered injury statistics from members of the Canadian

Ophthalmological Society. The frequency and distribution of eye injuries by age over a 10-year span are summarized in Table 28.3. The early data (1974–1975) demonstrated very vividly the need for both eye protection and standards for that protection in ice hockey. By 1977–1978, 1 year after the introduction of the facial protector standard, the eye injury frequency and the number of blind eyes had dropped substantially in the young age groups (10–20 years) where full facial protection was mandatory. In 1983–1984 there was a marked increase in the number of eye injuries to players in this age range (total of 46) but these injuries were not associated with organized hockey. They happened in non-organized games played on the street or frozen ponds and in which the players failed to wear facial protection.

The number of hockey-related eye injuries and blind eyes occurring in the age range of 21 years and older is truly cause for concern because facial protection is not mandatory for this age group. Facial protection is available for these players but they are reluctant to wear it. Even partial face protection can be useful in reducing injuries as was demonstrated by the work of Lorentzen et al. (1988) who showed that 52% of the facial lacerations occurring in a Swedish élite team over a 3-year period would have been prevented if the players had been wearing protective visors. Thus, when facial protection is worn in ice hockey, the risk of eye

and face injuries is small, but when it is not worn the likelihood of injury is very high.

RACQUET SPORTS

The use of biomechanical impact tests for evaluating eye protectors for the racquet sports has led directly to improved protection. Bishop et al. (1982) evaluated a number of lensed and lensless eyeguards by subjecting them to frontally directed ball impacts at speeds ranging from 22 to 49 m·s^{-1}. While the lensed protectors prevented headform eye contact in 98% of the cases, lensless eye protectors never prevented such contact even at low ball speeds. When a failure criterion of no eye contact was adopted in the eye protector standards, these lensless devices were essentially eliminated as certifiable products.

Even though there are standards for protective eye wear in the racquet sports, it is not mandatory for play, and as a result the proportion of racquet players wearing eye protectors is small. In a sample of Australian pennant squash players, only 8% used appropriate eye wear (Genovese et al. 1990) and the most common reason given for wearing eye protection was the occurrence of a previous injury to self or others.

While the efficacy of eye protectors in reducing serious eye injuries in the racquet sports is not well documented, it seems intuitive that

Table 28.3 Eye injuries in hockey by age. Adapted from Pashby (1985).

Age (years)	Number (and %) of cases									
	1974–1975	ULB	1976–1977	ULB	1977–1978	ULB	1978–1979	ULB	1983–1984	ULB
≤10	28 (12)	5	10 (11)	0	1 (2)	0	1 (2)	0	6 (5)	
11–15	76 (33)	6	18 (20)	1	5 (8)	0	3 (7)	0	18 (15)	
16–20	56 (24)	9	29 (32)	5	12 (24)	1	17 (41)	4	22 (18)	
≥21	69 (30)	13	33 (37)	5	31 (63)	7	20 (44)	7	78 (63)	
Unknown	24	4								
Total	253	37	90	11	49	8	41	11	124	13

ULB, unilateral legal blindness.

those devices intended to prevent ball or protector contact with the eye should be worn and that their use can and will substantially reduce the risk of serious eye injuries to the wearer.

Protecting the cervical spine

Although the cervical spine can be injured in a variety of ways, one of the most devastating cervical injuries is the burst or comminuted fracture of the vertebral body induced by axial compression and the associated cord trauma that results. Injuries of this type have been identified by McElhaney *et al.* (1979) in shallow water diving, by Torg *et al.* (1979) in football, and by Tator and Edmonds (1984) in ice hockey. The weight of both experimental and epidemiological evidence indicates that most severe injuries of this type occur in direct impacts in which the crown of the head strikes an unyielding surface such as the boards in an ice-hockey arena, a goalpost, the ground, another opponent, etc. The neck is usually partially flexed to about 30° so that the normal cervical lordosis is removed and the cervical column then bears a compressive load. The injuries produced in these situations are usually burst fractures/dislocations in the lower cervical spine (C4, C5, C6) often resulting in quadriplegia (Burstein *et al.*, 1982; Torg, 1985; Torg *et al.*, 1990).

Because of the seriousness of these injuries and the frequency of their occurrence in sporting and transportation situations, a great deal of research has been undertaken to determine both the mechanisms of injury and the load tolerance of the cervical spine. Among these are the works of Roaf (1960), Bauze and Ardran (1978), Nusholtz *et al.* (1981), Alem *et al.* (1984), Hodgson and Thomas (1980) and McElhaney *et al.* (1983, 1988) using human cadaver tissue; and Burstein *et al.* (1982) and Bishop and Wells (1986) using mechanical dummies coupled with computer models. Extensive reviews on the biomechanics of cervical injuries are also provided by Sances *et al.* (1984) and Yoganandan *et al.* (1990).

Biomechanical determination of cervical spine loading

Appropriate biomechanical evaluations are needed to understand the problem of cervical spine loading in crown-first collisions. There is a mistaken belief that the results of helmet drop tests have the potential to predict these devastating cervical spine injuries and that protective padding placed in the top of a helmet is an effective way to prevent their catastrophic results. However, these notions fail to consider the mechanical behaviour of the entire head–neck–torso system under impact.

Drop tests are used to evaluate the ability of the helmet to protect the head from blunt trauma. The effect of the torso on the head and neck in these impacts is minimal and the critical measure of helmet performance is usually the peak headform acceleration or the SI. Measuring the force required to stop the helmeted headform, rather than the acceleration, gives similar results. Using such a procedure to produce crown impacts to a football and hockey helmet, at an energy level of 54 J, resulted in a reaction force in excess of 10 000 N on the hockey helmet and in excess of 4300 N on the football helmet (Bishop & Wells, 1990) (Fig. 28.9).

In a head-first collision that produces axial loading of the cervical spine, the mechanism of injury is different from that of the head alone sustaining a blow. In such cases, the helmet usually functions as intended by minimizing the head acceleration and protecting the skull and brain. Simulated head-first collisions using an anthropometric test dummy (ATD) wearing a football helmet yielded peak headform accelerations of only 35–50 g but the compression forces on the dummy neck ranged from 6000 to 8000 N (Mertz *et al.*, 1978).

Bishop and Wells (1986) developed a simulation system which they have used to investigate cervical spine loading in crown-first collisions. The system includes a Hybrid III ATD which is propelled in free flight to strike a rigid barrier (Fig. 28.10). A six axis force trans-

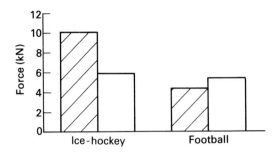

Fig. 28.9 Peak force experienced by an ice-hockey helmet and a football helmet subjected to a helmet drop test (▨) and to an anthropometric test dummy impact test (□). From Bishop & Wells (1990).

ducer measures three orthogonal forces and moments of force about the atlanto-occipital junction of the ATD. The force and moment data can be combined with positional information, obtained from digitizing the cinefilm of a given impact, and then processed using a computer model of the cervical spine. The output includes an estimate of the compressive force acting at several levels of the human cervical spine. Using this system travelling at 1.8 m·s^{-1}, with the dummy wearing the same football and hockey helmet used in the earlier drop tests, the compressive forces predicted at ATD level 5 (C6 in the human) are presented in Fig. 28.8. Thus, the extra protection afforded to the head by the football helmet (as shown in

the drop tests) was not effective in protecting the cervical spine.

In conducting the above simulations it was noted from the cinefilm that the ATD was not decelerated uniformly and the forward motion of the ATD torso continued for some time after the dummy headform came to a stop. Similar observations have been made by Burstein *et al.* (1982). Thus, the moving torso exerts a force on the neck and the neck in turn exerts an equal and opposite force to decelerate the torso. Clearly then, the critical measure for determining the potential for cervical spine injury is the load on the neck required to decelerate the mass of the torso and not the acceleration (or force) experienced by the headform.

Protective padding

Under conditions of axial compressive loading, then, the head and neck become trapped between two large masses moving toward each other (i.e. the object struck and the player's torso) and the force needed to reduce their relative velocities to zero is determined by the combined properties of the helmet or surface padding and the head–neck–torso system, and not by those of the helmet or padding material alone. The studies of Hodgson and Thomas (1980) and Burstein *et al.* (1982) have shown that only small reductions in compression can be achieved with helmets or padding and both

Fig. 28.10 System for conducting anthropometric test dummy impact tests against a fixed barrier. From Bishop & Wells (1986).

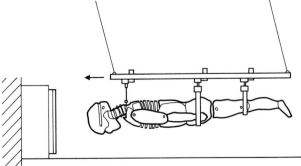

groups concluded that helmets are ineffective in head-first collisions because of the high energy levels and the relative stiffness of the helmet compared to the neck. The first condition leads to the second. The high energy causes the helmet liner to bottom out and become almost rigid before the large torso mass has been brought to rest.

Another way to consider this impact situation is to model the system as two springs in series, one representing the helmet and the other the neck. The total stiffness of the system will be equal to or less than the stiffness of the softest spring. The research cited above and that of Bishop and Wells (1986) strongly suggest that for conditions of axial compressive loading, the neck is a softer spring than the helmet. Thus, the forces experienced by the neck will be dictated principly by the properties of the neck and the helmet does not have a large influence. The helmet would have to be much less stiff than at present and would have to maintain that low stiffness under very high loads. This is difficult without making the helmet much larger than it is now as was demonstrated by Wells *et al.* (1987) using a computer model of the ATD under axial load. To produce a more uniform deceleration of the head—neck—torso system and to keep the force on the neck to a reasonable level of 2000 N, from an impact velocity of only 3 m·s^{-1}, would require a padding thickness of 13.4 cm. Obviously, this is not compatible with many sporting activities and other ways of providing protection against this type of injury situation must be sought.

Conclusion

This chapter has considered the requirements necessary for appropriate biomechanical evaluations of protective equipment for the head and face and has considered the complexity of protecting the cervical spine. Appropriate biomechanical evaluation requires test conditions that simulate as nearly as possible the actual injury-producing mechanism.

For sport helmets, several test protocols have

been developed that utilize different test rigs, headforms, energy levels and failure criteria. Where standards have been developed to evaluate the helmet's ability to protect against blunt trauma, it appears that the risk of head injury has been substantially reduced.

The use of dynamic tests for evaluating eye protectors in ice hockey and the racquet sports has likewise reduced the risk of serious eye injuries for those who wear the devices. Unfortunately, there are many players who do not wear eye or facial protection and serious injuries, including blindness, persist in this group.

The need for appropriate simulations and biomechanical evaluations is particularly important when considering protection of the cervical spine against excessively high compression forces. Attempting to predict neck forces on the basis of helmet drop tests or attempting to provide protection to the neck by increased padding materials placed in the crown of the helmet are not appropriate because both notions fail to consider the behaviour of the entire head—neck—torso system under impact. The forces needed to decelerate the torso in a crown-first impact are determined by the combined properties of the helmet or surface padding, the head, the neck and the torso and not by the helmet or padding materials alone. To maintain the compressive forces acting on the cervical spine in axial loading conditions within tolerable limits, the helmet would have to be much less stiff than at present and would have to maintain that low stiffness under very high loads. Both conditions are difficult to achieve without making the helmet disproportionately larger than it is now.

References

Alem, N.H., Nusholtz, G.S. & Melvin, J.W. (1984) Head and neck responses to axial impacts. In *Proceedings of the 28th Stapp Car Crash Conference*, Paper No. 841667. Society of Automotive Engineers, New York.

Bauze, R.J. & Ardran, G.M. (1978) Experimental production of forward dislocation in the human cervical spine. *J. Bone Joint Surg.* **60B**(2), 239–45.

Bishop, P.J. & Briard, B.D. (1984) Impact performance of bicycle helmets. *Can. J. Appl. Sport Sci.* **9**(2), 94–101.

Bishop, P.J., Kozey, J. & Caldwell, G. (1982) Performance of eye protectors for squash and racquetball. *Phys. Sportsmed.* **10**, 63–9.

Bishop, P.J. & Manton, J. (1987) *Injuries occurring in OUAA hockey during the 1986–87 season: a summary.* A report prepared for the Ontario Universities Athletic Association, Waterloo, Canada.

Bishop, P.J. & Wells, R.P. (1986) The Hybrid III anthropometric neck in the evaluation of head first collisions. In *Passenger Comfort Convenience and Safety Test Tools and Procedures*, Publication No. 174, pp. 131–40. Society of Automotive Engineers, Pennsylvania.

Bishop, P.J. & Wells, R.P. (1990) The inappropriateness of helmet drop tests in assessing neck protection in head first impacts. *Am. J. Sports Med.* **18**(2), 201–5.

Burstein, A.H., Otis, J.C. & Torg, J.S. (1982) Mechanics and pathomechanics of athletic injuries to the cervical spine. In J.S. Torg (ed) *Athletic Injuries to the Head, Neck and Face*, 1st edn, pp. 139–54. Lea & Febiger, Philadelphia.

Calvano, N.J. & Berger, R.E. (1979) Effects of selected test variables on the evaluation of football helmet performance. *Med. Sci. Sports* **11**(3), 293–301.

Clarke, K.S. (1991) An epidemiologic view. In J.S. Torg (ed) *Athletic Injuries to the Head, Neck and Face*, 2nd edn, pp. 15–27. CV Mosby, St Louis.

Corner, J.P., Whitney, C.W., O'Rourke, N. & Morgan, D.E. (1987) *Motorcycling and bicycle protective helmet requirements resulting from post crash study and experimental research.* Prepared for the Federal Office, of Road Safety, Canberra, Australia.

Cushman, R., Down, J., MacMillan, N. & Waclawik, H. (1990) Bicycle-related injuries: A survey in a paediatric emergency department. *Can. Med. Assoc. J.* **143**(2), 108–12.

Easterbrook, M. (1978) Eye injuries in squash: A preventable disease. *Can. Med. Assoc. J.* **118**, 298–305.

Easterbrook, M. (1981) Eye injuries in racquet sports: A continuing problem. *Phys. Sportsmed.* **9**, 91–101.

Fan, W.R. (1971) Internal head injury assessment. In *Proceedings of the 15th Stapp Car Crash Conference*, pp. 645–60. Society of Automotive Engineers, New York.

Fekete, J.F. (1968) Severe brain injury and death following minor hockey accidents: The effectiveness of the safety helmets of amateur hockey players. *Can. Med. Assoc. J.* **99**, 1234–9.

Gadd, C.W. (1966) Use of a weighted impulse criterion for estimating injury hazard. *Proceedings of the 10th Stapp Car Crash Conference*, pp. 164–74. Society of

Automotive Engineers, New York.

Gadd, C.W. (1972) *Report to society of automotive engineers sub committee.* Vehicle Research Department, General Motors Research Laboratory, Warren, Michigan.

Gennarelli, T.A. (1991) Cerebral concussion and diffuse brain injuries. In J.S. Torg (ed) *Athletic Injuries to the Head, Neck and Face*, 2nd edn, pp. 270–82. CV Mosby, St Louis.

Genovese, M.T., Lenzo, N.P., Lim, R.K., Morkel, D.R. & Jamrozik, K.D. (1990) Eye injuries among pennant squash players and their attitudes toward protective eyewear. *Med. J. Australia* **153**, 655–8.

Gerberich, S.G., Finke, R., Madden, M., Priest, J.D., Aamoth, G. & Murray, K. (1987) An epidemiological study of high school ice hockey injuries. *Child Nerv. System* **3**, 59–64.

Gurdjian, E.S., Hodgson, V.R., Hardy, W.G., Patrick, L.M. & Lissner, H.R. (1964) Evaluation of the protective characteristics of helmets in sports. *J. Trauma* **5**, 309–24.

Gurdjian, E.S., Roberts, V.L. & Thomas, L.M. (1966) Tolerance curves of acceleration and intracranial pressure and protective index in experimental head injury. *J. Trauma* **6**(5), 600–4.

Hodgson, V.R. (1957) National operating committee on standards for athletic equipment football helmet certification program. *Med. Sci. Sports* **7**(3), 225–32.

Hodgson, V.R. (1982) A standard for protective equipment. In J.S. Torg (ed) *Athletic Injuries to the Head, Neck and Face*, 1st edn, pp. 27–35. Lea & Febiger, Philadelphia.

Hodgson, V.R. (1983) Approaches and evaluative techniques for helmets. In D.A. Winter, R.W. Normen, R.P. Wells, K.C. Hayes & A.E. Patlo (eds) *Biomechanics IXB*, pp. 161–6. Human Kinetics, Champaign, Illinois.

Hogdson, V.R. (1989) *Prevention of focal and diffuse head injuries.* Presented at the 2nd Symposium on the Prevention of Catastrophic Sports and Recreational Injuries to the Spine and Head, Toronto.

Hodgson, V.R. (1991) Impact standards for protective equipment. In J.S. Torg (ed) *Athletic Injuries to the Head, Neck and Face*, 2nd edn, pp. 28–43. CV Mosby, St Louis.

Hodgson, V.R. & Thomas, L.M. (1972) Effect of long-duration impact on the head. In *Proceedings of 16th Stapp Car Crash Conference*, pp. 292–5. Society of Automotive Engineers, New York.

Hodgson, V.R. & Thomas, L.M. (1980) Mechanism of cervical spine injury during impact to the protected head. In *Proceedings of the 24th Stapp Car Crash Conference*, Paper No. 801300. Society of Automotive Engineers, New York.

Jørgensen, U. & Schmidt-Olsen, S. (1986) The epidemiology of ice hockey injuries. *Br. J. Sports Med.*

20(1), 7−9.

Lane, J.C. (1986) *Helmets for child bicyclists: Some biomedical consideration.* Prepared for the Federal Office of Road Safety, Canberra, Australia.

Long, G.J., Dowdell, B. & Griffiths, M. (1989) *Development of a localized loading test for pedal cycle helmets.* Prepared for the Road Safety Bureau, New South Wales.

Lorentzon, R., Wedren, H. & Pietila, T. (1988) Incidence, nature and causes of ice hockey injuries. *Am. J. Sports Med.* 16(4), 392−6.

McElhaney, J.H., Doherty, B.J., Paver, J.G., Meyers, B.S. & Gray, L. (1988) Combined bending and axial loading responses to the human cervical spine. In *Proceedings of the 33rd Stapp Car Crash Conference*, pp. 21−8. Society of Automotive Engineers, New York.

McElhaney, J.H., Paver, J.G., McCrakin, H.J. & Maxwell, G.M. (1983) Cervical spine compression responses. In *Proceedings of the 27th Stapp Car Crash Conference*, Paper No. 831615. Society of Automotive Engineers, New York.

McElhaney, J.H., Snyder, R.G., States, J.D. & Gabrielson, M.A. (1979) Biomechanical analysis of swimming pool injuries. In *The Human Neck: Anatomy, Injury Mechanisms and Biomechanisms*, Publication No. SP-438. Society of Automotive Engineers, New York.

Mertz, H.J., Hodgson, V.R., Thomas, L.M. & Nyquist, G.W. (1978) An assessment of compressive neck loads under injury producing conditions. *Phys. Sportsmed.* 6(11), 95−106.

Mill, N.J. (1990) Protective capability of bicycle helmets. *Br. J. Sports Med.* 24(1), 55−60.

Mohan, D., Bowman, B.M., Snyder, R.G. & Forest, D.R. (1979) A biomedical analysis of head impact injuries to children. *J. Biomech. Eng.* 101, 250−9.

Newman, J.A. (1975) On the use of the head injury criterion (HIC) in protective headgear evaluation. In *Proceedings from the 19th Stapp Car Crash Conference*, pp. 615−41. Society of Automotive Engineers, New York.

Norman, R.W. (1983) Biomechanical evaluations of sports protective equipment. In *Exercise and Sport Science Reviews*, Vol. 11, pp. 232−74. Franklin Institute Press, Philadelphia.

Nusholtz, G.S., Melvin, J.W., Huelke, D.F., Alem, N.M. & Black, J.G. (1981) Response of the cervical spine to superior-inferior head impact. In *Proceedings of the 25th Stapp Car Crash Conference*, Paper No. 811005. Society of Automotive Engineers, New York.

Ommaya, A.K. (1988) Mechanisms and preventive management of head injuries: a paradigm for injury control. In *32nd Annual Proceedings of the Association for the Advancement of Automotive Medicine*,

pp. 360−91. Society of Automotive Engineers, Worrendale, Philadelphia.

Pashby, T. (1977) Eye injuries in Canadian hockey. Phase II. *Can. Med. Assoc. J.* 117, 671−8.

Pashby, T. (1979) Eye injuries in Canadian hockey. Phase III: Older players now most at risk. *Can. Med. Assoc. J.* 121, 643−4.

Pashby, T. (1985) Eye injuries in Canadian amateur hockey. *Can. J. Ophthalmol.* 20(1) 2−4.

Pashby, T., Pashby, R.C., Chisholm, L.D.J. & Crawford, J.S. (1975) Eye injuries in Canadian hockey. *Can. Med. Assoc. J.* 113, 663−6.

Patrick, L.M., Lissner, H.R. & Gurdjian, E.S. (1963) Survival by design − Head protection. In *Proceedings of 7th Stapp Car Crash Conference*, pp. 171−82. Society of Automotive Engineers, New York.

Posch, E., Haglund, Y. & Eriksson, E. (1989) Prospective study of concentric and eccentric leg muscle torques, flexibility, physical conditioning and variation of injury rates during one season of ice hockey. *Int. J. Sports Med.* 2(10), 113−17.

Prasad, P. & Mertz, H.J. (1985) *The position of the United States delegation to the ISO Working Group 6 on the use of HIC in the automotive environment*, Technical Paper No. 851246. Society of Automotive Engineers, Philadelphia.

Roaf, R. (1960) A study of the mechanics of spinal injuries. *J. Bone Joint Surg.* 42B(4), 115−39.

Sances jr, A., Myklebust, J. & Marmain, D. (1984) Biomechanics of spinal injuries. CRC critical review. *Biomed. Eng.* 11, 1−76.

Schneider, R.C. & Nahum, A.M. (1972) *Impact studies of facial bones and skull*, Paper No. 720965. Research Laboratories, General Motors Co., Warren, Michigan.

Tator, C.H. & Edmonds, V.E. (1984) National survey of spinal injuries in hockey players. *Can. Med. Assoc. J.* 140, 875−80.

Thompson, R.S., Rivara, F.P. & Thompson, D.C. (1989) A case-control study of the effectiveness of bicycle safety helmets. *N. Engl. J. Med.* 320, 1361−7.

Torg, J.S. (1985) Epidemiology, pathomechanics and prevention of athletic injuries to the cervical spine. *Med. Sci. Sports Exerc.* 17(3), 295−303.

Torg, J.S., Truex, R., Quedenfeld, T.C., Burstein, A., Spealman, A. & Nichols, C. (1979) National football head and neck registry: Report and conclusions. *JAMA* 241, 1477−9.

Torg, J.S., Vegso, J., O'Neill, M. & Sennett, B. (1990) The epidemiologic, pathologic, biomechanical and cinematographic analysis of football induced cervical spine trauma. *Am. J. Sports Med.* 18(1), 50−7.

Versace, J. (1971) A review of the severity index. In *Proceeding of the 15th Stapp Car Crash Conference*, pp. 771–97. Society of Automotive Engineers, New York.

Vinger, P.F. (1981) Sports eye injuries — a preventable disease. *Ophthalmology* **88**, 108–13.

Vinger, P.F. & Toplin, D.W. (1978) Racquet sports: An occular hazard. *JAMA* **239**, 2575–7.

Wells, R.P., Bishop, P.J. & Stephens, M. (1987) Neck loads during head first collisions in ice hockey: experimental and simulations results. *Int. J. Sport Biomech.* **3**(4), 432–42.

Yoganandan, N., Scances, A., Pintar, F., Maiman, D., Cusik, J.F. & Larson, S.J. (1990) Injury biomechanics of the human cervical spine column. *Spine* **15**(10), 1031–9.

Chapter 29

Prophylactic Knee and Ankle Orthoses

JOHN L. PINKOWSKI AND LONNIE E. PAULOS

In sports the two most frequently injured joints are the knee and ankle. A proven orthotic device that would support these joints and limit or prevent injury without affecting sports performance would be a great benefit. In 1984, the American Academy of Orthopaedic Surgeons (AAOS) Sports Medicine Committee held a seminar to evaluate bracing (Drez, 1985). This committee recommended a classification of bracing as follows:

1 Prophylactic braces — those designed to prevent or reduce the severity of injury.

2 Rehabilitative braces — those designed to protect injured joints treated operatively or non-operatively.

3 Functional — those designed to provide stability for unstable joints.

Strict adherence to the above classification of braces has not always been possible. This is illustrated by the use of functional knee braces in an effort to prevent injury, thus by definition becoming a prophylactic brace.

The AAOS committee for evaluation of prophylactic braces developed seven ideal goals or qualities which these braces should strive for.

1 The brace should increase the stiffness of the knee to prevent injury from contact and non-contact stresses.

2 It should not interfere with normal function.

3 It should not increase injury elsewhere in the lower extremity.

4 It should adapt to various anatomical shapes and sizes.

5 It should not be harmful to other players.

6 It should be cost-effective and durable.

7 It should have documented efficacy in preventing injuries.

A brief description of brace design is helpful in understanding the differences among products. Most prophylactic knee braces are designed to protect the knee from a direct blow to the lateral aspect of the knee, thus shielding it from a valgus force. These braces are designed to reduce the resilient force on the collateral and cruciate ligaments. Most of these braces consist of a lateral bar with a single axis (Fig. 29.1a), dual axis (Fig. 29.1b) or polycentric hinge. However, experimentally no current hinge design simulates normal knee motion in all degrees of freedom (Regalbuto et al., 1989). Fewer braces incorporate medial and lateral bars with hinges and rigid plastic shells that encircle the thigh and calf (Fig. 29.2); an example of such a brace is the Iowa knee orthosis (Am Pro knee guard, American Prosthesis, West Branch, Iowa). This latter brace is larger and heavier than single-hinged braces without shells, and more closely resembles a rehabilitative or functional brace.

Some manufacturers place significant emphasis on the knee hinge design. It is important to note that accurate hinge placement in application of the brace is more important than hinge kinematics (Rarick et al., 1962). Lew (1982) found that there was greater variation in forces with reapplication of the brace than there was as a result of various hinge designs.

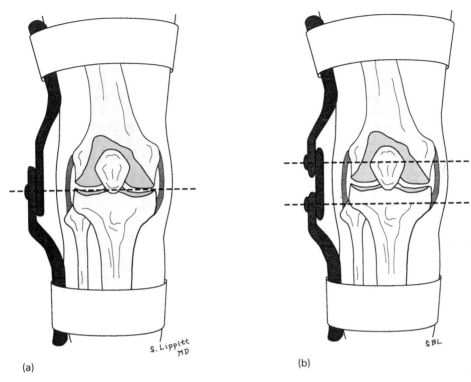

(a)   (b)

Fig. 29.1 (a) An example of a single-axis hinged prophylactic knee brace. (b) An example of a dual-axis hinged prophylactic knee brace. Courtesy of Dr S. Lippitt.

Most of the current literature on prophylactic braces focuses on the prevention of injuries of the knee due to a lateral impact. Fewer articles address prophylaxis of ankle injuries. The goal of this chapter is to evaluate the current information concerning the prevention of injury by the use of prophylactic knee and ankle orthoses. More importantly, the variables, materials, methods and statistics used in current research will be discussed to allow the reader to assess critically the value of continued research in this area.

Prophylactic knee braces

Prophylactic knee bracing is an issue clouded by flawed research, legal concerns, anecdotal testimony and emotions. Knee injuries can devastate a player for a prolonged period of time and may even herald an early end to an athletic career. In the 1980s several orthotic manufacturers developed braces that claimed to prevent knee injuries, specifically those injuries that occurred from a lateral impact. Without evidence of their effectiveness or safety, these prophylactic braces were marketed and gained popularity among athletes and teams. Some teams even mandated their use as a prerequisite to participation.

Current research continues to evaluate and develop protective gear in sports, with the desire to produce an orthotic that may prevent or reduce injuries to the knee. In this section, we will summarize the current knowledge on knee bracing. The difficulties in establishing a clear understanding of the effectiveness of prophylactic knee bracing will also be pointed out.

Most studies have evaluated brace usage in American football and can be divided into two

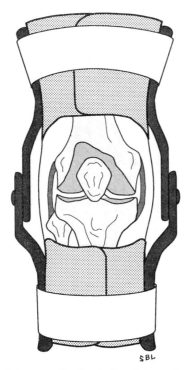

SBL

Fig. 29.2 An example of a single-axis hinged prophylactic knee brace with bilateral uprights and rigid plastic shells that encircle the thigh and calf, similar to the Iowa knee orthosis. Courtesy of Dr S. Lippitt.

broad categories: (i) clinical studies; and (ii) biomechanical studies.

Clinical studies

Several clinical and epidemiological studies have been published (Anderson *et al.*, 1979; Taft *et al.*, 1985; Whitesides *et al.*, 1985; Hewson *et al.*, 1986; France *et al.*, 1987; Garrick & Requa, 1987; Paulos *et al.*, 1987; Rovere *et al.*, 1987; Teitz *et al.*, 1987; Grace *et al.*, 1988; Sitler *et al.*, 1990). A review of the authors' conclusions would indicate that there is no agreement on the use of prophylactic bracing. Three studies found favourable results with brace use (Anderson *et al.*, 1979; Taft *et al.*, 1985; Sitler *et al.*, 1990), three studies found unfavourable results with brace use (Rovere *et al.*, 1987; Teitz

et al., 1987; Grace *et al.*, 1988), and one showed no significant differences with brace use (Hewson *et al.*, 1986).

After analysing each study carefully, a multitude of variables are found to exist which may invalidate conclusions drawn from these studies. Future reduction of these variables experimentally or statistically would yield more useful data and conclusions.

A standard definition of 'injury' is essential for comparing different studies. Definitions based on lost time from play can vary depending on the time period included. The time lost from games alone is different from the time lost from both practices and games. Alternatively, a significant injury may be defined by those needing surgery, which may be biased by the physician involved in treatment.

The timing of an injury may be critical in its inclusion in a study. For example, an injury that occurred on the last play of a game or the season may not fulfil a time lost criteria and therefore be excluded from analysis. Whitesides *et al.* (1985) feel that the 'time lost' method has an inherent deficiency because severe injuries occurring at the end of a season would not result in as many days lost as they would have if they occurred early in the season. Variable treatment time determined by the physician before returning the player to his or her sport can also introduce error in the time lost method.

Accurate assessment of the type of ligament injury and its severity are mandatory and require standardization. Even with standard grades of injury, there will still be interexaminer error. Injuries often are reported by a combination of trainers, coaches or physicians, each with varying levels of expertise.

Those studies examining injuries in different time periods are subject to errors stemming from changes in the coaching, equipment, rules, weather conditions, physicians and injury treatment methods in the different periods (Taft *et al.*, 1985; Hewson *et al.*, 1986; Rovere *et al.*, 1987).

Studies during the same time period must clearly indicate which players are receiving the brace and how they were selected (Teitz *et al.*, 1987; Grace *et al.*, 1988; Sitler *et al.*, 1990). Comparisons between braced and unbraced players should include matched controls in height, weight, skill level, player position, amount of time played, shoe type, manufacturer of the brace, and prior ligament injury history.

Several variables must be monitored in the braced group. A method of verifying compliance in the use and proper fit of the brace before and during the competition is imperative. The type of field turf, natural or artificial, field condition, and local weather conditions also influence injury rate analysis. The 'school effect' has been described (Teitz *et al.*, 1987) as biasing individuals from a particular school to the chance of injury. The probability of an injury occurring in a player is dependent on several circumstances unique to that school, such as specific coaching techniques, play formations and field conditions.

Finally, definition of terms and statistical analysis can often influence the outcome of a particular set of circumstances. The rate of injury is often defined as a function of player exposures, although the actual amount of playing time is unknown. To minimize this effect, matching two players at the same skill level and position should account for the same amount of playing time or exposure. Teams that switch to bracing after a high number of injuries in the prior season may statistically see less injuries the following year. This regression toward the mean may be due to a naturally occurring fluctuation in the incidence of injuries from year to year. This lower rate would have no real relationship to brace usage.

The above variables enlighten the interested observer about the difficulties of undertaking clinical studies to determine the true usefulness of prophylactic braces. Although the individual importance of any one of the above variables may be insignificant alone, in combination they may distort the end result.

STUDIES IN DETAIL

In 1979, Anderson described a single-sided, dual-hinged brace used to prevent reinjury in 9 élite football players (1979). Anderson concluded that this brace was effective because none of these players had a recurrence of injury in a cumulative total of 29 games. This sparked an interest in producing prophylactic knee braces to protect football players' knees from a lateral impact.

In a study presented at the American Orthopaedic Society for Sports Medicine in 1985, Taft *et al.* reported a decrease in the number of injuries in braced players at the University of North Carolina at Chapel Hill (1985). Two separate and unequal periods of brace and nonbrace wear were compared. This conclusion was based on a 70% decrease in surgically treated medial collateral ligament (MCL) injuries. Although the same physician provided care during this 7-year period, evolving differences in recommended treatment for MCL injuries could have biased the end results.

Another early study evaluating prophylactic braces in collegiate football was published in 1986 (Hewson *et al.*, 1986). Hewson *et al.* examined two sequential 4-year periods at the University of Arizona in Tucson. Only linemen, linebackers and tight ends were braced using the Omni Anderson knee stabler (Omni Scientific, Martinez, California). Each player participating in a practice or game was considered an exposure, for approximately 30 000 exposures in each 4-year period. Anterior cruciate ligament (ACL), MCL and meniscal injuries were evaluated. The final conclusion was that the overall number, type and severity of knee injuries was similar in both groups, and no statistically significant differences existed. It was determined that each player in the high-risk positions (linemen, linebackers and tight ends) encountered a 23% chance of knee injury each season.

Rovere *et al.* (1987) reviewed injury rates in football players at Wake Forest University, North Carolina. Two consecutive periods of time consisting of 2 years each were evaluated, one in which the Omni Anderson knee stabler was used and one in which a brace was not used. Injuries of the ACL, MCL, lateral collateral ligament (LCL), meniscus and patellar dislocations were included. The rates of knee injuries were higher with bracing than without. The number of ACL injuries was too small in both groups to be statistically analysed, but three occurred in the brace group compared to one in the unbraced group. The incidence rate for all knee injuries, was 6.1 per 100 unbraced players and 7.5 per 100 braced players. In this particular study, offensive players sustained most of the knee injuries, particularly the offensive linemen. The defensive backs had the lowest injury incidence. Of lesser importance, but still a concern for comfort and compliance, was the observation that the braced group had a higher incidence of muscle cramping in the gastrocnemius−soleus complex. The authors felt this was probably secondary to compression of the calf from tight wrapping of the brace.

In 1987, Teitz *et al.* published a large epidemiological, multicentre study analysing National Collegiate Athletic Association Division I schools' reported incidence of injuries in the braced and unbraced athlete. They felt that a large sample size would dilute other inherent biases, such as the school effect. Two separate years were analysed with 71 schools participating in 1984, and 61 schools in 1985. The players were grouped according to position and the authors compared the incidence, type, severity, mechanism of injury in relation to the playing surface, type of brace worn, distribution of braces among players of various skill levels, and history of previous knee injuries.

Uncontrolled variables in this study included the use of different braces, various skill levels of those braced, uncertainty in brace assignment, fit and compliance. The most important variable and a fatal design flaw was examiner variability.

Schools that required all athletes to wear braces were compared to those in which no athletes wore braces. Schools which switched

from no brace wear to brace wear the following year were analysed separately to minimize the school effect.

In the overall data set for the 1984 and 1985 seasons, players who wore braces had a significantly higher rate of injury than players who did not. In 1984, an 11% injury rate occurred in braced players compared to a 6% rate for unbraced players and in 1985, a 9.4% injury rate compared to 6.4%.

Playing surface, skill level, type of brace, and mechanism of injury had no significant influence on injury rates. There appeared to be no difference in the frequency of ACL, meniscal or combination injuries. The number of injuries requiring surgery also showed no difference.

The time lost for each individual injury was shorter among the braced group but overall time lost was increased due to the increase in total numbers of injuries.

As noted previously, schools that switched to bracing after having a high injury rate from the previous year may see a reduction in injuries due to the year to year variance. Those schools in this study actually had a slightly higher incidence of injury during the braced years.

Teitz *et al.* arrived at the overall determination that players who wore knee braces had significantly more knee injuries than unbraced players, but there was no difference in severity of the injuries. Therefore use of these braces, in an attempt to prevent injury to collegiate football players, could not be recommended by these authors.

Grace *et al.* (1988) reviewed the injuries of 580 high-school football players in a combined experience in Albuquerque and Santa Fe, New Mexico. Injuries were determined over the same two seasons for the braced and unbraced groups. The subjects were matched for height, weight, position and playing level (varsity or junior varsity) but not skill level. The decision to brace or not to brace was made by the participant's parents. There were 247 players who used a single-hinged brace and 83 who used a double-hinged brace. The unbraced players consisted of 250 players. The 53 injuries that occurred, recorded by the time lost method, were significantly more frequent in the group with a single-hinged brace (37 of 247; 15%) compared to the unbraced control group (11 of 250; 4%). More injuries also occurred in the double-hinged braced group (5 of 83; 6%) but the difference was not proven statistically significant. An increased number of injuries occurred in the braced players in all categories of injury severity except patellar subluxation. Another observation in this study was that the braced group suffered more foot and ankle injuries in the ipsilateral limb.

One of the most recent and best controlled clinical studies was performed at West Point Military Academy by Sitler et al. (1990). A prospective, randomized study was accomplished under rigidly regulated conditions. The study encompassed 1396 military cadets consisting of 21 570 athlete exposures in 1986 and 1987, where the playing surface, shoe type, athlete exposure, knee injury history and brace assignment were controlled either experimentally or statistically. All braced subjects utilized the same type of brace, the Don Joy protector knee guard (Don Joy, Carlsbad, California). Prior to each game or practice, each individual was checked for the brace, brace fit and shoe type. A knee injury constituted the inability to play football 1 day after injury. Sitler et al. concluded that the use of prophylactic knee braces significantly reduced the frequency of knee injuries, both in the number of MCL injuries and the total number of injured subjects. The frequency of knee injuries was 1.5 per 1000 exposures in the braced group compared to 3.4 per 1000 in the unbraced group. The reduction in the frequency of knee injuries was dependent on player position. Defensive players were seen to benefit most from bracing while no statistically significant differences were seen in the offensive players. Although the frequency of injuries was reduced in the defensive players, the overall severity of injuries was not significantly reduced with the use of prophylactic knee braces. Retrospec-

tively, Sitler et al. reviewed their injury data and did not observe any significant difference in the frequency of ankle injuries between the braced and unbraced groups.

Biomechanical studies

Since injuries to the MCL are quite common in contact sports, biomechanical investigations of the MCL with or without a lateral knee brace to decrease medial joint opening continue. These studies examine parametric data to determine the effectiveness of prophylactic braces in the laboratory, particularly those observations from lateral impact to the knee (Rarick et al., 1962; Baker et al., 1987; France et al., 1987; Paulos et al., 1987; Baker et al., 1989; Brown et al., 1990; France & Paulos, 1990). Most biomechanical studies investigate a specific loading condition. The test results are valid only under those conditions evaluated and cannot be extrapolated to other situations. Since there may be several mechanisms of injury to the knee, a brace designed according to one test condition may not be helpful in preventing injury under changing conditions of knee position, axial load and rotation. The test loads should simulate on the field conditions as closely as possible. Testing at low loads may not yield information useful enough to extrapolate to high-impact situations.

France et al. (1987) and France and Paulos (1990) produced a two-part study to determine the effectiveness of current braces. Part 1 of the study evaluated ligament tensions and joint displacements in cadaver knees at static, non-destructive valgus forces and low-rate destructive forces. They documented that the tension required to disrupt the MCL was higher or equal to ligament tensions in the ACL or posterior cruciate ligament (PCL). This indicates that a degree of ACL or PCL damage occurs at forces that disrupt the MCL. The amount of medial joint opening required to injure the MCL was found to be 7 mm and total disruption occurred at 15 mm. Hence, for a brace to be effective it must restrict the medial joint

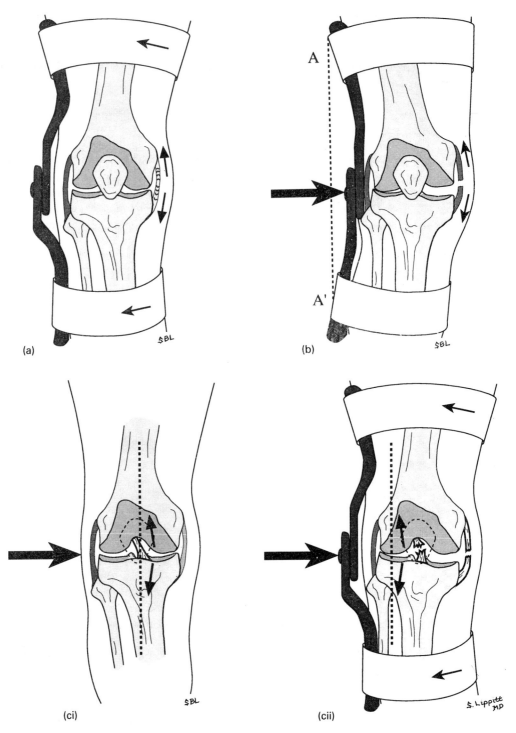

Fig. 29.3 (a) With the application of a prophylactic brace, an increase in the resting tension of the medial collateral ligament is seen. (b) Brace contact with the knee (large arrow) concentrates impact forces to the knee rather than allowing a broad distribution. This may lead to medial collateral ligament rupture (small arrows). (ci) In the unbraced knee, the axis of rotation to valgus stress (large arrow) occurs through the centre of the joint (small arrows). (cii) In the braced knee, the axis of rotation may be shifted to a lateral position (small arrows with dotted line), placing the anterior cruciate ligament under increased tension, perhaps leading to rupture.

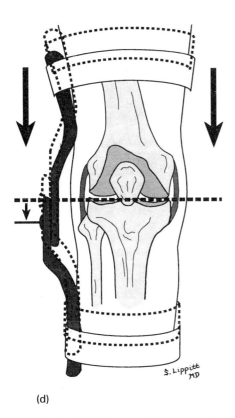

(d)

Fig. 29.3 *Continued* (d) Factors of ligament preload, premature joint line contact and centre axis shift may be worsened by slipping of the brace. Courtesy of Dr S. Lippitt.

opening below these values. After determining the contribution to valgus restraint of the individual ligaments, the effects of two prophylactic braces, the McDavid knee guard (MKG) (Clarendon Hills, Illinois) and the Omni Anderson knee stabler (Omni Scientific, Martinez, California), applied to cadaver knees were analysed. At low-rate dynamic loads, neither prophylactic brace provided significant protection. The two braces tested were not rigid enough to reduce the amount of medial joint line opening necessary to prevent ligament damage and were less rigid than the knee itself.

Four potentially adverse effects associated with the use of these braces were noted.

1 *Ligament preload*. This represented an increase in static MCL strain with brace application. Preload was seen in cadavers *without* axial load (Fig. 29.3a).

2 *Joint line contact*. The premature contact of the brace hinge or bar with the lateral aspect of the knee joint can concentrate forces directly into the knee joint rather than allowing a broader distribution without the brace (Fig. 29.3b).

3 *Centre axis shift*. The brace could produce a shift in the axis of valgus rotation from the centre of the knee to a lateral point, placing the ACL under tension sooner than in the unbraced knee. The significance of this effect would depend on how far lateral the axis shifted, the degree of brace stiffness and soft tissue motion under the brace (Fig. 29.3c).

4 *Brace slippage*. The brace design and fixation to limbs with various alignment could result in brace slippage. A poor fitting brace may not provide its intended function and could potentiate factors 1, 2 and 3 listed above (Fig. 29.3d).

In part 2 of this study, France *et al.* (1987) used sophisticated techniques and a surrogate limb to determine the characteristics of an ideal brace. Several braces were tested under impact loading. Particular attention was given to the above four potential adverse conditions to evaluate their significance. A validated surrogate limb allowed a wide array of parametric tests to be performed including higher strain rates than previous research, varied impactor masses, multiple knee flexion angles, and a constrained or free limb. This surrogate knee provided a reproducible way to perform several tests that could not have been performed on cadavers. Cadaver specimens are marred by their marked variability except in matched pairs. There are differences in age, size, gender and joint geometry.

The impact safety factor (ISF) was also defined by these authors:

$$\text{ISF} = \frac{\text{MCL peak tension, unbraced/impact momentum, unbraced}}{\text{MCL peak tension, braced/impact momentum, braced}}.$$

The higher the ISF, the safer the brace. For

example, an ISF of 1.5 indicates that there is an increase of 50% in the amount of force required to cause ligament failure.

Detailed examination of brace biomechanical properties was performed. Six braces were tested, the Omni Anderson knee stabler, the MKG, the Don Joy knee guard, the Mueller brace (Mueller Sports Medicine Inc., Praire du Sac, Wisconsin), the Renegade (Tru-Fit Inc., Hayes, Kansas), and the Stromgren brace (Stromgren-Scott Inc., Hayes, Kansas).

The following results were obtained. No brace was successful in maintaining joint line clearance during impact even though several continued to provide some resistance to valgus force. Some of the braces permanently deformed prior to joint line contact and therefore lessened any positive effect. Overall, the braces were least effective for smaller mass, higher velocity impacts with free hip and ankle motion and the knee at 30° of flexion. These trends were consistent for all braces tested. Variability in other biomechanical factors occurred. For example, the Omni Anderson brace had poor energy absorption characteristics and poor force distribution characteristics, but transmitted a large amount of the applied load. In contrast, MKG exhibited a high degree of energy absorption and only moderate to poor performance in force distribution and transmission. The most effective brace was the Don Joy protector knee guard (ISF 1.51) and the least effective was the MKG (ISF 1.18). The order of effectiveness as determined by the parametric tests performed by these authors was as follows: Don Joy, Tru-Fit, Omni Anderson and Stromgren, Mueller and MKG. No brace met minimum safety standards for all test conditions and some braces scored well in one category and poorly in another.

Several other conclusions were drawn from their work. First, MCL preload was found to be negated during joint compression forces in the four braces tested (MKG, Omni Anderson knee stabler, Don Joy and Stromgren). Second, by increasing the strain rate of the MCL, the failure force was found to increase progress-

ively. Third, on average only one brace tested exceeded the minimum ISF of 1.5 (Don Joy, ISF 1.51). Fourth, the current braces are best designed to protect the limb against high-mass, low-velocity injuries when the limb is fixed and near full extension. Whenever the limb is unconstrained and the knee is at 30° of flexion or more, the effects of bracing are negated. And last, it was discovered even under ideal conditions where a football player could see a lateral impact coming, a brace did not provide proprioceptive feedback to significantly protect the knee by muscular activation.

Paulos *et al.* concluded that a properly fit brace made of strong materials that did not slip or cause premature joint line contact, could be useful. Based on the braces tested in their study, they felt the braces provided limited protection against valgus injuries, and should not be routinely recommended to athletes. However, they would not deny access to properly designed braces if they were requested by the athlete, provided they are informed of the potential risks and have received proper instruction in application and fit.

Other authors have also evaluated prophylactic knee braces biomechanically. Brown *et al.* (1990) examined the Anderson, Am Pro (double upright), Magnum, Stromgren, Don Joy, MKG and Iowa (double upright). They found modest protection of the MCL by these braces. An increase in the failure loads of the MCL up to 20–30% was seen. The only significant difference in the braces was between the best performing (Omni Anderson) and the worst (MKG). The dual upright Iowa brace was found to perform better than the Am Pro, MKG and Don Joy in force to failure of the MCL. The Lenox Hill rehabilitative brace (Lenox Hill Brace Inc., Long Island City, New York) was found to have nearly twice the benefit than the prophylactic braces tested. The braces in this particular study were performed on the best situation for brace testing; knee in extension, foot fixed, hip partially constrained and high impactor mass.

Paulos *et al.* (1987), France *et al.* (1987) and

Brown *et al.* (1990) all found the MKG to provide substantially less protection than the other prophylactic braces tested.

Baker *et al.* (1989) examined several braces using cadaver knees. The functional braces evaluated were the CTi (Innovation Sports, Irvine, California), Don Joy, the Lenox Hill, PRO-AM (PRO-FIT Orthotics, Lynnfield, Massachusetts). The prophylactic braces tested were the Omni Anderson knee stabler and the MKG. The braces were tested under various conditions of knee flexion angle, foot fixation, impact masses and whether the knee had an intact or cut MCL. In the light of the deficiencies associated with cadaver models, several statements were determined by these experiments. Functional braces were found to have some capacity to control medial joint opening while prophylactic braces did not. The effect of the braces was less with the MCL cut. Oblique loading of the brace and knee flexion further reduced the capacity of the braces to provide a protective effect on the MCL. There was an increased ACL load above the measurement obtained without bracing. This suggests a preload effect on the ACL which may put it at risk for injury. Based on their results, Baker *et al.* could not advocate the prophylactic knee braces they tested.

As seen from the above clinical, epidemiological and biomechanical studies evaluating prophylactic knee braces, further research is necessary to define their true role in athletics. As we continue to learn more about the function of these braces with properly designed research, future generations of prophylactic knee braces will serve their intended purpose.

Ankle injury prophylaxis

The ankle is the second most commonly injured joint in sports, comprising 10–15% of all football injuries (Garrick, 1977). Ankle taping and ankle orthoses have been commonly used to help protect the ankle from injury (Fig. 29.4). Few studies have evaluated the effectiveness of these devices and these will be reviewed in the

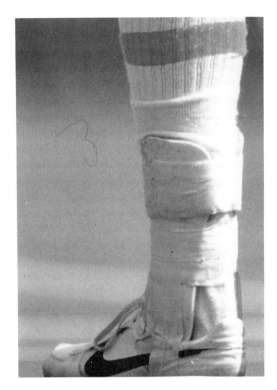

Fig. 29.4 Figure shows an example of an ankle orthosis used in an Olympic competition. Courtesy of the IOC archives.

following section. Further research is necessary to define their value and continued scientific investigation in this area is encouraged.

The research in examining the usefulness of ankle protectors has been primarily performed in a combination of clinical and biomechanical studies. The most commonly assessed parameter in these studies is ankle motion. It is thought intuitively that decreasing ankle motion will decrease ankle injuries. In order for motion data to be useful, the range of motion observed must be reproducible within the study and between studies. Range of motion should be determined in the pre-exercise, immediate post-taping or bracing, and post-exercise periods using standardized exercise routines. Most research describes the change in motion of the supported ankle but studies evaluating the on-field results are few. The sources of experimental error noted in the discussion of prophylactic knee braces can be applied to the following discussion of ankle injury supports.

In one of the earliest studies of ankle taping, Quigley *et al.* (1946) determined that taping could reduce the lateral mobility of the ankle without significantly affecting ankle dorsiflexion and plantar flexion. Rarick *et al.* (1962) determined that the taping technique with the greatest support was a combination of a basket weave, stirrup and heel lock pattern. This study noted that taping lost 40% of its initial support after 10 min of exercise. Malina *et al.* (1963) confirmed that after exercise for 5 min, there was a significant reduction in the protection provided by taping.

Other studies also confirm that the initial support provided by taping lessens during exercise. Glick *et al.* (1976) discovered that the talus was held firmly in the ankle mortise for no more than 20 min of exercise. Laughman *et al.* (1980) used electrongoniometers to measure the three-dimensional ankle motion of 20 subjects. Initial measurements indicated that taping does restrict motion associated with inversion ankle sprains. An average reduction in ankle motion by 18.6% was found between the untaped and taped ankle after 15 min of exercise in the motion parameters studied.

Fumich *et al.* (1981) used an Inman ankle device to measure several effort dependent motions of the ankle before taping, after taping, and after a 2.5–3-h football practice. Inversion with the ankle in the neutral or plantar flexed position had restriction of 50% of motion after exercise compared to pre-exercise. The sources of error in this particular study include the use of active instead of passive motion, which is effort dependent, and a lack of standardized exercise regimen. Myburgh *et al.* (1984) evaluated 12 squash players who competed in two matches with their ankles taped using a combination of basket weave, stirrup and heel lock taping applied to the skin. Two elastic ankle supports were also evaluated, which were the Futuro ankle brace (Jung Products, Cincinnati,

Ohio) and the Ace ankle support (Becton Dickinson, Rochelle Park, New Jersey). Prior to exercise, taping was found to provide up to 40% restriction of ankle motion but after 1 h of exercise, there was only up to 10% residual restriction of ankle motion. Maximal loosening occurred between 10 min and 1 h after exercise commenced. The elastic ankle supports did not provide significant support for any of the motions measured before, during and after exercise.

Hughes and Stetts (1983) reported that ankle taping and a custom, semirigid orthosis demonstrated a comparable decrease in support following 20 min of exercise. They did not compare differences between pre-exercise and postexercise motion or between postexercise motion and motion prior to application of the ankle support.

Bunch *et al.* (1985) attempted to evaluate the effectiveness of cloth and semirigid supports and taping. Tape offered the strongest initial support but there was no significant differences in motion between the supports after 305 inversion cycles to the ankles. Biomechanical testing using an instrumented foot ankle model showed that after a period of 20 min of cyclic stress there was a 21% reduction in support by taping, up to 8.5% reduction in support by cloth laced braces and no significant difference between the two.

Gross *et al.* (1987) compared ankle taping and a semirigid orthosis for restricting ankle motion using a Cybex II (Cybex, Division of Lumex Inc., Ronkonkoma, New York) apparatus. Postapplication and postexercise ankle motion were significantly less for both support systems compared with preapplication ankle motion. After 10 min of standardized exercise, inversion motion was significantly greater than pre-exercise motion for the ankle taping. The semirigid orthoses limited ankle motion significantly more than ankle taping following running.

Greene and Wight (1990) compared the support provided by the Aircast ankle training brace (Aircast Inc., Summit, New Jersey),

Swede-O-Universal ankle support (Swede-O-Universal, North Branch, Minnesota), and the ankle ligament protector brace before, during and after exercise. Their results indicate that the support provided by the Swede-O-Universal ankle support was reduced significantly following a 90-min softball practice. Most of the support loss occurred during the initial period of exercise. The ankle ligament protector brace demonstrated no loss of support with exercise. The Aircast ankle training brace demonstrated some loss of inversion support but no loss of eversion support. The investigators did not compare the preapplication and postexercise data to see if the support systems provided significant restriction of motion despite loosening that occurred during exercise. No comparisons were made among the postexercise data to clarify which support systems provided the greatest limitation of motion. The investigators also did not report what activities were involved in the 90-min softball practice. Different subjects were assigned to each of three ankle orthoses groups, and there was no assurance that the intensity and duration of stress imposition on the orthoses were equal among the groups.

Gross *et al.* (1991) compared two ankle orthoses Aircast sport stirrup and Swede-O-Universal ankle support and ankle taping in the restriction of eversion−inversion before and after exercise. 16 athletes had their ankle motion measured by Biodex (Biodex Corporation, Shirley, New York) testing without any support, and after the support was applied before and after exercise. All three support systems significantly reduced these ankle motions before and after exercise. Eversion was found to increase significantly in all types of support and inversion increased the most in the taped ankles. Eversion restriction was similar in all three supports after exercise. Inversion measurements following exercise were less (more restriction) for the tape and Aircast systems than the Swede-O-Universal system. The Aircast support provided more eversion support than tape and the Swede-O-Universal sys-

tems which were comparable to each other. Taping loosened significantly after exercise while the Swede-O-Universal and Aircast did not. However, taping restricted inversion motion most immediately after application. After exercise, the taping and Aircast systems provided equal restriction of inversion, which was greater than the Swede-O-Universal support. The Aircast system provided the most support against eversion immediately after application. The restriction of eversion was significant even though loosening occurred with exercise in all three supports. Therefore all systems provide equal support against eversion injuries.

With regard to actual injury prevention, Garrick and Requa (1987) found a reduced risk of ankle injuries in those players who taped their ankles prophylactically compared to the untaped players. The risk was even less in those athletes wearing high-topped shoes. Those players without previous injuries who were not taped showed an injury rate twice that of the taped players and in those players with previous injuries who were not taped there was an injury rate four times greater than those taped. Unfortunately those athletes braced, the position played, skill level and playing time were not clearly defined.

Rovere *et al.* (1988) retrospectively compared ankle taping and ankle stabilizers in preventing injuries. These authors assessed the effectiveness of a laced ankle stabilizer in preventing injuries and reinjuries over six college football seasons. There were several variables in this study including player choice of ankle support and type of shoe used. 297 players were subjected to 51 931 exposures over 6 years. Tape was worn by 233 players during 38 658 exposures to injury and orthotic stabilizers were worn by 127 players during 13 273 exposures. Tape had been applied when 159 injuries and 23 reinjuries occurred, and a stabilizer had been worn when 37 injuries and one reinjury occurred. Overall, a player wearing ankle stabilizers incurred about a 40% lower risk of injury than a player wearing tape. The data suggested that ankle orthotic stabilizers were relatively more effective in preventing injuries regardless of the type of shoes, and that low-top shoes were relatively more effective in preventing injury, regardless of the type of ankle support. The combination allowing the fewest injuries overall was low-top shoes and laced ankle stabilizers. Although still to be proven, this combination may allow the player to periodically retighten the lacer during the exposure, given easier access by a low-top shoe. The deficiencies noted in this study include its retrospective nature, lack of control of who wore which support, lack of matching for skill level and player position, and lack of comparison to an unsupported ankle.

It has been established that different support systems restrict ankle motion to some degree during exercise. Ankle orthoses are easier to apply and can be adjusted during the sporting activity, whereas taping is more time consuming and requires a skilled individual in application. Further investigation in the clinical application and statistical reduction in injuries is required before recommendations of the universal use of ankle prophylactic supports can be made.

References

Anderson, G., Seman, S.C. & Rosenfeld, R.T. (1979) The Anderson knee stabler. *Phys. Sportsmed.* **7**, 125–7.

Baker, B.E., VanHanswyk, E., Bogosian, S. *et al.* (1987) A biomechanical study of the static stabilizing effect of knee braces on medial stability. *Am. J. Sports Med.* **15**(6), 566–70.

Baker, B.E., VanHanswyk, E., Bogosian, S.P., Werner, F.W. & Murphy, D. (1989) The effect of knee braces on lateral impact loading of the knee. *Am. J. Sports Med.* **17**(2), 182–6.

Brown, T.D., Hoeck, J.E. Van & Brand, R.A. (1990) Laboratory evaluation of prophylactic knee brace performance under dynamic valgus loading using a surrogate leg model. *Clin. Sports Med.* **9**(4), 751–62.

Bunch, R.P., Bednarski, K. & Holland, D. (1985) Ankle joint support: A comparison of reusable laced-on braces with taping and wrapping. *Phys. Sportsmed.* **13**(5), 59–62.

Drez, D.J. Jr (ed) (1985) *Knee Braces.* Seminar report.

The American Academy of Orthopaedic Surgeons, Chicago.

France, E.P. & Paulos, L.E. (1990) *In vitro* assessment of prophylactic knee brace function. *Clin. Sports Med.* **9**(4), 823–42.

France, E.P., Paulos, L.E., Jayaraman, G., Rosenberg, T.D. & Jaen, J. (1987) The biomechanics of lateral knee bracing. Part II: Impact response of the braced knee. *Am. J. Sports Med.* **15**(5), 430–8.

Fumich, R.M., Ellison, A.E., Guerin, G.J. *et al.* (1981) The measured effect of taping on combined foot and ankle motion before and after exercise. *Am. J. Sports Med.* **9**, 165–70.

Garrick, J.G. (1977) The frequency of injury, mechanism of injury, and epidemiology of ankle sprains. *Am. J. Sports Med.* **5**, 241–2.

Garrick, J.G. & Requa, R.K. (1973) Role of external support in the prevention of ankle sprains. *Med. Sci. Sports Exerc.* **5**, 200–3.

Garrick, J.G. & Requa, R.K. (1987) Prophylactic knee bracing. *Am. J. Sports Med.* **15**(5), 471–6.

Glick, J.M., Gordon, R.B. & Nishimoto, D. (1976) Prevention and treatment of ankle sprains. *Am. J. Sports Med.* **4**, 136–41.

Grace, T.G., Skipper, B.J., Newberry, J.C. *et al.* (1988) Prophylactic knee braces and injury to the lower extremity. *J. Bone Joint Surg.* **70**(A), 422–7.

Greene, T.A. & Wight, C.R. (1990) A comparative support evaluation of three ankle orthoses before, during and after exercise. *J. Orthop. Sports Phys. Ther.* **11**, 453–65.

Gross, M.T., Bradshaw, M.K., Ventry, L.C. & Weller, K.H. (1987) Comparison of support provided by ankle taping and semirigid orthosis. *J. Orthop. Sports Phys. Ther.* **9**, 33–9.

Gross, M.T., Lapp, A.K. & Davis, J.M. (1991) Comparison of Swede-O-Universal ankle support and Aircast sport-stirrup orthoses and ankle tape in restricting eversion–inversion before and after exercise. *J. Orthop. Sports Phys. Ther.* **13**(1), 11–19.

Hewson Jr, G.F., Mendini, R.A. & Wang, J.B. (1986) Prophylactic knee bracing in college football. *Am. J. Sports Med.* **14**(4), 262–6.

Hughes, L.Y. & Stetts, D.M. (1983) A comparison of ankle taping and a semirigid support. *Phys. Sportsmed.* **11**(4), 90–103.

Laughman, R.K., Carr, T.A., Chao, E.Y. *et al.* (1980) Three-dimensional kinematics of the taped ankle before and after exercise. *Am. J. Sports Med.* **8**, 425–31.

Lew, J.L., Patrnchak, C.M., Lewis, J.L. & Schmidt, J. (1982) A comparison of pistoning forces in orthotic knee joints. *Orthot. Prosthet.* **36**(2), 85.

Malina, R.M., Plagenzz, L.B. & Rarick, G.I. (1963) Effort of exercise upon the measurement supporting strength of cloth and tape ankle wraps. *Res. Q.*

34, 158−65.

Myburgh, K.H., Vaughan, C.L. & Isaacs, B.K. (1984) The effects of ankle guards and taping on joint motion before, during and after a squash match. *Am. J. Sports Med.* 12, 441−6.

Paulos, L.E., France, E.P., Rosenberg, T.D., Jayaraman, G., Abbott, P.J. & Jaen, J. (1987) The biomechanics of lateral knee bracing. Part I: Response of the valgus restraints to loading. *Am. J. Sports Med.* 15(5), 419−29.

Rarick, G.L., Bigley, G., Karst, R. *et al.* (1962) The measurable support of the ankle joint by conventional methods of taping. *J. Bone Joint Surg.* 44A, 1183−90.

Regalbuto, M.A., Rovick, J.S. & Walker, P.S. (1989) The forces in a knee brace as a function of hinge design and placement. *Am. J. Sports Med.* 17, 535−43.

Rovere, G.D., Clark, T.J., Yates, C.S. *et al.* (1988) Retrospective comparison of taping and ankle stabilizers in preventing ankle injuries. *Am. J. Sports Med.* 16, 228−33.

Rovere, G.D., Haupt, H.A. & Yates, C.S. (1987) Prophylactic knee bracing in college football. *Am. J. Sports Med.* 15(2), 111−16.

Sitler, M., Ryan, J., Hopkinson, W., Wheeler, J., Santomier, J., Kolb, R. & Polley, D. (1990) The efficacy of a prophylactic knee brace to reduce injuries in football: A prospective, randomized study at West Point. *Am. J. Sports Med.* 18, 310−15.

Taft, T.N., Hunter, S.L. & Funderburk, C.H. (1985) *Preventive lateral knee bracing in football.* Presented at the 11th Annual Meeting of the American Orthopaedic Society for Sports Medicine, Nashville, Tennessee, July, 1985.

Teitz, C.C., Hermanson, B.K., Kronmal, R.A. & Diehr, P.H. (1987) Evaluation of the use of braces to prevent injury to the knee in collegiate football players. *J. Bone Joint Surg.* 69A, 2−9.

Whitesides, J.A., Fleagle, S.B., Kalenak, A. *et al.* (1985) Manpower loss in football: A 12-year study at the Pennsylvania State University. *Phys. Sportsmed.* 13(1), 103−14.

Chapter 30

Prophylactic Athletic Taping

GREGORY E. LUTZ, RONNIE P. BARNES, THOMAS L. WICKIEWICZ AND PER A.F.H. RENSTRÖM

For many years health-care professionals have recognized the value of using medical tape in the treatment and prevention of athletic injuries. Traditionally, certified athletic trainers, physical therapists and physicians have had to rely upon intuition and trial and error to design safe and effective taping methods. Because of an increased awareness of the biomechanical and kinesiological factors that contribute to athletic injuries, sound scientific principles are now being applied to this realm of sports medicine in the hopes of improving the medical care of the athlete.

Indications

Tape may be applied to almost any area of the body to treat a wide variety of muscular strains, tendinitises and joint instabilities (Reid, 1992). Acutely, tape provides support, pain relief and oedema control to an injured limb and/or extremity. Taping is also useful subacutely in compressing damaged tissue and reducing the tensile forces on the healing ligaments and soft tissue during rehabilitation, allowing for early protected mobilization. Additional uses of tape include holding wound dressings in place, or securing protective pads, braces and other types of athletic equipment.

Prior to taping for therapeutic purposes, a thorough evaluation of the extent of tissue damage and an accurate diagnosis is required. Premature taping of fractures, dislocations or ligamentous instabilities may give athletes a false sense of security and can potentially lead to further tissue damage. Prophylactic taping is not a substitute for the proper conditioning and strengthening necessary for athletic competition. The specific goals of taping should be clearly defined. Communication between the physician, the athletic trainer and/or physical therapist, and the patient is crucial to attain the best results. The success of taping does not only depend upon the materials or methods used, but also upon the willingness of the athlete to be taped. He or she must understand the purpose of taping, the length of time the segment will be taped and any necessary precautions. Regardless of the segments immobilized or supported, the tape should feel comfortable and should not cause skin problems, pressure neuropathies or circulatory disturbances.

Because of the high prevalence of ankle injuries and the substantial amount of player time lost (Garrick & Requa, 1988), methods to prevent these injuries have received considerable attention. Prophylactic taping has become one of the most common methods employed to prevent ankle injuries, despite questions regarding its efficacy. Opponents of ankle taping have stated that it is expensive, time-consuming and essentially useless due to the reduced skin adherence and changes in the strength of tape after only a few minutes of exercise (Ferguson, 1973; Andreasson & Edberg, 1983).

Other studies have shown that prophylactic

ankle taping may play a role in decreasing the incidence of injuries. Garrick and Requa (1973, 1988) reported a decreased incidence of ankle sprains among college basketball players whose ankles were taped, in comparison to those who were not taped. Although the method of taping, the number of participants with a previous history of ankle sprains, and the degree of instability present was not reported, they felt that ankle taping was effective in preventing ankle injuries. In a prospective study, Lindenberger et al. (1985) studied the effects of taping the ankles of handball players and found a significant reduction in the number of ankle injuries sustained in the taped group when compared to the untaped group.

At one university it has been estimated that the cost of medical taping was over US$50 000 (Anderson et al., 1992). Because of such a high cost in terms of time and materials, attempts have been made to identify alternative methods to prevent ankle injuries in athletes. Hughes and Stetts (1976) reported no difference between ankle taping and the use of a semirigid orthosis in limiting excessive ankle inversion. In a retrospective review of college football players, Rovere et al. (1988) found that a laced ankle orthosis was more effective than taping in the prevention of ankle injuries. Gross et al. (1987) compared the support provided by ankle taping and a semirigid orthosis and found that, after exercise, the semirigid orthosis provided a significantly greater restriction of joint motion. They felt that a semirigid orthosis offered the potential advantages of decreased expense, easier application and the ability to be periodically retightened after exercise.

Taping biomechanics

There are a variety of factors which play a role in the potential efficacy of medical tape when used to restrict joint motion and prevent injury. These factors include: (i) the tensile strength and adhesive properties of the tape used and how these change with exercise; (ii) the precise orientation of tape strips relative to the joint axes of motion; (iii) the degree of underlying joint instability; and (iv) the amount of soft tissue surrounding the joint.

Andreasson et al. (1983) studied the mechanical properties of tape and found that the tensile strength of tape is approximately $75 \text{ N} \cdot \text{cm}^{-1}$ width. The elastic modulus of the 'elastic' tapes averaged $269 \text{ N} \cdot \text{cm}^{-1}$ compared to $1280 \text{ N} \cdot \text{cm}^{-1}$ for 'stiff' tapes. Attarian et al. (1983) tested isolated individual bone–ligament–bone specimens and demonstrated the following maximum load : failure relationships: deltoid, 714 N; anterior talofibular ligament, 139 N; calcaneofibular ligament, 346 N; and posterior talofibular ligament, 261 N. This data reaffirms the need for tape of sufficient strength and width to provide protection from ligamentous injury. Tape strength that is lower than the ultimate strength of the anterior talofibular ligament (139 N) would provide little protection during inversion injuries. Pope et al. (1987) in a biomechanical study comparing ankle taping methods, concluded that only the figure-of-eight taping with three or more wraps would have enough strength theoretically to withstand the large moments $(420 \text{ N} \cdot \text{m})$ created at the ankle during athletic activities. They felt that the changes in tape strength after loading was more the result of shear failure at the skin surface rather than actual breakage of the tape.

Studies have shown that initially tape restricts motion, loosens after exercise and then provides some residual restriction (Rarick et al., 1962; Laughman et al., 1980; Andreasson & Edberg, 1983; Fumich et al., 1983). Rarick et al. (1962) demonstrated that as much as 50% of the original supporting strength of medical tape is lost after only 10 min of exercise. In a three-dimensional kinematic analysis of ankle taping before and after exercise, Laughman et al. (1980) demonstrated that tape does restrict those motions associated with inversion ankle injuries; however, postexercise evaluations revealed generalized loosening of the tape. Whether or not the amount of residual restriction remaining after exercise is enough to provide adequate protection for the ankle ligaments is unknown. Theoretically, since the degree of injury may range from microtears of the collagen bundles to complete ligamentous rupture, even loosened tape may provide enough restriction of joint motion to limit injury severity. Certainly the clinical findings of Garrick and Requa (1973) would support this theory.

In general, because a wide range of plantar flexion is necessary to perform athletic activities, the goal of taping is to restrict motion in the frontal rather than sagittal plane. In theory, such restriction would reduce the varus or valgus moments at the subtalar axis, thereby reducing ligamentous stress during athletic activities. Wilkerson (1991) performed a biomechanical study that showed planar motion could be selectively affected depending upon the taping method used. It was shown that the addition of a subtalar sling to standard taping methods was twice as effective in restricting frontal plane motion as compared to sagittal plane motion. Although sagittal plane motion was also more restricted with this technique, he felt that for the ankle with chronic instability, the benefit of having nearly twice as much residual restriction of inversion would outweigh any decrease in performance that might be caused by the addition of a subtalar sling. In support of this statement, Larsen (1984) found that the best stabilizing effects of ankle taping were obtained in those ankles with the greatest degree of instability. Clearly a balance must be achieved between providing enough support to prevent joint injury, while allowing enough motion to perform high level athletic activities. These variables are highly dependent upon the skill and knowledge of the health-care professional applying the tape. Tape applied incorrectly might not only lead to a decrease in performance, but also may predispose the athlete for injury to the joint immobilized or other joints along the kinetic chain.

Tape correctly applied to a joint may act as an external ligament which aids in restricting excessive joint motion. The tape, like a ligament, is dependent upon its adherence at its origin and insertion. Areas such as the hand and ankle, where there is a minimum of soft tissue, favour maximum tape adherence. To attain maximum support and protection with taping, the joint must be positioned anatomically to counteract forces that contribute to injury patterns. For example, at the onset of normal stance, eversion is initiated creating a valgus moment at the subtalar joint (Perry, 1983). If the ankle were positioned in an inverted position, a varus moment would be created, which would be resisted by active contraction of the everting muscles. If these muscles are not strong enough to resist the moment or are delayed in recruitment, the tensile strength of the lateral ligaments may be exceeded, resulting in injury. One of the ways to prevent an inversion plantar–flexion ankle injury is to tape the joint in a neutral position with slight eversion. Based on this information, an athlete with calcaneovarus alignment would be at a higher risk for inversion ankle injuries and should be taped prophylactically.

Taping mechanisms

The exact mechanism or mechanisms behind the beneficial effects of taping have not been clearly defined. It is felt that joint instability cannot be defined on a purely mechanical basis. Studies have shown that patients with chronic ankle instability may also exhibit deficits in dynamic control (Freeman, 1965; Loos & Boelens, 1984; Karlsson & Andreasson, 1992). A differentiation is made between mechanical instability (due to pathology of the bony, cartilagenous and ligamentous structures) and functional instability (due to muscle weakness or delay in recruitment from proprioceptive abnormalities) (Freeman, 1965; Karlsson & Andreasson, 1992).

Karlsson and Andreasson (1992), in an electromyographic and mechanical analysis, found that the reaction time of the peroneal muscle group was significantly slower in patients with a history of ankle instability. The addition of tape to these ankles resulted in a significant improvement in the reaction time of the pero-neal muscles, particularly in those patients with the greatest degree of instability. The authors concluded that the mechanisms behind the function of ankle taping were to restrict not only extremes of joint motion, but also to en-hance proprioceptive feedback mechanisms and to shorten the recruitment time of the dynamic ankle stabilizers. This confirmed find-ings previously reported of the effectiveness of tape in facilitating peroneal muscle activity (Loos & Boelens, 1984).

Types of tapes

Medical tape is manufactured in various colours, widths and strengths. White and brown are the standard colours and the widths are usually 0.5 in (1 cm), 1 in (2.5 cm), 1.5 in (4 cm) and 3 in (7.5 cm). The strength of the tape is dependent upon the material used and the thread count (the number of threads per inch). The higher quality tapes are stronger, less affected by environmental conditions and, consequently, are usually more expensive. The tapes most commonly used for the treatment and prevention of athletic injuries are zinc ox-ide impregnated, rubber-backed linen that are either non-stretch or stretchable elastic. Some woven or fabric-backed tapes are used as surgical tapes and are considered to be hypoallergenic.

The linen non-stretch tape is traditionally used to tape ankles, feet, toes, wrists, hands and fingers. The elastic stretchable tapes are more commonly used to tape shoulders, arms, elbows and knees. These tapes are manufac-tured to be adaptable, contouring, lightweight and waterproof. All of these tapes unroll easily from a cardboard or plastic core of approxi-mately 1 in (2.5 cm) diameter. This design al-lows the health-care professional to place his or her fingers through the roll of tape to facilitate application. Tape is sensitive to extreme heat, cold and humidity and may not always unroll evenly. This may affect the modulation of press-ure by the person applying the tape and can

lead to a tourniquet effect. Tape should always be stored in a cool, dry place.

Tape should be applied directly to the skin to provide maximum support. Repeated daily taping may require the use of a thin polyester urethane foam underwrap to decrease skin ir-ritation. In either case, it is important to clean the skin with soap and water before applying tape. Dirt and debris can contribute to skin irritation. Body oils and preparations, such as lotions and petroleum jelly, will inhibit tape adherence. Hair removal from the area to be taped is also essential for good tape adherence. The area can be shaved with a safety razor or with electric hair shears or clippers. Hair should be removed even if underwrap is used.

A formula containing tincture of benzoin can be used to make the skin tacky and assist in prolonged tape adherence. These formulae are referred to as skin tougheners or tape adherents and are relatively safe. Occasionally an allergic reaction may occur, but these instances are rare.

Friction points, such as the dorsum of the foot and the Achilles tendon area, can be pro-tected with petroleum jelly and a 4 × 4 gauze or polyethylene pads applied to the area prior to the application of the underwrap. Tape should be applied neatly with a minimum of wrinkles which can lead to irritation and/or blisters.

Taping precautions

1 Tape should not be applied to individuals with known sensitivities to tape, its com-ponents or preparation items such as tape underwrap and tape adherents that contain tincture of benzoin.
2 Caution should be used in applying tape to individuals with circulatory insufficiency. Distal extremities may be prone to vascular compromise in these individuals. Taping a swollen extremity may also impede circulation.
3 The elderly and individuals with certain skin conditions may be prone to skin stripping or trauma to the stratum corneum or underlying tissues that may lead to secondary infection.

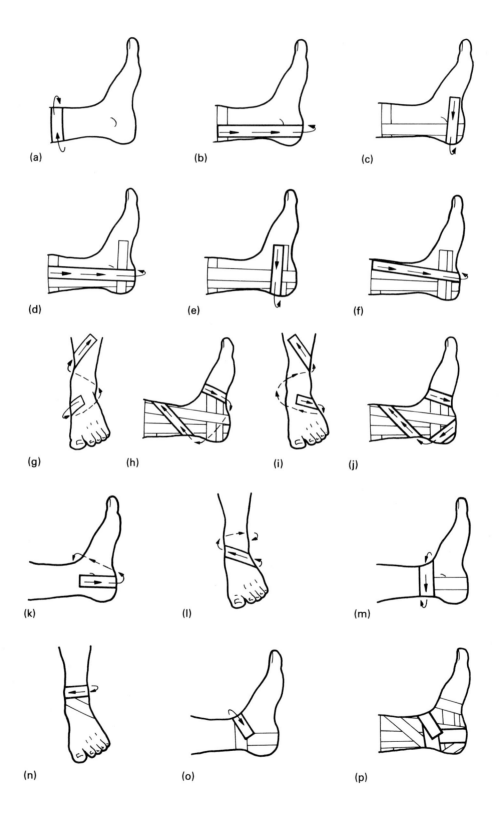

(a)   (b)   (c)

(d)   (e)   (f)

(g)   (h)   (i)   (j)

(k)   (l)   (m)

(n)   (o)   (p)

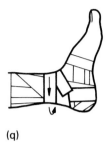
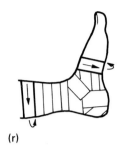

(q)　　　　　　　　　　　　　　(r)

Fig. 30.1 (*Left and above*) Basketweave ankle strapping. See text for details.

4 Taping can inhibit sweating and cause anhidrosis. Prolonged use of tape should be monitored for skin effects. The environment of prolonged tape application may encourage the growth of bacterial flora of the skin.

5 Significant restriction to the range of motion of joints may predispose an athlete to injury and impede performance.

6 Tape should never be applied to fractures or severely ruptured ligaments to allow athletes to participate prematurely.

7 Tape should always be removed with care and pulled slowly away from the skin to prevent skin trauma.

Taping methods

There are a variety of taping techniques used to treat and prevent athletic injuries (Reid, 1992). The following taping techniques are presented in a simple, step-by-step manner to promote ease of tape application. They are by no means all inclusive, but represent some of the taping techniques commonly used.

Basketweave ankle strapping

Purpose: Prevention of inversion ankle sprains.
Tape: 1.5 in (4 cm) or 2 in (5 cm) white zinc oxide linen non-stretch tape.
Comment: The tape is to be applied snugly, but not too tight with as few wrinkles as possible. Tape should overlap by 0.5 in (1 cm) to avoid gaps. At least one half the width of the tape should be applied to the skin. The use of tape adherent facilitates the tape to stick properly. Underwrap may be used.

TECHNIQUE

1 Anchor strip on leg (Fig. 30.1a) applied at the level of the musculotendinous junction of the Achilles tendon.

2 The first stirrup (Fig. 30.1b) begins on the medial side of the leg at the level of the anchor strip, proceeding under the heel and up the lateral side of the leg to the anchor strip. The leading edge of the tape should bisect the medial and lateral malleoli.

3 The first lateral strip starts at the midpoint of the arch of the foot medially (Fig. 30.1c), proceeds parallel to the sole of the foot around the back of the heel, ending laterally at the midpoint of the arch of the foot.

4 The second stirrup begins at the anchor medially (Fig. 30.1d), proceeding in the same direction as the first stirrup, but overlapping the first stirrup one half the width of the tape in the initial stirrup.

5 The second lateral strip starts medially at the same point as the first, the midpoint of the arch of the foot and follows the same route as the first lateral, but overlapping the first by one half the width of the tape (Fig. 30.1e).

6 The third stirrup begins medially at the anchor step one half the width of the second stirrup and proceeds under the calcaneus, making sure the leading edge of the tape does not go beyond the calcaneus. This may require angulation of the tape as shown in the figure

(Fig. 30.1f). The stirrup is ended on the lateral side of the leg at the level of the anchor strip and overlapping one half the width of the tape of the second strip.

7 The next strip is the first of two heel locks which begins on the dorsum of the foot at the instep (Fig. 30.1g), proceeds under the arch and side of the heel, behind the heel towards the anterior portion of the leg and ends on the leg above the ankle (Fig. 30.1h).

8 The second heel lock proceeds in the same manner as the first, but in the opposite direction (Fig. 30.1i,j).

9 A figure-of-eight is the next strip, beginning on the medial malleolus (Fig. 30.1k), going under the foot to the lateral side, up the instep (Fig. 30.1l), around the back of the ankle (Fig. 30.1m,n) to the instep, and ends on the medial aspect of the ankle (Fig. 30.1o,p).

10 The remaining strips are the lace-up and final anchors. Overlapping one half the width of the tape, starting just above the malleoli, the lace proceeds until the level of the top of the stirrups is reached (Fig. 30.1q). The last lace-up

strip is the final anchor on the top and one anchor around the instep (Fig. 30.1r).

Ankle pre-wrap application

Ordinarily, a pre-tape wrap is used prior to the application of the tape. A polyester urethane pre-wrap material is available commercially that should be applied after the limb has been shaved from the level of the musculotendinous junction of the Achilles tendon to the midfoot.

TECHNIQUE

1 Begin on instep and bisect the heel (Fig. 30.2a)

2 Return back to the instep and behind the heel (Fig. 30.2b)

3 Proceed under the heel and across the instep (Fig. 30.2c)

4 Go behind the heel on the other side of the foot and under the heel (Fig. 30.2d)

5 Going back to the instep and spiralling up the leg to the desired height (Fig. 30.2e).

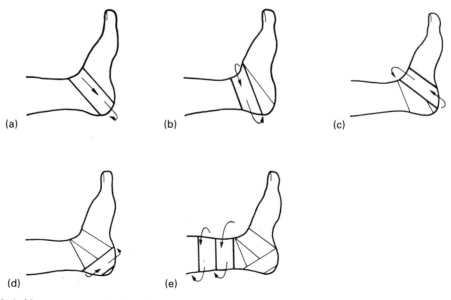

Fig. 30.2 Ankle pre-wrap application. See text for details.

Longitudinal arch taping

Purpose: To give general support to the longitudinal arch of the foot.

Tape: 1.5 in (4 cm) white, zinc oxide, linen, non-stretch tape (1 in (2.5 cm) tape for smaller feet).

Comment: Can be helpful taping for shin splints and arch strains. Athlete should curl the toes to relax the arch during application.

TECHNIQUE

1 The plantar surface of the foot should be sprayed with the tape adherent. Start the first strip of tape on the ball of the foot below the 1st metatarsalphalangeal joint (Fig. 30.3a). While holding the end of the tape firmly to the ball of the foot, apply the tape diagonally across the arch, around the heel, over the side of the foot, ending the strip just below the first toe.

2 The second strip of tape is then applied in a similar manner with the exception of applying the strip under the 5th metatarsalphalangeal joint, and ending on the lateral aspect of the foot (Fig. 30.3b).

3 Cross-strips are applied over the two anchor strips starting at the heel and working towards the toes (Fig. 30.3c,d). These strips should anchor on the sides of the foot. They are applied with even pressure, but should not cause the foot to crease. Each cross-strip should overlap the other by one half.

4 Apply two strips on the dorsum of the foot and end on the plantar surface (Fig. 30.3e). These strips secure the taping to allow for putting on socks and shoes. Very little pressure is used when applying these strips. A cover strip or anchor can be applied around the heel from the 1st to the 5th metatarsalphalangeal joint region to secure the ends of the cross-strips.

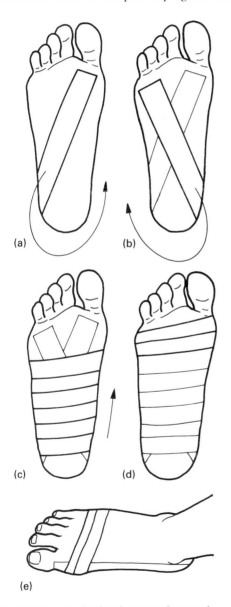

Fig. 30.3 Longitudinal arch taping. See text for details.

Diamond basketweave knee taping

Purpose: To support the collateral ligaments of the knee.

Tape: 1.5 in (4 cm) white, zinc oxide, linen, non-stretch tape or 3 in (7.5 cm) elastic tape.

Comment: Skin should be shaved around the lower half of the quadriceps muscles down to the mid-gastrocnemius region. Underwrap may be used. The knee should be taped with the knee in slight flexion. This can be achieved by placing a 2 in (5 cm) elevation beneath the heel.

TECHNIQUE

1 Two anchor strips should be placed around the quadriceps and the gastrocnemius.

2 A strip of tape is then applied from the lateral thigh extending to the medial shin anchor. Another strip is placed from the posterior lateral calf to the lateral thigh. These strips should cross and form an X over the medial joint line.

3 Two more individual strips of tape are placed in the same manner posterior to the previous strips and overlapping them half-way.

4 Again, the strips are placed individually posterior to the previous strips and overlapping them by one-half. These strips should continue to cross at the joint forming a fan effect.

5 The steps described in points 2–4 should be repeated over the lateral aspect of the knee, creating a lateral fan.

6 The taping patterns should create a diamond effect around the patella.

7 The ends of all strips are covered with three or more additional anchors over the completed diamonds. Care should be taken not to secure them too tightly. This should be done around the thigh and calf. They can be applied from the top of the taping to just above the knee, and from the bottom of the calf to just below the knee.

Conclusion

There are many unique variations of taping which can be employed to treat or prevent athletic injuries. In addition to ingenuity, anatomical, kinesiological and biomechanical knowledge are all required to maximize the potential benefits of taping. Ongoing scientific investigation is needed to understand more completely both the mechanical and non-mechanical effects of taping, as well as the cost-effectiveness of taping compared to other methods of injury prevention.

References

Anderson, K., Wojtys, E.M., Loubert, P.V. & Miller, R.M. (1992) A biomechanical evaluation of taping and bracing in reducing knee joint translation and rotation. *Am. J. Sports Med.* **20**, 416–21.

Andreasson, G. & Edberg, B. (1983) Rheological properties of medical tape used to prevent athletic injuries. *Textile Res. J.* **53**, 225.

Attarian, D.E., McCrackin, H.J. & Devito, D.P. (1985) Biomechanical characteristics of human ankle ligaments. *Foot Ankle* **6**, 54–8.

Ferguson, A.B. (1973) The case against ankle taping. *Am. J. Sports Med.* **1**, 46–7.

Freeman, M.A.R. (1965) Instability of the foot after injuries to the lateral ligament of the ankle. *J. Bone Joint Surg.* **47B**, 669–77.

Fumich, R.M., Ellison, A.E., Guerin, G.J. *et al.* (1983) The measured effect of taping on combined foot and ankle motion before and after exercise. *Am. J. Sports Med.* **9**, 165–71.

Garrick, J.G. & Requa, R.K. (1973) The role of external support in the prevention of ankle sprains. *Med. Sci. Sport Exer.* **5**, 200–3.

Garrick, J.G. & Requa, R.K. (1988) The epidemiology of foot and ankle injuries in sports. *Clin. Sports Med.* **7**, 29–36.

Gross, M.B., Bradshaw, M.K., Ventry, L.C. *et al.* (1987) Comparison of support provided by ankle taping and semirigid orthosis. *J. Orthop. Sports Phys. Ther.* **9**, 33–9.

Hughes, L.Y. & Stett, D.M. (1976) A comparison of ankle taping and a semirigid support. *Phys. Sportsmed* **11**(2), 99–103.

Karlsson, J. & Andreasson, G. (1992) The effect of external ankle support in chronic lateral ankle instability: an electromyographic study. *Am. J. Sports Med.* **20**, 257–61.

Larsen, E. (1984) Taping the ankle for chronic instability. *Acta Orthop. Scand.* **55**, 551–3.

Laughman, R.K., Carr, T.A., Chao, E.Y.S. *et al.* (1980) Three-dimensional kinematics of the taped ankle before and after exercise. *Am. J. Sports Med.* **8**, 425–31.

Lindenberger, U., Reese, D., Andreasson, G., Renström, P. & Peterson, L. (1985) *The effect of prophylactic taping of ankles.* PhD Thesis, Chalmers University of Technology, Goteborg, Sweden.

Loos, T. & Boelens, P. (1984) The effect of ankle tape on lower limb muscle activity. *Int. J. Sports Med.* **5**, 45.

Perry, L. (1983) Anatomy and biomechanics of the hindfoot. *Clin. Orthop.* **177**, 9–15.

Pope, M.H., Renström, P., Donnermeyer, D. & Morgenstern, S. (1987) A comparison of ankle taping methods. *Med. Sci. Sports Exer.* **19**, 143–7.

Rarick, G.L., Bigley, G., Karst, R. *et al.* (1962) The measurable support of the ankle joint by conventional methods of taping. *J. Bone Joint Surg.* **44A**, 1183−90.

Reid, J.C. (1992) *Sports Injury Assessment and Rehabilitation*. Churchill Livingstone, New York.

Rovere, G.D., Clarke, T.J., Yates, C.S. *et al.* (1988) Retrospective comparison of taping and ankle stabilizers in preventing ankle injuries. *Am. J. Sports Med.* **16**, 228−33.

Wilkerson, G.B. (1991) Comparative biomechanical effects of the standard method of ankle taping and a taping method designed to enhance subtalar stability. *Am. J. Sports Med.* **19**, 588−95.

Chapter 31

Sport Shoe Construction: Orthopaedic and Biomechanical Concepts

BERNARD SEGESSER AND BENNO M. NIGG

Before the early 1960s, analysis of human movement during locomotion and physical activity was not a widespread scientific activity. However, appropriate methodologies were developed to quantify the kinematics (Carlet, 1872; Muybridge, 1887; Fischer, 1895; Marey, 1895), and the kinetics of the human body (Carlet, 1872; Basler, 1929; Elftman, 1934, 1938) which, subsequently, were used to estimate internal forces and moments (Bresler & Frankel, 1950; Paul, 1965). With the unprecedented growth of sporting activity, especially running (Cavanagh, 1980), analysis of human movement during physical activity became popular. Several sport medicine clinics and research centres started projects studying the connection between sport activities and the occurrence of sport injuries (Subotnick, 1975; James et al., 1978; Segesser et al., 1978; Clement et al., 1981) and/or the influence of footwear on movement and load characteristics (Unold, 1974; Nigg et al., 1977; Bates et al., 1979; Cavanagh, 1980). Results from these studies were often applied to the development of sport shoes.

Sport shoes which are not appropriate for the individual needs of a runner may force the lower extremities into movement patterns which overload specific structures, resulting in chronic pain and/or injuries. In the attempt to help athletes avoid such injuries, orthopaedic research concentrated on the basic understanding of functional anatomy (Inman, 1976; Hamilton & Ziemer, 1983; Hargens et al., 1984; Debrunner, 1985), on the analysis of typical

injuries as related to sport shoes and sport surfaces (Segesser & Nigg, 1980; Andreasson & Peterson, 1986), and on the epidemiological analysis of sport injuries (James et al., 1978; Clement et al., 1981).

Biomechanical research concentrated on the analysis of external and internal forces acting on and in the locomotor system (Mann & Hagy, 1980), on the analysis of how sport shoes influence external and internal forces (Nigg et al., 1977; Cavanagh, 1980; Robbins & Gouw, 1990) and on the determination of ultimate stress and strain for the most endangered biological structures (Akeson et al., 1985).

After approximately two decades of sport shoe-related research (Nigg, 1986; Cavanagh, 1990) it seems appropriate to summarize the knowledge and developments in this area and to attempt to synthesize the understanding in concepts which are based on anatomical, orthopaedic and biomechanical considerations. The purpose of this chapter is to discuss (i) functional orthopaedic and epidemiological information; and (ii) biomechanical concepts as they relate to sport shoe construction.

Functional considerations

Definition of terms

Various terms are inconsistently used to describe the movement of the foot and leg or of parts of them (Inman, 1976; Mann & Hagy, 1980; Hamilton & Ziemer, 1983; Hamilton,

1984; Debrunner, 1985; Sarrafian, 1987). Consequently, the terms used in this chapter are defined in the following paragraphs.

FOOT AXIS

1 Anteroposterior (AP) axis of the foot: axis from the centre of the calcaneus to the contact between the second and the third phalanges, parallel to the plantar surface of the foot.
2 Mediolateral (ML) axis of the foot: axis from the medial to the lateral side of the foot, parallel to the plantar surface of the foot.
3 Inferosuperior (IS) axis of the foot: axis from the plantar to the dorsal surface of the foot perpendicular to the plantar surface of the foot. Sometimes, this axis is labelled 'vertical' or 'longitudinal' axis.

MOVEMENT DESCRIPTION: GENERAL

1 Functional. A movement description is called *functional* if it relates to actual joint axes and/or coordinate systems which are related to actual anatomical functions.
2 Clinical. A movement description is called *clinical* if it relates to arbitrarily defined axes and/or coordinate systems. Clinical movement descriptions are often introduced in situations where a functional movement description is difficult or even impossible. The functional description of movement has the advantage of describing the actual movement with respect to rotation in actual joints. However, it often has the disadvantage that it cannot be quantified easily. The clinical description has the advantage that movement can be quantified easily with sufficient accuracy in clinical and research settings. However, it has the disadvantage that it does not indicate actual joint motion.

MOVEMENT DESCRIPTION: THE FOOT

1 Plantar-dorsiflexion. Rotation of the foot around an ML axis through the foot. Plantar-dorsiflexion is a clinical movement description.
2 Ab-adduction. Rotation of the foot around an IS axis through the foot. Ab-adduction is a clinical movement description.
3 In-eversion. Rotation of the foot around an AP axis through the foot. In-eversion is a clinical movement description.
4 Pro-supination. Rotation of the foot around the subtalar joint axis (Manter 1941; Inman, 1976). Pro-supination and supination are a combination of in-eversion, plantar-dorsiflexion and ad-abduction in clinical terms (Ensberg & Andrews, 1987) and are functional movement descriptions.
5 Torsion. Rotation of the forefoot with respect to the rearfoot around an AP axis of the foot (Fig. 31.1). Torsion is a clinical movement description. The expression 'torsion' in a biomechanical sense was introduced by Steindler as a movement 'of the forefoot against the back part' (1955). The movement occurs in the midtarsal joint. However, this is not a true joint in a mathematical sense since it is composed by various joint contact areas. The term 'torsion' is currently used for movement analysis with sport shoes (Segesser *et al.*, 1989; Stacoff *et al.*, 1989).

Forces in biological structures

Forces in biological structures act in different loading modes such as tension, compression and shear. Ligaments, capsules and tendons are primarily exposed to tension; muscles to tension, compression and shear; cartilage to compression and shear; and bone to tension, compression and shear. The forces acting on biological structures can have positive or negative effects. Positive reactions include an increase in the density of the collagen structure in all biological materials (Akeson *et al.*, 1985; Hargens & Akeson, 1986). Negative reactions include a decrease in collagen structure or, in acute cases, ruptures or fractures (Hargens *et al.*, 1984; Lachmann, 1988). The ultimate stresses and strains for specific structures depend on loading mode, loading history, age, gender and nutrition.

The mechanical properties of biomaterials

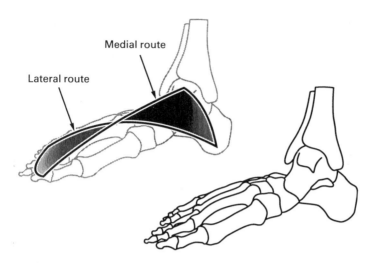

Fig. 31.1 Schematic illustration of the foot construction subdivided into a medial and a lateral route. Adapted from Hamilton & Zierner (1983).

describe their mechanical reaction to acting forces. Each biological structure has typical force–deformation or stress–strain relationships, indicating elastic range, ultimate stress and ultimate strain. Chronic and/or acute injuries to the locomotor system occur when ultimate stress–strain limits are exceeded (Segesser *et al.*, 1983). However, ultimate stress–strain limits are different for chronic and acute injuries.

Aetiological considerations

The determination of factors influencing the aetiology of specific sport injuries is difficult. Most clinical data banks contain limited information to connect the aetiology of specific injuries with the use of specific sport shoes. Injuries which appear several years after the actual sport activity can often not be related to previous sport activities and/or sport shoes used. Additionally, statistical information gathered in medical clinics may be contaminated by the expertise of a clinic specializing in knees, for instance. Thus, analysis and interpretation of statistical information for this purpose should be treated carefully.

GENERAL EPIDEMIOLOGICAL FACTS

It has been reported that between 27 and 70% of runners or joggers are injured in a period of 1 year (Clement *et al.*, 1981; Brody, 1982; Engsberg & Andrews, 1987; Warren & Jones, 1987; Bahlsen, 1988; Marti *et al.*, 1988), and that between 21 and 50% of tennis players are injured per season (Biener & Caluori, 1977; Kuhland *et al.*, 1979; Nigg & Denoth, 1980). It is speculated that many of these injuries occur due to excessive forces rather than due to insufficient material properties of the human biomaterial (Nigg & Bobbert, 1990).

The initial contact of the foot with the ground results in an impact force. High impact forces and/or impact loading have been speculated or shown to be related to cartilage degeneration (Radin *et al.*, 1973, 1982), fatigue fractures and shin splints (James *et al.*, 1978; Clement *et al.*, 1981; Andreasson & Peterson, 1986), Achilles tendon problems (Jørgensen, 1985) and haematological changes (Falsetti *et al.*, 1983). Additionally, results of a prospective study showed an increased frequency of overuse injuries for soldiers with low shock absorbency in the heel pad (Jørgensen & Hansen, 1989). However, prospective studies, analysing the association of external and/or internal impact forces with the aetiology of sport injuries are not known.

SPECIFIC EPIDEMIOLOGICAL FACTS

For the following discussion, information from the data bank of the Sport Medical Clinic

'Rennbahnklinik' (Muttenz, Switzerland) is used. The data bank includes 10 496 cases registered between 1981 and 1990. For this analysis, 5932 injuries which occurred during sporting activities were included. The discussion concentrates on injuries to the lower extremities.

The incidence of injuries to specific structures is summarized in Table 31.1 for running (n = 1903), European handball (n = 736), volleyball (n = 537), racquet sports (n = 790) and soccer (1966). The specific sports are individually discussed in the following paragraphs.

Running. The lower extremities accounted for 79% of all injuries which occurred in running. The knee region accounted for 25%, the leg for 32%, the ankle joint complex (AJC) for 15% and the foot for 7% of all injuries diagnosed in runners. Tendon injuries were frequent in

structures around the knee and leg. It is speculated that several tendon injuries were related to excessive eversion (Bahlsen, 1988) and/or eversion velocity (Stacoff *et al.*, 1988) of the foot. Possible suggested mechanisms are as follows. The muscle–tendon units of the tibialis posterior and the flexor digitorum longus are exposed to high tensile forces during excessive eversion of the foot. Shoes with excessive eversion are, therefore, assumed to increase the forces in these structures and are the reason for tendinitis, bursitis and tenovaginitis. Possible problems resulting from increased forces include injuries to the origin of the tibialis anterior or the flexor digitorum longus at the crest of the tibia. It is speculated that the development of attachment injuries is not a static but a dynamic problem. Flat feet, for instance, are not necessarily connected to excessive

Table 31.1 Structures and sites injured for selected groups of athletes in percentages of all the specific sites and structures based on data from 5713 patients. The column 'All' includes all the sport injuries diagnosed in the Rennbahn Klinik, Muttenz.

Site	Structure	All (%)	Running (%)	Team handball (%)	Volleyball (%)	Racquet sports (%)	Soccer (%)
Knee	Ligament	14	8	21	19	11	22
	Cartilage	4	4	4	7	5	5
	Tendon	7	13	4	11	4	2
	Bone	1	0	0	0	0	1
Lower leg	Ligament	0	0	0	0	0	0
	Cartilage	9	0	0	0	0	0
	Tendon	0	28	4	7	10	5
	Bone	1	4	4	3	1	2
AJC	Ligament	14	12	18	23	12	17
	Cartilage	1	1	2	2	1	1
	Tendon	1	2	4	1	1	1
	Bone	1	0	0	0	0	1
Foot	Ligament	2	1	2	1	3	3
	Cartilage	1	0	0	1	0	1
	Tendon	1	4	2	2	3	2
	Bone	2	2	3	3	1	2
Other		41	21	32	20	48	35
Total		100	100	100	100	100	100

AJC, ankle joint complex.

pronatory movement during locomotion. Feet with 'normal' static structures, on the other hand, may be excessive pronators in a dynamic situation and subsequently be exposed to excessive stresses at origins and insertions of tendons.

Excessive foot movement also influences the positioning of the calcaneus with respect to the leg. Excessive rotation of the calcaneus will increase the asymmetry of the force distribution in the Achilles tendon and may be the reason for injuries to the Achilles tendon including microscopic or partial strains.

Cartilage injuries represented only about 5% of the diagnosed and treated runner population. It is speculated (Radin *et al.*, 1973, 1982; Falsetti *et al.*, 1983; Nigg *et al.*, 1990; Radin *et al.*, 1991) that long-term degeneration and wear of cartilage may be associated with running, high impact forces and/or high impact loading. However, conclusive evidence supporting this speculation has not been provided yet.

Ball games. The term 'ball games' includes the sports of soccer, European handball and volleyball. The lower extremities accounted for 71% of all injuries diagnosed. Most frequent injuries occurred in the knee and ankle joint regions primarily to ligaments and capsules. Compared to running, ball games include at least two additional movement elements, rotations and side movements during jumps and shuffles. During sideward movements the lateral ligaments of the AJC, e.g. the weak fibular ligaments, are exposed to stress. Consequently, injuries may occur to those ligaments when the movement becomes excessive, for instance, when the foot rolls over the lateral shoe wedge. The structures injured in such excessive movements include the ligamentum talofibular (anterius and less often posterius) and the ligamentum calcaneofibular. In those cases the protection mechanism of the peroneus longus and brevis is not sufficient.

Cartilage injuries in ball games accounted for about 6% of all diagnosed injuries and it is speculated that a significant number of these were related to excessive impact forces. However, conclusive evidence for this speculation is unavailable.

Racquet sports. The term 'racquet sports' includes the sports of tennis, squash and racquetball. The number of lower extremity injuries included 52% of the total number of diagnosed injuries. This percentage agrees with earlier published epidemiological data from questionnaires (Nigg & Denoth, 1980). Muscle—tendon injuries had about the same frequency as ligamentous injuries. Myogelosis (hardening of an area of a muscle) and insertion tendinosis of the peroneus brevis and longus occurred more often than in the running population. This may be related to additional supination control of this muscle during lateral movement, especially during sliding in tennis on clay (Stuessi *et al.*, 1987). The frequently occurring Achilles tendon problems may indicate a maladjustment between the leg and the calcaneus, suggesting that the alignment of the calcaneus with the leg must be maintained in prosupinatory and supinatory movements.

Cartilage was injured in racquet sports in 6% of all diagnosed injuries. The distribution was in the same order of magnitude as in running and ball games and similar considerations are appropriate for the potential correlations between excessive impact forces and those cartilage injuries.

Consequences for sport shoe construction

The results of the injury analysis suggest that, from an orthopaedic and epidemiological point of view (with no regard for performance-related criteria), sport shoes should be constructed to:
1 Support the function of the foot.
2 Take into account the physiological ranges of motion of the foot.
3 Avoid excessive rotation movement of the shoe due to excessive moment arms for moments resulting from ground reaction forces.
4 Avoid, in general, excessive forces.
Shoes constructed in such a way are assumed

to restrict motion and to avoid excessive movement in the joints. Consequently, the internal structures should be less strained and stressed and the injury frequency should be reduced. However, these are theoretical considerations and experimental evidence that sport shoes constructed using these criteria are associated with less injuries is still unavailable (Nigg & Bobbert, 1990).

Biomechanical concepts

Sport activities such as running, tennis and skiing are so different in their movements and functions that specific sets of concepts may be required for the optimal construction of a sport shoe for each of these activities. In the following, a biomechanical concept is presented which is limited to sports where conventional sport shoes are used such as running, tennis, court games, volleyball and basketball. Sport shoes for Alpine and cross-country skiing, skating, bobsledding and golfing, for instance, are not included in this specific set of concepts.

Two principal aspects are of importance for a sport shoe from a biomechanical perspective: (i) prevention of excessive load and related injuries; and (ii) improvement of performance. A sport shoe should be constructed to prevent excessive load acting on structures of the human body and/or to support the achievement of the best possible performance. Note that these two concepts (prevention of injuries and improvement of performance) can be mutually exclusive.

Concepts for prevention of excessive load

The concept 'prevention of excessive load' results from the observation that sport activities are often associated with sport injuries. It is assumed that the frequency of injuries may be reduced if a sport shoe is constructed to:
1 Limit the impact forces during landing.
2 Support the foot during the stance phase.
3 Guide the foot during the final phase of ground contact.

In the terminology used in sport shoe research the reduction of the impact force peak is called cushioning. This definition includes any method resulting in reduced impact forces, shoe construction and/or changes in movement such as increased knee flexion during impact. However, in this chapter the aspect of cushioning due to sport shoe construction is discussed. A concept applicable for all sport shoes included in this chapter is that sport shoes should be constructed to provide adequate cushioning of impact forces. Inversion and/or eversion has been shown in prospective studies to correlate with the aetiology of injuries (Luethi et al., 1986; Bahlsen, 1988). A concept applicable for all sport shoes included in this chapter is that sport shoes should be constructed to provide adequate support for the foot during the stance phase. In the terminology of sport shoe research the function of the shoe in the positioning of the foot during the final part of ground contact is called 'guidance'. The term guidance includes that rotational motion in the AJC and in the foot should be limited to avoid possible excessive forces in internal structures. A concept applicable for all sport shoes included in this chapter is that sport shoes should be constructed to provide guidance during the final part of ground contact.

Previous research supporting the three (preventive) concepts does not provide a full understanding of cushioning, support and guidance as they relate to load reduction and injury prevention. Research on cushioning concentrated primarily on the assessment of external impact forces. Further research needs to concentrate on internal impact forces and their mechanical and biological effects, two aspects which are currently not well understood. It is possible that changes in cushioning properties of a shoe relate rather to comfort than to injury prevention. Research on support and guidance needs to address the correlation between excessive foot movement, related leg and thigh movement, and possible mechanical and biological effects.

The three concepts, cushioning, support and

guidance, provide a framework which is based on the current knowledge. It can be applied for technical solutions to control movement and, consequently, to reduce internal forces. It is suggested that each concept can be achieved with two technical options: material properties or construction (Table 31.2).

TECHNICAL SOLUTIONS

Various materials (gaseous, fluid or solid) have been used to improve the cushioning properties of the sport shoe. The material properties of the midsole may, for instance, influence the defor-

mation of the midsole during a movement and, consequently, have an effect on the cushioning properties. Special shoe constructions have been used to provide support and/or guidance. A medial support in a running shoe, for instance, reduces the maximal eversion and eversion velocity of the shoe (Nigg et al., 1986). However, there have been suggestions that similar or even better results may be achieved by changing the sensory input into the foot. This may be achieved by using 'small rigid irregularities to flat, fairly rigid insoles' (Robbins & Guow, 1991). The result of such a strategy would be a change of movement

Table 31.2 Schematic representation of a set of possible concepts for sport shoe construction for running, tennis, court sports, basketball, volleyball and similar sport activities.

Goal	Concept	Technical options	Examples
Control of movement and load	Cushioning	Material	Air Gel Dual density Hydroflow Viscoelastic insoles
		Construction	Flare Soft cell Torsion Cantilever Air compartments Sensory insoles
	Support	Material	Density variations
		Construction	Orthotic devices Sole width Stable shaft Bandages Heel counters Heel stabilizer Air compartments Air pump Stability elements Sensory insoles
	Guidance	Material	Density variations
		Construction	Orthotic devices Thread in sole Torsion Bandages Sensory insoles

induced by an altered perception as a result of changes in the sensory feedback.

Concepts for performance

Performance is defined as the result of a physical activity measured in time, distance, work or a similar quantity. Performance in running, for instance, could be defined as the time from start to finish or the energy needed to run a defined distance. In high jumping it may be defined as the height of the jump.

Performance can be quantified by measuring the oxygen consumption during a defined activity such as treadmill running. One of the most surprising results in such measurements is that running with running shoes requires on average about 3–5% more energy than running without running shoes (unpublished results of own measurements with eight subjects and three trials per footwear condition). Part of this additional work can be explained by the additional work required to lift, accelerate and decelerate the additional mass of the shoe. However, this does not explain the whole difference.

Energy-related research in sport shoes is not well developed. Only few publications report results describing the connection between sport shoes (Catlin & Dressendorfer, 1979; Frederick et al., 1980; Clement et al., 1982; Hayes et al., 1983) or sport surfaces (McMahon & Green, 1979) and energy aspects. They do not provide, however, a comprehensive base for the development of concepts for performance. Consequently, the concepts which are discussed here are based on intuition and/or theoretical considerations. Two possible concepts are discussed: (i) a concept describing the requirements for energy return from a sport shoe; and (ii) a concept describing the energy conservation through a sport shoe.

For energy return with sport shoes it is suggested that energy must be returned at the right location, time and frequency. Forces which should return energy through the shoe–foot interface must act at the right location. If

take-off occurs at the forefoot of the right foot, forces must act between shoe and foot of the right forefoot. Forces acting between the shoe and foot of the left leg or forces which act between the shoe and the heel of the right foot while the heel is in the air are internal forces and are not able to produce work which can be used to return energy.

Forces which should return energy through the shoe–foot interface must act at the right time. If the deformation of the shoe sole during landing should be used for the subsequent take-off, the sole should be constructed as a spring-like structure which deforms for the first half and restores for the second half of the contact time.

Forces which should return energy through the shoe–foot interface must act with the right frequency. Assume a contact time for the foot of 0.25 s. A shoe sole acting with the right frequency would compress during the first 0.125 s and restore in the second 0.125 s. This would correspond to a frequency of 2 Hz. This is obviously unrealistic.

The principles of optimal energy return are well illustrated with a championship diver on a diving board. However, there are problems when attempting to return a relevant amount of energy from a shoe sole to a runner. The maximally possible energy return, E_{max}, can be estimated by considering the shoe sole as an ideal spring and by calculating the energy stored in the spring:

$$E_{max} = 0.5 \times f \times d^2$$

where f = spring constant of the shoe sole, and d = maximal deformation. The formula illustrates that energy return increases with increasing spring stiffness of the shoe sole and/or with increasing deformation, two effects which are in opposite directions. Assuming a maximal deformation of the shoe sole of 1 cm (heel) and a spring constant of the shoe of 10^5 N·m (Denoth, 1980, p. 63) provides a maximally possible returned energy per step of:

$$E_{max} = 0.5 \times 10^5 \text{ N·m} \times 10^{-4} \text{ m}^2$$
$$= 5 \text{ J}.$$

This maximally possible returned energy for each step can be compared with the total energy needed during a step. The assumed total energy needs during a marathon are about 10×10^6 J. This number can be divided by an assumed number of steps during a marathon (20 000) which provides a total energy per step. E_{tot}, of about 500 J. Consequently, the maximally possible returned energy from the deformation of the shoe sole in this example is only about 1%. This is, however, a conservative estimate. The shoe sole is not an ideal spring. Denoth (1980) documented a loss of energy in a running shoe sole of about 30–40%. Additionally, the deformation of the heel cannot be transferred into the forefoot and the actual deformation of the forefoot is much smaller than 1 cm. Taking all these factors into account leads to the conclusion that the actually returned energy, E_{act}, is much smaller than 1%. Consequently, return of energy seems not to be an appropriate concept in sport shoe construction to improve performance. However, it is suggested that energy return can play a major role in sport surfaces (McMahon & Green, 1979) because sport surfaces have a higher spring constant and allow more deformation.

The second concept, addressing the energy balance question is: if the energy requirements are of interest one should concentrate on strategies to minimize the loss of energy. Possible shoe-related factors affecting energy loss include:

1 Work against gravity (weight of shoe).
2 Work against gravity (centre of mass).
3 Work for acceleration (weight of shoe).
4 Work due to cushioning.
5 Work to stabilize joints.
6 Work due to changes in movement.

Two of these aspects will be discussed in more detail.

The additional work, ΔE_1, to accelerate the additional shoe mass, Δm, from no movement during ground contact to a maximal foot speed, v, can be estimated as:

$$\Delta E_1 = 0.5 \times \Delta m \times v^2.$$

This additional work can be compared with the actual work during one step, E_{act}, which was discussed earlier. The results of this estimation (Fig. 31.2) indicate that an additional shoe mass of 100 g corresponds to additional required work of about 1% for a maximal foot speed of 10 m·s^{-1} which corresponds to a running speed of about 5–7 m·s^{-1}. Additionally, changes in shoe construction may influence the movement of the path of the centre of mass. It is suggested that the vertical movement of the centre of mass, H, increases with decreasing stiffness of the midsole of a shoe. Such changes affect the amount of energy spent. The additional energy, ΔE_2, can be estimated as:

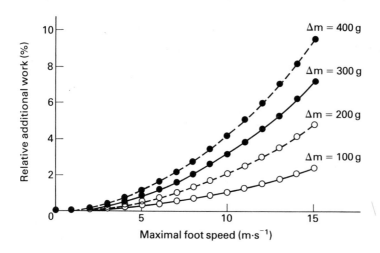

Fig. 31.2 Estimated relative additional work due to acceleration of the additional shoe mass as a function of the maximal speed of the foot.

$\Delta E_2 = m_{tot} \times g \times H.$

A rough estimate suggests additional work of 1–2% for additional vertical movement of the centre of mass of 5 mm.

The two estimated amounts of energy lost, however, do not explain the total difference of up to 5% between running barefoot and running with running shoes. Further research is needed to understand the difference in energy requirements for barefoot and shod running. It is suggested that further insight may be gained by studying the factors relevant to minimize the loss of energy.

Current sport shoe construction

Current sport shoe construction uses several strategies to achieve the goals of the 'preventive concepts' cushioning, support and guidance. It would be another (possibly quite interesting) project to compare each single strategy with the claimed function. However, it is suggested that excessive inversion and eversion due to faulty shoe construction has been reduced in the last decade as a result of the application of the 'preventive concepts' of support and guidance.

The strategies used in current sport shoe construction to optimize energy aspects use a reduction of weight and constructions which are claimed to return energy. Based on the discussions in this chapter, the weight reduction approach is appropriate and relevant differences are expected from shoes with less weight. However, the claim to return energy with special shoes seems unfeasible and it is proposed that 'energy returning shoes' should not show different energy balances than normal shoes.

Imaging techniques in the construction of sport shoes

The practical implementation of biomechanical concepts in the construction of sport shoes requires that constructional elements be designed in accordance with the anatomical and functional structures of the foot. For this purpose, imaging techniques may be used (Segesser et al., 1989). Characteristics to be investigated on the sport shoe are specially identified with lead oxide or marked with lead strips (Fig. 31.3).

In the region of the heel, cushioning must take place where the bony parts of the calcaneus may be close to the ground. Cushioning elements affect the stability of the calcaneus. Consequently, an incorrect alignment of the stabilizing heel cap may mechanically irritate the Achilles tendon in push-off (Fig. 31.4).

In the region of the tarsal bones, pronation can be counteracted by compaction of material or by a supporting insole under the sustentaculum tali. The material of the uppers, and if necessary the heel cap for pronation control, must be considered so that no movement of the foot into the lateral material of the shoes is possible. The uncoupling between the rear foot and forefoot must be attained by alterations in the construction and the material technique in the shoe in the region of the tarsal bones and the base of the metatarsals (Fig. 31.5).

The constructional characteristics of the shoe in the forefoot, such as the form of the last, material compaction, sole profile, etc., ensure correct flexion of the ball of the foot and push-off movement. The push-off movement is supported under the middle rays of the foot by flexion grooves and/or by the profile arrangement for release of rotation at the level of the head of the metatarsals (Fig. 31.6).

Three-dimensional computer tomography enables imaging of the constructional elements on the sole and on the material of the uppers, so that the uppers (heel cap, laces, etc.) can be designed even better in accordance with the anatomy of the foot (Fig. 31.7).

Application of the sport shoe for therapy

Research has shown that movement pattern can be forced onto the foot and leg by the sport shoe and that incorrect movement pattern can

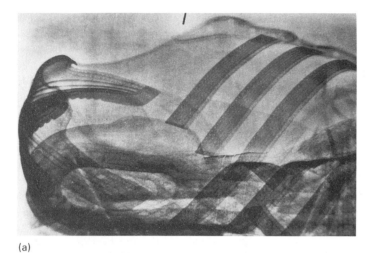

(a)

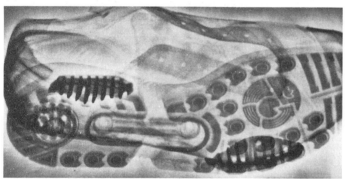

(b)

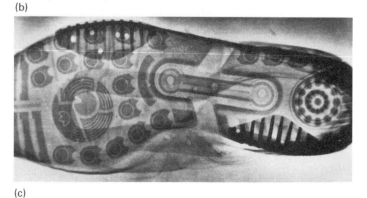

(c)

Fig. 31.3 Important constructional elements of the shoe are rendered visible for radiological imaging techniques with lead oxide. (a) Bandage system of the upper material of the shoe. (b) Medial rearfoot and lateral forefoot reinforcement. (c) Rearfoot cushioning, midfoot torsion bar and forefoot rotation structure.

be corrected by alterations in or on the sport shoe (Subotnick, 1975; Segesser et al., 1978; Segesser & Nigg 1980; Clement et al., 1981; Nigg & Segesser, 1988; Stacoff et al., 1988). Moreover, we know from investigations on the rehabilitation of injuries to the locomotor apparatus that a more rapid orientation of the collagen fibres and a better tissue nutrition is to be expected from moderate tension and pressure strain of the injured tissue with a

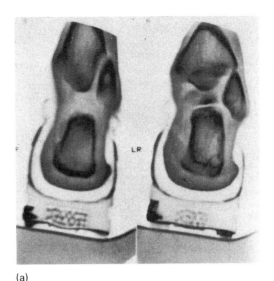

(a)

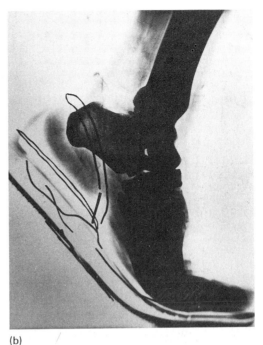

(b)

Fig. 31.4 Arrangement of cushioning elements and the heel cap imaged in (a) the computer tomogram and (b) with conventional X-rays.

limited movement (Akeson *et al.*, 1985; Hargens & Akeson, 1986; Lachmann, 1988).

It is therefore appropriate to apply knowledge from sport shoe research in early functional rehabilitation of sport injuries and to construct therapeutic sports shoes. These should be designed to ensure an optimum movement support providing appropriate forefoot flexion and prevent excessive strain on the injured tissue. This form of functional immobilization reduces possible symptoms typical for plaster cast immobilization. This treatment modality has beneficial psychological aspects and enables more rapid social reintegration.

In some countries in Europe, the functional follow-up treatment of fibular ligament injuries with or without operation has become established. Precondition for an early functional conservative or postoperative follow-up treatment is on the one hand an adequate supination protection, and on the other hand a limitation of movement with support of forefoot flexion during flexure of the ball of the foot in walking. Tension measurements on the fibular ligament

show that a moderate tension stimulus without damaging stress of the injured ligament is possible with movement of the ankle joints from dorsal to plantar of 10−0−20 without an additional pronation and supination component and that this is reasonable for the therapeutic procedure in fibular ligament injuries (Wirth *et al.*, 1978; Segesser *et al.*, 1983; Paessler, 1986; Segesser *et al.*, 1986).

This requirement is only fulfilled when the upper of the shoe is drawn up at least 4−5 cm above the ankle joint axis to the calf with a rigid connection between the upper and the ankle cap fixed with the sole (Fig. 31.8). Otherwise, the lever of the sole is more effective in inducing a supination distortion than the supination deceleration of the shoe uppers, as shown by the slight prophylactic effect of high-upper training shoes in various kinds of sport.

Limitation of movement, supination protection and support of flexure of the ball of the foot allow walking under full body weight as early as 8−10 days later in surgically or conservatively treated fibular ligament injuries or

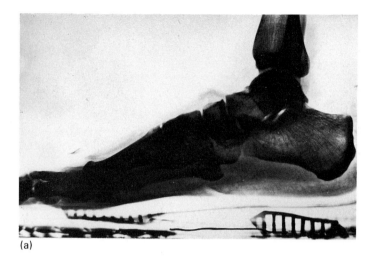
(a)

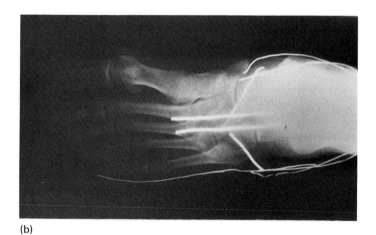
(b)

Fig. 31.5 (a) Material compaction under the sustentaculum tali for control of pronation. (b) Position of elements to ensure torsion in the region of the tarsal bones.

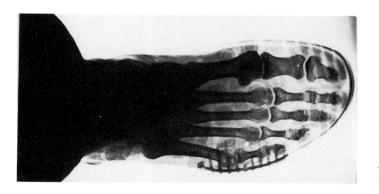

Fig. 31.6 Imaging of the form of the last, profile and material compaction in the forefoot region.

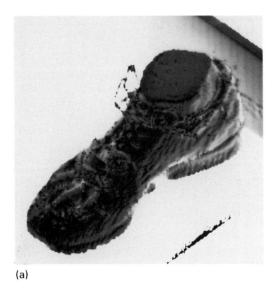
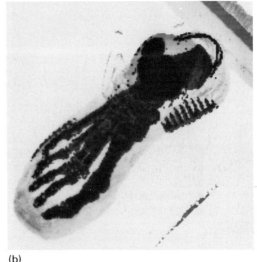

(a)   (b)

Fig. 31.7 Three-dimensional computer tomography for appraisal of the sole and material of the uppers (a) with regard to the anatomy of the foot (b).

ligament reconstructions; symmetrical gait characteristics are attained within 2–3 days (Segesser *et al.*, 1987; Stuessi, 1987). These advantages of gait support make it possible to use the stabilization shoe in other orthopaedic and neurological conditions such as arthrosis or arthodesis of the ankle joint, ankle fractures, flexor muscle weakness, etc.

For early functional follow-up treatment of surgically or conservatively treated Achilles tendon rupture, Zwipp *et al*. (1990) have developed a shoe with uppers extending to the proximal calf with variable stabilizability and a heel height which can be varied by up to 2 cm (H.H. Paessler, personal communication; Schierink, 1990). With ventral tongue strengthening and lateral stabilizers, a force transmission from the foot to the lower leg is possible with adequate relief of the Achilles tendon, so that this shoe can already be worn a few days after an Achilles tendon rupture (Fig. 31.9).

Our own investigations on the gait characteristics after early functional treatment of operated Achilles tendon ruptures and partial ruptures show that gait characteristics supported by the shoe can be attained which enable forefoot flexion in walking and push-off movement with minimal tensile strain of the Achilles tendon in the high-upper Achilles tendon shoe. The moderate tension stimulus acting on the tendon ensures a more rapid restoration of force transmission to the foot via the plantar reflexors, so that normalization of the push-off movement occurs within a few days after taking off the shoe.

Modified training shoes with variable restrictions of movement and biomechanically demonstrable function support of flexure of the ball of the foot in walking (Fig. 31.10) are an effective measure for treatment of fibular ligament injuries and injuries of the Achilles tendon and in orthopaedic and neurological problems which require support of the movement sequence of the foot (arthrodesis, arthrosis, peroneal pareses, etc.). The early functional follow-up treatment ensures moderate loading stimuli on the tissue with elimination of tension peaks, thus enabling a shorter rehabilitation time with minimal inactivity atrophy and thus a more rapid reintegration into everyday life.

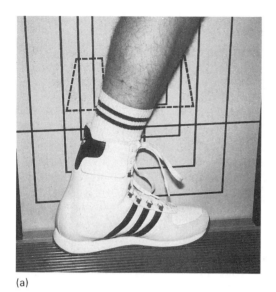

(a)

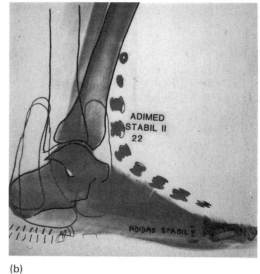

(b)

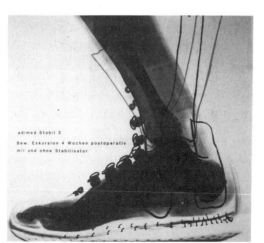

(c)

Fig. 31.8 Limitation of the extent of movement (a and b) and active and passive supination protection characterize the rehabilitation shoe ADIMED STABIL 2. (c) After taking off one of the stabilizers, the scope of movement is increased.

Conclusion

Two possible concepts which are important for the construction of sport shoes on the basis of anatomical, orthopaedic and epidemiological criteria are presented. The first concept has the objective of reducing excessive force. It comprises cushioning, support and guidance, which can be achieved by tuning of the material properties or constructional characteristics of the sports shoe. The other concept comprises the improvement of performance; this can be achieved by reduction of the loss of energy. Modern technology and imaging techniques may be used to support decision-making processes in shoe construction. Products of such procedures may be used in therapeutic and/or rehabilitation applications.

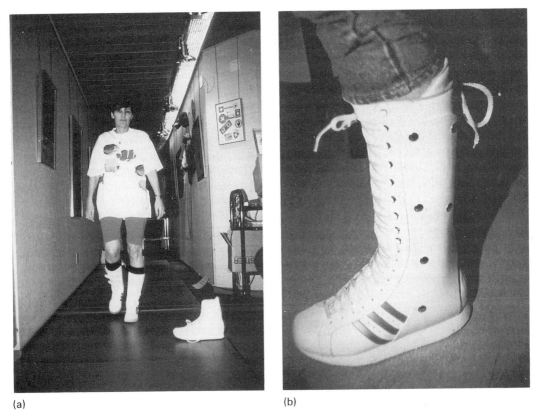

(a)   (b)

Fig. 31.9 (a) Subject during locomotion 3 weeks after surgical treatment of an Achilles tendon rupture. (b) High upper-Achilles tendon shoe for rehabilitation after ruptures and partial ruptures.

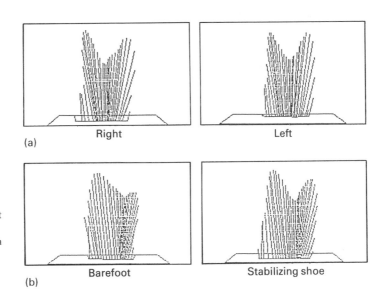

Fig. 31.10 Illustration of the application of force vector diagrams in the control of functional support. (a) Vector diagrams for a stabilizing shoe for walking for a fibular ligament reconstruction (both sides after 7 days). (b) Vector diagrams for a foot 5 weeks after Achilles tendon surgery, barefoot (left) and in a stabilizing shoe (right).

References

Andreasson, G. & Peterson, L. (1986) Effects of shoe and surface characteristics on lower limb injuries in sports. *Int. J. Sports Biomech.* **2**, 202−9.

Akeson, W.H., Frank C.B., Amiel, D. & Woo, S.L.-Y. (1985) Ligament biology and biomechanics. In: G. Finermcia (ed) *Symposium on Sports Medicine, The Knee*, pp. 111−51. CV Mosby, St Louis.

Bahlsen, H.A. (1988) *The etiology of running injuries*. Unpublished thesis, University of Calgary, Calgary.

Basler, A. (1929) *Das Gehen* (gait). Canton.

Bates, B.T., Osternig, L.R., Mason, B.R. & James, S.L. (1979) Functional variability of the lower extremity during the support phase of running. *Med. Sci. Sports Exerc.* **11**, 328−31.

Biener, K. & Caluori. P. (1977) Tennissportunfaelle (Sports injuries in tennis). *Med. Klinik* **72**, 754−7.

Bresler, B. & Frankel, J.P. (1950) The forces and moments in the leg during level walking. *ASME Transactions* **72**, 27−36.

Brody, D.M. (1982) Techniques in the evaluation and treatment of the injured runner. *Orthop. Clin. N. Am.* **13**, 541−58.

Carlet, M. (1872) *Essai experimental sur la locomotion de l'homme* (Human locomotion experiments). Annales des Sciences Naturelles, 1872.

Catlin, M.E. & Dressendorfer, R.H. (1979) Effect of shoe weight on the energy cost of running. *Med. Sci. Sport Exerc.* **11**, 80.

Cavanagh, P.R. (1980) *The Running Shoe Book*. Anderson World Inc., California.

Cavanagh, P.R. (ed) (1990) *Biomechanics of Distance Running*. Human Kinetics, Illinois.

Clement, D.B., Taunton, J.E., Smart, G.W. & McNicol, K.L. (1981) A survey of overuse running injuries. *Phys. Sports Med.* **9**, 47−58.

Clement, D.B., Taunton, J.E., Wiley, J.P., Smart G.W. & McNicol, K.L. (1982) Investigation of metabolic efficiency in runners with and without corrective orthotic devices. *Int. J. Sports Med.* **2**, 14−15.

Debrunner, H.U. (1985) *Biomechanik des Fusses* (Biomechanics of the foot). Enke, Stuttgart.

Denoth, J. (1980) Materialeigenschaften (Material properties). In B.M. Nigg & J. Denoth (eds) *Sportplatzbeläge*, pp. 54−67. Juris Verlag, Zurich.

Elftman, H. (1934). A cinematic study of the distribution of pressure in the human foot. *Anat. Rec.* **59**, 481−90.

Elftman, H. (1938) The force exerted by the ground in walking. *Arbeltsphysiologie* **10**, 485−91.

Engsberg, J.R. & Andrews, J.G. (1987) Kinematic analysis of the talocalcaneal/talocrural joint during running support. *Med. Sci. Sports Exerc.* **19**, 275−84.

Falsetti, H.L., Burke, E.R., Feld, R., Frederick, E.C. & Ratering, C. (1983) Hematological variations after endurance running with hard and soft soled running shoes. *Phys. Sports Med.* **8**, 118−27.

Fischer, O. (1895) Der Gang des Menschen (The human gait). In *Abhandlungen der saechsischen Gesellschaft der Wissenschaft*. B.G. Teubner, Leipzig.

Frederick, E.C., Howley, E.T. & Powers, S.K. (1980) Lower O_2 cost while running on air cushion type shoe. *Med. Sci. Sport Exerc.* **12**, 81−2.

Hamilton, W.C. (1984) Anatomy. In W.C. Hamilton (ed) *Traumatic Disorders of the Ankle*, pp. 1−12. Springer-Verlag, New York.

Hamilton, J.J. & Ziemer, L.K. (1983) Functional anatomy of the human foot and ankle. In K.A. Johnson (ed) *The Foot and Ankle*, pp. 1−14. American Academy of Orthopaedic Surgeons Symposium. CV Mosby, St Louis.

Hargens, A.R. & Akeson, W.H. (1986) Stress effects on tissue nutrition and viability. In A.R. Hargens (ed) *Tissue Nutrition and Viability*, pp. 1−24. Springer-Verlag, New York.

Hargens, A.R., Akeson, W.H., Garfin, S.R., Gelberman R.H. & Gershuni, D.H. (1984) Compartment syndromes. In J. Denton (ed) *Practice of Surgery*, pp. 1−18. Lippincott, Philadelphia.

Hayes, J., Smith, L. & Sanpietro F. (1983) The effects off orthotics on the aerobic demands of running. *Med. Sci. Sport Exerc.* **15**, 169.

Inman, V.T. (1976) *The Joints of the Ankle*. Williams & Wilkins, Baltimore.

James, S.L., Bates, B.T. & Osternig, L.R. (1978) Injuries to runners. *Am. J. Sports Med.* **6**, 40−50.

Jörgensen, U. (1985) Achillodynia and loss of heel pad shock absorbency. *Am. J. Sports Med.* **13**, 128−33.

Jörgensen, U. & Hansen, C.P. (1989) *The significance of heel pad shock absorbancy for the development of overuse injuries*. Unpublished thesis, University of Linkoping, Linkoping.

Kuhlund, D.N., McCue, F.C., Rockwell, D.A. & Gieck, J.H. (1979) Tennis injuries: Prevention and treatment. *Am. J. Sports Med.* **7**, 249−53.

Lachmann, S. (1988) *Soft Tissue Injuries in Sport*. Blackwell Scientific Publications, Oxford.

Luethi, S.M., Frederick, E.C., Hawes M.R. & Nigg, B.M. (1986) Influence of shoe construction on lower extremity kinematics and load during lateral movement in tennis. *Int. J. Sports Biomech.* **2**, 156−65.

McMahon, T.A. & Green, P.R. (1979) Influence of track compliance on running. *J. Biomech.* **12**, 893−904.

Mann, R.A. & Hagy, J. (1980) Running, jogging and walking: A comparative electromyographic and biomechanical study. In J.E. Bateman & A.W. Trott (eds) *The Foot and Ankle*, pp. 167−75. Decker,

Stuttgart.

Manter, J.T. (1941) Movements of the subtalar and transversal joints. *Anat. Rec.* **80**(4), 397–409.

Marey, E.J. (1895) *Movement*. Arno, New York.

Marti, B., Vader, J.P., Minder, E.C. & Abelin, T. (1988) On the epidemiology of running injuries: The 1984 Bern Grand Prix Study. *Am. J. Sports Med.* **16**, 285–94.

Muybridge, E. (1887) *Animal Locomotion*, Vols 1–11. University of Pennsylvania, Philadelphia.

Nigg, B.M. (ed) (1986) *Biomechanics of Running Shoes*. Human Kinetics, Illinois.

Nigg, B.M., Bahlsen, A.H., Denoth, J., Luethi, S.M. & Stacoff, A. (1986) Factors influencing kinetic and kinematic variables in running. In B.M. Nigg (ed) *Biomechanics of Running Shoes*, pp. 139–59. Human Kinetics, Illinois.

Nigg, B.M. & Bobbert, B.M. (1990) On the potential of various approaches in load analysis to reduce the frequency of sports injuries. *J. Biomech.* **23**(Suppl. 1), 2–12.

Nigg, B.M. & Denoth, J. (1980) *Sportplatzbelaege* (Playing Surfaces). Juris, Zurich.

Nigg, B.M., Eberle, G., Frei, D. & Segesser, B. (1977) Biomechanische Analyse von Fussinsuffizienzen (Biomechanical analysis of foot insufficiencies). *Med. Orthop. Techn.* **6**, 178–80.

Nigg, B.M. & Segesser, B. (1988) The influence of playing surfaces on the load on the locomotor system and on football and tennis injuries. *Sports Med.* **5**, 375–85.

Paessler, H.H., Berger, R. & Maerz, S. (1986) Gips oder Spezialschuh zur Nachbehandlung operierter frischer fibulaerer Bandlaesionen (Cast or special shoe as treatment after surgery of acute ankle ligament injury). *Prak. Sporttraumatol. Sportmed.* **4**, 50–4.

Paul, J.P. (1965) Bioengineering studies of the forces transmitted by joints. In R.M. Kennedy (ed) *Engineering Analysis, Biomechanics and Related Bioengineering Topics*, pp. 369–80. Pergamon Press, Oxford.

Radin, E.L., King, H.Y., Riegger, C., Kish, V.L. & O'Connor, J.J. (1991) Relationship between lower limb dynamics and knee joint pain. *J. Orthop. Res.* **9**, 398–405.

Radin, E.L., Orr, R.B., Kelman, J.L., Paul, I.L. & Rose, R.M. (1982) Effect of prolonged walking on concrete on the knees of sheep. *J. Biomech.* **15**, 487–92.

Radin, E.L., Parker, H.G., Pugh, G.V., Steinberg, R.S., Paul, I.L. & Rose, R.M. (1973) Response of joints to impact loading. *J. Biomech.* **6**, 51–7.

Robbins, S.E. & Gouw, G.J. (1990) Athletic footwear and chronic overloading. A brief review. *Sports Med.* **9**, 76–85.

Robbins, S.E. & Gouw, G.J. (1991) Athletic footwear:

Unsafe due to perceptual Illusions. *Med. Sci. Sports Exerc.* **23**, 217–24.

Sarrafian, S.K. (1987) Functional characteristics of the foot and plantar aponeurosis under tibiotalar loading. *Foot Ankle* **8**, 4–18.

Schievink, B. (1990) Variabler Therapieschuh fur fruhfunktionelle Behandlung — Eine gute Alternative (Variable therapy shoe for early functional treatment). *OST* **6**, 20–3.

Segesser, B., Jenoure, P., Feinstein, R. & Vogt-Sartori, S. (1986) Wirkung aeusser Stabilisationshilfen (Tape, Bandage, Stabilschuh) bei fibulären Distorsionen (Effects of external stabilizers for fibular distorsion). *OST* **7**, 342–56.

Segesser, B., Jenoure, P., Michel, P., Stuessi, E. & Luethi, S. (1987) Gang- und Laufanalyse am Beispiel der Sporttraumatologie (Analysis of walking and running in examples of sports traumatology). *Swiss Med.* **3B**, 43–7.

Segesser, B. & Nigg, B.M. (1980) Insertionstendinosen am Schienbein, Achillodynie und Ueberiastungsfolgen am Fuss — Aetiologie, Biomechanik, therapeutische Moeglichkeiten (Tibial insertion tendinoses, Achillodynia and damage due to overuse of the foot — aetiology, biomechanics, therapeutic possibilities). *Orthopaede* **9**, 207–14.

Segesser, B., Ruepp, R. & Nigg, B.M. (1978) Indikation, Technik und Fehlermoeglichkelten einer Sportschuhkorrektur (Indication, technique and error possibilities in sport shoe correction). *Orthop. Praxis* **11**, 834–7.

Segesser, B., Stacoff, A. & Nigg, B.M. (1983) Die Belastbarkeit der Sprunggelenke aus biomechanisch-klinischer Sicht (Load capacity of the ankle joint complex from a biomechanical and clinical perspective). *Med. Sport* **23**, 1–13.

Segesser, B., Stuessi, E., Stacoff, A., Kaelin X. & Ackermann. R. (1989) Torsion, ein neues Konzept im Sportschuhbau (Torsion and new concepts for sport shoe construction). *Sportverietzung-Sportschaden* **3**, 167–82.

Segesser, B., Wiggli, U. & Vogt-Sartori. S. (1989) *Bildgebende Verfahren im der Sportschuhforschung* (Torsion: A new concept in the design of a sports shoe). Internal Report, Adidas.

Stacoff, A., Denoth, J., Kaelin, X. & Stuessi, E. (1988) Running injuries and shoe construction: Some possible relationships. *Int. J. Sports Biomech.* **4**, 342–57.

Stacoff, A., Kaelin, X., Stuessi, E. & Segesser, B. (1989) The torsion of the foot in running. *Int. J. Biomech.* **5**(4), 375–89.

Steindler, A. (1955) *Kinesiology of the Human Body*. Charles C. Thomas, Illinois.

Stuessi, E. (1989) Was heisst Ganganalyse? (What is good analysis?) *Swiss Med.* **3B**, 8–13.

Stuessi, E., Stacoff, A. & Tiegermann, V. (1987) Schnelle Seitwaertsbewegungen im Tennis (Fast sideward movements in tennis). In B. Segesser & W. Pfoerringer (eds) *Der Schuh im Sport*, pp. 56–64. Perimed, Erlangen.

Subotnick, S.I. (1975) Orthotic foot control and the overuse syndrome. *Phys. Sports Med.* 3, 75–9.

Warren, B.L. & Jones, C.J. (1987) Predicting plantar fasciitis in runners. *Med. Sci. Sports Exerc.* 19, 71–3.

Wirth, C.J., Kueswetter, W. & Jaeger, M. (1978) Biomechanik und Pathomechanik des oberen Sprunggelenks (Biomechanics and pathomechanics of the ankle point). *Hefte Unfallheikunde* 131, 10.

Chapter 32

Orthotics in Injury Prevention

NEIL CRATON AND DONALD C. MCKENZIE

Regular physical activity continues to be a significant pastime for people throughout the world. For several years, government agencies, the medical community and fitness enthusiasts from a number of disciplines have been urging the populace to engage in regular aerobic exercise in order to benefit their health and increase their sense of well-being. This multifaceted campaign has been extremely successful, and has resulted in ever increasing numbers of fitness participants. An unfortunate but predictable sequela of this increased dedication to the pursuit of physical activity has been an increase in the number of musculoskeletal injuries, particularly those of the lower extremity, often associated with overuse. The aetiology of these injuries can be traced to errors in training, inadequate strength and flexibility, an inappropriate surface, altered biomechanics and poor footwear. Of these, biomechanical factors frequently make a substantial contribution to overuse conditions. The sports medicine clinician is commonly called upon to address these biomechanical issues and to take appropriate measures to correct these aetiological factors. Often, the physician will utilize an orthotic device as part of the overall treatment regimen. Furthermore, the opinion of the sports medicine practitioner is often sought by patients who are questioning the use of orthotic devices in the prevention of injuries. This review will focus on orthotic devices and their contribution to the prevention and treatment of sports injuries.

Orthotics

Orthotics are appliances used to support, align, prevent or correct and improve the function of moveable parts of the body. Those frequently used in the prevention and treatment of disorders of the lower extremity in sports medicine are inserted into the patient's footwear. In this discipline, orthotics serve three primary functions. First, they are used to maintain the foot in a position of subtalar neutral through the support phase of gait. In theory, this will minimize the individual's tendency to either excess pronation or supination and the attendant injuries associated with these foot movements. The ability to maintain the subtalar joint in the neutral position is frequently used in the definition of an orthotic. Second, orthotic devices can be used to dissipate the energy associated with foot strike, in essence functioning as auxillary shock absorbers. Third, specially designed and manufactured orthotics can be used to treat specific patterns of biomechanical disadvantage by unloading the injured areas of the lower extremity.

There are numerous forms of orthotics, ranging from simple adhesive felt, to sophisticated expensive devices, custom made from a cast of the patient's foot. While there are commercially available, prefabricated orthotics, these frequently fail to maintain the individual's foot in the position of subtalar neutral. These products tend to be cheaper than their custom-made counterparts, and are widely available. However, they may not provide adequate control of motion or correction of alignment to treat or prevent injury. Generally, a thorough biomechanical assessment by a duly qualified practitioner will define the problem precisely, to a degree which can rarely be matched with commercially available devices.

Orthotics have traditionally been divided into categories based on their density, from soft, semisoft, semirigid to rigid. Soft orthotic devices are constructed to specifications from premade 'blanks'. They can be posted as required. They tend to be less expensive than semirigid orthotics, provide greater shock absorption, are easily adjusted to, and can often obviate the need for semirigid orthotics. Anatomically, they extend under the entire foot, mimicking the shoe's insole.

Semirigid orthotics are constructed with flexible plastics such as polyethylene, polypropylene, polyvinyl chloride, or materials such as rohadur. They usually extend from the posterior aspect of the calcaneus to the midportion of the metatarsals. They provide a more flexible platform than rigid acrylic orthotics, and hence are less likely to break when subjected to extreme forces (Micheli et al., 1986). These devices are manufactured from negative casts of the patient's foot in the subtalar neutral position. They tend to be expensive and require a period of gradual adaptation to the biomechanical alterations. They have the advantages of being more durable than soft orthotics and provide better control of subtalar motion due to their superior density. This form of orthotic is generally manufactured at laboratories under the supervision of a well-trained orthotist or podiatrist.

Biomechanical considerations

As a preface to the discussion of orthotics as preventative and therapeutic agents, the biomechanics of running, as well as the commonly identified patterns of stance and lower limb morphology which contribute to injury, should be considered.

The biomechanics of running have been well documented (Bates et al., 1979; Subotnick, 1985). Researchers from numerous disciplines have demonstrated the wide variability in running styles that contribute to the uniqueness of each person's locomotion. In addition, they have identified certain patterns of alignment which predispose the individual to a specific group of injuries. The fluid motion of running can be subdivided into alternate support and airborne phases, each of which can be further divided into component parts (Fig. 32.1).

At the beginning of the contact phase (often erroneously referred to as heel strike) the foot is typically in a supinated position, with external rotation of the tibia. The position of supination consists of subtalar inversion, ankle

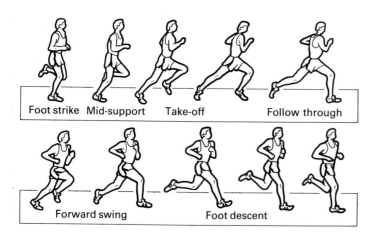

Foot strike Mid-support   Take-off   Follow through

Forward swing   Foot descent

Fig. 32.1 Biomechanics of running. From Subotnick (1985).

joint plantar flexion and forefoot adduction (Taunton *et al.*, 1988). In this position, the midtarsal joint is locked, stabilizing the fore-foot. As the foot is loaded secondary to ground contact, it begins to pronate and the tibia rotates internally. The movement of pronation is characterized by subtalar joint eversion, ankle dorsiflexion and forefoot abduction. During pronation the midtarsal joint is unlocked. This increases the flexibility of the foot and allows it to accommodate to the running surface, with a simultaneous dissipation of the energy imparted from ground strike. Pronation is, therefore, a normal and integral segment of the support phase of running gait. As the foot strikes the ground, there is a synchronous extension of the hip and flexion of the knee. There is progressive ankle dorsiflexion and knee flexion for the first half of the support phase of gait to facilitate further shock absorption (McKenzie *et al.*, 1985). The body continues to move forward over the fixed foot into the midstance of gait and the airborne leg passes the stance leg. This is associated with external rotation of the femur and tibia in concert with resupination of the foot and locking of the midtarsal joint, which stabilizes the longitudinal arch of the foot. This series of events creates a rigid lever to allow efficient propulsion, powered by forceful contraction of the gastrocnemius and soleus muscles with continued knee and hip extension.

As walking is a popular fitness activity, it is worthwhile briefly considering its biomechanical profile. In walking, the ground reactive force is essentially equal to body weight, whereas in running it approximates three times body weight, on a level surface (Cavanagh & Lafortune, 1980; Subotnick, 1985). The gastrocnemii contract to stabilize the ankle in walking, whereas in running they are active propulsive agents. The walking gait is broad-based in contrast to the running gait where each foot lands in close proximity to the midline of the body (Fig. 32.2). In running, the feet tend to point straight ahead or are slightly internally rotated. However, in walking, it is characteristic

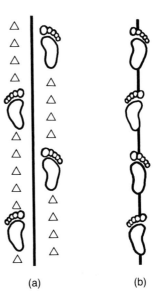

(a)   (b)

Fig. 32.2 Foot placement during (a) walking; (b) running. From Schamberger (1983).

for the feet to be externally rotated. The stance phase is similar in walking and running, albeit three times longer in walking. As walking velocity increases, the stance phase is progressively decreased, and the float phase (where both feet are air-borne) develops and is correspondingly increased (Table 32.1).

Clinical biomechanical assessment

A simple and clinically useful method of classifying an individual's biomechanical profile is by the configuration of the longitudinal arch of the foot. Using this schema, three foot types have been defined: (i) the normal foot; (ii) the high-arched cavus foot; and (iii) the flat plano-valgus foot (Fig. 32.3). Individuals with a neutral foot are said to be the most efficient and least likely to experience injuries secondary to biomechanical factors (Micheli *et al.*, 1986). The person with a flat or planovalgus foot type tends to undergo prolonged pronation, which extends into the propulsive phase of gait (Fig. 32.4). This can also be caused by excessive tibial varum, subtalar or forefoot varus, and

Table 32.1 Gait differences between walking and running. From Subotnick (1985).

Walking	Running
Single/double support phase	Single/double float phase
Ground reactive force equals body weight	Ground reactive force equals three times body weight
Musculature stabilizes ankle during propulsion	Active plantar flexion of the ankle during propulsion
Broad base of gait (feet externally rotated)	Gait progression midline of body (feet mildly internally rotated)
Stance phase 740–800 ms	Stance phase 250 ms
Foot lands in front of centre of gravity	Foot lands directly under centre of gravity

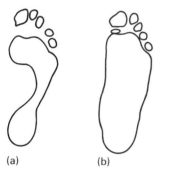

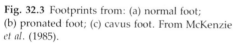

Fig. 32.3 Footprints from: (a) normal foot; (b) pronated foot; (c) cavus foot. From McKenzie *et al.* (1985).

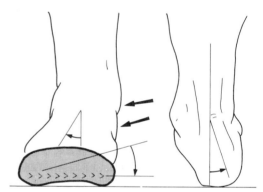

Fig. 32.4 Hyperpronation causes secondary effects such as increased tension on the medial aspect of the ankle and foot, valgus deviation of the calcaneus, oblique traction of the calcaneus tendon and increased internal rotation of the tibia. This hyperpronation can be prevented by use of orthotics. From Renström (1988).

many other common biomechanical factors (Taunton *et al.*, 1988). This excessive pronation is associated with a compensatory excessive and prolonged internal rotation of the tibia. This increased tibial rotation is translated up the kinetic chain to the femur, the hips, the pelvis and even to the lumbosacral spine. As such, the runner with excessive foot pronation may consequently suffer from a myriad of disorders involving the lumbar spine and entire lower extremity (Renström & Johnson, 1985). This foot type is very effective at dissipating the energy associated with ground strike and acting as a shock absorber.

The other end of the biomechanical spectrum is characterized by the high-arched cavus foot. Runners with this type of foot architecture have

decreased subtalar motion following ground strike, and hence, less energy is dissipated within the foot itself. Similarly, there is loss of the internal tibial rotation which is usually associated with subtalar movement. With foot strike, the heel remains in varus and the midtarsal joint fails to unlock. Due to these factors, the longitudinal arch remains rigid and energy is transmitted through the lateral foot to the knee without being significantly absorbed.

In the broadest biomechanical terms, the planovalgus foot is characterized by excellent shock absorption with excessive motion and the cavus foot by inferior shock absorption and limited subtalar motion.

Athletic footwear

The evolution of running shoes in recent years has been substantial. The major developments of modern athletic footwear involve features for motion control, shock absorption and the rigid cavus foot. These represent qualities which were initially only obtained with the use of orthotics but for the last few years have been found with increasing frequency in athletic shoes.

There are many factors included in modern shoes to enhance motion control. The use of thermoplastic heel counters is probably the single most important part of the stability system. The heel counter cradles the calcaneus and minimizes movement at the subtalar joint. This effectively limits excessive pronation (McKenzie, 1987). Additional motion control is gained by enhancing the torsional stability around the longitudinal axis of the shoe. This is typically achieved by the use of firm materials placed between the upper of the shoe and its midsole. This is referred to as board-lasting and is another factor designed to limit pronation. Furthermore, the medial aspect of the shoes' midsole is often reinforced with a material which has a higher density than that utilized in the lateral aspect. This helps to prevent medial collapse of the shoe and again serves to control excessive pronation. The final aspect of shoe construction used to limit pronation is straight-lasting of the sole; this eliminates the usual gentle 7 or 8° medial curve characteristic of earlier athletic shoes (Fig. 32.5).

All shoe manufacturers have invested substantial time and money to develop shoes with augmented shock-absorbing capabilities. This research has seen the development of a host of innovations which serve to diminish the forces transmitted to the foot and leg associated with the ground strike phase of gait. Air-filled chambers, gels and other similar materials and

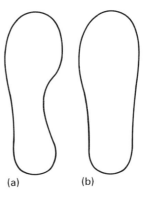

Fig. 32.5 Configuration of the last of a running shoe: (a) curved; (b) straight. From Schamberger (1983).

methods have greatly decreased the energy transmitted to the leg with running, and theoretically can decrease the incidence of injuries associated with impact loading (Macintyre *et al.*, 1991).

The third category of general shoe construction deals with those designed for the rigid cavus foot. As alluded to previously, this type of foot is characterized by limited subtalar motion and poor shock absorption. Therefore it requires features which are designed to enhance motion and dissipate energy. This is achieved by using a curved last which increases the pronation of the foot. The second tactic used to increase shoe flexibility is called slip-lasting. The upper of the shoe is constructed like a moccasin and is sewn into the midsole of the shoe with no intervening material. This augments longitudinal torsion and again, increases flexibility. The third factor in shoes for the cavus foot is the inclusion of an effective shock-absorbing midsole as outlined previously. The final way shoes for the cavus foot maximize energy dissipation is to use a narrow heel width with a minimal flare (Fig. 32.5). This again maximizes pronation and consequent energy dissipation.

It is evident that the footwear currently available has numerous biomechanical advantages over the prototypical sneaker of yesterday. Many of the previous indications for orthotic use have been addressed by these developments. As such, the running shoes of the 1990s are effective agents in the prophylaxis of overuse injuries of the lower extremity associated with athletic activity.

Orthotic prescription

Orthotics are used both as therapeutic and prophylactic agents. Whatever the indication for their use, orthotics must be prescribed only after a thorough history and physical examination with careful attention to the patient's biomechanical parameters. This assessment begins with an inspection of the patient's standing gait. Factors such as muscular asymmetry, femoral neck anteversion, genu varum or valgum, patellar squinting, patella alta, excessive Q angle, tibial varum, pes planus and pes cavus are important to note. A functional assessment of the patient's gait should also be conducted to see if active movement significantly alters the patient's biomechanical profile. Patients frequently have more functional pronation than that seen in the standing position (Schamberger, 1983). With regard to orthotic use, the position of the subtalar joint is of the utmost significance. Ideally, when the subtalar joint is in the neutral alignment, the central axes of the tibia, talus and calcaneus are in direct alignment, and this axis is perpendicular to the horizontal axis of the metatarsals (Subotnick, 1985) (Fig. 32.6).

Subtalar alignment is most easily appreciated with the patient in the prone position, while the examiner palpates the medial and lateral aspects of the talus (Fig. 32.7). With equal talar protrusion on each side of the ankle joint, the subtalar joint is said to be in the neutral position. Next, a line is drawn that bisects the longitudinal aspect of the calcaneus. The angle created by this line and the line bisecting the tibia, is referred to as the rearfoot or subtalar angle. It is commonly oriented in a slight varus fashion (Fig. 32.7); Taunton et al. (1981) assert that the 'normal' subtalar varus angulation is 3°. The relative alignment of the forefoot is then determined. Standard practice involves placing a plantar force on the 4th and 5th metatarsals until resistance is felt. The plane which is defined by the metatarsal heads in this position is compared with the plane perpendicular to the line bisecting the calcaneus (Fig. 32.8). Again a slight varus deviation of approximately 2° is considered normal (Taunton et al., 1981). It is evident that this is not an exact science; the precise angles are debatable and often practitioner dependent. Substantial increases in either rearfoot or forefoot varus often necessitate increased and prolonged subtalar pronation during the running gait.

Once the patient's alignment has been thoroughly assessed and measured, the practitioner must decide on the appropriate orthotic posting. The posting is the precise angulation that the orthotic is intended to impart to the rearfoot and forefoot. Conservative posting is recommended to minimize adaptation difficult-

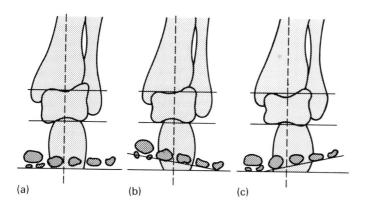

(a)   (b)   (c)

Fig. 32.6 Lower extremity rearfoot and forefoot relationships: (a) normal forefoot; (b) forefoot varus; (c) forefoot valgus. From Subotnick (1985).

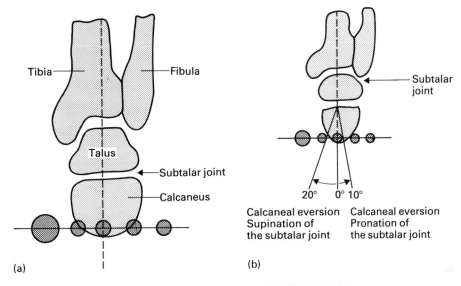

Tibia

Fibula

Talus

Subtalar joint

Calcaneus

(a)

Subtalar joint

20°   0° 10°

Calcaneal eversion
Supination of
the subtalar joint

Calcaneal eversion
Pronation of
the subtalar joint

(b)

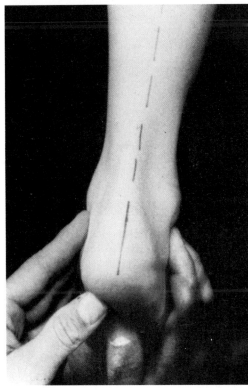

(c)

Fig. 32.7 (a) Neutral subtalar joint; (b) motion about the subtalar joint; (c) determining the neutral position. From Franz (1988).

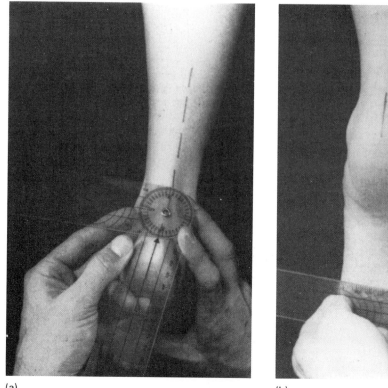

(a)

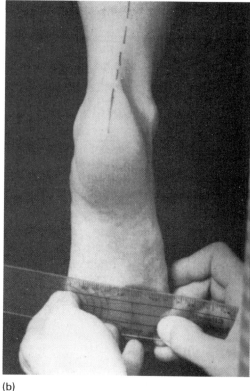

(b)

Fig. 32.8 Measurement of (a) subtalar; and (b) forefoot deviations from the neutral position. This athlete has a mild varus alignment of both the subtalar and forefoot.

ies and prevent overcorrection. Varus posting which is too aggressive frequently leads to lateral foot, leg and knee pain as lateral structures are placed under excessive traction. In addition, excess varus posting can increase the frequency of lateral ankle sprains. The sport the patient is involved in needs to be considered. Sports with a high risk of lateral ankle sprains, such as volleyball and basketball, necessitate conservative posting, while sports such as distance running can use more aggressive posting. The patient's footwear must also be addressed, as different shoes can have vastly different biomechanical properties. Also, the prescribing physician must be aware of potential biomechanical differences between feet and measure each foot independently (Taunton *et al.*, 1988).

General consequences of orthotic use

The majority of sports medicine practitioners and athletes are satisfied with the clinical benefits afforded by orthotic devices (McKenzie, 1987). Numerous investigators have demonstrated that orthotics are effective at reducing both the extent and velocity of pronation as well as limiting calcaneal eversion (Bates *et al.*, 1979; Smith *et al.*, 1983; Taunton *et al.*, 1985). Clement *et al.* (1984) have also shown that orthotics do not substantially alter the oxygen cost of running.

Medical practitioners who prescribe orthotics must inform their patients that the device is not a 'cure' for their biomechanical problems, and is only worthwhile when it is being used.

This requires long-term commitment on the part of the patient. Unfortunately, the biomechanical features which orthotics control are often not affected by other forms of therapy.

A review of the literature indicates that more than 75% of injured athletes treated with orthotics as part of their therapeutic protocol returned to their previous level of activity (James *et al.*, 1978; Clement *et al.*, 1981). One must remember, however, that the orthotic was only one part of a comprehensive rehabilitation programme in these studies, and therefore, undue reliance cannot be placed on these devices.

Specific indications for orthotics

Orthotic use in sports medicine has to be viewed as an endeavour which is both therapeutic and prophylactic. When a practitioner treats a patient with an orthotic for an injury, he or she is also attempting to prevent a recurrence of that injury. The patient's biomechanics obviously are involved in the aetiology of the condition, and by virtue of their correction, the injury will, in theory, be less likely to recur.

The indications for orthotic use have traditionally fallen under two broad categories, paralleling the extremes of foot morphology. Simply stated, the planovalgus foot requires orthotics to stabilize the subtalar joint, while the cavus foot requires additional shock absorption. As mentioned previously, improvements in modern athletic footwear have decreased the need to prescribe orthotics for modest biomechanical abnormalities (Macintyre *et al.*, 1991). In fact, the knowledgeable physician can now prescribe specific shoes in an effort to compensate for abnormal alignment. However, there are still many conditions which will benefit from definitive orthotic prescription.

While biomechanical problems are only one of a host of intrinsic factors leading to overuse injury, there is an association between foot type and injury. Disorders associated with each type of foot and those common to both are listed in Table 32.2.

Clinical situations

Most injuries associated with the hypermobile planovalgus foot benefit from the use of semirigid orthotics (James *et al.*, 1978; D'ambrosia, 1985). These offer superb motion control without increasing shock absorption. In this situation, soft orthotics are often used as an interim step prior to the construction of semirigid orthoses (James *et al.*, 1978). In children, soft orthotics can be used instead of semirigid orthotics. This decreases the expense of frequently making new semirigid orthotics as the child's foot continues to grow.

The posterior tibialis tendon is important in decelerating the motion of the foot in the transverse plane, as well as supporting the medial arch. Hence, it is particularly vulnerable in individuals with planovalgus feet. In the runner, repeated episodes of overpronation can lead to irritation and subsequent tendon injury. Preventing the excess subtalar eversion and supporting the medial longitudinal arch with a semirigid orthotic can be of dramatic benefit.

Tibial stress syndrome generally has a multifactorial aetiology. A substantial contribution

Table 32.2 Common overuse injuries with reference to foot type.

Cavus foot	Both	Planovalgus foot
Metatarsalgia	Iliotibial band friction syndrome	Posterior tibial tendonitis
Peroneal tendonitis	Plantar fasciitis	Tibial stress syndrome
Tarsal stress fractures	Achilles tendonitis	Morton's neuroma
Metatarsal stress fractures	Patellar tendonitis	
Fibular stress fractures	Patellofemoral pain syndrome	

is made by prolonged pronation which results in internal rotation of the tibia. This syndrome can be treated with semirigid orthotics to minimize this excessive motion. Some researchers have documented a decreasing incidence of tibial stress syndrome (Macintyre *et al.*, 1991) and hypothesized that biomechanical corrections in footwear are at least partially responsible. This represents a good example of injury prophylaxis by addressing the role of alignment in the origin of injury.

Conditions associated with the cavus foot are listed in Table 32.2. These have traditionally been considered less amenable to orthotic correction. Metatarsalgia, metatarsal and tarsal stress fractures typically require augmented shock absorption or methods to unload the painful area. Orthotics toward the soft end of the spectrum are generally used in these clinical situations.

The exact anatomical configuration of the metatarsal heads represents an area of some controversy. Some authors state that a 'transverse metatarsal arch' does not exist (Basmajian & Slonecker, 1989), yet biomechanical studies have shown that the majority of weight is borne by the 1st and 5th metatarsal heads (James *et al.*, 1978; Schamberger, 1983), and the concept of a transverse metatarsal arch is useful clinically. If this arch is poorly defined, or 'collapsed', the patient will typically bear excessive weight on the 2nd, 3rd and 4th metatarsals, bones which are structurally ill-suited to weight-bearing. Frequently this leads to callous formation in the plantar aspect of the 2nd, 3rd and 4th metatarsal heads. Protracted stress can lead to metatarsalgia and metatarsal stress fractures. This is particularly significant in the case of the 2nd metatarsal which is firmly anchored proximally in the mortice of the cuneiforms and therefore, relatively immobile. Furthermore, the narrowing of the space between the metatarsals can lead to pressure on the interdigital nerve. This frequently leads to the formation of a Morton's neuroma, most commonly in the space between the 3rd and 4th metatarsals. Here, the interdigital nerve receives contributions from both the medial and lateral plantar nerves, and substantial interdigital mobility at this site can lead to neural irritation and eventual neuroma formation.

To benefit these conditions, the practitioner may prescribe a metatarsal pad. This simple device is shaped like a small cookie and is placed just proximal to the plantar surface of the metatarsal heads (Fig. 32.9). This serves two functions. First, it augments the transverse metatarsal arch and thereby increases the space between the metatarsals, decreasing the mechanical neural irritation (Schamberger, 1983).

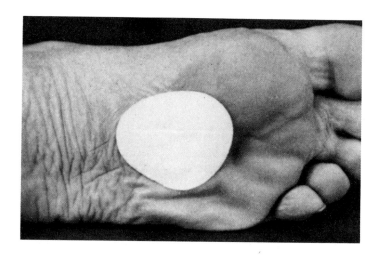

Fig. 32.9 Placement of a metatarsal pad.

Second, it diverts some of the force associated with ground strike away from the metatarsal heads. Care must be taken when placing this pad. If it is too close to the metatarsal heads, it will increase the metatarsalgia; if it is too far removed, it will not be effective.

Another valuable orthotic modification can be used in the treatment of sesamoiditis. This is the 2–5 metatarsal bar. This entails using a band of firm material placed under the 2nd to 5th metatarsal heads. In the case of sesamoiditis, the area under the painful bones is cut out. Theoretically this unloads the painful area. Investigators have reported good results with this tool (Clement, 1987).

Treatment of iliotibial band friction syndrome can involve both the more classic semi-rigid varus posted orthotic or a different form of orthotic modification. In one form, forefoot overpronation and the consequent internal tibial rotation, places excess traction on the tibial attachment of the band, leading to increased friction at the lateral femoral epicondyle and the development of pain. Pain can also be experienced over the greater trochanter of the femur, and into the gluteal musculature. This type is treated with the more traditional semi-rigid orthotic to decrease subtalar motion. In cases of iliotibial band friction syndrome when the patient has a rigid type of cavus foot and genu varum, excessive force is transmitted through the foot to the knee. Here, excessive traction develops over the lateral femoral epicondyle, again leading to pain (Garrick & Webb, 1990). To address these factors, lateral foot posting is used to decrease the traction along the lateral leg structures while simultaneously decreasing the varus alignment at the knee. Such unconventional lateral posting has been used for other lateral leg conditions such as fibular stress fractures, peroneal tendonitis and trochanteric bursitis (Schamberger, 1983).

A Morton's extension is another modification which can be made to standard orthotics to address specific biomechanical problems. This is used to treat patients with hallux valgus and 'Morton's foot' with secondary metatarsalgia.

In these conditions, the 1st metatarsal is adducted, medially rotated, and appears shortened. This causes the 2nd metatarsal to appear longer than the first. This can cause the 2nd metatarsal head to bear an inappropriate amount of weight. Furthermore, hallux valgus is thought to be exacerbated by forefoot overpronation. Therefore, an orthotic limiting subtalar motion can be of benefit to these conditions and prevent their progression. In addition the orthotic can incorporate an extension under the base of the 1st metatarsophalangeal joint. This allows more weight to be borne in this area during the propulsive phase of gait, and hence, can alleviate the discomfort associated with these entities.

Orthotics as preventive therapy

In sports medicine, as in all medical disciplines, prevention of injury and illness is of the utmost importance. Appropriate training protocols, strength and flexibility exercises, protective equipment, prudent coaching, modern footwear, good nutrition, adequate supervision, sanctioned officiating and safe environments all make substantial contributions to the safety of the participants. Given this desire to prevent injuries, the sports medicine practitioner is often faced with the decision of whether or not to prescribe orthotic devices to the individual with obvious biomechanical aberrancy who has not yet suffered injury as a result of these factors. To answer this question, appropriately, the sports medicine practitioner must be aware of several salient facts. First, biomechanical factors are only one of the potential aetiological considerations in any disorder. It is wise to view biomechanical factors as contributory to, not causative of, injury. They represent only one of a host of intrinsic and extrinsic causes of musculoskeletal problems; however, they can be a very significant factor (Hess et al., 1989). Second, orthotics cannot be viewed as a panacea, and must be incorporated into a comprehensive preventive or rehabilitative programme, as alluded to previously. Furthermore, the athletic footwear of the 1990s is designed to address most moderate biomechanical problems.

Given the above, it seems prudent to encourage appropriate footwear for the patient or athlete with obvious malalignment, and to stress a sensible training regimen. The prescription of orthotics based only on anatomical factors is a controversial issue and can be of considerable expense. In addition, as with all forms of therapeutic and prophylactic endeavours, there are potential unwanted side-effects with these devices. Further study into the aetiology and prevention of overuse athletic injury may allow more precise recommendations in the future.

References

Basmajian, J. & Slonecker, C. (1989) *Grant's Method of Anatomy. A Clinical Problem Solving Approach.* Williams & Wilkins, Baltimore.

Bates, B., Osternig, L., Mason, B. & James, L. (1979) Foot orthotic devices to modify selected aspects of lower extremity mechanics. *Am. J. Sports Med.* **7**, 338–42.

Cavanagh, P. & Lafortune, M. (1980) Ground reaction forces in distance running. *J. Biomech.* **13**, 397–406.

Clement, D. (1987) Stress fractures of the foot and ankle. In R.J. Shephard & J.E. Taunton (eds) *Foot and Ankle in Sport and Exercise*, pp. 56–70. Karger, Basel.

Clement, D., Taunton, J., Smart, G. & McNicol, K. (1981) A survey of overuse running injury. *Phys. Sportsmed.* **9**, 47–58.

Clement, D., Taunton, J., Wiley, P., Smart, G. & McNicol, K. (1984) The corrective orthotic devices effect on O_2 uptake during running. In Bachl, Porkop & Suckert (eds) *Current Topics in Sports Medicine*, pp. 930–40. Urban & Schwartzenberg, Baltimore.

D'ambrosia, R. (1985) Orthotic devices in running injuries. *Clin. Med.* **4**, 611–18.

Franz, W. (1988) Overuse syndromes in runners. In M.B. Mellion (ed) *Office Management of Sports Injuries and Athletic Problems*, pp. 289–310. Hanley & Belfus, Philadelphia.

Garrick, J. & Webb, D. (1990) *Sports Injuries: Diagnosis and Management.* WB Saunders, Philadelphia.

Hess, G., Cappiello, W., Poole, R. & Hunter, S. (1989) Prevention and treatment of overuse tendon injuries. *Sports Med.* **8**, 371–84.

James, S., Bates, B. & Osternig, L. (1978) Injuries to runners. *Am. J. Sports Med.* **6**, 40–9.

Macintyre, J., Taunton, J., Clement, D., Lloyd-Smith, R., McKenzie, D. & Morrell, R. (1991) Running injuries: A clinical study of 4173 cases. *Clin. J. Sport Med.* **1**, 81–7.

McKenzie, D. (1987) The role of the shoe and orthotics. In R.J. Shephard & J.E. Taunton (eds) *Foot and Ankle in Sport and Exercise*, pp. 30–8. Karger, Basel.

McKenzie, D., Clement, D. & Taunton, J. (1985) Running shoes, orthotics and injuries. *Sports Med.* **2**, 334–47.

Micheli, L., Santopietro, F. & Sohn, R. (1986) Athletic footwear and modifications. In J. Nicholas & E. Hershman (eds) *The Lower Extremity and Spine in Sports Medicine*, pp. 584–601. CV Mosby, St Louis.

Renström, P. (1988) Diagnosis and management of overuse injuries. In A. Dirix, H.G. Knuttgen & K. Tittel (eds) *The Olympic Book of Sports Medicine*, pp. 446–68. Blackwell Scientific Publications. Oxford.

Renström, P. & Johnson, R. (1985) Overuse injuries in sports: A review. *Sports Med.* **2**, 316–33.

Schamberger, W. (1983) Orthotics for athletes: Attacking the biomechanical roots of injury. *Can. Fam. Phys.* **29**, 1670–80.

Smith, L., Clarke, T., Hamill, C. & Santopietro, F. (1983) The effects of soft and semi-rigid orthoses upon rearfoot movement in running. *Med. Sci. Sports Exerc.* **15**, 171.

Subotnick, S. (1985) The biomechanics of running; Implications for the prevention of foot injuries. *Sports Med.* **2**, 144–53.

Taunton, J., Clement, D., Smart, G., Wiley, P. & McNicol, K. (1985) A triplanar electrogoniometer investigation of running mechanics in runners with compensatory overpronation. *Can. J. Appl. Sport Sci.* **10**, 104–15.

Taunton, J., Clement, D. & Webber, D. (1981) Lower extremity stress fractures in athletes. *Phys. Sportsmed.* **9**, 77–86.

Taunton, J., McKenzie, D. & Clement, D. (1988) The role of biomechanics in the epidemiology of injuries. *Sports Med.* **6**, 107–20.

Taunton, J. & Moore, P. (1990) *Running Shoes for the '90s: Technological Advances.* Sports Aider, Sport Medicine Council of British Columbia, Canada.

Chapter 33

Heat in Injury Prevention and Care

DAVID F. MARTIN AND WALTON W. CURL

The use of heat in its various forms to increase tissue temperature is called thermotherapy. Numerous agents can be used to raise tissue temperature, either in a general fashion or in localized areas. Although, classically, heat is used in the late stages of athletic injury rehabilitation, increased tissue temperature throughout preparticipation warm-up has proved to be of value, and therefore thermotherapy is being investigated as a means of preventing injury (Cox *et al.*, 1989; Prentice & Malone, 1990). Understanding the effects of heat on various tissues, heat transfer and the modes of heat delivery to tissues, will allow the sports medicine specialist to use thermotherapy to prevent injury, to treat injury, to rehabilitate injury and to prevent reinjury.

Effects of heat on tissues

In addition to increasing local tissue temperature, heat has a number of physiological effects that may be important to injury prevention. Classically, thermotherapy has been used in the later stages of injury rehabilitation, but an in-depth look at its physiological effects may reveal applications for heat in the prevention of athletic injury as well. One such effect is vasodilatation, which results in an increase in blood flow to warmed tissues, and a concomitant increase in capillary permeability, which, in turn, increases the removal rate of metabolic wastes. The vasodilatation occurs both in arterioles and in capillaries and results in over-

all increased blood flow to the body part or tissue that is being treated. This increased blood flow may well be responsible for many of the beneficial physiological effects of thermotherapy (Cox *et al.*, 1989).

Thermotherapy is also analgesic, and as such, has been used for thousands of years in the management of athletic injuries (Marino, 1986; Peterson & Renström, 1986). The analgesic effects of heat are not well understood, but experience has shown its useful effect on pain mediated by inflammation. Cox *et al.* (1989) have shown that heat can act selectively on free nerve endings and peripheral nerve fibres to increase the pain threshold. Heat also is believed to play a role in decreasing sensory nerve conduction velocities and in activating descending pain inhibitory systems. Concomitantly, heat-mediated vasodilatation can reduce pain by removing the waste products from injured tissue — prostaglandins, bradykinins and histamines (Cox *et al.*, 1989). Finally, heat can directly affect γ fibres of muscle spindles, decreasing their activity and sensitivity to stretch, and thereby decreasing muscle spasm and reducing pain.

A second physiological effect of heat is to increase local tissue metabolism. Heat increases blood flow, which increases the delivery of oxygen, phagocytes and enzymes to tissues, which, in turn, increase the metabolic rate. With a 10°C rise in temperature, a cell's chemical activity and metabolic rate become two to three times normal (Cox *et al.*, 1989). This increase in tissue metabolism may have a protective effect, allowing tissues to withstand increased stresses and demands before it is injured.

The most important effect of heat in thermotherapy is its effect on connective tissues, specifically collagen. Collagen has both viscous and elastic properties, so the faster it is loaded, the stiffer it becomes (Peterson & Renström, 1986). The application of thermal energy alters these visco-elastic properties, making the collagen more extensible by increasing both elasticity and plasticity. Because tendons, joint capsules and muscles have a high collagen content, heat can increase their flexibility and perhaps decrease their risk of injury (Peterson & Renström, 1986; Cox et al., 1989; Strickler et al., 1990). Passive warming by 4°C has been shown to increase the amount of elongation of a muscle before its rupture. This protective effect lends credence to the preventive value of a warm-up before any athletic activity (Safran et al., 1988; Strickler et al., 1990). With heated collagen fibres being more extensible, heat can be used to prepare and protect injured tissues in an athlete during rehabilitative exercises.

In summary, then, muscles function better when they are warmed to levels slightly above body temperature — strength, speed and developed power are maximized when muscle temperature is increased. Connective tissue viscosity is lowered and elasticity is increased, resulting in reduced tissue friction and less resistance to muscle contraction. The increased blood flow secondary to increased temperature brings vital oxygen more quickly and speeds removal of the waste products of muscle contraction. Elevated tissue temperature speeds the chemical reactions necessary for contraction of muscles and results in greater strength, decreased fatigue, quicker recovery and decreased postexercise soreness (Solomonow & D'Ambrosia, 1987). The importance of this improved muscle function to both injury prevention and injury rehabilitation should not be overlooked.

The scientific basis for these physiological effects of thermotherapy is sound in some

areas, weak and tenuous in others (Cox et al., 1989). More research is needed to determine specific tissue responses to different types of heat; much more data are needed concerning timing and dosages of heat in relation to the above tissue responses.

Heat transfer

Heat can be delivered to tissues by way of four main mechanisms: (i) conduction; (ii) convection; (iii) radiation; and (iv) conversion. When using the various means of transferring heat, it is important to know which mechanism is being used and which tissues are being heated. Deeper tissues may be damaged without the skin being burned, so depth of heat penetration and anatomical knowledge are extremely important. Thermotherapy is often utilized around joints; peripheral nerves in those areas can be subjected to significant heating because there is minimal subcutaneous tissue covering and insulating them from harm.

Conduction is the exchange of heat through surface contact. In conduction, one body transfers thermal energy to another by direct physical contact. Energy flows from the warmer object to the cooler object and equalizes the temperatures, thereby warming the cooler body, especially at the point of contact. An example of thermotherapy by conduction is the use of hot packs. Heat transfer by conduction is primarily superficial, because the thickness of overlying subcutaneous tissues, muscles and fat limits the passage of heat to the deeper tissues.

Convection is the transfer of thermal energy to a body part as air or water molecules flow across that part. With thermotherapy, warm−hot water or air is circulated past a joint or a limb, imparting thermal energy to that part and causing a rise in its temperature. An example of heat transfer by convection is the whirlpool. Although convection involves direct contact just as conduction does, it is the flow and movement of the heating medium across the body that truly characterizes convection.

Radiation is the transfer of thermal energy from a warmer source to the body or body part through a conducting medium such as air (Cox *et al.*, 1989). Electromagnetic energy is emitted from a specific source to heat an area of the body's surface. While conduction and convection require a transport medium, radiation does not (Prentice & Malone, 1990). An example of radiation thermotherapy is the heat lamp. The medium that separates the body from the source (air, in the case of the heat lamp) does affect the energy exchange and therefore is important in judging how much heat is imparted to the body surface.

Conversion is the transformation of one form of energy into another. In thermotherapy, this usually involves shortwave or ultrasound (i.e. non-thermal forms of energy). Heat is produced as these forms of energy are converted to thermal energy in the tissues. As electrical and sound wave energy penetrates the tissues, it is converted to thermal energy and produces heat (Prentice & Malone, 1990). Conversion can be effective at depths up to 5 cm and thus is useful in the treatment of deeper tissues. Unlike conduction and radiation, which depend solely on temperature differences to deliver thermal energy, and convection, which depends both on temperature differences and on mass transport of the warmer medium, conversion thermotherapy does not depend on temperature differences between the heat source and the body (Prentice & Malone, 1990).

In understanding and utilizing thermotherapy, these mechanisms of heat transfer are extremely important. For example, not all therapeutic thermal energy is absorbed by superficial tissues — it can be reflected *or* transmitted to deeper layers. This can be critical when heat-sensitive structures are near the area or body part being treated with thermotherapy. Selec-

tive heating is desirable, but not always attainable because conduction, convection, radiation and conversion are not always precise in their transfer of thermal energy to tissues.

It must be remembered that in addition to gaining heat and being warmed as a result of three of these mechanisms — conduction, convection and radiation — a body part or area can lose heat through these mechanisms as well. Also, heat can be dissipated through evaporation as sweat changes from liquid to vapour on the skin, but this mechanism is not important in thermotherapy (Prentice & Malone, 1990).

Exercise and subsequent muscle activity also can lead to heating. An exercising muscle at maximal activity can generate more than 20 times as much energy as that at rest, thereby leading to increased heat in both the muscle and the nearby tissues (Mellion & Shelton, 1990). This thermal energy not only is transferred to surrounding joints and tissues, but also is transferred to circulating blood. In addition, the increase in basal metabolic rate during exercise contributes to a rise in body temperature. Blood has a high capacitance for heat and can transport a relatively large heat load with only a moderate increase in its temperature (Mellion & Shelton, 1990). An understanding of these mechanisms is important in evaluating warm-up, both as a treatment and as an injury prevention tool.

Methods of heat delivery

The superficial application of heat increases the temperature of the skin and immediate underlying tissues, with a concomitant increase in circulation to a depth of 1 cm (Cox *et al.*, 1989; Poole *et al.*, 1991; Saliba *et al.*, 1991). The most common forms of superficial thermotherapy are contrast whirlpools, warm whirlpools, paraffin wax, hydrocollator packs and infrared heat. These transfer thermal energy by conduction, convection and radiation.

Deeper heating is generally achieved through the mechanism of conversion and the two most common forms are diathermy (using high-frequency electromagnetic currents) and ultrasound (using high-frequency sound waves to vibrate and thus to heat tissues). These deep-heating modalities can heat effectively to depths of 2–5 cm (Marino, 1986).

Superficial heating

The application of superficial heat causes a sudden rise in skin temperature of approximately 5°C. The body then increases blood flow in an attempt to dissipate the heat with cooling blood — these vasodilatation effects are mediated by local axon reflexes to the skin, the release of chemical mediators and local spinal reflexes (Saliba et al., 1991). Reduction in pain, relaxation of muscle spasm, and increased flexibility result from superficial thermal energy transfer. Indications for superficial heating include subacute injury, muscle spasm, decreased range of motion and use in warm-up before exercise. Contraindications to the use of superficial heating include impaired skin sensation, poor circulation, poor thermal regulation, haemophilia and bony or soft tissue tumours (Cox et al., 1989; Saliba et al., 1991).

Whirlpools can be used for pure warming or as contrast baths. They apply heat circumferentially, and have the added advantage of the buoyant properties of water. This can aid in pain relief and muscle relaxation, and the fact that the athlete can perform active movements or exercises in the whirlpool can further warm the tissues. Thermal energy can be exchanged through both conduction and convection (Poole et al., 1991). The temperature of the water for simple thermotherapy should stay between 36 and 43°C; for contrast baths, the warm water temperature should be between 40 and 43°C; and the cold water temperature between 10 and 15°C.

The duration of warming whirlpool baths is 15–30 min; if contrast baths are used, the warm-water cycle is shortened and the cold-water cycle interspersed as 1–2 min immersions (Cox et al., 1989). As a source of superficial heat, whirlpools are especially useful in facilitating exercise. In addition, they provide even, circumferential, controllable heating (Poole et al., 1991).

Paraffin wax can provide localized superficial heat, especially in small joints such as those about the wrist, fingers, ankle and foot. Mineral oil is added to the paraffin to lower its melting point, and the bath is kept at 52–54°C. The body part being treated is then successively placed into the bath and removed to allow coats of paraffin to harden on the skin. The coated body part is then wrapped with towels or plastic to insulate and sustain the heating (Saliba et al., 1991), and the wax remains in place for 15–30 min before being removed. Care must taken with this form of superficial heat, because there is decreased control of the increase in temperature and thus an increased risk for skin burns (Cox et al., 1989).

Hydrocollator packs, or hot packs (Fig. 33.1), deliver thermal energy by conduction and are used at temperatures between 50 and 70°C. The packs generally consist of canvas pouches of petroleum distillate (Prentice, 1986). The packs are immersed until they are used and are then wrapped in towels before being applied to the body. This insulation is important and should be at least 2 cm thick to prevent burns of the skin (Cox et al., 1989). Treatment time is generally 15–20 min. Hydrocollator packs are commercially available and can be reused. The athlete should not lie directly on a hydrocollator pack because this can damage the pack as well as burn the skin.

Infrared heat penetrates only 2–3 mm into the skin, but it can be used to elevate local temperature quite rapidly and it does not come into contact with the skin. Burning of the skin can be avoided by the use of moist towels over the area being treated and the use of dry towels to protect surrounding areas (Cox et al., 1989). The moist towels trap the heat build up and allow greater blood to tissue heat exchange (Prentice, 1986).

Superficial heating results in increased circulation, greater flexibility, decreased pain and

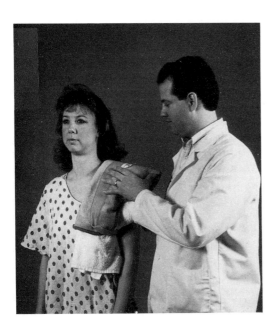

Fig. 33.1 Application of a hot pack for superficial heating. (Method: conduction; depth: <2 cm; type: increased skin temperature and vasodilation; heat: up to 5°C.)

decreased muscle spasm. The mechanisms of these changes are not fully understood, but they may well be tissue-protective. Further investigation will be needed to ascertain their appropriate place in the prevention of athletic injuries.

Deep heating

Diathermy and ultrasound (Fig. 33.2) are the two ways that heat can be delivered to deeper tissues. Both cause temperature changes through conversion, and function at depths of 2–5 cm. It is important to remember that while they function locally at these depths, their thermal energy can be transferred more widely through tissue-to-tissue direct conduction. Anatomical relationships must be remembered so that appropriate tissues can be heated without surrounding structures being damaged.

Diathermy is the use of high-frequency electromagnetic currents to induce deep heating through vibration and distortion of

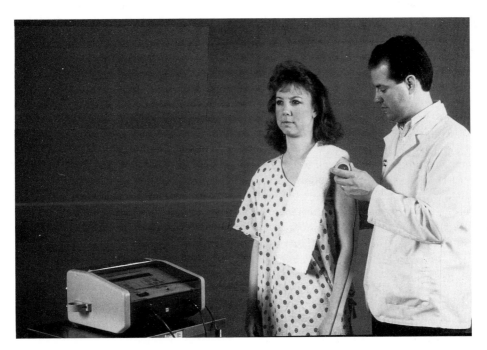

Fig. 33.2 Application of ultrasound for deep heating. (Method: conversion; depth: 2–5 cm; type: high-frequency sound waves and vasodilation; heat: up to 2°C.)

tissue molecules. It has been in clinical use since the 1920s. Shortwave diathermy can penetrate somewhat more deeply (3–5 cm) than microwave diathermy, although tissues with high water content (fat, muscle) are heated preferentially (Cox *et al.*, 1989). Diathermy provides deep, dry heating, but if used inappropriately may cause subcutaneous fat necrosis. Studies on the effectiveness of diathermy have not shown it to be significantly more useful than hot packs (DATTA, 1983). The value of applying diathermy in athletic injury treatment and prevention remains unclear, but it should be studied further because diathermy is an effective method of heating deep tissues (Poole *et al.*, 1991).

Ultrasound uses waves with a frequency of greater than 20 000 c.p.s. to generate heat by tissue vibration (Peterson & Renström, 1986). This high-frequency sound energy can heat tissues as deep as 5 cm (Saliba *et al.*, 1991). Research into the use of ultrasonic waves dates back to the early 1800s, but the first published report of its therapeutic use came in 1938 (Cox *et al.*, 1989). Ultrasound does not involve electromagnetic radiation as do the other forms of deep heating, and it is also unique because it is not significantly attenuated by fat. Sound waves are well absorbed by tissues with high protein content, such as muscle and connective tissues, and can heat tissues up to 2°C to a depth of 5 cm. Ultrasound also has other non-thermal effects, including micromassage through vibration, alterations in cell permeability, alterations in sodium/potassium diffusion, and accelerated enzyme activity (Cox *et al.*, 1989; Saliba *et al.*, 1991). Ultrasound has been shown to be effective in reducing the pain associated with inflammation, and current therapeutic indications include sprains, strains, tendinitis, bursitis, tenosynovitis, pain secondary to inflammation, muscle spasm, joint stiffness and contracted scar tissue. Ultrasound can also be used to deliver medications through the skin, a process known as phonophoresis.

Contraindications to ultrasound include its use over open growth plates in children, in skin problems, around suspected malignant tumours, around the eyes or heart, and around a cardiac pacemaker (Marino, 1985; Cox *et al.*, 1989; Poole *et al.*, 1991; Saliba *et al.*, 1991).

The use of ultrasound for injury prevention in the athlete has not been investigated, but it remains the mainstay of deep thermotherapy in the treatment of athletic injuries. The effects of ultrasound are promising in athletic injury prevention due to the ability to deliver heat to deep tissues, resulting in perhaps more joint motion, greater flexibility and more efficient muscle function during warm-up before athletic participation. More research is needed to evaluate ultrasound as an effective tool for injury prevention.

Heat retainers

None of the heat-transfer techniques discussed thus far can be used during athletic competition. A heat retainer, however, can be used during competition, as well as during training and at rest. Heat retainers (Fig. 33.3) are manufactured from synthetic materials designed to generate and retain heat. They generally are used to offer support, tactile feedback and circumferential wrapping/heating to various areas in the limbs, especially the joints (ankles, knees, thighs, wrists, elbows) (Peterson & Renström, 1986). The most effective heat retainer is porous, has minimal absorptive capacity, and has good insulation to retain body heat. Examples include neoprene knee sleeves, ankle wraps and elbow sleeves. Early studies on the use of these devices to prevent athletic injuries show them to be an effective form of 'active' thermotherapy (Peterson & Renström, 1986).

Implications for injury prevention

Thermotherapy has been used for centuries to treat various types of pain. Increasing superficial and deep tissue temperature can increase blood flow, promote healing, enhance metabolism and increase collagen (and therefore

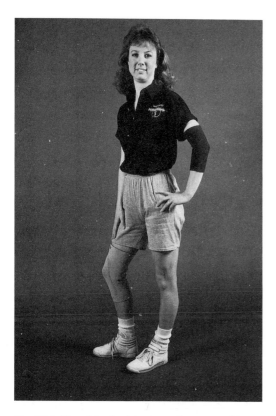

Fig. 33.3 Use of heat retainers on the arm and leg.

muscle and tendon) elasticity and flexibility. In contrast, the application of heat to prevent injuries in athletes is new.

Warm-up has been shown to decrease athletic injuries (Ekstrand, 1982), and it is now believed that a portion of this benefit may well be due to tissue warming. The fact that heating collagen can increase its elasticity and flexibility, coupled with the ability of heated muscles to absorb more energy, may indeed make thermotherapy an effective mode of injury prevention (Strickler *et al.*, 1990). Perhaps if tissues, either superficial or deep, that are at risk for injury are heated, those tissues will be protected by some of the above effects on their physiology and function. An athlete could then use a heat-retainer to keep the tissues warm and protected during athletic activity. However, no sound research currently demonstrates these effects.

Conclusion

The sports medicine specialist needs to be aware of the various forms of thermotherapy — their application before activity may not only be protective, but may also improve performance. The use of heat to ensure appropriate range of motion and flexibility before athletic activity can decrease joint stiffness and muscle spasm; coupled with a heat-retaining device used during activity, this thermotherapy can result in reduced risk of injury.

References

Cox, J.S., Andrish, J.T., Indelicato, P.A. & Walsh, W.M. (1989) Heat modalities. In D. Prez (ed) *Therapeutic Modalities for Sports Injuries*, pp. 1−24. Year Book Medical Publishers, Chicago.

DATTA (Diagnostic and therapeutic technology assessment) (1983) Diathermy (questions and answers) *J. Am. Med. Assoc.* **250**, 540.

Ekstrand, J. (1982) *Soccer injuries and their prevention*. Linkoping University Medical Dissertation No. 130, Linkoping, Sweden.

Marino, M. (1986) Principles of therapeutic modalities: Implications for sports injuries. In J.A. Nicholas & E.B. Hershman (eds) *The Lower Extremity and Spine in Sports Medicine*, pp. 195−214. CV Mosby, St Louis.

Mellion, M.B. & Shelton, G.L. (1990) Safe exercise in the heat and heat injuries. In M.B. Mellion, W.M. Walsh & G.L. Shelton (eds) *The Team Physician's Handbook*, pp. 59−69. Harvey & Belfus, Philadelphia.

Peterson, L. & Renström, P. (1986) *Sports Injuries: Their Prevention and Treatment*, pp. 153−5. Year Book Medical Publishers, St Louis.

Poole, R.M., Lee, B.C. & Blackburn, T.A. (1991) Physical modalities in rehabilitation. In B. Reider (ed) *Sports Medicine: The School-Age Athlete*, pp. 67−87. WB Saunders, Philadelphia.

Prentice, W.E. (1986) *Therapeutic Modalities in Sports Medicine*. Times Mirror/Mosby College Publishing, St Louis.

Prentice, W.E. & Malone, T.R. (1990) Thermotherapy. In W.B. Leadbetter, J.A. Buckwalter & S.L. Gordon (eds) *Sports-induced Inflammation: Clinical and Basic Science Concepts*, pp. 455−62. American Academy of Orthopaedic Surgeons, Park Ridge, Illinois.

Safran, M.R., Garrett Jr, W.E., Seaber, A.V., Glisson, R.R. & Ribbeck, B.M. (1988) The role of warm-up in muscular injury prevention. *Am. J. Sports Med.* **16**,

123–9.

Saliba, E.N., Grieck, J.H. & Foreman, S.A. (1991) Therapeutic modalities for the treatment of athletic injury. In W.A. Guama & A. Kalenak (eds) *Clinical Sports Medicine,* pp. 277–312. WB Saunders, Philadelphia.

Solomonow, M. & D'Ambrosia, R. (1987) Biomechanics of muscle overuse injuries: a theoretical approach. *Clin. Sports Med.* **6**(2), 241–57.

Strickler, T., Malone, T. & Garrett, W.E. (1990) The effects of passive warming on muscle injury. *Am. J. Sports Med.* **18**, 141–5.

Further reading

Feiring, D.C. & Derscheid, G.L. (1989) The role of preseason conditioning in preventing athletic injuries. *Clin. Sports Med.* **8**(3), 361–72.

Gieck, J.H. & Saliba, E.N. (1987) Application of modalities in overuse syndromes. *Clin. Sports Med.* **6**(2), 427–66.

Stanish, W.D., Curwin, S.L. & Bryson, G. (1990) The use of flexibility exercises in preventing and treating sports injuries. In W.B. Leadbetter, J.A. Buckwalter & S.L. Gordon (eds) *Sports-induced Inflammation: Clinical and Basic Science Concepts,* pp. 731–46. American Academy of Orthopaedic Surgeons, Park Ridge, Illinois.

Williford, H.N., East, J.B., Smith, F.H. & Burry, L.A. (1986) Evaluation of warm-up for improvement in flexibility. *Am. J. Sports Med.* **14**, 316–19.

Chapter 34

Initial Management of Acute Injuries

WALTON W. CURL AND DAVID F. MARTIN

Treatment of the acute injury in an athlete is extremely important — the initial management of a sports injury can speed recovery, protect an athlete from further injury, and enhance performance upon the athlete's return to play. Delayed or inappropriate treatment can have a deleterious effect on recovery, recovery time and future performance. The sports medicine specialist must work with athletes, referees, officials, coaches and administrators to ensure swift treatment when athletes sustain injuries. Injury recognition and prompt initiation of appropriate therapy is critical to reduce potentially long-term ill effects that can occur with complex athletic trauma.

Athletic injuries can involve muscles, tendons, ligaments, bones and joints along with surrounding soft tissues. When these structures are injured, the body's initial response is related to the bleeding that occurs when blood vessels around the structures are torn (Peterson & Renström, 1986). The bleeding quickly spreads to surrounding tissues, increasing the zone of injury. Those tissues can be damaged secondary to local pressure effects and by their own inflammatory response to the pain and pressure. This early phase can lead to a large area of inflammation and therefore swift action, first to identify the area of injury and then to modulate tissue damage and response can greatly reduce healing time.

Damage to blood vessels from an acute athletic injury can lead to a large amount of local bleeding. This haemorrhage spreads to surrounding tissues and causes pressure changes as noted above. These changes lead to pain, which increases local oedema, thereby increasing pressure on tissues and delaying healing and rehabilitation. In the acute phase, this bleeding can continue until clotting occurs. Although this is not usually a long period of time, the clearing and removal of this haematoma and surrounding oedema can be a lengthy process. Therefore, immediate treatment to control bleeding and interrupt this cycle is imperative for early return to athletic activity following an injury. Swift and appropriate treatment to stop the initial bleeding, protect surrounding tissues from pressure damage, reduce the size of the zone of injury, and decrease the inflammatory response are the most important factors in determining recovery time (Peterson & Renström, 1986; Walsh et al., 1990; Leadbetter, 1990).

Overuse injuries, while not causing a local bleeding response, can lead to the same type of cyclical tissue injury. The classic overuse injury is caused by microtrauma to a structure that is repeated by continued activity. Although the bleeding characteristic of an acute injury usually does not occur, the inflammatory response does, and it leads to tissue damage. Similar to an acute injury in the sense that local swelling leads to more tissue injury, more pain and subsequently more swelling, the overuse injury primarily causes an inflammatory response that ultimately is what damages tissues. Therefore, even though in the overuse injury setting acute bleeding does not occur, the early treatment of the inflammatory response caused by repetitive microtrauma is important for recovery. The principles of treating acute injuries where the initial response is bleeding following by inflammation can also be applied to overuse injuries where the inflammation is the primary event.

Inflammation is manifested in tissues as swelling, increased temperature, erythema, pain and loss of function (Curl, 1990). It is the pain and tenderness that can limit an athlete's function and delay rehabilitation, hinder recovery, and impair performance. The inflammatory response is the body's reaction to injury or destruction of vascularized tissues. Inflammation relating to acute sports injuries can result from undue pressure on soft tissues, friction between soft-tissue planes, repetitive overload of soft tissues, or trauma sufficient to cause local injury and bleeding (Peterson & Renström, 1986; Curl, 1990; Leadbetter, 1990). This inflammation is a time-dependent process mediated by vascular, cellular and chemical events leading to tissue repair or scar formation (Leadbetter, 1990). Because prolonged inflammation can lead to increased scarring, early treatment must be initiated to prevent that outcome. As the inflammation is treated, it must be remembered that the inflammation not only is the body's initial response to injury, but also is an initial part of the healing process. The sports medicine specialist should attempt to modulate the inflammatory process to guide its outcome to the athlete's benefit. Described outcomes include spontaneous resolution, fibroproductive healing, regeneration and a chronic inflammatory response (Leadbetter, 1990). Interrupting the inflammatory cycle is important and the initial management of an athletic injury cannot only identify and remove the causes of inflammation, but can also modulate the process to enhance healing and recovery.

Bleeding that occurs after an acute injury provokes an inflammatory response. Once the bleeding is controlled, it is that response that enables the body to remove the blood from the tissues. This is done mainly through the lymphatic system (Peterson & Renström, 1986). Scarring may develop as this process occurs. Early intervention can reduce the amount of scarring and resultant reinjury when the weaker scar tissue is subjected to load on return to activity. Initial injury management is critical in controlling initial bleeding, decreasing local swelling, modulating the inflammatory response, inhibiting pain, beginning early rehabilitation, minimizing scar formation and shortening recovery time.

Several factors are important in the initial management of athletic injury. The first aspect is the initial approach to the athlete and his or her injury. Emergency treatment must be available when necessary, and criteria to determine when an athlete should be returned to the playing field also are important once initial evaluation of the injury is completed. A method of quickly and efficiently assessing an acute athletic injury will be presented, followed by a discussion of initial treatment.

Approach to injury

The sports medicine specialist plays many roles in caring for the athlete. Preparation is paramount to both injury prevention and treatment (Whiteside, 1991). The health-care team for an athlete or an athletic event can include coaches, referees/officials, trainers, therapists and physicians. Each member of the team must be dedicated both to learning from and to teaching the other individuals contributing to the care of injuries. Cooperation is a must and the approach one uses when an acute injury occurs is important to maximize the speed and quality of recovery. As members of the sports medicine team function to treat acute injuries, they must be aware of six areas that encompass all facets of sports medicine participation and care: (i) presence/availability; (ii) management; (iii) observation; (iv) history; (v) physical examination; and (vi) disposition (Table 34.1) (Whiteside, 1991). By considering each of these

Table 34.1 Six facets of sports medicine participation.

Presence/availability
Management
Observation
History
Physical examination
Disposition

areas, acute injuries can be evaluated within an organized framework and appropriate treatment and prevention modalities can be initiated.

Presence/availability

The sports medicine specialist must be sure that by his or her presence, appropriate care is always available for athletes at risk. Injuries occur during practice as well as at games, so appropriate medical personnel and equipment must be available to treat injuries at all times. This can be done through communication with coaches and educational seminars covering the basic initial treatment when injuries occur. In addition to being available, the sports medicine specialist also has the responsibility of being knowledgeable concerning sport-specific mechanisms of injury. This information is useful in injury prevention and also in anticipating both acute and overuse injuries. 'Presence' refers not only to physical presence during practice and contests, but also to presence for the coaches and athletes to develop trust and rapport — an athlete needs to know that the sports medicine specialist is available and must be able to trust in his or her dedication and abilities.

In addition to acute injury care during the season, appropriate athletic injury management includes appropriate preseason preparation and diligent postseason evaluation. Before the season begins, medical records must be obtained from each athlete and a physical examination must be performed. This may include determination of fitness and should involve identification of risk factors for injury. Preseason preparation also includes obtaining and maintaining medical supplies necessary for injury treatment. Postseason evaluation should cover all athletes injured during the season and repeat examination of the injured areas to ensure valuable off-season rehabilitation to prevent reinjury. In addition, the entire sports medicine programme and team should be evaluated each season and improved upon as needed.

Management

This area involves equipment, playing surfaces, scheduling and venues. The sports medicine specialist in a position to deal with athletic injuries must ensure that equipment, especially protective gear, is in good condition and is fit properly to the athlete. Equipment that does not fit can cause injury or can place an athlete at increased risk, and often the coach and the athlete are unaware of what safety features are important in various pieces of sporting equipment. As playing surfaces change, injury patterns will vary, and it is important to be prepared for the types of injury that are most common with the surface in use.

Scheduling plays an important role in injury prevention by allowing time for appropriate rest, nutrition and warm-up. In addition, any specific treatments that acute injuries may require must be scheduled when they are needed — the first 48 h following an injury are critical, and facilities and medical personnel to treat injuries within that time frame must be available. Venues for practice, play and lodging are important, and the safety of the athlete must be kept in mind. Although these functions may seem more administrative than medical, members of the medical team must evaluate the athletic operation as part of their treatment of athletic injuries and provide remedies when problems or risk factors are identified (Whiteside, 1991).

Observation

The sports medicine specialist will best be prepared to handle acute injury situations by carefully observing the athlete in action. This involves not only game or contest performance, but also warm-up and cool-down periods. It is important for the sports medicine specialist to know an athlete's personality, reaction to adversity, response to pain and other distinctive habits or characteristics (Whiteside, 1991).

Each sport has aspects that place specific athletes and specific body parts at risk. It is helpful to know and to understand each sport and to observe the contest carefully to identify potential injury mechanisms. Then, when an injury occurs, the treatment plan can be placed into action quickly. When an injury occurs under direct observation, the information gained by being able to see precisely the stresses that tissues and other structures are subjected to is invaluable — both to treatment and to injury recognition.

History

An acutely injured athlete is often in significant distress, often screaming and writhing in pain. Even under such adverse conditions, some history must be obtained because it is extremely important. The nature and location of pain can be elicited easily, particularly when the athlete and physician have already established good lines of communication. An athlete's description of what was seen, felt and heard from his or her perspective can be important in delineating what structures are actually injured. Taking the time to establish and verify the history and mechanism of injury can pay great dividends in starting proper treatment promptly.

Physical examination

The examination of an acute injury before the onset of swelling and establishment of a significant inflammatory response is extremely valuable. Before an injury occurs, the sports medicine team must have designated the individuals responsible for history taking, examination and transport — the individual responsible for the initial physical examination also should be involved in the early treatment of the injury, because the information gained from the first examination is quite accurate. Protective equipment must be removed carefully to allow a thorough examination (Peterson & Renström, 1986; Whiteside, 1991). This might require transport of the athlete to a locker room or training room after the on-field evaluation for critical injury.

The initial examination should be geared toward establishing a preliminary diagnosis and determining participation status (Whiteside, 1991). Communication to the athlete and the coach is important when playing status is being considered. Once a diagnosis is developed and playing status is determined, immediate treatment and/or rehabilitation should be started. This initially may involve only protection from further injury, but having available the appropriate modalities for acute treatment is the sports medicine specialist's responsibility, as outlined in the management section.

Disposition

The final aspect of this six-pronged approach to sports injuries is disposition. This involves the management of an acute injury from the playing field to the treatment room. Further work-up may be necessary — radiographs, repeat examination, scanning — and this must be scheduled promptly while treatment is in progress and being modulated constantly as new information becomes available. The athletic trainer may be able to tape or brace an injury to allow return to play. This again must be modulated along with ongoing treatment. Constant observation is the key and if an athlete is able to return to play, re-evaluation of the injured area as it responds to the stresses of play is important. Return to play criteria are essential and will be discussed below; suffice it to say here that the member of the team responsible for making this decision must have a good understanding of those criteria before injury occurs.

Disposition following an acute injury is important as an athlete leaves the playing (or practice) field. Both the athlete and coach must clearly understand the treatment plan and its implementation. The first 48–72 h are too important in acute injury treatment to leave this disposition to chance. Members of the sports medicine team must agree on a plan and ensure that it is carried out. In an institutional or team setting, a weekly injury report detailing injuries, current treatment, and prognosis can be an invaluable communication tool among the sports medicine team, coaches, and athletes (Fig. 34.1).

Initial treatment

With utilization of the above approach, injuries can be minimized, but when they do occur, their prompt treatment is ensured. What is the appropriate initial treatment? This section will cover proper initial treatment with a proven plan. Cryotherapy is the mainstay of this plan and will be covered in depth.

Emergency evaluation and treatment

The sports medicine specialist must be prepared for all types of emergencies (Fig. 34.2). Head, neck and chest injuries can all lead to cardiovascular collapse in the athlete. A plan to utilize the ABCs of airway, breathing and circulation is important. Methods of establish-

Weekly injury report			
14 January 1992			
NAME	**SPORT**	**INJURY**	**COMMENTS**
John Doe	FB	R. syndesmosis injury	Much improved, still has pain occasionally when climbing and descending stairs
Tracy Jones	FB	Unstable L. trapeziometa-carpal joint	Improved; able to lift weights with hand
Georgia Brown	WBKB	L. thumb — fracture distal phalanx	Doing well
Bill Smith	MBKB	L. knee — meniscal tear	To see doctor in TR, not complaining of pain

Fig. 34.1 An example of a weekly injury report. Courtesy of Guilford College Sports Medicine. FB, football; L, left; MBKB, men's basketball; R, right; TR, training room; WBKB, women's basketball.

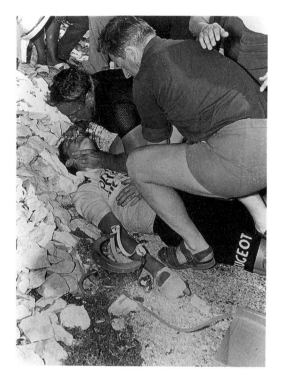

Fig. 34.2 A correct acute evaluation is important for suitable treatment. Courtesy of the IOC archives.

ing an adequate airway and maintaining ventilation and circulatory support through basic or advanced cardiac life support are essential tools for all individuals responsible for the care of athletes.

An emergency treatment plan (see Appendix 34.1) is very useful in educating all members of the sports medicine team — this plan should include step-by-step instructions for each potential emergency and assigns each responsibility to a specific individual. The plan should also include listings and locations of necessary equipment and maps of athletic venues. Emergencies that should be covered by this plan include severe head or neck injuries, cardiac arrest and heat stroke (Fig. 34.3).

Immediate injury care

Once it has been established that an injury is not life-threatening, a functional assessment of the injured area should be performed (Fig. 34.4). This should include evaluation for soft-tissue defects, muscle function deficits, joint motion deficits, swelling and tenderness (Peterson & Renström, 1986; Whiteside, 1991). If function is impaired to the point of precluding athletic activity, treatment should begin immediately.

Basic first aid of an athletic injury comes

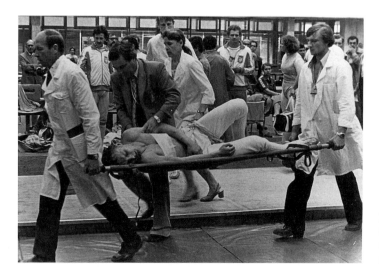

Fig. 34.3 A backboard should be used if a serious injury is suspected. Courtesy of the IOC archives.

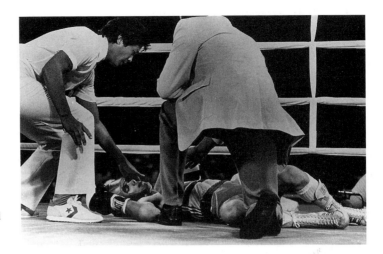

Fig. 34.4 In some sports an experienced physician is needed to make the initial examination. Courtesy of the IOC archives.

from the mnemonic PRICES (Shelton, 1990; Walsh *et al.*, 1990): protection, rest, ice, compression, elevation and support (Table 34.2).

PROTECTION

The protection portion of first aid to athletic injuries refers to a number of types of protection. Primarily, the athlete must be protected from making the injury worse. In addition, intact structures surrounding the injured structures must be protected and supported. Finally, other athletes must be protected from possible injury as an injured athlete returns to participation, so devices used for protection should not have sharp edges and must have a soft covering.

Protection can come in many forms. The use of splints or slings to immobilize extremities is common. Crutches prevent the lower ex-

Table 34.2 Acute injury care via the mnemonic PRICES.

Protection
Rest
Ice
Compression
Elevation
Support

tremities from the stresses of weight-bearing. Additional support can be gained from taping, bracing or strapping. Pain should be the guide used to judge whether or not an area is sufficiently protected as an athlete is moved.

REST

It is difficult to enforce rest in an injured athlete. Therefore, two types of rest have been developed: absolute and relative (Shelton, 1990). Absolute rest involves complete cessation of activity and is usually indicated in the first 24 h after an injury. Relative rest allows activity that involves only uninjured areas or systems but do not stress the injured areas. Cardiovascular conditioning should be maintained in the injured athlete and this can be ensured by using extremities not involved with injury. In addition, once acute inflammation has subsided, gentle range of motion movements and exercise can be started in the injured extremity to avoid stiffness and to speed rehabilitation. The rest period is critical, though, in order to avoid prolonging the inflammatory phase.

ICE

The next step in the treatment of an acute injury is the application of ice or cold, i.e. cryotherapy. Cold can control pain and oedema and can help prevent further tissue damage at the site of the injury (Saliba *et al.*, 1991). Cryotherapy as a therapeutic modality is one of the oldest known forms of treatment, having been used by Hippocrates (400 BC) to reduce swelling and pain by producing numbness (Poole *et al.*, 1991). In the seventeenth century, the application of snow was used as a form of anaesthesia during amputations (Marino, 1986). The use of cold in treating acute athletic injuries is widespread because cold is simple to use, inexpensive and effective (Poole *et al.*, 1991). Cold has beneficial effects on soft-tissue injuries, not only in the first 48 h after injury, but also during rehabilitation by decreasing pain and muscle spasm to allow better mobilization (Grana *et al.*, 1989).

Acute musculoskeletal injuries lead to bleeding, resultant inflammation, oedema, muscle spasm and pain. Without appropriate therapy, these effects can cause loss of motion, disuse, deconditioning and decreased return of function (Grana *et al.*, 1989). Cold treatment is extremely important in the interruption of this cycle. Methods of reducing soft-tissue temperatures include cold compresses, ice, ice packs, ice massage, ice immersion, coolant sprays and gel refrigerant packs. A cooling depth of approximately 4 cm has been reported (Grana *et al.*, 1989; Poole *et al.*, 1991).

The two physical principles commonly used to lower tissue temperature are conduction and evaporation, with conduction being the more common (Poole *et al.*, 1991). Conduction leads to direct loss of tissue heat by contact of the tissues with a colder body. The magnitude of cooling is affected by temperature difference, exposure time, the mode of cryotherapy being used, and the surface area involved. Skin temperature decreases within minutes of cold application, whereas cooling of subcutaneous tissues and muscles can take up to 20–30 min. Adipose tissue is an excellent insulator, so the amount of fat over injured tissues must be considered when cryotherapy is used.

Evaporation is the cooling principle used when chemical sprays are applied to the skin.

Temperature decreases as these liquids evaporate from the skin, but there is negligible cooling of subcutaneous tissues and muscles (Marino, 1986; Peterson & Renström, 1986; Poole *et al.*, 1991).

Cryotherapy has multiple beneficial physiological effects in addition to the decrease in temperature. These include decreases in inflammation, metabolic rate, circulation and muscle spasm, and an increase in tissue stiffness (Knight, 1990). Collectively, these changes result in decreased pain and quicker recovery.

Cryotherapy appears to delay inflammation by decreasing the effects of histamine on the vascular membranes, on neutrophil activation and on leukocytes (Grana *et al.*, 1989; Knight, 1990).

The decrease in metabolism effected by cold application reduces enzymatic function, which in turn may aid in pain inhibition, and decrease swelling and oxygen consumption in the tissues surrounding the injured area. By these mechanisms, marginally viable cells at the periphery of the zone of injury may be able to survive, thereby reducing necrosis and necrotic tissue and decreasing formation of scar tissue (Poole *et al.*, 1991).

The vasoconstriction caused by cryotherapy results in decreased blood flow to the zone of injury. This can have some effect on initial bleeding if the cold is applied quickly, and it acts as well to decrease swelling and to prevent haematoma formation. The phenomenon of cold-induced vasodilatation has been described in the fingers, but there is no evidence that it occurs as well around other joints or in larger tissue masses such as lower extremity muscles (Grana *et al.*, 1989). Cold application increases blood viscosity, and thus should help decrease haemorrhage in the acute injury setting as well (Saliba *et al.*, 1991).

The above effects appear to produce a decrease in local oedema, but there are no objective data that demonstrate any effect of cold on tissue permeability. Because cold is used in conjunction with compression and elevation (see below), it is probably those mechanisms that are the most likely source of decreased oedema (Grana *et al.*, 1989).

Cryotherapy inhibits pain in two ways:
1 Sensory transmissions of pain impulses are slowed or blocked.
2 Muscle spasm is decreased.
Afferent nerve conduction velocities and δ pain fibre transmissions are decreased; transmissions across sensory fibre synapses are blocked. These can result in analgesia and even anaesthesia in areas of cold application (Grana *et al.*, 1989; Saliba *et al.*, 1991). Muscle spasm is reduced by a direct effect of cold on the muscle spindle, which inhibits the stretch reflex.

All these effects combine to make cryotherapy extremely valuable in treating acute athletic injuries. Continuous cooling in the first 2–3 h after injury is important, and the treatments should be used intermittently over the first 48 h. Thereafter, cryotherapy can be used in conjunction with rehabilitative exercises to ease return of motion and strengthening by decreasing pain, inflammation and muscle spasm (Grana *et al.*, 1989).

COMPRESSION

The early use of compression can support an injured area while decreasing oedema. Once the injury has been evaluated, the involved area can be wrapped, which can decrease oedema and pain by allowing the tissues to stabilize and coagulation to develop in injured vessels.

ELEVATION

Along with ice and compression, elevation of an injured extremity is useful, because it can decrease swelling by decreasing blood flow thereby increasing the drainage of soft-tissue oedema. The importance of elevation cannot be overstressed. The athlete must be persuaded to elevate the injured extremity, something that is difficult to do when he or she wishes to return to play immediately during a competition. However, it will pay dividends in minimizing

the initial tissue insult and thus in speeding recovery.

SUPPORT

The final aspect of athletic injury first aid is support. This intervention helps to stabilize the injured tissues and to prevent further injury. If adequate support can be gained, the athlete can return to competition. Taping, wrapping or bracing can aid in compression as well as in support, but they also greatly decrease pain — an injury that is immobilized can be remarkably painless. Use of early immobilization combined with the above modalities reduces oedema, pain and inflammation so that the all-important mobilization can be started earlier and more effectively.

Return to play

The final consideration in treating the acute athletic injury is deciding when the athlete can return to play. This is a fundamental question for the sports medicine specialist because it involves sports morbidity and mortality (McKeag, 1991). This not only is a question of deciding on a return to play, it also is a question of judging an athlete fit to 'begin to play', the latter by appropriate preseason screening (McKeag, 1991). Once an injury occurs, the sports medicine specialist is responsible for establishing a diagnosis and beginning treatment. Once this is done, returning the athlete to competition depends on three factors:
1 The athlete will not make the existing injury worse.
2 The athlete will not be at increased risk of other injuries.
3 The athlete can perform at a level so as to protect himself or herself and not place other competitors at risk.
If these criteria are met, return to play should be *considered*.

In that 'consideration', factors to be taken into account include the situation of the athletic contest — its importance, the time remaining, future scheduling and playing conditions. The athlete can then be subjected to functional sideline testing. An athlete unable to perform simulated activities for the sideline sports medicine team will not do better in actual competition. If return to play must be delayed, the injury should be reassessed frequently so that the athlete can return to competition as soon as possible. Treatment and/or rehabilitation should not be neglected during the time an athlete is not participating, whether that be minutes on the sidelines or months following a serious injury.

An athlete who is returned to competition after an acute injury must be observed carefully for assurance that no further damage is taking place and no undue risks are being taken. Continued reassessment and postseason evaluation with appropriate off-season rehabilitation are critical to the prevention of reinjury.

Return to play judgments must be individualized, but the health of the athlete always must take precedence over the desires of the injured athlete, the other athletes, the coaches, the relatives and the fans (Peterson & Renström, 1986; McKeag, 1991).

Conclusion

The sports medicine specialist will come into contact with many acute injuries. Preparation is the key to proper evaluation, management, treatment and speedy recovery. The key is to develop a plan and an approach, and to have the resources to place these into action. This will enable athletes to participate more safely, and when injuries do occur, their treatment will be appropriate not only to shorten recovery time, but also to improve function and to prevent reinjury.

Appendix 34.1 An example of an emergency treatment plan*

Sports emergencies

The sports medicine staff at Guilford College consists of the head athletic trainer, the assistant athletic trainer, student athletic trainers and the team physician. These individuals provide health care to athletes participating in the intercollegiate sports programme at Guilford College. During the course of practice sessions and games, medical problems or injuries may occur which necessitate emergency care or transport. The following guidelines and action plans outline those steps to be taken in the event of emergency.

General guidelines

1 The most senior athletic training staff member present will be the team leader.
2 High Point Rescue will provide an emergency medical system (EMS) unit for all home football games.
3 Communication steps to be taken to access EMS units:
   (a) hand-held radios to Guilford College Security (channel 1). Security will telephone EMS and meet them at campus entrance and escort them to the site of emergency,
   (b) during practices, a hand-held radio will provide communication between the practice area and the staff trainers. Channel 2 is to be used by sports medicine and intramural athletics. Channel 1 is only to be used to contact security. Two radios are available. These will be used by the staff trainer in charge and by the trainer (or student trainer) at the most distant or appropriate athletic venue (practice or game),
   (c) cellular telephone. This will be available

* Courtesy of Guilford College Sports Medicine, Mary N. Broos, W. Dickson Schaefer and Herb Appenzeller.

on the Guilford College sideline at all home football games,

(d) press box telephone. This is the second line of telephone communication available at home football games,

(e) the telephone at the physical education centre desk will be the back-up to the hand-held radio at home basketball and volleyball games, and

(f) as a back-up to the hand-held radio, when the Haworth Fields are being used, the telephone in Dana House will be accessible. The access/equipment should be checked by the trainer covering the venue.

4 Venue access for EMS vehicles:

(a) football/lacrosse field. Fieldhouse end of the field, gate will be open (see map),

(b) Ragan Brown fieldhouse. Competition courts: down gravel road to the right of the building to the back entrance of the fieldhouse (see map). Training room: parking lot adjacent to baseball field (see map),

(c) Haworth fields. Drive off New Garden Road near rest-room building to field (see map),

(d) baseball field. EMS unit will be directed to the fieldhouse/baseball field parking lot. Injured athletes will need to be transported from fields to the gate at the left field foul pole (see map), and

(e) departure. Security can unlock gate behind Dana Auditorium for EMS unit exit from campus, to avoid speed bumps (see map).

Action plans for specific occurrences

HEAD/NECK INJURY

1 Senior staff person stabilizes head/neck and is team leader.

2 Cervical collar will be kept in the football/lacrosse splint bag and available for all practices/games.

3 Backboard will be on field for football games and will be kept in the training room at all other times.

4 An injured athlete will not be placed on a backboard by Guilford College staff unless the athlete is prone in which event he or she will be rolled onto the backboard.

5 Helmet and shoulder pads will be left on and the face mask removed.

6 Lacrosse helmets will be left on.

7 One student trainer or athlete will be sent to direct EMS unit to the field and the athlete.

8 In the event of an injury in the absence of the staff trainer or team physician, the student trainer in charge will stabilize the head and neck and maintain basic life support.

9 A staff trainer will be called to the area and EMS activated by appropriate methods as listed in the communication section (number 3 under general guidelines).

MEDICAL EMERGENCY

1 Senior staff person (or the training staff member in charge at the time) will administer first aid and be the team leader.

2 The second responder will assist in first aid as needed and access the emergency care system through communication lines as outlined above.

3 The team leader will designate an individual to handle transport consideration: this will include meeting the EMS unit and ensuring that field access is available and well marked.

HEAT INJURY

1 Senior staff person (or the training staff member in charge at the time) will administer first aid and be the team leader.

2 The second responder will access the emergency care system through communication lines as outlined above.

3 Water/cooling is available at the following sites:

(a) football/lacrosse field: at 50-yard line on press box side of field, there is a water hose (in ground box),

(b) Ragan Brown fieldhouse: men's locker room shower or women's volleyball/tennis locker room shower. These are located adjacent to the training room and the trainer in charge is responsible for access, and

(c) Haworth fields: water is taken from the locker room to the field. Dana House showers are available in an emergency. The trainer in charge is responsible for checking/ensuring availability of water/cooling.

(d) Baseball field: men's locker room adjacent to the training room.

References

Curl, W.W. (1990) Clinical relevance of sports-induced inflammation. In W.B. Leadbetter, J.A. Buchwater & S.L. Gordon (eds) *Sports-induced Inflammation*, pp. 149–54. American Academy of Orthopaedic Surgeons, Park Ridge, Illinois.

Grana, W.A., Curl, W.W. & Reider, B. (1989) Cold modalities. In D. Drez (ed) *Therapeutic Modalities in Sports Injuries*, pp. 25–32. Year Book Medical Publishers, Chicago.

Knight, K.L. (1990) Cold as a modifier of sports-induced inflammation. In W.B. Leadbetter, J.A. Buchwatter & S.L. Gordon (eds) *Sports-induced Inflammation*, pp. 463–77. American Academy of Orthopaedic Surgeons, Park Ridge, Illinois.

Leadbetter, W.B. (1990) An introduction to sports-induced soft-tissue inflammation. In W.B. Leadbetter, J.A. Buchwatter & S.L. Gordon (eds) *Sports-induced Inflammation*, pp. 3–23. American Academy of Orthopaedic Surgeons, Park Ridge, Illinois.

McKeag, D.B. (1991) Criteria for return to competition after musculoskeletal injury. In R.C. Cantu & L.J. Micheli (eds) *ACSM's Guidelines for the Team Physician*, pp. 196–204. Lea & Febiger, Philadelphia.

Marino, M. (1986) Principles of therapeutic modalities: Implications for sports injuries. In J.A. Nicholas & E.B. Hershman (eds) *The Lower Extremity and Spine in Sports*, pp. 195–244. CV Mosby, St Louis.

Peterson, L. & Renström, P. (1986) *Sports Injuries: Their Prevention and Treatment*, pp. 42–70. Year Book Medical Publishers, St Louis.

Poole, R.M., Lee, B.C. & Blackburn, T.A. (1991) Therapeutic modalities in rehabilitation. In B. Reider (ed) *Sports Medicine: The School-Age Athlete*, pp. 67–87. WB Saunders, Philadelphia.

Saliba, E.N., Grieck, J.H. & Foreman, S.A. (1991) Therapeutic modalities for the treatment of athletic injury. In W.A. Grana & A. Kalenak (eds) *Clinical Sports Medicine*, pp. 277–311. WB Saunders, Philadelphia.

Shelton, G.L. (1990) Comprehensive rehabilitation of the athlete. In M.B. Mellion, W.M. Walsh & G.L. Shelton (eds) *The Team Physician's Handbook*, pp. 259–78. Hanley & Belfus, Philadelphia.

Walsh, W.M., Hald, R.D. & Peter, L.E. (1990) Musculoskeletal injuries in sports. In M.B. Mellion, W.M. Walsh & G.L. Shelton (eds) *The Team Physician's Handbook*, pp. 251–8. Hanley & Belfus, Philadelphia.

Whiteside, J.A. (1991) Field evaluation of common athletic injuries. In W.A. Grana & A. Kalenak (eds) *Clinical Sports Medicine*, pp. 130–51, WB Saunders, Philadelphia.

Further reading

Bell, G.W. (1986) Infrared modalities. In W.E. Prentice (ed) *Therapeutic Modalities for Sports Medicine*, pp. 79–117. Times Mirror/CV Mosby College Publishing, St Louis.

Harvey, J. (1991) First aid of injuries in sports. In R.C. Cantu & L.J. Micheli (eds) *ACSM's Guidelines for the Team Physician*, pp. 159–62. Lea & Febiger, Philadelphia.

Hunter-Griffin, L.Y. (1991) *Athletic Training and Sports Medicine*, pp. 775–811. American Academy of Orthopaedic Surgeons, Park Ridge, Illinois.

Puffer, J.C. (1991) Organizational aspects. In R.C. Cantu & L.J. Micheli (eds) *ACSM's Guidelines for the Team Physician*, pp. 95–100. Lea & Febiger, Philadelphia.

Chapter 35

Tendon Overuse Injuries: Diagnosis and Treatment

WAYNE B. LEADBETTER

Tendon injuries represent a frequent diagnostic and therapeutic challenge in sports medicine, capable of producing either devastating sudden loss of function or potentially chronic recurrent disability. Tendon injuries are the result of a variety of forces and loads enforced upon tendon tissue during sports performance. These sport-induced cell-matrix responses of tendon tissue are characterized by a broad spectrum of histological and biochemical adaptations. And while there is a statistical association with the aging athlete, tendon damage acquired from abusive training, maladaptations or structural predispositions often strike the younger athlete in the prime of competition. There is growing evidence that basic pathohistological and pathophysiological differences distinguish the acute and chronic (overuse) forms of tendon injury. This chapter will define some of these distinguishing features as well as provide observations on overall clinical therapeutic principles.

The spectrum of soft-tissue sports injuries — a definition of terms

Sport-induced soft-tissue injuries, of which tendon injury is a typical example, are characterized by a spectrum of cell-matrix responses represented by the interrelated processes of inflammation, repair and degeneration (Leadbetter, 1992). It is helpful to define these terms in order to more fully understand the observed clinical problems.

Sports 'injury' (from the Latin *injure*, to make unjust, not right) is the loss of cells or extracellular matrix resulting from sport-induced trauma. Injury represents a failure of cell-matrix adaptation to load exposure. All sport-related connective tissue injury responses can be categorized in two interrelated categories: (i) macrotraumatic—acute tissue destruction; and (ii) microtraumatic—chronic abusive load or use (Leadbetter, 1990a).

In tendons, the mechanism of injury has much to do with the subsequent pathohistological pattern. Overuse and overload may not be synonymous terms, because injury can result from excessive and rapid change in use without significant change in resistance—hence, the origin of the term cumulative trauma disorder, or as the author prefers 'cumulative cell-matrix adaptive response'. Synovial structures such as the tendon sheath as well as peritenon structures are prone to this form of stress response. Injuries can further be divided into acute and chronic patterns according to rate of onset.

1 *Acute injuries* are typified by a sudden crisis followed by a fairly predictable, although often lengthy, resolution. In tendons, an acute injury often consists of midsubstance ruptures occurring either through aberrant tissue or as the result of high strain rates (Butler *et al.*, 1978; Amadio, 1992).

2 *Chronic injuries* are characterized by slow, insidious onset, implying an antecedent subthreshold spectrum of structural damage. Eventually this leads to a crisis episode that is often heralded by pain and/or signs of inflammation. Chronic injuries may last months or even years and are distinguished by a persistence of symptoms without resolution. Paratenonitis and tendinitis are typical of such complaints.

There appears to be some overlap between acute and chronic injuries, with the bridging stage at 4–6 weeks termed the subacute stage of injury. Another perspective on the acute versus chronic process would define a chronic injury as an acute injury occurring in association with some impairment to healing (T.K. Hunt, personal communication). In the athlete, there are both intrinsic and extrinsic factors that can impair recovery.

It is difficult to define sports injuries clinically. Furthermore, because tendon injury falls within the domain of an athletic soft-tissue complaint, the athlete's injury is often defined solely by the amount of pain and the inability to perform. Proper therapy often depends on defining the exact anatomical extent and occurrence of tissue injury (Noyes *et al.*, 1988). Classic signs of inflammation after injury are *not* always present or identifiable as a reliable guide. A complaint is not so much identified with a specific structure as within an anatomical area. It is a painful shoulder, not a painful biceps tendon; it is a painful knee, not a painful patella tendon. And although the immediate onus on the examiner is to be competent and accurate in making the physical diagnosis, the elicitation of pain does not necessarily shed light on the exact pathology or mechanism of injury. Hence, tendon injury relating to occult joint instability or dynamic tendon stress overload as may be present with the hyperpronating foot, may be revealed only

by further analysis. Of all the clinical signs, it is loss of function (functi laesa) that provides the necessity for treatment of tendon injury, indeed for all sports injuries.

Rovere's attempt to define tendinitis in a study of theatrical dance students exemplifies this difficulty. He defined tendinitis as 'a syndrome of pain and tenderness localized over a tendon, usually aggravated by activities that bring the particular muscle tendon unit into play, usually against resistance ... The syndrome is inclusive of tenosynovitis and tenovaginitis as well as actual inflammation of the tendon substance itself' (Rovere *et al.*, 1983).

Sport-induced inflammation (from the Latin *inflammare*, to set on fire) is a localized tissue response initiated by injury or destruction of vascularized tissues exposed to excessive mechanical load or use. It is a time-dependent evolving process characterized by vascular, chemical and cellular events leading to tissue repair, regeneration or scar formation (Fig. 35.1). Clinically observed pathways of sport-induced soft-tissue inflammation include spontaneous resolution, fibroproductive healing, regeneration or chronic inflammatory response (Leadbetter, 1990a). The four cardinal signs of acute inflammation were defined by Celsus (AD 14–37) in the often quoted phrase 'rubor et tumor cum calore et dolore' (redness and swelling with heat and pain) (Table 35.1). It is important to note that this was probably a description of an empyema and fistula of the chest (Majno, 1975). Based upon such historic tradition, pain has assumed a disproportionate importance in the clinical definition of inflammation, so that any painful structure is immediately presumed inflamed. It has taken the

Table 35.1 Recognition of the 'cardinal signs' of inflammation.

Heat, *Calor*—metabolic radiant energy
Redness, *Rubor*—increased vascularity (angiogenesis) and blood flow
Swelling, *Tumor*—extracellular oedema and matrix changes
Pain, *Dolor*—stimulation of afferent nerve endings by noxious mediators
Loss of function, *Functi laesa*—decreased performance caused by direct damage
   or inhibiting pain, oedema

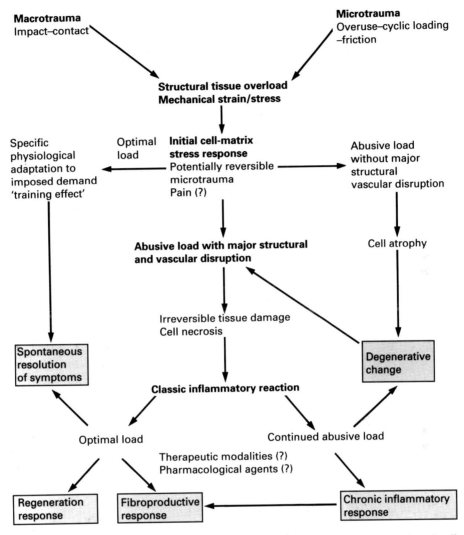

Fig. 35.1 The theoretical pathways of sport-induced inflammatory responses. With permission from Leadbetter (1990a).

advent of more accurate non-invasive assessment techniques such as magnetic resonance imaging (MRI) and the accumulation of surgical biopsy evidence to correct what may be an improper clinical emphasis. As will be further discussed, the source of connective tissue pain is now known to be multifactorial (Hargreaves, 1990).

Repair of soft-tissue injury has been defined as replacement of damaged or lost cells and extracellular matrices with new cells and matrices (Woo & Buckwalter, 1988). Regeneration is a form of repair that produces new tissue that is structurally and functionally identical to normal tissue (Cohen *et al.*, 1992). Repair by scar is the postnatal mammalian response to injury, unlike in the fetal wound, which is capable of healing without exuberant scar formation (Adzick & Longaker, 1992). Acutely injured tendon repair by scar deposition never exactly replicates the histological or biomechanical properties of the original structures (Woo & Buckwalter, 1988; Weiss et al., 1991). Regeneration is often seen as the ideal wound healing response; whereas the response of tendon healing may result in either an adequate response or inadequate response, depending on the athlete's demands.

Degeneration describes a change in tissue from a higher to a lower or less functionally active form (Leadbetter et al., 1990). Such weakened structures are then more vulnerable to sudden dynamic overload or cyclic overloading leading to mechanical fatigue and failure. A prominent source of degeneration is cell atrophy, which is the decrease in the size and/or function of a cell in response to a presence (or lack of) an environmental signal (Rubin & Faber, 1988). Such down-regulation involves decreased protein synthesis and a decrease in such activities as energy production, replication, storage and contractility. In sports injury, immobilization is a prominent cause of cell atrophy in the tendon (Woo et al., 1975; Frank et al., 1991). Additional causes include decreased nutrition, diminished endocrine hormonal influence, persistent inflammation, aging and denervation. Reversal of the degenerative process is not a typical feature in degenerative conditions beyond an undefined cell-matrix limit. Ultimately, degeneration represents a profound imbalance in cell-matrix homeostasis (Fig. 35.2).

Chronic inflammation involves the replacement of leukocytes by macrophages, plasma cells and lymphocytes in a highly vascularized and innervated loose connective-tissue milieu at the site of injury. Although findings of chronic inflammation are typical in sites such as the lateral epicondylar lesions of the elbow (Nirschl & Pettrone, 1979), such responses are not found in all chronic sports injuries (Pudda et al., 1976; Kannus & Jozsa, 1991). The mechanism that converts an acute inflammation to a chronic inflammatory process is not known; continued abusive load and irritation may stimulate the local release of cytokines, resulting in both autocrine (cell self-stimulation) and

paracrine (stimulation of adjacent cells) modulation of further cell activity (Bailey et al., 1973; Clark & Henson, 1988; Almekinders et al., 1992).

Thus, inflammation, degeneration and repair form a functional spectrum of cell-matrix responses with the predominance of any one response depending upon the mechanism of injury and the homeostatic balance of the tendon tissue.

Acute macrotraumatic tendon injury

Acute tendon injury may occur from a sudden deforming eccentric strain, crush from extrinsic pressure or laceration. The insult may result in a lesion in continuity or a total disruption. A critical element defining acute tendon injury response is the accompanying vascular disruption and initiation of an acute phase response signalled by activation of the clotting mechanism and platelet activation. In most bodily wounds, what follows is an orderly progression, or cascade, of overlapping processes that under ideal circumstances is 'predictable' including: (i) inflammation; (ii) cell replication; (iii) angiogenesis; (iv) matrix deposition; (v) collagen protein formation; (vi) contraction, i.e. remodelling; and in cases of exposed wounds (vii) epithelialization (Hunt & Dunphy, 1979). In fact, this represents an ideal sequence of events influenced not only by the type of insult but also such factors as age, vascularity, nutrition, genetics, hormonal changes, innervation and activity level. The literature contains many excellent and exhaustive reviews of the vascular, cellular and biochemical events in this process (Hunt & Dunphy, 1979; Clark & Henson, 1988; Adzick & Longaker, 1992) (Fig. 35.3).

Acute connective tissue injury can further be classified into three phases (Leadbetter, 1991).

Phase I: Acute vascular and inflammatory response

This phase is characterized by activation of the clotting mechanism and the aggregation of

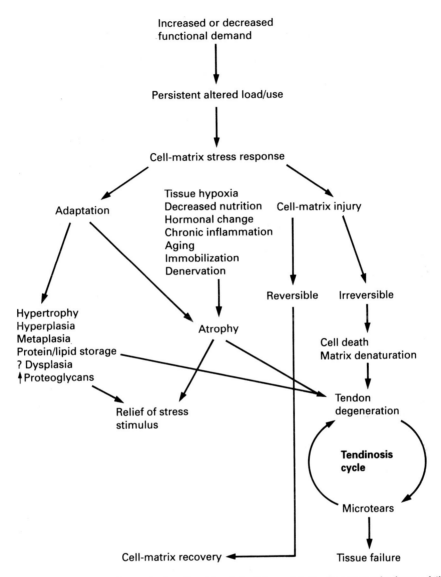

Fig. 35.2 Cell-matrix response to change in functional level. In this model, tendinosis results from a failed cell-matrix adaptation to excessive changes in load use. Such failure is modified by both intrinsic and extrinsic factors.

platelets in clots that release a variety of growth factors, notably platelet-derived growth factor (PDGF), transforming growth factor (TGF βI and βII), which together with the formation of fibrin clots provide the initial scaffold and chemotactant influence on reparative cell migration. This inflammatory dominant phase lasts only a few days and is characterized by the influx of neutrophils followed by the migration of circulating monocytes from the vasculature into the tissues where they constitute the tissue macrophage population responsible for almost all the cell signalling of the many subsequent events in fibroplasia, cell proliferation and eventual wound remodelling. During this phase, damaged tissue is removed

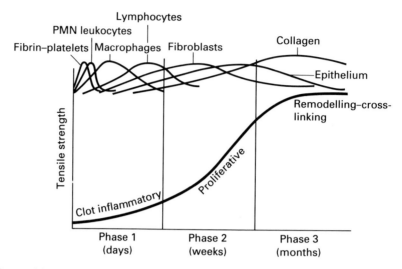

Fig. 35.3 Ideal wound-healing model. Originally derived from the study of skin lacerations, a variety of factors may distort the actual healing sequence in tendons. Although this diagram is an accurate portrayal of cell-matrix wound-healing events, note that the temporal relationship of the various phases is such that the duration of phase 1 is measured in hours or a few days, but phase 3 may extend indefinitely. Normal tendon is not regenerated, however. PMN, polymorphonuclear cell. Adapted with permission from Gamble (1988).

and the stage is set for cell proliferation and reparation. The arachidonic acid cascade is an enzymatically driven sequence leading to the production of prostaglandins, thromboxanes, leukotrienes, eicosanoids and slow reacting substance of anaphylaxis (SRS-A). This cascade is one of the primary chemical events producing the cardinal signs of inflammation (Rubin & Faber, 1988).

Phase II: Repair—regeneration

Beginning at 48 hours and lasting up to 6–8 weeks, this phase is characterized by the presence of tissue macrophages derived from circulating monocytes that have migrated into the injury area. In acute lacerated tendons, there is some evidence that the epitenon tenocyte or synoviocyte may also act as such a pluripotential cell to catalyse wound repair. Once activated, tenocytes behave as modified fibroblasts carrying out collagen production and supplying additional protein mediators of repair and as a source of production for matrix proteoglycan replenishment. Endotenocyte

tendon cells (residing within the tendon) are less metabolically active in this process than epitenocytes. Initially, type III collagen in a woven pattern is rapidly deposited, characterized by small fibrils deficient in cross-linking. The remainder of the repair process is characterized by a shift to the deposition of type I collagen which continues for an indeterminate period during the final maturation phase (Gamble, 1988; Rubin & Faber, 1988).

Phase III: Remodelling—maturation

This is characterized by a trend towards decreased cellularity and an accompanying decrease in synthetic activity, increased organization of extracellular matrix and a more normal tissue biochemical profile. While collagen maturation and functional fibril linear realignment can be seen as early as 2 months after injury, final biomechanical properties can be reduced by as much as 30%, despite this remodelling effort (Woo & Buckwalter, 1988). Biochemical differences in collagen type and arrangement, water content, DNA content and

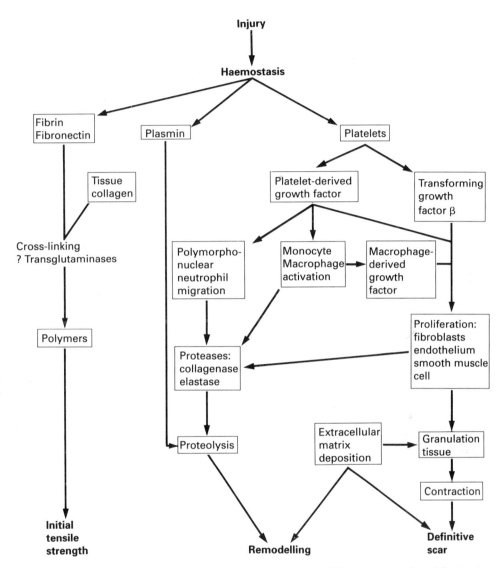

Fig. 35.4 Summary of events in the macrotraumatic wound response. With permission from Martinez-Hernandez (1990).

glycosaminoglycan content persist indefinitely, and the material properties of these scars never equal those of the intact tendon (Amadio, 1992) (Fig. 35.4).

Chronic microtraumatic tendon injury

A microtraumatic tendon injury is distinguished by the observation that degenerative changes are a prominent histological feature, especially in cases of spontaneous tendon rupture (Arner & Lindhold, 1959; Kannus & Jozsa, 1991). This degenerative tendinopathy is thought to be the result of a hypoxic stress response involving both tenocyte and matrix components (Kannus & Jozsa, 1991). Inflammatory cell infiltration and the orderly phased wound repair as seen in macrotrauma seem to be absent or aborted.

Histopathological changes proceeding spontaneous rupture of tendon in a study of 891 patients (397 Achilles tendons, 302 biceps brachii tendons, 40 extensor pollicis longus tendons, 82 quadriceps tendons and patellar ligaments and 70 other tendons), found 97% were affected with prior pathological changes (Kannus & Jozsa, 1991). The mean patient age was 49 years. Also of interest was the finding of similar pathological changes in 34% of the otherwise asymptomatic control population.

Such observations have led to a histological classification of tendon injury and to the coining of the term tendinosis: a focal area of intratendinous degeneration that is initially asymptomatic (Puddu *et al.*, 1976; Clancy, 1982; Leadbetter, 1992). Based upon the anatomy of the tendon and its surrounding tissues, it is possible to describe four pathological conditions: (i) paratenonitis; (ii) paratenonitis with tendinosis; (iii) tendinosis; and (iv) tendinitis. This classification emphasizes the distinction between peritenon or synovial inflammation and the increasing involvement of the tendons' substance reflecting failed adaptation to physical load and use; it emphasizes the variable stress responses of tendon structure (Table 35.2).

Surgical findings in adult athletes with overuse tendon injuries involving the Achilles tendon, posterior tibial tendon, digital finger flexor tendon, lateral elbow extensors, medial elbow flexor, patella tendon or triceps displayed varying degrees of the following: (i) tenocyte plasia; (ii) a blast-like change in morphology from normal tenocyte appearance; (iii) prominent small vessel in-growth with accompanying mesenchymal cells; (iv) paravascular collections of histiocytic or macrophage-like cells; (v) endothelial hyperplasia and microvascular thrombosis; (vi) collagen fibre disorganization with mixed reparation and degenerative change; and (vii) microtears and collagen fibre separations (Figs 35.5–35.9). Inflammatory cell populations were prominent in the synovium and peritendinous structures, as well as the surrounding areas of intratendinous calcification, and at sites of previous intratendinous steroid injection.

Reparative cells were evident in patients with tendinosis and tendinitis pathology despite the coexistent findings of cell-matrix degeneration. Polymorphonuclear cells and lymphocytes were minimally present (Leadbetter, 1992).

The synovial sheath and paratenon are also involved in microtraumatic injury, especially as the result of friction with persistent perturbation of the synovial cells (Almekinders *et al.*, 1992). A study of 16 athletes presenting with peritendinitis revealed increased enzyme activities mainly found in the fibroblast, inflammatory cells and vascular walls within peritenon. The results indicated marked metabolic changes which occur with an increased catabolism, lowered pH and decreased oxygenation of the inflamed areas. Typical findings include fibroexudation with deposition of fibronectin and fibrinogen, proliferation of blood vessels, and in some cases marked endothelial hyperplasia with obliteration of microarterioles (Kvist *et al.*, 1987). Growth factors have been substantiated to modulate this process (Joyce *et al.*, 1992) (Fig. 35.10).

Badalamente *et al.* (1992) in studying the biopsy tissues of typical cumulative trauma disorders including trigger-finger, de Quervain's disease and carpal tunnel syndrome, identified fibrocartilaginous metaplasia in the trigger-finger and de Quervain's conditions but not a synovitis. A chondroid metaplasia stress response appeared to be present. Both chondroid metaplasia in the pully A1 tissue as well as synovitis in the tenosynovium were found. In the carpal tunnel syndrome, a proliferation of type B secretory synovial cells were present in the tendon sheath. There exists an *in vitro* capability of the human internal tendon fibroblast to produce inflammatory mediators including prostaglandin E_2 and leukotriene (LTB4) in response to repetitive motion (Almekinders *et al.*, 1992). This provides a potential source of pain symptoms in tendon injury that may be distinct from fibre disruption.

In flat tendons, such as the extensor carpi radialis brevis of the lateral elbow, there are similar findings of intratendinous degeneration

Table 35.2 Terminology of tendon injury. Adapted from Clancy (1990) and Puddu *et al.* (1976).

New	Old	Definition	Histological findings	Clinical signs and symptoms
Paratenonitis	Tenosynovitis Tenovaginitis Peritendinitis	An inflammation of only the paratenon, either lined by synovium or not	Inflammatory cells in paratenon or peritendinous areolar tissue	Cardinal inflammatory signs: swelling, pain, crepitation, local tenderness, warmth, dysfunction
Paratenonitis with tendinosis	Tendinitis	Paratenon inflammation associated with intratendinosis degeneration	Same as above, with loss of tendon collagen fibre disorientation, scattered vascular ingrowth but no prominent intratendinous inflammation	Same as above, with often palpable tendon nodule, swelling and inflammatory signs
Tendinosis	Tendinitis	Intratendinous degeneration due to atrophy (aging, microtrauma, vascular compromise, etc.)	Non-inflammatory intratendinous collagen degeneration with fibre disorientation, hypocellularity, scattered vascular ingrowth, occasional local necrosis or calcification	Often palpable tendon nodule that can be *asymptomatic*, but may also be point tender. Swelling of tendon sheath is absent
Tendinitis	Tendon strain or tear	Symptomatic overload of a tendon with vascular disruption and inflammatory repair response	Three recognized subgroups: each displays variable histology from purely inflammation with acute haemorrhage and tear, to inflammation superimposed upon pre-existing degeneration, to calcification and tendinosis changes in chronic conditions. In chronic stage there may be: 1 Interstitial microinjury 2 Central tendon necrosis 3 Frank partial rupture 4 Acute complete rupture	Symptoms are inflammatory and proportional to vascular disruption, haematoma, or atrophy-related cell necrosis. Symptom duration defines each subgroup: 1 Acute (<2 weeks) 2 Subacute (4–6 weeks) 3 Chronic (>6 weeks)

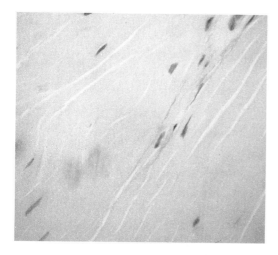

Fig. 35.5 Normal appearance of the Achilles tendon. Note the sparse histological cellularity, subtle crimp and linear fibre array.

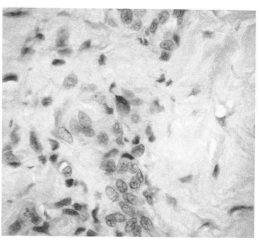

Fig. 35.7 Microscopic appearance of granulation tissue seen at sites of chronic tendon injury and tendinosis (from lateral epicondyle).

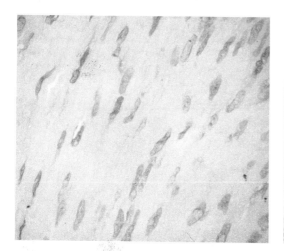

Fig. 35.6 Microscopic appearance of a tendinosis site in an Achilles tendon. Note fibroplasia and blastula morphology in the vacuoles with probable lipid accumulation; this is evidence of cell stress.

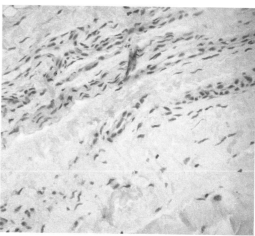

Fig. 35.8 Microscopic appearance of a tendinosis site in an Achilles tendon. Note the disorganized collagen array with incomplete scar depositions.

with a gray immature oedematous and friable scar tissue (Nirschl & Pettrone, 1979). This tissue is essentially characteristic in histological appearance to that of chronic granulation tissues seen in various sites throughout the body. The term angiofibroblastic hyperplasia, so coined to describe these findings, does not merit recognition as a distinct pathological

entity. Additional characteristics of this granulation tissue include many small fibre sensory nerves and presumably a high concentration of cytokine nociceptor stimulators.

The electronic microscopic appearance of microtraumatic tendon degeneration reveals alterations in the size and shape of mitochondria in the nuclei of the tenocyte. Intra-

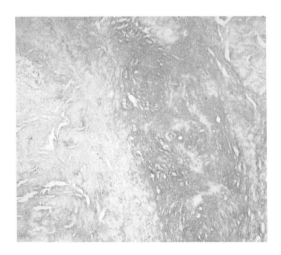

Fig. 35.9 Microscopic appearance of severe tendon degeneration in an Achilles tendon. Note total disorganization, hypocellularity and early dystrophic calcifications (darker stain).

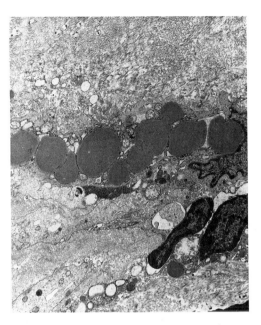

Fig. 35.11 Electron micrograph of a tendinosis lesion (×6210). Note the lipid depositions, cellular necrons and swollen mitochondria.

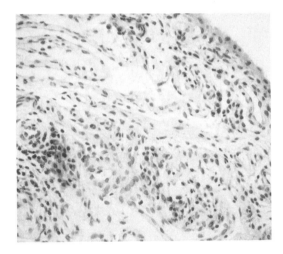

Fig. 35.10 Microscopic appearance of paratenonitis (posterior tibial tendon). Note the pronounced inflammatory cell response and villous hypertrophy.

cytoplasmic or mitochondrial calcification may be seen. Dystrophic calcium phosphate salts precipitate in degenerative tendon tissue as a result of mitochondrial injury. The resulting calcification is deposited in the collagen matrix as chalky-appearing hydroxyapatite crystals,

the 'tombstones' of tendon injury (Leadbetter, 1992). Cytoplasmic vacuoles, lipid deposition and cell necrosis changes are thought to result from relative hypoxia (Kannus & Jozsa, 1991) (Fig. 35.11). Similar changes have been documented in reparative cells after tendon laceration (Manske et al., 1984). Changes in the collagen fibres include longitudinal splitting, disintegration, angulation with a unique bent-fibre appearance (knicking) and abnormal variations in fibre diameters (Kannus & Jozsa, 1991).

The existence of this form of microtraumatic response in the very young athlete remains controversial. The advantage of youth with respect to the efficiency of cellular repair and unique matrix characteristics may account for the clinical absence in the author's experience of the tendinosis lesion. Alternatively, tissue failure may be occurring differently. However, the profound exposure in youth endurance sports and the prevalence of complaints invites further investigation.

Acute versus chronic clinical injury profiles

In addition to the histopathological pattern of cell response to injury, acute and chronic injuries are distinguished by their clinical injury profiles. The acute injury profile is characterized by a defined time of onset with the trauma episode generally observed as a sudden catastrophic occurrence, such as a collision or contact injury, or in the case of a tendon, a spontaneous midsubstance disruption. At the moment of injury, pain is likely to be severe. This is typically followed by a period of gradually decreasing pain as inflammation is treated intensively. Pain eventually falls below an arbitrary threshold at which time the patient will feel well. When pain is no longer inhibiting, the athlete will request a return to activity; however, when the biological curve of wound healing is plotted versus the subjective pain response over time, a potential period of reinjury vulnerability appears. The duration of this period of vulnerability is proportional to the original severity of the structural damage, the rate of healing of the given individual (which is likely to be slower with age), the nature of the target tissue that was injured, and lastly the expected demand or load exposure upon return to sports. The period of vulnerability after an acute injury would, in theory, be lengthened by any raising of the

arbitrary pain threshold of the athlete or by any rapid removal of the subjective pain (for example, with aggressive anti-inflammatory treatment or analgesic treatment). It would be lengthened by the adverse effects of any inappropriate immobilization; but it would be shortened by functional rehabilitation or protective bracing that would either hasten fibrogenesis or decrease tensile load on a tendon. Because research has suggested that an injured connective tissue may attain only 70–80% of original structural and biomechanical integrity after as much as 12 months, the period of vulnerability in these injuries can be lengthy, implying the need for protected activity despite the absence of pain and an ongoing rehabilitation programme to improve muscular support (Fig. 35.12).

Chronic soft-tissue injuries differ from acute injuries in several important ways. The moment of injury, in the athlete's perception, may be a moment of noxious pain. This often occurs after overexertion (such as a long-distance run or intense throwing), resulting in pain becoming insidiously inhibiting over a period or explosively disabling hours or days after the event. Muscle, tendon and synovial structures typically evidence this type of stress response to sports activity. The examiner's inquiry about the preinjury training patterns and cumulative load exposures is critical to understanding why this type of tissue response has been triggered.

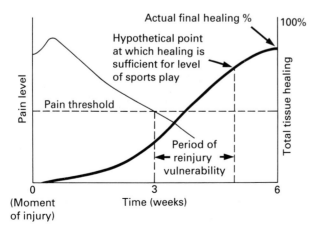

Fig. 35.12 Hypothetical profile of acute macrotraumatic tissue injury. This profile is typical of an acute partial tendon strain or the pattern of healing in other acutely injured connective tissues such as a lateral–collateral ligament sprain in the ankle. Thin solid line, pain; heavy solid line, tissue healing.

For instance, a careful history in a marathon-distance runner might reveal that an inadequate amount of time was spent in prerace preparation and that several weeks of mild, but not inhibiting, pain symptoms had been generated by abusive training before the actual moment of injury. This is the transitional injury pattern. In theory, subclinical injury and dysfunction (e.g. microtrauma) precede the moment of conscious injury. The implication is that damage has been accumulating for a long time before the first opportunity for medical treatment. This is distinct from acute injury, in which the onset of injury and initial treatment often closely coincide. The accumulation of repetitive scar adhesions, degenerative change and adverse effects in chronic microtrauma imply that a recovery will be slower. Again, a period of vulnerability to reinjury results, which is increased when conventional anti-inflammatory measures and reduction pain are applied without regard for the lack of adequate structural integrity. In chronic inflammatory injury it is the history that provides a proper recommendation and adjustment of activity (Fig. 35.13).

The principle of transition

The principle of transition states that a 'sports injury is most likely to occur when the athlete experiences any change in mode or use of the involved part' (Leadbetter, 1990a). Transitional injury is rate dependent. Sudden ill-timed activity changes are more injurious. Whether in training or during injury recovery, the result is an undesired breakdown response that may outstrip tissue morphostatic efforts by imposing overload or overuse demands on the cell-matrix environment. There is growing evidence for a cellular disuse transitional response, as well as an overuse breakdown response (Harper *et al.*, 1991). Factors correlating with the incidence of jumper's knee are hard playing surfaces and an increased frequency of training sessions (Colosimo & Bassett, 1990). A relationship between complete rupture of the Achilles tendon and a sedentary lifestyle has been noted; although the issue is not specifically addressed in the report, it is likely that many of these injuries occurred in the transition from inactivity to activity (Jozsa *et al.*, 1989). A study on Achilles tendinitis and peritendinitis ident-

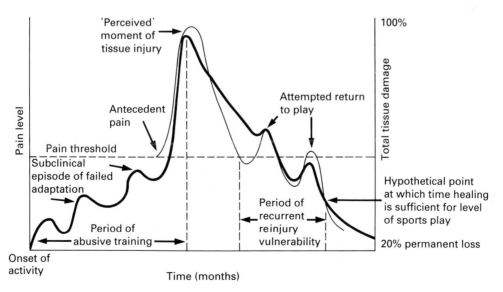

Fig. 35.13 Profile of chronic microtraumatic soft-tissue injury. This profile is typical of overuse tendon injury. Thin solid line, pain; heavy solid line, percentage of tissue damage.

ified a training error as the primary aetiological factor in more than 75% of all cases (Clement *et al.*, 1984). Of these, the majority represented a sudden increase in mileage. Too rapid a return to activity was also noted as a prime cause of reinjury (Clement *et al.*, 1984). Ilizarov (1989), in an attempt to determine the influence of rate and frequency of osseous distraction on cellular behaviour, identified a window of tolerable distraction rate of 1 mm·day^{-1} with as many as 60 incremental lengthenings, thereby creating a gradual transition stress response. He found the rate effects proportional to the growth of the fascial fibroblast and capillary ingrowth. Examples of transitional risks include any attempt to increase performance level, improper training, changes in equipment, enviromental changes such as new surfaces or different training attitudes, alterations in frequency, intensity and duration of training, attempts to master new techniques, return to sport too soon after injury, and even body growth itself. Transition theory correlates with current recommendations on periodization in athletic training (Fig. 35.14).

Wolff's law of soft tissue

Tendon structures are subject not only to tensile load but also to high compressive forces. Such compression occurs extrinsically at sites of pulleys and bony prominences; intrinsic compression is the result of a cyclic torque load seen secondary to pronation of the foot in the Achilles tendon, in the anterior cruciate ligament during the rotatory movement of the knee and in the rotator cuff during torque about the shoulder. An accumulation of large-molecular-weight proteoglycans has been demonstrated in regions of human posterior tibial tendon posterior to the medial malleolus, implying a synthetic stress response as a physiological adaptation to compressive forces (Vogel, 1991). Similar findings were noted in the anterior cruciate ligament tissue, as well as in the bovine flexor tendons, where fibro-cartilaginous-matrix metaplasia is a common finding (Koob *et al.*, 1991). Woo, in analysing the mechanical properties of tendon and ligaments, has theorized an ideal homeostatic level of stress and strain duration to maintain mech-

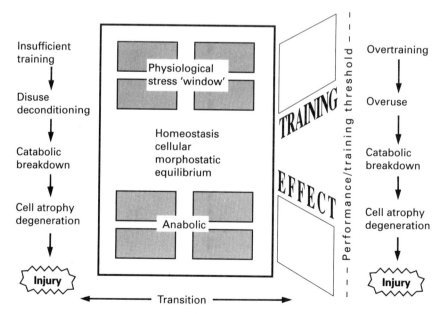

Fig. 35.14 The principle of transition: the more rapid the transition, the greater the risk. With permission from Leadbetter (1991).

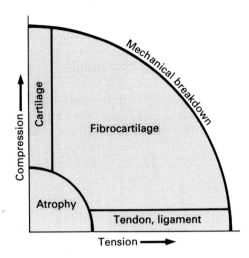

Fig. 35.15 Theoretical schema for Wolff's law of soft tissue. From Amadio (1992).

anical properties and tendon mass (Woo & Buckwalter, 1988). The cells, collagen and matrix in tensile and pressure zones of different tendons may differ. Whether these effects are mediated by cytoskeletal deformation or are due to as yet unproven local piezoelectrical effects of matrix on cells is unknown (Frank et al., 1991). Based upon such observations, a theoretical model has been suggested for Wolff's law of soft tissue (Amadio, 1992) (Fig. 35.15).

Epigenetic and genetic influences on tendon cell-matrix response

There are both epigenetic and genetic influences on tendon cell-matrix response.

Epigenetic factors

Epigenetic factors are defined as those factors that can influence the phenotypic expression (i.e. protein production) of the cell without altering the genome. Vascularity, hormonal influence and rest may exert epigenetic influence on tissue injury healing. Aging may be considered to have both an epigenetic and genetic role in injury response.

AGING

Aging is best characterized by a failure to maintain homeostasis under conditions of physiological stress. The salient characteristic of aging is not so much a decrease in basal functional capacity as a reduced ability to adapt to environmental stress (Rubin & Faber, 1988).

There is evidence to suggest that the tendon collagen fibre possesses all of the cross-linkages it will ever have shortly after its synthesis (Menard & Stanish, 1989). During maturation, reducible cross-linkages gradually stabilize. This results in a less compliant collagen fibre subject to shear stress injury. Aging is also accompanied by a significant decrease in tendon glycosaminoglycan concentration. There are extensive data on the aging of cells in vitro (Hayflick, 1980). Collagen synthesis has long been thought to decrease with age; however, this decrease may be overcome in the presence of ascorbic acid. Generally, aging results in changes in the matrix integrity and in the rate of wound healing, although aging does not prevent adequate clinical wound healing, which can be stimulated by physical training. There are documented morphological, immunological and biochemical aging changes. With aging, collagen fibres increase in diameter, vary more in thickness, and there may be an overall increase in soluble collagen. These morphological changes correspond to biochemical changes that include a decrease in proteoglycans and water content. Parallel changes in elastic fibres also occur (Ippolito et al., 1980). With age, adaptation requires a longer interval of rest and recovery. This is presumably related to the documented down-regulation in the cellular biology of the older athlete. With injury, however, the biochemical and morphological character of tendon tissue may change. In comparing an area of tendon degeneration in a 25-year-old adult with spontaneous Achilles tendon rupture with that of a normal 24-year-old, Ippolito noted that in the area of tendinosis there was a 34% loss of collagen and an increase in proteoglycans of more than 100%, with a significant increase in water and glycoprotein content (Ippolito et al., 1975).

VASCULARITY

Vascularity has long been thought to play a prominent role in tendon degeneration, especially in the supraspinatus portion of the rotator cuff, in the Achilles tendon and at sites of extrinsic bone pressure (Uhthoff & Sarkar, 1991). Since the injection study of Rathbun and McNab (1970), a watershed area in the distal supraspinatus tendon had been offered as an explanation of the aetiology of rotator cuff degeneration. However, there is evidence that the vascularity in the critical zone of the supraspinatus tendon is actually hypervascular, secondary to a low-grade inflammatory incitation with neovascularization after mechanical irritation (Chansky & Iannotti, 1991). Brooks et al. (1992) likewise came to the conclusion that no significant difference existed between the vascularity of the supraspinatus portion of the rotator cuff, and that factors other than vascularity were important in the pathogenesis of supraspinatus tendon rupture.

These assertions tend to shed a different light on the theory of hypoxic intratendinous degeneration and the aetiology of tendinosis. Focal load influences on cell-matrix metabolism may play as great a role as any proposed diminished vascularity. Wilson and Goodship (1992) have measured a core temperature increase of 5–9°C secondary to hysteresis energy losses in the equine superficial digital flexor tendon during exercise. This radiant energy equals 10% of the lost elastic energy upon unloading and is thought to be potentially cytotoxic. Further research is needed to resolve this question. There is evidence for a diminished microvascular supply in the central core of the round tendon and in the distal third of the Achilles tendon (Schatzker & Branemark, 1969).

HORMONAL INFLUENCE

Hormonal influence on tendon biology primarily relates to oestrogen and insulin. It has been suggested that diminished oestrogen levels, premature menopause or premenopausal hysterectomy may be associated with incidence of tendinosis in women; no other data are available to support this contention (Nirschl, 1969). In addition, diabetics are known to heal with some difficulty (Madden & Aren, 1991).

REST

Rest has long been clinically recognized to aid a patient with a tendon injury. The beneficial role of rest in the therapeutic intervention of the inflammation repair process is imperical and undefined. Although it may be said that rest does not heal, theoretically, cell reparative efforts may catch up during rest. The effects of rest are probably multifactorial and may include improved vascularity in the tendon at rest or represent an improved morphostatic balance between matrix degradation and production. Different forms of rest include total abstinence, protected activity or altered activity. Such classifications imply a modulation in cell-matrix load signal and load recovery phase. There is evidence that repetitive motion and variation of frequency (i.e. cycles) may create a positive reparative signal post-injury (Gelberman et al., 1988). Absolute rest or abstinence does not de facto increase the athlete's potential to tolerate renewed load during participation. Modified load rehabilitative prescription has been shown to be important to any successful return to sports performance (Curwin & Stanish, 1984; Teitz, 1989).

Genetic influences

Genetic influences are implicated in the modulation of tendon cell-matrix response based primarily on clinical observations. The mesenchymal syndrome may be a genetically determined cause of failed healing (Nirschl, 1969;

1990). Tendinosis appears in multiple sites in approximately 15% of such patients and in sites not necessarily subjected to obvious overuse. An association among lateral epichondral extensor carpi radialis brevis tendinosis, rotator cuff degeneration, carpal tunnel syndrome, cervical and lumbar disc degeneration, plantar fasciosis, de Quervain's syndrome and trigger-finger tendinosis has been observed (Nirschl & Pettrone, 1979; Leadbetter, 1992). Blood type O has been statistically related to tendon rupture (Jozsa et al., 1989). It is interesting that Achilles tendon rupture in children is uncommon and has been encountered only in children whose parents have experienced tendon rupture (Singer & Jones, 1986). Young adult herniated disc syndrome is often seen in the presence of a familial history (W.B. Leadbetter, personal observation). An underlying collagen diathesis has been suggested. The significance of the mesenchymal theory is in the early recognition of the patient who presents with frequent tendon complaints disproportionate to the level of activity. In addition to ruling out systemic disease, these patients are unusually vulnerable and must be counselled as to proper participation and moderation in their activity.

The factors leading to potential failed healing response are both intrinsic and extrinsic and are summarized in Table 35.3.

Sources of pain in tendon injury

The sources of tendon pain are multifactorial and include both paratenon as well as intrinsic cellular and biomechanical deformation sources (Fig. 35.16). The synoviocyte is capable of secreting a wide array of inflammatory mediators, in particular interleukin-1 and prostaglandin E_2 (Fox et al., 1989). How movement and friction activate these cells is not known, but particles of cartilage and the degradation of other protein molecules may incite a synovial reaction (Rodosky & Fu, 1990). The intrinsic tendon fibroblast is capable of producing inflammatory mediator proteins under repetitive stress (Almekinders et al., 1992). Elongation under load of the tendon beyond its elastic limit may trigger nociceptors as well as myotendinous reflexes. There would appear to be a distinction between the pain due to inflammation and that due to degeneration (W.B. Leadbetter, personal observation). The pain of inflammation may evolve when excessive loading results in immediate cell-matrix and capillary vessel damage, producing the onset of the acute inflammatory cascade typically seen in macrotraumatic or synovial irritation. Degenerative pain may evolve from excessive cyclic microloading, which results in matrix molecular alterations, loss of tissue strength, resultant increased strain deformation with loading and stimulation of pain mechanoceptors.

Grading schemes for musculoskeletal pain

Table 35.3 Factors leading to failed tendon healing.

Intrinsic	Extrinsic
Vascular vulnerability	Overt
Limited cell function potential	Continued self-abuse
Limited cellularity	Improper training (overstimulus or inadequate stimulus)
Aging	Improper technique
Genetic predisposition (mesenchymal syndrome,	Improper equipment
collagen cross-linking, etc.)	Harsh environment
Irreversible change, cystic calcific degeneration	Covert
Hormonal	Joint instability
Other (autoimmunity, etc.)	Extrinsic pressure
	Biomechanical fault

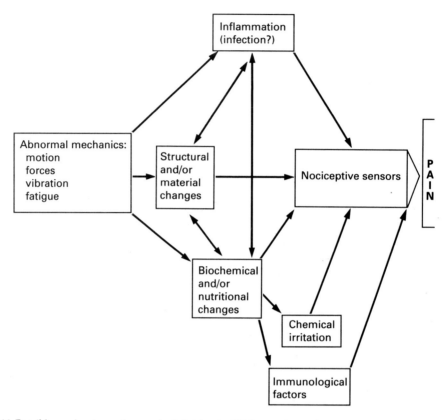

Fig. 35.16 Possible mechanisms of musculoskeletal pain. With permission from White (1989).

are applicable to tendon injury and provide a useful subjective therapeutic guideline (Brody, 1982; Leadbetter, 1990a) (Table 35.4).

Principles in the treatment of tendon injury

Initial assessment and non-operative care

It is important to recognize that the patient presenting with a tendon complaint often brings a legacy of many weeks or months of abusive overuse or overload activity, most probably as a result of overtraining. This can best be summarized by the 'rule of too's' — too often, too hard, too soon, too much, too little, too late, etc. In this respect the patient's presentation as 'injured' is only the tip of an injury iceberg that grows into a clinical crisis when symptoms have finally become intolerable and performance inhibited. Upon initial presentation, the history is critical in chronic overuse injury to determine any evidence of overtraining. The physical examination is important in identifying the anatomical and functional maladaptation patterns that must be unravelled to achieve satisfactory recovery. Initial plain roentgenograms are important to rule out coincident bone and musculoskeletal conditions. So-called sports tumours are sometimes presented as athletic injuries. Since, for the most part, initial plain roentgenograms are negative, a common error is not repeating the plain roentgenograms 6–12 weeks after the initial visit, especially for revealing stress reactions in bone as well as periosteal stress reactions at muscle–tendon attachments.

After the initial evaluation, a variety of

Table 35.4 The clinical grading of sport-induced soft-tissue inflammations. Adapted from Leadbetter *et al.* (1990).

Grade	Subjective pain pattern	Physical signs	Tissue damage	Healing potential	Relevant therapeutic measures
I	Pain after activity only. Duration of symptoms <2 weeks. Spontaneous relief within 24 hours	Non-localized pain	Microinjury		Proper warm-up and conditioning. Avoidance of abrupt transition in activity level
II	Pain during and after activity, but no significant functional disability. Duration of symptoms >2 weeks, <6 weeks	Localized pain. Minimal or no other signs of inflammation		Potential spontaneous resolution	Analysis of technique and efficiency. Decrease transitional abuse and improve training — Training, coaching and self-help measures often effective
III	Pain during and after sport lasting for several days despite rest with rapid return upon activity. Significant functional disability. Duration of pain >6 weeks. Night pain may occur	Intense point tenderness with prominent inflammation (oedema, effusion, erythema, crepitus, etc.)	Macroinjury		Medical assessment of structural vulnerability (e.g. flat feet, inflexibility, muscle weakness, etc.) Protected activity (e.g. bracing). Modification or substitution of different exercises to avoid excessive load on injured part
IV	Continuous pain with sport and daily activity. Total inability to train or compete. Night pain common	Grade III symptoms plus tissue breakdown, atrophy, etc. Impending or actual tissue failure		Permanent scar and residual tissue damage more likely	Surgical treatment often indicated to stimulate fibrous scar and repair or create structural alteration such as releases or decompression, potential permanent withdrawal from activity (e.g. degenerative joint disease) — Medical diagnosis and opinion valuable

specific measures should be prescribed to the athlete. Remember the mnemonic REST'M (*Rest* and *Rehabilitation*, *Education*, *Support* of the injured part, *Training* and *Technique*, *Modification* of activity, *Modalities* and *Medication*). These principles are not unique and have been proposed and refined by many sports medicine authors (Brody, 1982; Chayter & Stanish, 1992; Kibler *et al.*, 1992; Leadbetter *et al.*, 1992; O'Connor *et al.*, 1992). Rest may not cure, but its value in the initial treatment of overuse tendon injury is legion. Rest plays a vital role in cell-matrix homeostasis, especially with aging. Although absolute immobilization is harmful, the concept of protected activity and preventing force overload should be promoted whenever possible. Many authors point out the pitfall of recommending surgical alternatives by default in the face of an inadequate rehabilitation programme. In this regard a great deal of time must be spent in educating the athlete to alter abusive behaviour (Kibler *et al.*, 1992; Leadbetter, 1992). Support of the injured part through various bracing measures and orthotics, improved alterations in training and technique, and modification of activity all help to decrease the overload and overuse of the involved anatomical structure.

As to specific modalities, ice remains the single most useful intervention. Its availability, lack of expense, margin of safety and the ability of the athlete to self-treat immediately after activity add to its appeal. We find the use of most physical modalities to lack sufficient sub-stantiation as to a clinically *significant* effect on the promotion of soft-tissue healing. Generally, it seems functionally useful to cool down inflamed and swollen structures, especially after exercise rehabilitation or activity. Medication is prescribed in as simple and cost-efficient form as possible. We have found little difference in efficacy among non-steroidal preparations. Individual prescription is based on the athlete's tolerance and response. Medication is never a solution by itself, because it treats only the initial inflammatory symptoms of the underlying injury; it is, however, useful in a limited way to allow compliance with the remainder of the therapeutic programme. Corticosteroid injection therapy remains controversial as to its tissue effect and ability to promote healing. There is no question that in synovial structures with prominent immunological and inflammatory activity, corticosteroid injection has a dramatic impact, e.g. as in isolated paratenonitis or paratenon bursitis. The clinician should review guidelines for the appropriate use of corticosteroid injection (Leadbetter, 1990b) (Table 35.5).

Most athletes seem to lose patience with a non-operative programme after 6–12 weeks if they are not making some appreciable progress. In situations in which disability is prominent from the onset and the physical examination implies that significant structural injury has already been accumulated, appropriate supplemental radiological imaging, such as the MRI, arthrogram, bursagram or tri-phase bone

Table 35.5 Use and abuse of corticosteroid injections. From Leadbetter *et al.* (1990).

Proper use	Improper use
6-week preinjection trial of rest, adjusted level of play and conditioning	Acute trauma
	Intratendinous injection
Discrete, palpable site of complaint	Infection
Peritendinous or inflammatory target tissue (avoid tendon)	Multiple injections (more than three)
Limit of three injections, spaced weeks apart, given only if first led to demonstrated improvement	Injection immediately before competition
	Frequent intra-articular injections
Rest (protection) for 2–6 weeks after injection	
Avoidance of contributing mechanical cause (e.g. equipment, conditioning)	

scan, may be useful in further screening of the athlete's complaint. These tests may be done earlier if the athlete needs to know when he or she is likely to return to play; this urgency is more intense in the highly competitive or professional athlete. Although a reliance on extensive radiological assessment in the absence of a carefully carried out history and physical examination is inappropriate, early focusing on the exact extent of the athlete's injury and ideally eliminating some concern often improves compliance, builds confidence and establishes rapport with the athlete while providing further insight. Allowing the athlete to participate in the decision-making of the trial-and-error process that is involved in the clinical treatment of soft-tissue injury and tendinitis can be a wise strategy. After all avenues have been exhausted but before secondary disuse and deconditioning have become prominent, surgical treatment is recommended based upon the severity of the pain. Surgery is more likely in cases demonstrating rest pain, nocturnal pain or loss of performance. A word of caution: malicious diagnoses, particularly neoplasms, can cause the same symptom presentation as tendinitis. Radiological screening is always prudent.

In the recovery phase after tendon injury or surgery, it is critical to protect against abrupt transition and to emphasize adequate retraining. The observations of Clement *et al.* (1984) in the management of non-operative Achilles tendinitis apply well in the recovery of tendon injury as well as in postoperative management, in that an asymptomatic recovering patient can easily precipitate a severe relapse if he or she returns to activity too suddenly. This is further understandable given the known persistent structural and biomechanical changes in the injured or operated tendon. Also important is an analysis of contributing structural dynamic dysfunctions in the kinetic chain affecting the injured tendon. This applies both to the overhead (throwing and racquet sports) and running athlete. For instance, without appropriate attention to deficient technique or scapula

stabilization in the overhead athlete, or proper support of dynamic lower leg dysfunction with an appropriate orthotic or shoe modification in the running athlete, initial treatment is likely to fail. Schemes such as the return to running transitional programme proposed by Brody (1982) exemplify proper sports medicine prescription after injury or surgery (Table 35.6). Such programmes can be created for any sports activity at any level of competition. The overall approach to the perioperative assessment of the tendon-injured athlete is summarized by the algorithm in Fig. 35.17.

Operative treatment of tendon injury

An analysis of currently recommended surgical procedures in chronic overuse tendon injury reveals a variety of surgical goals (Leadbetter *et al.*, 1992).

1 To alter the tissue structure and restore strength by inducing scar repair.
2 To remove a nidus of offending aberrant tissue, e.g. chronic granulation tissue, degenerative tendon, hypertrophic synovium or calcific deposit.
3 To encourage revascularization of tendon tissue.
4 To relieve extrinsic pressure, either bony or soft tissue.
5 To relieve tensile overload.
6 To discover and repair gross interstitial tendon rupture.
7 To replace or augment injured tendon structure, e.g. transfers or grafts.

These objectives are achieved through such techniques as: (i) intratendinous or paratendinous excision; (ii) decompression; (iii) synovectomy or bursectomy; (iv) multiple linear tendon incisions, a procedure we have called longitudinal internal tenotomy; (v) tensile 'release'; (vi) direct repair of partial interstitial rupture; and (vii) tendon transfer or graft.

There are many limitations inherent in present surgical approaches. The main problem in the diagnosis of sport-induced soft-tissue injury and tendinopathy is that the exact nature and extent of the pathology is difficult to assess

Table 35.6 Return to running after injury. Running schedule given in miles with approx. kilometre distances in brackets. From Brody (1982).

The runner must be free of pain and tenderness, with normal daily activities before resuming his or her training programme. (On a scale of 0 to 10, on which 0 is normal and 10 is the worst, the runner is asked to rate his or her pain with normal activities; they must be at 0.)

1 If 0: Run every other day for 2 weeks, then a maximum of 5 days·week^{-1} for the next 4 weeks. If the previous level was 4–6 miles·session^{-1} (6.5–9.5 km·session^{-1}) begin with 1 mile (1.5 km). (If previous level per session was <4, begin with 0.5 mile·session^{-1} (0.8 km·session^{-1}).) If no pain with running, follow the following weekly mileage schedule:

1 (1.5)	0 (0)	1 (1.5)	0 (0)	1 (1.5)	0 (0)	2 (3)
0 (0)	2 (3)	0 (0)	2 (3)	0 (0)	3 (4.5)	0 (0)
3 (4.5)	2 (3)	0 (0)	3 (4.5)	3 (4.5)	0 (0)	4 (6.5)
3 (4.5)	0 (0)	4 (6.5)	4 (6.5)	0 (0)	5 (8)	4 (6.5)
0 (0)	5 (8)	5 (8)	0 (0)	6 (9.5)	5 (8)	0 (0) etc.

2 If you have short intervals of pain with running:
  A No running for 2 weeks.
  B 10-min total workout, alternating 4-min run and 1-min walk. If no pain, add 5 min every 3 days, working up to 30 min, then progress to the next step. If you experience pain, cut back 5 min and work up.
  C 15 min total workout, alternating 4.5-min run and 0.5-min walk. If no pain, add 5 min every 3 days, working up to 30 min, then progress to next step. If you experience pain, cut back 5 min and work up.
  D Run steadily for 15 min, adding 5 min every 3 days. If you experience pain, cut back 5 min and work up.

3 If you have pain after running:
  A Cut your workout by 50% and progress by adding 10% a week.
  B If you cut your workout 50% and still have pain, cut it by 50% again and progress by adding 10% a week.

4 Running routine:
  moist heat (5 min) → stretch → run as prescribed → ice massage (10 min)
  At night:
  moist heat (20 min) → stretch, weight lift, back exercises

until the time of surgery. Ideally, aberrant pathological tissue is eradicated and the healing environment of the tendon improved; however, the process of inflammation and scar repair after surgical wounding leads to a poorly regulated scar response and not a true regeneration (i.e. identical replacement of tissue by new tissue) (Gelberman *et al.*, 1988). Surgery obviously necessitates the disruption of normal tissue while gaining access to the abnormal tissue. The creation of surgical adhesions is a common, undesired risk. It is simplistic to claim that a 'bad scar' is replaced by a 'good scar' as a result of surgical intervention. More often, structurally inadequate, excessively inflamed tissue or degenerated tissue is replaced by an initial woven, immature and disorganized collagen fabric; this may eventually evolve to be adequate but is not normal tissue even after many months. Placed under the repetitive demands of sports performance, such tissue may be very sensitive to transitional stress and display vulnerable durability.

There are four fundamental aetiological criteria in sport-induced chronic soft-tissue injury surgery.

1 The movement and strain patterns specific to the different kinds of sports or training.

2 Structural weaknesses of the human anatomy, e.g. critical zones of vascularization, tendon

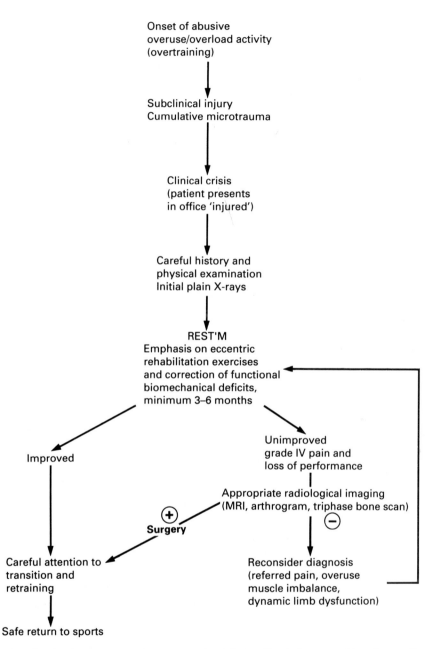

Fig. 35.17 Algorithm for the treatment of overuse tendon injuries. Surgical treatment is only one alternative in an extensive therapeutic plan.

tunnels or muscular compartments with potential risk of ischaemia.

3 Structural variations in human anatomy, e.g. anomalous tendon structure, persistent femoral anteversion, hyperpronation of the foot, abnormal configuration or abnormal variation in the subacromial arch.

4 Biomechanical insufficiency of certain soft

Table 35.7 Common surgical techniques in the treatment of overuse tendon injuries.

Technique	Typical application
Intratendinous or paratendinous excision	Persistent ossicle in Osgood–Schlatter disease Rotator cuff calcific tendinosis Debridement chronic granulation tissue (e.g. lateral elbow epicondyle, subacromial space) Retrocalcaneal bursectomy Excision of accessory tarsal navicular
Decompression	Subacromial impingement syndrome Haglund's syndrome De Quervain's tenovaginitis Trigger-finger release Achilles paratenonitis (fibrosheath inflammation)
Synovectomy–bursectomy	Subacromial impingement Retrocalcaneal bursectomy Tenovaginitis
Longitudinal internal tenotomy (linear tendon incision)	Achilles tendinosis Patella tendinosis Elbow extensor or flexor origin injury
Tensile 'release'	Plantar fasciitis (fasciosis)
Repair	Rotator cuff Elbow extensor or flexor origin injury Achilles tendon interstitial tear
Drilling or scarification of bone tendon attachment	Elbow extensor or flexor origin injury Patella bone (Sinding–Larsen–Johansson)
Tendon transfer	Posterior tibial tendinosis with attenuation

tissues, e.g. regeneration limits in dense connective tissue or aging characteristics (Schneider, 1982).

In addition to the compromised cell function and matrix degenerative changes documented in microtraumatic injury, there are significant variations in the intrinsic healing ability of dense connective tissue. Variations in cell ultrastructure, proliferative capacity, phenotypic expression *in vitro*, as well as the gross morphology of tendon and ligament have been reported (Lyon *et al.*, 1991; Chandrasekharam *et al.*, 1992; Clark & Harryman, 1992). Repair and functional improvement, given these con-

ditions, can be unpredictable. Despite these limitations a variety of useful surgical techniques have been described (Table 35.7).

Longitudinal internal tenotomy is often employed in the treatment of refractory tendinosis, such as seen in lesions of the Achilles tendon, patella tendon, extensor carpi radialis brevis and posterior tibial tendon. Typically, one or two incisions are made along the course of the involved tendon to allow exposure of the internal degenerative tendon tissue or chronic granulation area. Typically, the area of failed healing is excised and an exuberant scar response ensues which results in a two to threefold increase in the diameter of the operated tendon. Despite the previously documented abnormal characteristics of repair scar, the shear bulk of this acute wounding response improves the tensile strength and performance capability of the injury site over time (Leadbetter *et al.*, 1992). The reader is referred to specific references in the literature for a full discussion of the application of this technique: Achilles tendon (Leadbetter *et al.*, 1992; Mahan & Carter, 1992); patella tendon (Blazina *et al.*, 1973; Kelly *et al.*, 1984; Colosimo & Bassett, 1990; Feretti *et al.*, 1983); chronic lateral epicondyle extensor digitorum comus tendon injury or tennis elbow (Nirschl & Pettrone, 1979; Yeager & Turner, 1985); posterior tibial tendinosis (Leadbetter *et al.*, 1992; Johnson, 1983).

Conclusion

Once thought to be biologically inert, tendons are best appreciated as a heterogeneic group of structures with variations in cell character, collagen orientation, collagen cross-linking, vascular supply, configuration, load pattern, biomechanical profile, shape, and the presence or absence of a synovial lining. Tendons have the potential to manifest one of several stress-adaptation behaviours depending upon the mechanism of injury and the nature of the continuing sports demand. Statements that tendon healing progresses in a typical pattern regardless of the mechanism of injury (Chaytor & Stanish, 1992) are untenable in the light of previous discussions. Similarly, the body's immediate and long-term responses to physical trauma are not always the same for all types of athletic injuries; nor are tissue responses always inflammatory. There are many extraneous factors which may alter the clinical course of tendon healing in the athlete; of these, aging and transition in activity would appear to be most important.

Van der Muelen (1982) has identified at least three important questions that help determine the therapeutic approach and timing of return to athletic activity after injury: (i) an accurate diagnosis must be established; (ii) the severity of the injury must be fully assessed; and (iii) the relationship between the cause of the injury and its effect must be determined. When a slight load creates serious soft-tissue damage, it may be assumed that the damaged tissue was less resistent or had increased vulnerability. Abusive overtraining or inadequate conditioning are often implicated. Treatment of tendon overuse injuries should include treatment of the acute crisis; elimination of abusive technique; graduated and protected return to activity; and proper reconditioning and retraining for competition. Immediate symptomatic relief is never a substitute for a more lasting and comprehensive solution. A sport-specific and injury-specific programme is always required for full athletic recovery.

References

Adzick, N.S. & Longaker, M.T. (1992) *Fetal Wound Healing*. Elsevier, New York.

Almekinders, L.C., Banes, A.J. & Ballinger, C.A. (1992) Inflammatory response of fibroblasts to repetitive motion. *Trans. Ortho. Res. Soc.* **17**, 678.

Amadio, P.C. (1992) Tendon and ligament. In I.K. Cohen, R.F. Diegelmann & W.J. Lindblad (eds) *Wound Healing: Biochemical and Clinical Aspects*, pp. 384–95. WB Saunders, Philadelphia.

Arner, O. & Lindhold, A. (1959) Subcutaneous rupture of the Achilles tendon: A study of 92 cases. *Acta Chir. Scand.* **239**(Suppl.), 1–51.

Badalamente, M.A., Sampson, S.P., Dowd, A. *et al.* (1992) The cellular pathobiology of cumulative trauma disorders/entrapment syndromes: Trigger finger, de Quervain's disease and carpal tunnel syndrome. *Trans. Orthop. Res. Soc.* **17**, 677.

Bailey, A.J., Bazin, S. & Delaunay, A. (1973) Changes in the nature of the collagen during development and resorption of granulation tissue. *Biochem. Biophys. Acta* **328**, 383–90.

Blazina, M.E., Kerlan, R.K. & Jobe, F.W. *et al.* (1973) Jumper's knee. *Orthop. Clin. N. Am.* **3**(4), 665–78.

Brody, D.M. (1982) Techniques in the evaluation and treatment of the injured runner. *Orthop. Clin. N. Am.* **13**, 541–58.

Brooks, C.H., Revell, W.J. & Heatley, F.W. (1992) A quantitative histological study of the vascularity of the rotator cuff tendon. *J. Bone Joint Surg.* **74B**, 151–3.

Butler, D.L., Groodes, E.S., Noyes, F.R. *et al.* (1978)

Biomechanics of ligaments and tendons. In R.S. Hutton (ed) *Exercise and Sports Sciences Reviews*, pp. 125–81. Franklin Institute Press, Washington.

Chandrasekharam, N.N., Amiel, D., Green, M.H., Berchuck, M. & Pikeson, W.H. (1992) Characterization of the intrinsic properties of the anterior cruciate and medial collateral ligament cells: An *in vitro* cell culture study. *J. Ortho. Res.* **10**, 465–75.

Chansky, H.A. & Iannotti, J.P. (1991) The vascularity of the rotator cuff. *Clin. Sports Med.* **10**, 807–22.

Chayter, R. & Stanish, W.D. (1992) Clinical treatment of tendinitis. *Sports Med. Digest* **14**, 2.

Clancy, W.G. (1982) Tendinitis and plantar fascitis in runners. In R. D'Ambrosia & D. Drez (eds) *Prevention and Treatments of Running Injuries*, pp. 77–87. Charles B Slack, Thorofare, New Jersey.

Clancy, W.G. (1990) Tendon trauma and overuse injuries. In W.B. Leadbetter, J.A. Buckwalter & S.L. Gordon (eds) *Sports-Induced Inflammation: Clinical and Basic Science Concepts*, pp. 609–18. American Academy of Orthopaedic Surgeons, Park Ridge, Illinois.

Clark, J.M. & Harryman, D.T. (1992) Tendons, ligaments, and capsule of the rotator cuff — gross microscopic anatomy. *J. Bone Joint. Surg.* **74A**, 713–25.

Clark, R.A.F. & Henson, P.M. (eds) (1988) *The Molecular and Cellular Biology of Wound Repair*. Plenum Press, New York.

Clement, D.B., Taunton, J.E. & Smart, G.W. (1984) Achilles tendinitis and peritendinitis: Etiology and treatment. *Am. J. Sports Med.* **12**, 179–84.

Cohen I.K., Deigelmann, R.F. & Linzlas, W.J. (eds) (1992) *Wound Healing: Biochemical and Clinical Aspects*. WB Saunders, Philadelphia.

Colosimo, A.J. & Bassett III, F.H. (1990) Jumper's knee: Diagnosis and treatment. *Orthop. Rev.* **19**, 139–49.

Curwin, S. & Stanish, W. (1984) *Tendinitis: Its Etiology and Treatment*. Collamore Press, Lexington, Massachusetts.

Feretti, A., Ippolito, E., Mariani, P. *et al.* (1983) Jumper's knee. *Am. J. Sports Med.* **11**, 58–62.

Fox, R.J., Lotz, M. & Carson, D.A. (1989) Structures and function of synoviocytes. In D.J. McCarty (ed) *Arthritis and Allied Conditions: A Textbook of Rheumatology*, 2nd edn, pp. 273–87. Lea & Febiger, Philadelphia.

Frank, C., MacFarlane, B., Edwards, P. *et al.* (1991) A quantitative analysis of matrix alignment in ligament scars: A comparison of movement versus immobilization in an immature rabbit model. *J. Ortho. Res.* **9**, 219–27.

Gamble, J.G. (1988) The musculoskeletal system: Physiological basics: In L.Y. Hunter-Griffin (ed) *Athletic Training and Sports Medicine*, 2nd edn.

Raven Press, New York.

Gelberman, R., Goldberg, V., An, K.N. *et al.* (1988) Tendon. In S.L.-Y. Woo & J.A. Buckwalter (eds) *Injury and Repair of the Musculoskeletal Soft Tissue*, pp. 1–40. American Academy of Orthopaedic Surgeons, Park Ridge, Illinois.

Hargreaves, K.M. (1990) Mechanisms of pain sensation resulting from inflammation. In W.B. Leadbetter, J.A. Buckwalter & S.L. Gordon (eds) *Sports-Induced Inflammation: Clinical and Basic Science Concepts*, pp. 383–92. American Academy of Orthopaedic Surgeons, Park Ridge, Illinois.

Harper, J., Amiel, D. & Harper, E. (1991) Changes in collagenase and inhibitor in ligaments and tendon during early development of stress deprivation. *Trans. Orthop. Res. Soc.* **16**, 114.

Hayflick, L. (1980) Cell ageing. *Ann. Rev. Gerontol. Geriatrics* **1**, 26–67.

Hunt, T.K. & Dunphy, J.E. (eds) (1979) *Fundamentals of Wound Management*. Appleton-Century-Crofts, New York.

Ilizarov, G.A. (1989) The tension–stress effect on the genesis and growth of tissues: II. The influence of the rate and frequency of distraction. *Clin. Orthop. Rel. Res.* **239**, 263–85.

Ippolito, E., Natali, P.G., Postacchini, F. *et al.* (1980) Morphological, immunological, and biochemical study of rabbit Achilles tendon at various ages. *J. Bone Joint Surg.* **62A**, 583–93.

Ippolito, E., Postacchini, F. & Riccardi-Pollini, P.T. (1975) Biomechanical variations in the matrix of human tendons in relation to age and pathological conditions. *Ital. J. Orthop. Traumatol.* **1**, 133–9.

Johnson, K.A. (1983) Tibialis posterior tendon rupture. *Clin. Orthop.* **177**, 140–7.

Joyce, M.E., Pruitt, D.C. & Manske, P.R. (1992) Synthesis and *in situ* localization of TGF-B1, TGF-B2, PDGF-A, PDGF-B, and SFGF during flexor tendon healing. *Trans. Orthop. Res. Soc.* **17**, 680.

Jozsa, L., Balint, J.B., Kannus, P. *et al.* (1989) Distribution of blood groups in patients with tendon rupture. *J. Bone Joint Surg.* **71B**, 272–4.

Jozsa, L., Kvist, M., Balint, B.J. *et al.* (1989) The role of recreational sport activity in Achilles tendon rupture. A clinical, pathoanatomical and sociological study of 292 cases. *Am. J. Sports Med.* **17**, 338–43.

Kannus, P. & Jozsa, L. (1991) Histopathological changes preceding spontaneous rupture of a tendon. *J. Bone Joint Surg.* **73A**, 1507–25.

Kelly, D.W., Carter, V.S., Jobe, F.W. *et al.* (1984) Patellar and quadriceps tendon ruptures. Jumper's knee. *Am. J. Sports Med.* **12**, 357–80.

Kibler, W.B., Chandler, T.J. & Stracener, E.S. (1992) Musculoskeletal adaptations and injury due to over training. In J.O. Holloszy (ed) *Exercise and Sports*

Sciences Reviews, Vol. 20, pp. 99–126. Williams & Wilkins, Baltimore.

Koob, T.J., Vogel, K.G. & Thurmond, F.A. (1991) Compression loading *in vitro* regulates proteoglycan synthesis by fibrocartilage in tendon. *Trans. Orthop. Res. Soc.* **16**, 49.

Kvist, M., Jozsa, L., Jarvinen, M.J. *et al.* (1987) Chronic Achilles paratenonitis in athletes: A histological and histochemical study. *Pathology* **19**, 1–11.

Leach, R.E. & Schepsis, A.A. (1992) When hindfoot pain slows the athlete. *J. Musculoskeletal Med.* **9**(4), 106–24.

Leadbetter, W.B. (1990a) An introduction to sports-induced inflammation. In W.B. Leadbetter, J.A. Buckwalter & S.L. Gordon (eds) *Sports-Induced Inflammation: Clinical and Basic Science Concepts*, pp. 2–23. American Academy of Orthopaedic Surgeons, Park Ridge, Illinois.

Leadbetter, W.B. (1990b) Corticosteroid injection therapy in sports injuries. In W.B. Leadbetter, J.A. Buckwalter & S.L. Gordon (eds) *Sports-Induced Inflammation: Clinical and Basic Science Concepts*, p. 527. American Academy of Orthopaedic Surgeons, Park Ridge, Illinois.

Leadbetter, W.B. (1991) Physiology of tissue repair. In L.Y. Hunter-Griffin (ed) *Athletic Training and Sports Medicine*, 2nd edn, pp. 96–123. Raven Press, New York.

Leadbetter, W.B. (1992) *The pathohistology of overuse tendon injury in sports.* Exhibit at American Academy of Orthopaedic Surgeons Annual Meeting, Washington, DC, 20 February 1992.

Leadbetter, W.B., Buckwalter, J.A. & Gordon, S.L. (eds) (1990) *Sports-Induced Inflammation: Clinical and Basic Science Concepts.* American Academy of Orthopaedic Surgeons, Park Ridge, Illinois.

Leadbetter, W.B., Mooar, P.A., Lane, G.J. *et al.* (1992) The surgical treatment of tendinitis. Clinical rational and biologic basis. *Clin. Sports Med.* **11**(4), 679–712.

Lyon, R.M., Akeson, W.H., Amiel, D., Kitabayashi, L.R. & Woo, S.L.Y. (1991) Ultrastructural differences between the cells of the medial collateral and the anterior cruciate ligaments. *Clin. Ortho. Rel. Res.* **272**, 279–80.

Madden, J.W. & Aren, A.J. (1991) Wound healing: biologic and clinical features. In D.C. Sabiston (ed) *Textbook of Surgery*, 14th edn, pp. 164–77. WB Saunders, Philadelphia.

Mahan, K.T. & Carter, S.R. (1992) Multiple ruptures of the tendon Achilles. *J. Foot Surg.* **31**(6), 48–59.

Majno, G. (1975) *The Healing Hand: Man and Wound in the Ancient World.* Harvard University Press, Cambridge, Massachusetts.

Manske, P.R., Gelberman, R.H., Vande Berg, J.S. *et al.* (1984) Intrinsic flexor–tendon repair: A morpho-

logical study *in vitro*. *J. Bone Joint Surg.* **66A**, 385–96.

Martinez-Hernandez, A. (1990) Basic concepts in wound healing. In W.B. Leadbetter, J.B. Buckwalter & S.L. Gordon (eds) *Sports-Induced Inflammation: Clinical and Basic Science Concepts*, p. 78. American Academy of Orthopaedic Surgeons, Park Ridge, Illinois.

Menard, D. & Stanish, W.D. (1989) The ageing athlete. *Am. J. Sports Med.* **17**, 187–96.

Nirschl, R.P. (1969) Mesenchymal syndrome. *Virginia Med. Monthly* **96**, 659–62.

Nirschl, N.P. (1990) Patterns of failed healing in tendon. In W.B. Leadbetter, J.A. Buckwalter & S.L. Gordon (eds) *Sports-Induced Inflammation: Clinical and Basic Science Concepts*, pp. 577–85. American Academy of Orthopaedic Surgeons, Park Ridge, Illinois.

Nirschl, R.P. & Pettrone, F.A. (1979) Tennis elbow. The surgical treatment of lateral epicondylitis. *J. Bone Joint Surg.* **61A**, 832–9.

Noyes, F.R., Lindenfeld, T.N. & Marshall, M.T. (1988) What determines an athletic injury (definition)? Who determines an injury (occurrence)? *Am. J. Sports Med.* **16**(Suppl.), 565–6.

O'Connor, F.G., Sobel, J.R. & Nirschl, R.P. (1992) Five step treatment for overuse injuries. *Phy. Sports Med.* **20**(10), 128–42.

Puddu, G., Ippolito, E. & Postacchini, F. (1976) A classification of Achilles tendon disease. *Am. J. Sports Med.* **4**, 145–50.

Rathbun, J.B. & McNab, I. (1970) The microvascular pattern of the rotator cuff. *J. Bone Joint Surg.* **52B**, 540–53.

Rodosky, M.W. & Fu, F.H. (1990) Induction of synovial inflammation by matrix molecules implant particles and chemical agents. In W.B. Leadbetter, J.A. Buckwalter & S.L. Gordon (eds) *Sports-Induced Inflammation: Clinical and Basic Science Concepts*, p. 357. American Academy of Orthopaedic Surgeons, Park Ridge, Illinois.

Rovere, G.D., Welsh, L.X., Gristina, A.G. *et al.* (1983) Musculoskeletal injuries in theatrical dance students. *Am. J. Sports Med.* **11**, 195–8.

Rubin, E. & Faber, J.L. (eds) (1988) *Pathology.* JB Lippincott, Philadelphia.

Schatzker, J. & Branemark, P.I. (1969) Intravital observation on the microvascular anatomy and microcirculation of the tendon. *Acta Orthop. Scand.* **126**(Suppl.), 1–23.

Schneider, P.G. (1982) Indications for surgical treatment of chronic soft tissue injuries. *Int. J. Sports Med.* **3**(Suppl.), 15–17.

Singer, K.M. & Jones, D.C. (1986) Soft tissue conditions of the ankle and foot. In J.A. Nicholas & E.D. Hershman (eds) *The Lower Extremity and Spine in Sports Medicine*, p. 148. CV Mosby, St Louis.

Teitz, C.C. (1989) Overuse injuries. In C.C. Teitz (ed) *Scientific Foundation of Sports Medicine*, p. 299. BC Decker, Toronto.

Uhthoff, H.K. & Sarkar, K. (1991) Classification and definition of tendinopathies. *Clin. Sports Med.* **10**, 707–20.

Van der Meulen, J.C. (1982) Present state of knowledge on processes of healing in collagen structures. *Int. J. Sports Med.* **3**(Suppl. 1), 4–8.

Vogel, K.G. (1991) Proteoglycans accumulate in a region of human tibialis posterior tendon subjected to compressive force *in vitro* and in ligaments. In *Transactions of the Combined Meeting of the Orthopaedic Research Societies of USA, Japan and Canada*, 21–23 October 1991, p. 58.

Weiss, J.A., Woo, S.L.-Y., Obland, K.J. *et al.* (1991) Evaluation of a new injury model to study medical collateral ligament healing: Primary repair versus inoperative treatment. *J. Orthop. Res.* **9**, 516–28.

White III, A.A. (1989) The 1980 symposium and beyond. In J.W. Frymoyer & S.W. Gordon (eds) *New Perspectives in Low Back Pain*. American Academy of Orthopaedic Surgeons, Park Ridge, Illinois.

Wilson, A.M. & Goodship, A.E. (1992) Hysteresis energy losses in the equine superficial digital flexor tendon during exercise produce a local temperature sufficient to damage fibroblasts *in vitro*. *Trans. Orthop. Res. Soc.* **17**, 679.

Woo, S.L.-Y. & Buckwalter, J.A. (eds) (1988) *Injury and Repair of Musculoskeletal Soft Tissues*. American Academy of Orthopaedic Surgeons, Park Ridge, Illinois.

Woo, S.L.-Y., Matthews, J.V., Akeson, W.H. *et al.* (1975) Connective tissue response to immobility. Correlative study of biomechanical measurements of normal and immobilized rabbit knees. *Arthritis Rheum.* **18**, 257–64.

Yeager, B. & Turner, T. (1985) Percutaneous extensor tenotomy for chronic tennis elbow: American Office Procedures. *Orthopaedics* **8**, 1261–3.

Index